Human Molecular Biology

An Introduction to the Molecular Basis of Health and Disease

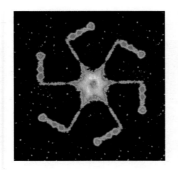

Human Molecular Biology is an introduction to health and disease for the new generation of life scientists and medical students. By integrating cutting-edge molecular genetics and biochemistry with the latest clinical information, the book weaves a pattern that unifies biology with syndromes, genetic pathways with disease phenotypes, and protein function with drug action. From the origins of life to the present day, a narrative is traced through the workings of genomes, cells and organ systems, culminating in the linking of laboratory technologies to future research. Lavishly illustrated throughout with two-color diagrams and full color clinical pictures, this text brings the complexities and breadth of human molecular biology clearly to life. By merging the fields of molecular biology and medicine, this groundbreaking account launches the reader into a new dimension where health and disease are seen to be complementary components of the same biomolecular spectrum.

Richard J. Epstein, M.D., Ph.D, is Deputy Director of the National Cancer Centre, and Associate Professor at the National University of Singapore. He began life in Sydney and has held medical school teaching posts at Cambridge, Harvard, and London.

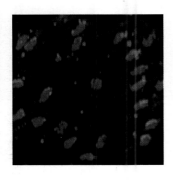

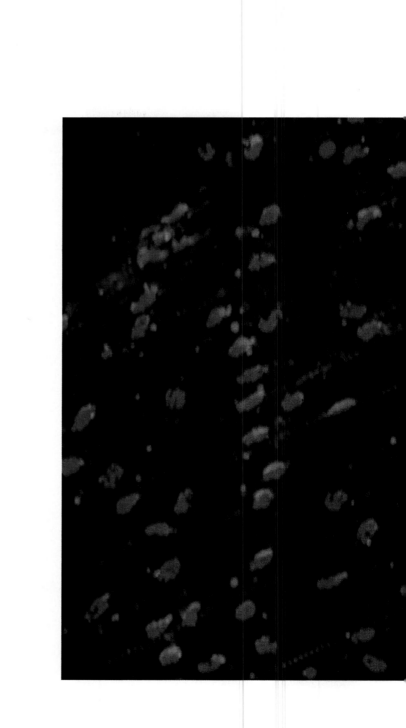

Human Molecular Biology

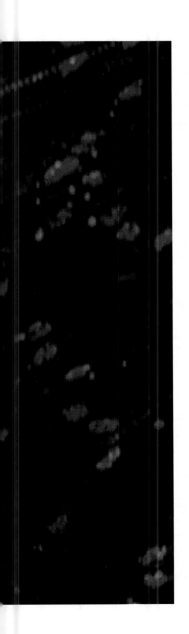

An Introduction to the
Molecular Basis of Health and Disease

Richard J. Epstein

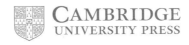

CAMBRIDGE
UNIVERSITY PRESS

PUBLISHED BY THE PRESS SYNDICATE OF THE UNIVERSITY OF CAMBRIDGE
The Pitt Building, Trumpington Street, Cambridge, United Kingdom

CAMBRIDGE UNIVERSITY PRESS
The Edinburgh Building, Cambridge CB2 2RU, UK
40 West 20th Street, New York, NY 10011–4211, USA
477 Williamstown Road, Port Melbourne, VIC 3207, Australia
Ruiz de Alarcón 13, 28014 Madrid, Spain
Dock House, The Waterfront, Cape Town 8001, South Africa

http://www.cambridge.org

First published 2003

Printed in Italy by G. Canale & C. S.p.A.

Typeface Utopia 9/13 pt.   *System* QuarkXPress™   [SE]

A catalogue record for this book is available from the British Library

Library of Congress Cataloguing in Publication data

Epstein, R. J.
    Human molecular biology : an introduction to the molecular basis of health and
    disease / Richard J. Epstein.
        p.   cm.
    Includes bibliographical references and index.
    ISBN 0 521 64285 X (hardcover) – ISBN 0 521 64481 X (pbk.)
    1. Molecular biology. 2. Pathology, Molecular. 3. Human biology. I. Title.
    QH506 .E66 2001
    612–dc21   2001035238

ISBN 0 521 64285 X hardback
ISBN 0 521 64481 X paperback

The publisher and author welcome feedback from all readers of this book.
Please e-mail your comments and suggestions to the *Human Molecular Biology*
e-mail address at: hmb@cambridge.org

Contents in brief

Contents in detail

▌ From molecular biology to human genetics

1 Biomolecular evolution   9

IV From molecular cell biology to human physiology

Preface

Good health is a matter of having the right molecules in the right place at the right time. This may seem self-evident, but the idea that health is determined *mainly* by molecules has only gained acceptance in recent years.

Consider this in historical perspective. A century ago health was regarded as a function of body parts – if you had a regular bowel and a strong heart you were OK. This anatomic model of health was superseded in due course by models based on organ function, the so-called system-based (physiologic) approach. But physiologic systems are interdependent: you can't have an effective gastrointestinal system without a nervous system, or a competent immune system without a hemopoietic system, or a responsive cardiovascular system without an endocrine system. This limitation has so far prevented even the most integrated biomedical curricula from communicating a wholly holistic view of human biology.

A popular response to such difficulties has been the proposal that students of the twenty-first century should no longer be force-fed so much information. Facts have become unfashionable, an irrelevance to the higher goal of imbuing trainees with creative insights and self-learning potential. What is needed, many believe, is a way of transmitting broad scientific principles without the burden of detail.

Sadly, this goal is no more feasible than that of teaching music without instruments. Details – facts – are essential for illustrating both general principles and instructive exceptions. A glut of detail may impair learning, but it is not the details per se that are at fault. Rather, it is the lack of a recurring *pattern* to those details which frustrates student and teacher alike.

The realization is now dawning that what is needed is not to teach less, but to teach more skillfully; not to memorize more facts but to assimilate more patterns. To do so it is essential to identify themes of structure and function within life, themes that have been collectively dubbed molecular biology by the uninitiated – for many of whom, one suspects, the word "molecular" may mean "incomprehensible". The good news is that this problem is now solved: there is no longer any such thing as molecular biology.

All biology is now about molecules. Molecular biology is little more than a buzzword from a bygone era in which technical change outpaced public understanding. The transition to a new biological world order is almost complete: technologies have matured, seed concepts are crystallizing, and a critical mass of knowledge is nearing accrual. The biological basis of health and disease has become inescapably molecular.

Human Molecular Biology is about molecules. This book is intended as a language primer for the life sciences – a translation aid for students seeking to decipher the Rosetta stone of *Homo sapiens*. In these pages an attempt has been made to portray molecular structure and function in the frame of human health and disease, such that:

- Biomedical science is taught *from the molecules up* rather than *from the diseases down* – that is, the molecular basis of health is used to predict and elucidate disease rather than vice versa, with disease serving mainly as a teaching aid to illustrate normal molecular function.
- Diseases are presented not as invariant clinicopathologic entities (spot diagnoses or syndromes) but rather as dynamic molecular processes which overlap in time, degree, and quality with normal biology.
- The emphasis on understanding disease has shifted away from the anatomy of bones and veins and towards the anatomy of genes and proteins.

Human Molecular Biology is not a comprehensive catalog of medicine or molecular biology, nor is it a textbook of biochemistry or physiology. It doesn't embrace prokaryotic genetics or genealogical charts, and includes no name-dropping anecdotes from biohistory. Rather, it presents a beginner's guide to the language of human biology – a molecule-by-molecule account of life and its problems. Note that the term "molecule" here includes proteins, sugars, and lipids as well as the more fashionable nucleic acids. For DNA is only half the story: it is the interconnected workings of genes, proteins, and intermediary molecules which define health and disease.

Most attempts to translate cutting-edge research into textbooks suffer from prematurity, oversimplification, outdatedness, errors, irrelevance . . . and *Human Molecular Biology* is unlikely to prove immune to all these faults. You shouldn't expect to become a handle-turning molecular biologist by reading this book, since to do that you need to work in a laboratory for several years; a hand-waving familiarity with the basics of biomedical science is a more realistic goal. The placement of molecular biology methodology at the end of this book emphasizes that an encyclopedic knowledge of laboratory techniques is no longer a prerequisite for understanding molecular biology.

How much training will the biomedical professional of the twenty-first century need to understand the language of life? It is as crazy to insist that everyone is equally familiar with Okazaki fragments and 14-3-3 proteins as it would be for all of us to learn stereotactic brain surgery. Yet it is not too much to expect that future biomedical graduates will, for example:

- Know what is meant by terms such as **transcription factor, tumor suppressor, leucine zipper, homeobox gene, RFLP,** and **G-protein.**
- Be able to explain the principles behind methodologies such as **PCR, nuclear magnetic resonance, gene knockout,** and **DNA microarray.**
- Comprehend the difference between **candidate gene** and **positional cloning** approaches to identifying disease genes.
- Have at least a vague familiarity with **homologous recombination, post-translational modification, polyadenylation, linkage disequilibrium, protein trafficking, evolutionary conservation,** and **molecular chaperones.**
- Understand in broad outline processes such as **immunoglobulin gene rearrangement, developmental hemoglobin switching, long-term potentiation** and **reverse cholesterol transport.**
- Have at least heard of terms such as **snurp, signal peptide, cyclin-dependent kinase, topoisomerase, Alu, p53, Ras,** and **Tat.**
- Be aware of technologies such as **recombinant protein production, subtractive hybridization, two-dimensional gel electrophoresis, retroviral gene transfer** and **antisense oligonucleotides.**

Demystification is the key to fluency in the molecular biosciences. The grammar of this language involves notions of hydrophobicity and hydrogen bonding and hybridization, of aromaticity and electrophilicity, of splicing and insertion and ligation and recombination, of randomness and repetition, of reversibility and commitment. But the vocabulary required for this grammar need not be exhaustive.

Human Molecular Biology is organized to cater for readers of different levels. Newcomers should begin at the beginning, whereas others may consult specific areas of interest. Each chapter is punctuated by sandwich sections called *Clinical Keynotes, Molecular Minireviews, Pharmacologic Footnotes,* and *Superfamily Spotlights.* The details of laboratory practice are left until the final section.

This is a great time to be a student in the biomedical sciences. A page-turning molecular narrative is beginning to displace the hypnotic anatomic/physiologic lectures so familiar to students of earlier decades. Biomedical education is thus presented with a challenge on the one hand and an opportunity on the other: to formulate a coherent body of knowledge such as our forefathers would not have dreamed possible, while using this knowledge to reinvent biomedical education from the inside out. Today's students and teachers need to decide for themselves whether it is riskier to surf this tidal wave of knowledge or to paddle aside and watch it disappear over the horizon of the twenty-second century. *Human Molecular Biology* is an invitation to catch the wave.

Acknowledgements

Many people assisted in the birth of this book. My gratitude goes to Julia Alberta, Ab Guha, Scott Pomeroy, and Gillian Smith for commenting upon early chapter drafts, as well as to anonymous reviewers for their encouraging comments on the original proposal. I also thank Peter Silver of Cambridge University Press for his steady guidance of the project from start to finish; Jane Fallows for her talented renderings of decidedly untalented sketches; Kate Whitley and Julie Dorrington of the Wellcome Medical Photographic Library for invaluable help in sourcing illustrations; Sarah Price for her energetic but tactful editing of my error-ridden prose; and Jane Williams and Lucille Murby for outstanding design and production. Thanks must also go to my mentors, without whom I would have long ago given up chasing paper, getting nowhere – so thanks in particular to Tony Basten, Paul Smith, Chuck Stiles, Tom Frei, Ed Newlands, and Steve Bloom for their unstinting support over the years. And of course I thank Anne, Julia, Catherine, Helen, and Alec, for tolerating the many empty evenings and weekends; may they come to regard this labor of love as a fruit of their own. Last but not least, I thank Geri and Jules, for everything.

Read me first . . .

Everything in molecular biology is connected to everything else. It is therefore tempting to support a text of this nature by including every conceivable citation, and by cross-referencing every mention of a molecule or malady. However, since the resulting rash of references would mesmerize most readers, a range of remedies has been instituted:

1. Journal citations have been omitted. This is not an attempt to deny credit to the biomedical storm troopers who first captured the information that has been rearranged herein. Rather, the task of using citations to credit even a proportion of these pioneers overwhelmed this writer's best efforts early on, and surrender became unconditional on realizing that tens of thousands of attributions would be needed.

2. The book is organized as a narrative. Any given section of the text thus assumes knowledge of the foregoing sections, obviating the need to include retrospective page references. The book can still be used as a reference (rather than programmed) text, but the appearance of unreferenced allusions should prompt the interested reader to consult the index for an earlier reference.

3. Page cross-references are not always included for text items emphasized by either **blue** or **bold type**. In such instances, the index provides references.

4. In the figures, disease pathways are marked as filled red triangles (▲), whereas medicinal treatments are indicated using filled red capsules (◉).

When used for the first time, or on reintroducing a major concept in a new section of the text, molecular names and concepts are indicated in **bold**. A passing reference to a new molecule or concept will usually be accompanied by a forward page reference, but under these circumstances the name may be left visually unemphasized.

Finally, names of diseases and toxins are highlighted in **sans serif**, whereas names of drugs are shown in **sans serif blue**. Eponymous disease names are used without apostrophe (e.g., **Parkinson disease**). Gene names are rendered in *italics*. Human molecules are usually indicated by a capital first letter, whereas genes and proteins of lower organisms are shown in lower case.

Select glossary of confusing terms and abbreviations

ABH	blood group antigens
ABO	blood groups
ADH	alcohol dehydrogenase
ADH	antidiuretic hormone (vasopressin)
AID	activation-induced deaminase
AIDS	acquired immunodeficiency syndrome
a.k.a.	also known as
AKAP	A-kinase anchoring protein
ALA	5-aminolevulinate (δ-aminolevulinic acid)
Ala	alanine
ALAS	δ-aminolevulinate synthetase
ALDH	acetaldehyde dehydrogenase
anti-idiotype	antibody directed against an idiotope
anti-idiotypic antibody	antibody directed against an anti-idiotype
antisense	oligonucleotide sequence which binds complementary nucleic acid
AP	alkaline phosphatase
AP	amyloid P (fibril)
AP	apurinic/apyrimidinic (site)
AP1	activator protein-1 (Jun-Fos heterodimer)
APC	activated protein C
APC	adenomatous polyposis coli (gene)
apo (a)	plasminogen-like apoprotein of Lp(a)
apo A	apolipoprotein A (includes apoAI, apoAII)
araC	cytosine arabinoside
araC	gene-activating protein in *E. coli*
Bcl	oncogene family first associated with *B-c*ell *l*ymphomas
Bcr	*B*reakpoint *c*luster *r*egion gene activated by Philadelphia chromosomal translocation interrupting the *Abl* gene in chronic myeloid leukemia
BNP	"brain natriuretic peptide"; most abundant in *heart*
bp	base pair (one nucleotide length)
CAM	cell adhesion molecule
CaM kinase	calcium/calmodulin-dependent protein kinase
cAMP-dependent kinase	protein kinase A
cap (lymphocyte)	plasma membrane modification
cap (mRNA)	modification (methylation) of 5' end of transcript
CAP	catabolite activator protein
CaR	calcium (-sensing) receptor
CAR	constitutive androstane receptor
CAT (assay)	*c*hloramphenicol *a*cetyl *t*ransferase technique for measuring promoter strength by inserting this bacterial gene downstream of the promoter in question and measuring the amount of CAT mRNA transcribed
CAT (box)	(var., CAAT, CCAAT) DNA-binding upstream element

neu	carcinogen-induced rodent oncogenic homolog of ErbB2
NF1	neurofibromatosis-associated tumor suppressor gene
NF1	nuclear factor 1; an adenovirus replication protein
NFAT	nuclear factor of activated T cells
NFκB	*n*uclear *f*actor which transactivates the immunoglobulin κ light chain enhancer in *B* cells
nitric oxide	endogenous vasodilator and neurotransmitter
nitrous oxide	laughing gas
nonsense	mutation which terminates transcription
NSAID	nonsteroidal anti-inflammatory drug
p14^{ARF}	human Cdk4 inhibitor with *a*lternate *r*eading *f*rame to p16^{INK4}
p19^{ARF}	murine homolog of p14^{ARF}
PARP	poly(ADPribosyl) polymerase
PCNA	proliferating cell nuclear antigen
PCP	phencyclidine (angel dust)
PCR	polymerase chain reaction
PCT	porphyria cutanea tarda
PD-ECGF	platelet-derived endothelial cell growth factor
PDGF	platelet-derived growth factor
phosphatidylserine	membrane lipid
phosphoserine	post-translationally modified amino acid
PI3K	phosphatidylinositol-3′-kinase (PI-3′-kinase)
PIP$_2$	phosphatidylinositol bisphosphate
PIP$_3$	phosphatidylinositol trisphosphate
PLA$_2$	phospholipase A$_2$
Pl^{A2}	platelet A2 polymorphism of the GPIIIA integrin subunit
platelet-activating factor	arachidonate derivative produced by and for platelets
platelet factor IV	an antiangiogenic platelet-derived coagulation cofactor
platelet-derived growth factor	mesenchymal growth factor produced by platelets for stromal cells
P-loop	structural motif within nucleotide phosphatases (e.g., GTPases)
protein C	endogenous circulating anticoagulant
protein kinase C	signaling molecule family with multiple isoforms
P-site	adenyl cyclase domain that interacts with purine ring of adenosine
PTC	human homolog of *patched* gene
PTC	papillary thyroid cancer
P-type	(ATPase) in which active site is activated by (auto)phosphorylation
q.v.	which see
RACE	rapid amplification of cDNA ends
RANTES	*r*egulated on *a*ctivation *n*ormal *T* cell *e*xpressed and *s*ecreted (chemokine)
SAA	serum amyloid A
SAGE	serial analysis of gene expression
SAP	serum alkaline phosphatase
SAP	serum amyloid P (fibril)
SAP	SLAM-associated protein
SLAM	signaling lymphocyte-activation molecule (CDw150)
SLAP	Src-like adaptor protein
spp.	species (e.g., of microorganism)
SRE	serum response element
SRF	serum response factor
SRP	(ribosomal) signal recognition particle
syndrome X	obesity syndrome
tandem genes	contiguous runs of multi-copy genes, e.g., encoding histones

tandem repeats	highly repetitive DNA sequences (satellite DNA)
TAP	transporter associated with antigen processing
TAP	trypsinogen activator peptide
Tar	bacterial aspartate (chemotaxis) receptor
TAR	*trans-a*ctivation *r*esponsive RNA sequence in HIV
Tat	HIV1-encoded trans-activating protein
TAT	tyrosine aminotransferase
TBG	thyroxine-binding globulin
TGB	thyroglobulin
TPA	tetradeconyl phorbol ester acetate
tPA	tissue plasminogen activator
V1R	vomeronasal organ (pheromone) receptor type 1
VR1	vanilloid (spicy taste or pain) receptor type 1
Veg1	*Xenopus* morphogen
vegetable	neither animal nor mineral
vegetal	inferior end of embryo, opposite animal pole
VEGF	vascular endothelial growth factor ("vascular permeability factor")
VP-16	etoposide (cytotoxic drug)
VP16	herpes simplex transcription factor

Introduction: A disease for every gene?

Most of the time we take our health for granted. "Health" is often equated with lack of disease, but defining disease is not straightforward. Is ageing a disease? Acne? Fatigue? How about loose-jointedness? Senile irritability? Dandruff, say, or color-blindness? Obesity? What about depression? Homosexuality? Hypersexuality? Hyperintelligence? Or baldness, or hirsutism? And even plain ugliness? – we do, after all, train plastic surgeons to treat it.

Doctors often portray diseases as syndromes, living illustrations of which are labeled cases. That students often perceive diseases as puzzles to be solved is therefore unsurprising. However, away from the ivory tower of Grand Rounds, diseases may not be so clearly bar-coded. Patients recover or die without a diagnosis, overlap syndromes occur, multiple pathologies coexist, spontaneous and functional phenomena are freely invoked. The notion of disease as a pure clinicopathologic entity is thus blurred in practice.

In recent years this muddle has been clarified by the insight that genetic mutations may contribute to a disease phenotype; for example, the discovery of mutations in the rhodopsin gene transformed retinitis pigmentosa from a Corridor Curiosity to a Textbook Tutorial. This change in outlook has brought science and medicine together. Articles concerning human disease now flood into scientific journals, just as gene sequence depositions are drifting into medical journals. In clinical textbooks molecular explanations are supplanting bedside descriptions, whereas primers of molecular biology often use human diseases to enliven their bloodless subject matter. Does this mean that the overburdened student must assimilate even more information than did their predecessors? The answer is yes – and no.

Yes, because there is no way to reverse the growth of knowledge. There *is* more information now, and biomedical education needs to produce graduates able to sift such data and communicate it to an internet-befuddled public. No, because at long last more information is being translated into less confusion – a change that reflects the substitution of crystal-clear concepts for the disparate vagaries of more venerable curricula. There is far more to learning medicine than just acquiring information, of course, but significant time and effort still needs to be reserved for this activity.

Of the many problems confronting life science students today, learning the jargon can be one of the most frustrating: novices may find it difficult to appreciate the lake's glassy reflection due to the murky rivers of nomenclature discoloring it (Figure 1). Molecules are named on virtually any basis:

- Structure; e.g., **titin, fibrillin**.
- Function; e.g., **scatter factor, perforin, survivin, defensin**.
- Cell location; e.g., **nucleolin, intercellular adhesion molecule-1, caveolin**.
- Disease link; e.g., **dystrophin, neurofibromin, azoospermia factor**.
- Tissue distribution; e.g., **epidermal growth factor, ubiquitin, Pit-1**.
- Historical association; e.g., **transforming growth factor-β**.

Figure 1 Pathways to learning the language of biomedicine. Force-fed facts obscure scientific insights, whereas presentation of reproducible patterns tends to crystallize such insights.

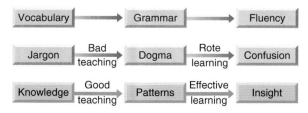

- Discoverers' whim; e.g., *mothers against decapentaplegic* (**Mad**).
- Wishful thinking; e.g., **tumor necrosis factor, mammostatin**.

Proteins with labels suggesting specific functions may have distinct roles in different phases of life as well as in different tissues or species. Some molecules are named after their interaction with synthetic drugs – the morphine, benzodiazepine and cannabinoid receptors, and the multidrug transporter come to mind. Similarly, one could be forgiven for believing that the cystic fibrosis transmembrane conductance regulator has nothing to do with normal ion channel function. Only by constantly hearing and speaking the vocabulary of molecules – their structures and functions, that is, rather than their names – can we hope to become fluent in the modern language of biology.

Medicine is now about molecules

It is impossible to understand disease without first understanding health. One cannot understand bleeding without first understanding coagulation; scarring, without understanding healing; or cancer without understanding cell growth and differentiation. Understanding normal processes provides a way of integrating medical concerns with molecular themes – receptors, polymerization, adhesion, phosphorylation, ionic selectivity, and so on. The recent acquisition of this understanding makes the goal of a seamless biomedical syllabus feasible for the first time.

Somewhere between 30 000 and 35 000 genes are now believed to inhabit the human genome. Many of these are dysregulated in more than one disease, just as many diseases are associated with the dysregulation of more than one gene. The possibility that each gene may come to be associated with at least one disease is thus unnerving for those aspiring to biomedical scholarship. To illustrate the complexity of structure–function relationships involved, consider the following:

1. Mutations affecting the cell surface receptor **Ret** may cause diseases as diverse as **thyroid cancer** and **congenital aganglionic megacolon**.
2. **Osteopetrosis** (marble bone disease) is inducible in mice by germline mutations affecting either growth factors, enzymes or DNA-binding proteins.
3. Clinically distinct infantile weakness syndromes may result from the same muscle gene product being affected by severe gene mutations (**Duchenne dystrophy**) or mild gene mutations (**Becker dystrophy**), or even by mutations affecting associated glycoproteins (**Fukuyama disease**).

Many other examples could be cited: the numerous disorders resulting from gene mutations affecting the **β-globin** protein, for example. Yet although fewer than 10 000 genetic diseases have been characterized, more information already exists than any individual can assimilate. Even as today's gene hunters race to fit genotypes to phenotypes, tomorrow's researchers will seek phenotypes for orphan genotypes. We are thus entering a new era in which genes, regulatory sequences, and their polymorphisms will be in search of a disease. For just as the identification of a phenotype now suggests a variety of candidate genotypes, so may a conserved genotypic variant come to imply the existence of a clinical phenotype.

Disease phenotypes of the future may be far more subtle, however, than those of the past. An average metabolic process involves 20–100 molecules; for example, glucose homeostasis involves glycolytic enzymes, glucose transporters, glycogen synthetases, disaccharidases, gluconeogenetic enzymes, and so on. Similar cascades are involved in DNA replication, RNA splicing,

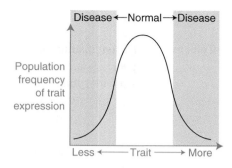

Figure 2 Disease defined as a variation from the normal distribution. Irrespective of whether a trait is under- or overexpressed, either extreme can be regarded as abnormal.

tissue-specific gene regulation and almost every other biological process – including mating, which involves the activation of about 100 genes (at least in yeast). Not only is there a multiplicity of mutable target molecules in these processes, but also a spectrum of error severity for each step. These errors range from drastic lesions such as gene deletions and frameshifts through to more covert defects such as upstream regulatory sequence mutations, intron variants, splicing aberrations, mutations affecting post-translational modification, and so on. Genetic alterations of these types may come to explain interindividual differences currently viewed as constitutional or polymorphic rather than disease-associated (Figure 2).

Molecules are easy to understand

Molecules like DNA are simple – if they weren't, we wouldn't be here. Nonetheless, there are a lot of molecules out there, and trying to commit each one to memory is unrealistic. Put another way, our biology (which has evolved over hundreds of millions of years) may be quantitatively too complex for any individual to comprehend in its entirety. Certain internal contradictions of biology may complicate learning:

1. Biomolecular interactions tend to be specific
   - Despite this, such interactions often also exhibit (apparent) redundancy, promiscuity and degeneracy.
2. Biomolecular pathways tend to be hierarchical
   - Despite this, pathways are often also highly combinatorial, random, oscillatory and/or reversible.

Biological specificity creates the impression of large numbers of molecules interacting in a complex manner, but this disguises the underlying simplicity: combinatorial interactions are unified by homologous modular subunits which represent the building blocks of structure and function. Specificity and promiscuity are thus two sides of the same biological coin, repetition and variation of a common genetic theme. The hierarchy of biologic processes – i.e., the tendency of one stimulus to dominate another – reflects Nature's abhorrence of a stalemate, but a strictly hierarchical system lacks flexibility.

The human mind is limited by its ability to focus on only one thing at a time. This handicaps our understanding of biology: life occurs as much in parallel as in sequence, and moving goalposts are hard to keep in focus. Biomolecules are constantly phosphorylated and dephosphorylated, sequestered and mobilized, cleaved and ligated, denatured and refolded, reduced and oxidized, hydrolyzed and synthesized. Yet behind this haze of biological connexity lies a simple logic – for every yes there is a no; for every stop, a go; for every accelerator, an airbag.

Biology, then, is basically binary. Complexity is all too often a euphemism for confusion – half of science is incorrect, but we don't know which half. This is as true today as a century ago; the main difference is that progress in biology now more closely resembles the filling-in of a jigsaw puzzle than the application of tiny brushstrokes to a blank canvas. Yet biology remains a digital system: as patterns blend and trends appear, principles will emerge from hitherto nebulous data, and the unifying themes of biomedical science will crystallize into human consciousness. Molecules will be mysterious no more.

Summary

Medicine is now about molecules. Molecules are easy to understand.

From molecular biology to human genetics

1 Biomolecular evolution

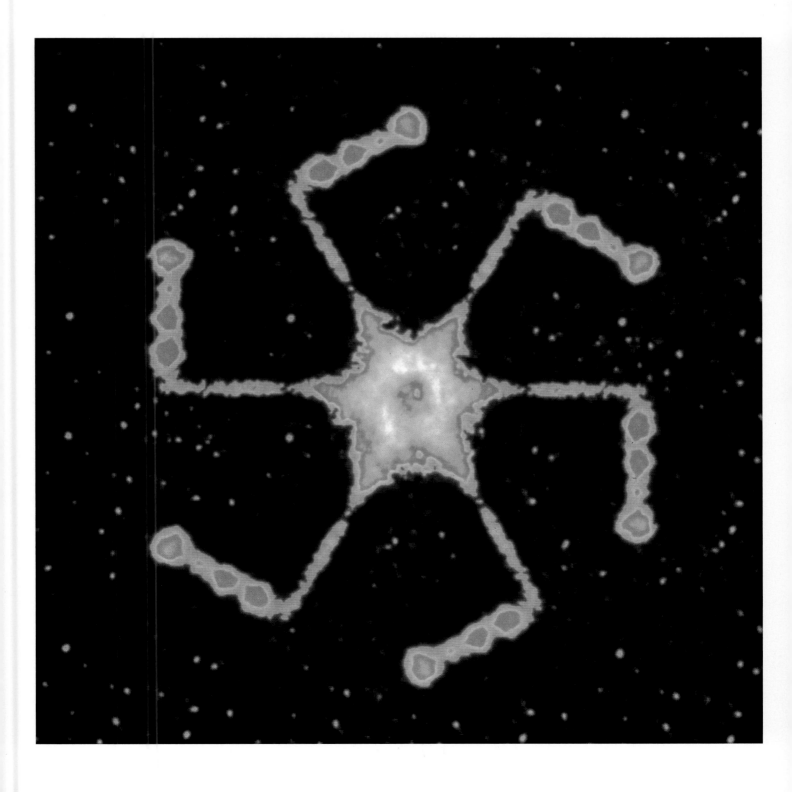

Figure 1.1 (*previous page*) The interface between the living and the inanimate: a virus (T7 phage) particle (National Medical Slide Bank, no. 13253).

This opening section introduces the terms and concepts needed to understand the topics covered later. We begin by reviewing the fundamentals of molecular action, and then examine how molecules give rise to living systems. The defining structural features of genes and proteins are presented, and the role of these molecules in evolution addressed. Finally, molecular mechanisms contributing to genomic change and adaptation are examined.

Atoms and elements

Sunlight supplies energy for life on Earth

Time began with the Big Bang 14 billion years ago. To begin with all was hydrogen; the next three minutes saw the birth of deuterium and helium through energy-releasing fusion reactions, unleashing the primordial fireball. The resultant formation of stars created a focus for helium consumption, and hence for the energy-dependent intrastellar synthesis of carbon and oxygen.

Ten billion years then passed, during which time our planet formed from the gravity-dependent accretion of asteroidal debris spinning around the Sun. For the next billion years or so there were gales, floods, volcanic eruptions and earthquakes on the Earth – but no life. So why should the miracle of life have since taken root in this humble backwater of the universe?

In fact, there is nothing miraculous about life. The development of life on Earth was probably inevitable; trapped in a stable orbit at a temperate distance from the Sun, the Gaia-like milieu of the planet simply happened to be suitable for molecules to self-select. Given the size and age of the universe, the development of life beyond our solar system seems all but certain.

The Sun was fainter back in those early days of planetary history, and the surface of the Earth cooler. Life as we know it may therefore have originated within the retained warmth of the Earth's crust, where subterrestrial iron could react with water to liberate hydrogen through hydrothermal vents to enter the biospheric haze of nitrogen, yielding ammonia. The greenhouse effect so created would have elevated surface temperatures, enabling nascent thermophilic life forms to convert ambient chemicals to useable nutrients and polymers.

Such fixation reactions probably began about 3.5 billion years ago, by which time the energy to drive them was increasingly obtainable from sunlight. Today's Sun is even stronger, converting 700 million tons of hydrogen to 695 million tons of helium every second: the missing 5 million tons is converted to radiant energy which speeds across the galaxy. For this reason the light-absorbing pigments of blue-green algae (cyanobacteria) would have been among this planet's founding biomolecules. Humans today also express light-absorbing pigments, mainly in their skin and retinas.

The transformation of Earth to a green planet was central to the evolution of animal life. Absorption of sunlight via the green pigment chlorophyll releases charged particles which propel biochemical reactions in a controlled fashion; in this way plants harness solar energy to drive the synthesis of chemical energy stores. Since the evolution of animal life depended upon ingestion of herbaceous foodstuffs – and given that even oil and coal represent transformed plant materials – most energy-requiring processes on Earth are ultimately driven by the battery power of the Sun. A key step in the biological conversion of atmospheric gases to chemical energy (photosynthesis) is the

A.

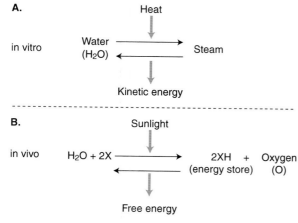

B.

Figure 1.2 Energy transfer reactions. *A*, When a kettle boils, heat energy is converted into the kinetic energy of water molecules (such as can be harnessed by steam engines). Hence, the energy of the heat source is transferred to the water molecules. *B*, Energy transfer via chemical reactions. In an uphill (energy-requiring) reaction, green plants absorb solar energy to split water into oxygen (O), which is excreted as waste, and hydrogen (H), which is used to modify the substrate molecule X. In the reverse (downhill) reaction in animals, the modified substrate XH represents a chemical energy store that releases free energy when disrupted.

use of sunlight to split **water** into its constituent **atoms**, an energy transfer reaction not unlike boiling a kettle to create steam (Figure 1.2).

MOLECULAR MINIREVIEW

Atoms and subatomic particles

Atoms are the fundamental subunits of matter. Atoms contain a core of electrically positive particles (**protons**) adjacent to neutral particles of similar mass (**neutrons**); this core is surrounded by a cloud of tiny negatively charged **electrons** which whiz around the proton-neutron nucleus. The orbits of these electrons comprise a series of concentric **shells** with increasing energy content: the maximum number of electron pairs in each shell increases quadratically as the shell diameter increases from 1 to 4 to 9 to 16.

An atom is said to be in its **ground state** when all of its electrons are in their home shells. Absorption of energy leads to an **excited state** in which one or more electrons jump a shell. The number of protons defines the **atomic number** of a specific **element**, and equals the number of electrons. With the exception of the first element hydrogen, which lacks a neutron, elemental atoms contain the same number of neutrons as protons; this makes the **atomic weight** (in **daltons** or **Da**) twice the atomic number. About 100 elements make up the natural universe.

Atoms containing the same number of protons but different numbers of neutrons are termed **isotopes**. For example, the addition of one or two neutrons to a hydrogen atom yields the hydrogen isotopes deuterium (^{2}H) and tritium (^{3}H) respectively. Unstable isotopes are **radioactive**, and are used as tracers in experimental work. Radioactive isotopes undergo **exponential decay**, and the time taken to lose half of the radioactivity is termed the **half-life** ($t^{1/2}$) of the isotope.

Molecules are formed by covalent bonding of atoms

Chemistry is defined by the formation and destruction of bonds between atoms. An atom with an unequal number of protons and electrons contains a net **charge** and is termed an **ion**; oppositely charged ions attract each other, giving rise to relatively weak **ionic** (electrovalent) **bonds** linking the two ions (e.g., Na$^+$Cl$^-$, or table salt). However, atoms stick most tightly to other atoms by forming electron-sharing **covalent** (combining) **bonds**. A **molecule** is a single particle containing a covalently bonded assortment of atoms in a characteristic ratio and configuration, and can comprise one or more atoms of one or more elements. When a molecule takes on a stable three-dimensional arrangement with a fixed internal atomic structure, a **crystal** is said to be created.

The number of covalent bonds that an atom can form depends upon the number of **unpaired electrons** in its outer shell (Figure 1.3). This number is termed the **valence**, or combining power, of the atom. When two atoms share one electron pair, a **single** (covalent) **bond** is formed between them; the sharing of two electron pairs represents a **double bond**, whereas the sharing of three electron pairs represents a **triple bond**. An atom with one or more unpaired electrons (such as may occur, for example, following excitation by an external energy source) is termed a **free radical**. Electrons may move back and forth or **resonate** between two adjacent bonds, creating an alternating bond structure stabilized by **resonance**.

All chemistry is dynamic. The outcome of a chemical reaction represents the **equilibrium** between several competing reactions of different speeds, some of

Figure 1.3 The formation of covalent intramolecular bonds through sharing of electron pairs. Hydrogen atoms have one unpaired electron, whereas oxygen atoms have two in their outer electron shell. A stable water molecule can thus form by the combination of two hydrogens and one oxygen, since all three atoms now contain fully paired electron shells (the number of electrons needed to complete shell number $n = 2 \times n^2$).

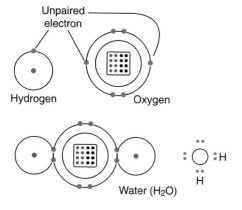

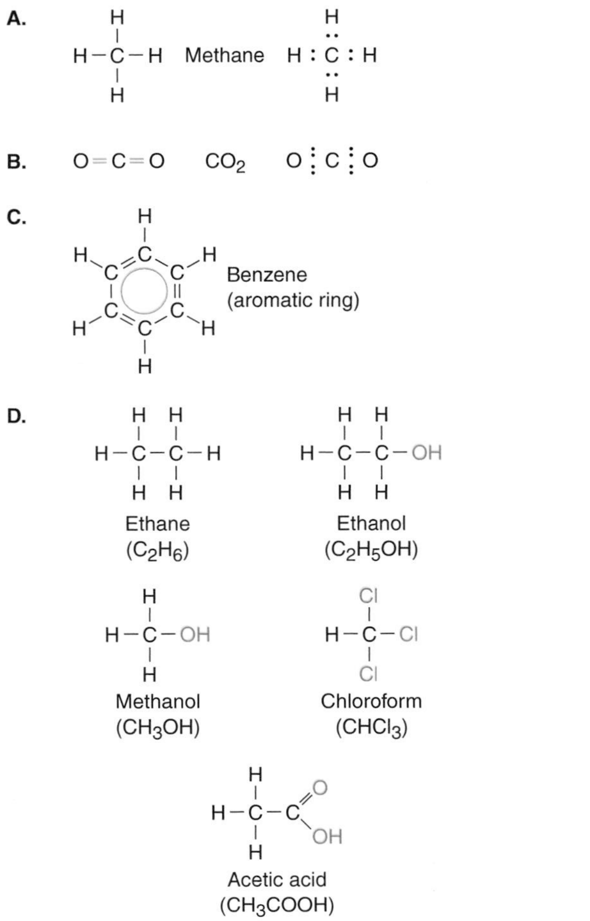

A.

B.

C.

Benzene
(aromatic ring)

D.

Ethane
(C_2H_6)

Ethanol
(C_2H_5OH)

Methanol
(CH_3OH)

Chloroform
($CHCl_3$)

Acetic acid
(CH_3COOH)

Figure 1.8 Bonding conformations of carbon compounds. *A, B,* Comparative structures of methane and carbon dioxide. When carbon is fully reduced and saturated, it forms methane (*A*); when it is fully oxidized and unsaturated, it forms carbon dioxide (*B*). *C,* Structure and representation of the (aromatic) six-carbon benzene ring. *D,* Structures of other carbon compounds mentioned in the text.

rich in oxygen and nitrogen tend to be polar and hence soluble. In contrast, molecules that are unusually carbon rich tend to be nonpolar and insoluble; the longer the carbon **chain length**, the lower tends to be the water solubility. Hydrocarbons such as octane (eight carbons; found in petroleum) are immiscible in water, for example, as are the longer fatty acids. Similarly, large insoluble molecules such as starch require digestive hydrolysis to smaller sugars for absorption into the bloodstream. Carbon chain length is indicated by the name of the molecular subclass: a **pentose** is a five-carbon sugar (-ose), for example. Carbon chains need not always be linear, however, and may instead form a **ring** in which double bonds alternate between adjacent carbons by resonance. Ringed compounds are often termed **aromatic** since some have a sweet petrol-like smell (Figure 1.8*C*).

MOLECULAR MINIREVIEW

Chirality

Human beings are asymmetrical. Most of us have our heart on the left and our liver on the right, and favor the use of one eye, ear and hand. This spatial paradigm of **handedness** can be applied to other asymmetric three-dimensional structures including molecules.

Viewed along a single axis, carbon-based molecules composed of similar linear subunits may display differential twist or **chirality**. This asymmetry is defined by convention using the orientation of the most distant carbon in the molecule relative to the chemical group defining the molecular family (e.g., an aldehyde group). Earthly life is based largely on the L- (**left-handed**) configuration of such molecules. The only **right-handed** (D-; from the Latin *dexter*) molecules are:

1. The genetic material.
2. Sugars (mono- and polysaccharides).

Numerous explanations have been advanced as to why we live in a left-handed biomolecular world, including theories based on the Earth's magnetic field and the polarization of sunlight. The default hypothesis is that enantioselectivity breeds enantioselectivity, and it just happened to start out left-handed . . .

The term **steric** denotes the conformational properties of a molecule which constrain its structural interactions with other molecules. If the L-form of molecule A normally interacts with the L-form of molecule B, for example, it may fail to interact with the D-form of molecule B due to **steric hindrance**.

PHARMACOLOGIC FOOTNOTE

Organic therapeutics

Carbon compounds in which all free electrons are paired off in different directions, i.e., in which all the intramolecular carbon links are single covalent bonds, are said to be **saturated**. In contrast, compounds containing higher-energy double or triple carbon bonds are **unsaturated**. Double/triple bonds are under greater strain and hence release more energy when ruptured; for example, the triple bond of acetylene (C_2H_2) allows it to burn at temperatures hot enough to cut metal. Saturated carbon compounds tend to be nonpolar, making these molecules lipophilic and hence capable of penetrating fatty body compartments such as nerve sheaths and brain; examples include anesthetics such as **ether**.

Table 1.1. Structural classification of amino acids

	Essential (dietary)	Nonessential (synthesized)
Acidic		Aspartate (Asp, or D)
		Glutamate (Glu, E)
Basic	Lysine (Lys, K)	Arginine (Arg, R)
Uncharged hydrophilic	Histidine (His, H)	Tyrosine (Tyr, Y)
	Threonine (Thr, T)	Serine (Ser, S)
		Asparagine (Asn, N)
		Glutamine (Gln, Q)
Hydrophobic	Valine (Val, V)	Glycine (Gly, G)
	Leucine (Leu, L)	Alanine (Ala, A)
	Isoleucine (Ile, I)	Proline (Pro, P)
	Phenylalanine (Phe, F)	Cysteine (Cys, C)
	Methionine (Met, M)	
	Tryptophan (Trp, W)	

The properties of a carbon compound are further dictated by its **side chains**. Substituting a hydroxyl group for hydrogen, for example, converts ethane into water-soluble ethanol – the popular recreational drug – whereas swapping three chlorines for hydrogens converts methane to the anesthetic **chloroform**. If we replace a single methane hydrogen with a carboxyl (COOH) group, the result is the tasty two-carbon compound, vinegar (acetic acid; Figure 1.8*D*).

Compounds having the same number of elemental atoms but a different spatial arrangement of side chains are termed **isomers**. For example, the sugars glucose and galactose are isomers: they have the same chemical formula, but their properties differ because of the dissimilar orientation of one of their hydroxyl groups. Isomers that are exact mirror-images of each other are termed **enantiomers** (from the Greek *enantios*, meaning opposite). Drugs may be isomeric (e.g., **L-DOPA**, **D-penicillamine**) and mixtures of such isomers are described as **racemic**.

Organic molecules

Proteins are functional amino acid chains

The most diverse group of carbon-based biomolecules are **proteins**. More than 50% of nonaqueous human body mass is accounted for by this molecular species. Proteins may be extremely large, reflecting either the serial incorporation of functional subunits termed **domains** or the polymerization of repeated structural **motifs**. Most human proteins have a molecular weight between 5000 and 400 000 Da (5–400 kDa), but some are megadaltons in size.

Proteins are synthesized as a linear polymeric sequence of carbon-containing **amino acids**, each of which has a molecular weight around 100 Da. A short amino acid sequence – short enough, say, to be artificially synthesized by a machine in a laboratory – is termed a **peptide**. Most peptides are fewer than 50 amino acids in length; such molecules may transmit signals within the body, but tend to be too small to serve a structural role. Larger proteins are termed **polypeptides**, some of which may be modified by the addition of moieties such as metal ions or fats. An "average" protein contains somewhere in the order of 10 000 atoms.

Twenty amino acids are sufficient to synthesize all known proteins (Table 1.1). Nine of these amino acids – histidine, isoleucine, leucine, lysine, methionine, phenylalanine, threonine, tryptophan and valine – cannot be synthesized by the body, and must therefore be ingested in the diet as **essential amino acids**. Amino acids are so-called because they have an amine ($-NH_2$) group at one end, and a carboxyl ($-COOH$) group at the other. These two groups can be linked in series to form a chain which grows into a peptide or polypeptide. The first amino acid in the chain retains its unbound NH_2 group, whereas the last retains a free COOH group; hence, the biosynthetic start site of a protein is termed the **amino-** or **N-terminal**, whereas the completion site is the **carboxy-** or **C-terminal** (Figure 1.9).

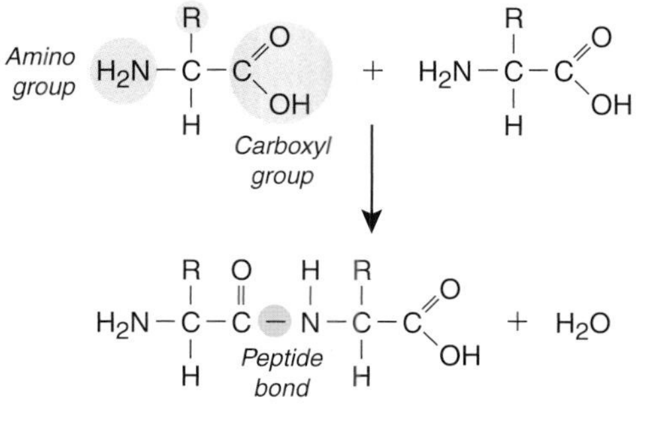

As the polypeptide chain lengthens, the nascent protein folds into its functional three-dimensional conformation. Protein folding is influenced by the spatial and chemical properties of the amino acid side-chains which confer properties such as acidity, aromaticity and hydrophobicity. For example, charged (basic or acidic) residues are highly polar and hence tend to position themselves on the exterior of proteins rather than embedded within the

Figure 1.9 Joining of two amino acids via formation of a peptide bond. The basic amino acid structure is that of a carbon chain with amino- and carboxy-termini, with the side-chain (R) determining the specific attributes. The energy-dependent elimination of a water molecule permits the formation of a peptide bond between the amino (NH_2) and carboxyl (COOH) groups of adjacent amino acids; hence, this bond can in turn be hydrolyzed to yield energy.

Table 1.2. Distinguishing functional features of amino acids

Distinguishing feature	Amino acid
Aromatic ring	His (H), Phe (F), Trp (W), Tyr (Y)
Sulfhydryl (SH) group	Cys (C) (two SH groups form one disulfide bond
Sulfur-containing (no SH)	Met (M)
Imino (not amino) acid group	Pro(P) (bends molecules)
Phosphorylation substrates	Ser (S), Thr (T), Tyr (Y) (all contain hydroxyl group)
Neurotransmitters	Gly (G) (inhibitory) Glu (E), Asp (D) (excitatory)

Figure 1.10 The biological role of phosphorylation. *A*, Structure of mono- and polyphosphates. Phosphate groups coalesce to form polyphosphate bonds by eliminating two hydrogen atoms and one oxygen (i.e., one water molecule) to create a phosphoanhydride bond, which can in turn be subjected to hydrolysis. *B*, Oxidative phosphorylation. High-energy polyphosphate bonds are created by the coupled NADH-dependent reduction of oxygen to water during respiration, with food molecules $(CH_2O)_n$ providing the energy input.

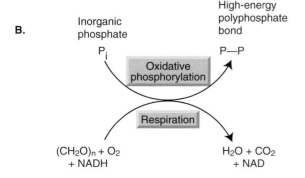

hydrophobic core of the molecule. Amino acids thus represent an alphabet of chemical letters for spelling out both the linear and three-dimensional language of proteins.

Protein synthesis is an energy-dependent process. In a reaction that yields a water molecule, the NH_2 group of one amino acid forms a **peptide bond** with the COOH group of the next amino acid during protein synthesis (Figure 1.9). Conversely, hydrolysis of the peptide bond liberates free energy. Much of life is spent either creating or hydrolyzing these peptide bonds, with the former process occurring most spectacularly during embryogenesis and the latter during severe illness or terminal decline.

These alterations in the body's rate of protein synthesis and destruction define the kinetics of **metabolism**. A class of "doing proteins" termed **enzymes** are in charge of metabolic processes such as the energy-dependent cleavage of downstream **substrate** proteins. Enzymes are themselves often the downstream effectors of **receptor** molecules which are activated by the specific binding of **ligands**. One of the most important functions of enzymes is to move **phosphate** groups on and off neighboring proteins, thereby modulating the behavior of those proteins and transducing a chemical signal down a multi-molecular biochemical pathway.

MOLECULAR MINIREVIEW

Phosphorus

What is it about phosphorus which makes this nonmetal of such unique importance in regulating protein function? The first clue relates to its luminosity, or phosphorescence, which derives from the readiness of phosphorus to absorb energy and thus trap electrons into a metastable energy level. A second clue is apparent on striking a match: the phosphorus on the match head burns readily on exposure to oxygen. Hence, this is an excitable element which avidly combines with oxygen, even at room temperature – like oxygen, phosphorus hates to be alone. Indeed, the only place where residual free phosphorus may be found in the natural environment is on meteorite debris ("shooting stars") from outer space.

Phosphate groups transfer energy between proteins

Phosphate, the oxide of phosphorus, has two critical functions in biology:
1. **Energy storage** due to its ready incorporation into bond-rich polyphosphates which can be subsequently hydrolyzed to yield free energy.
2. **Signaling** via the transfer of its electronegative charge to phosphate-accepting amino acids (Table 1.2); the acidic, and thus polar, nature of the phosphate group alters the external conformation of proteins.

A phosphate group contains four oxygens in a tetrahedral arrangement around a central phosphorus atom. With five electrons in its outer shell, phosphorus shares two electrons with one double-bonded oxygen and one electron each with three further O^- atoms (Figure 1.10*A*). This **orthophosphate** (PO_4^{3-}), or **inorganic phosphate** (P_i), may be reduced to form phosphoric acid (H_3PO_4); more often, however, the phosphate combines with an organic group to form a **phosphate ester** or **phosphodiester** bond. This interaction confers a large negative charge on the phosphorylated molecule which now carries a phosphoryl group (PO_3^{2-}); it is this negative charge which is responsible for intermolecular binding events.

Phosphate can bind other phosphate groups to form di- and triphosphates. In humans this accumulation of **polyphosphates** is driven by the oxidation of NADH to NAD which in turn scavenges electrons from food (e.g., from sugars) then transfers them back (from NADH) to oxygen. Oxidation of NADH drives the formation of **phosphoanhydride bonds** between phosphate groups, creating storable chemical energy; the efficiency of this energy transfer is almost 50%, which is formidable compared with that of a car engine (about 10%). Subsequent hydrolysis of these bonds yields free energy, reflecting the ability of monophosphates to undergo further oxidation. The poison **arsenic**, which also binds four oxygens, mimics a phosphate group and thus prevents phosphate-dependent energy transfer.

Polyphosphates represent the main free energy store for all living things. The respiratory electron transfer reactions which we use to convert food to energy are a prime example of high-energy phosphate fuel storage. This critical metabolic process, termed **oxidative phosphorylation** (Figure 1.10*B*), results in the minting of the body's free energy currency (pp. 165–6). Enzymes that catalyze the addition of phosphates to substrate molecules are termed **kinases**, whereas enzymes that catalyze the removal of phosphate groups are termed **phosphatases**.

CLINICAL KEYNOTE

Anabolism and catabolism

The sum total of chemical reactions occurring within a living organism – its metabolism – includes the biosynthesis and hydrolytic degradation of carbon-based molecules including (but not restricted to) proteins. The size and complexity of carbon-based molecules hint at both the energy required for their synthesis and that derivable from their breakdown: these processes are termed **anabolism** and **catabolism** respectively. As a rule of thumb, most complete metabolic reactions in human biology involve between 20 and 50 proteins.

Anabolic processes cause organisms to grow, whereas catabolism is associated with wasting. Disorders such as progressive cancer, fulminant infections and uncontrolled diabetes may be associated with **cachexia** – a severe catabolic state which reflects both the inadequate intake and utilization of nutrients, and the breakdown of structural molecules as a way of making extra nutrients available to the stressed body.

Catabolic efficiency depends upon the tissue availability of oxygen. In the absence of O_2, sugars such as glucose are incompletely catabolized (by anaerobic **glycolysis** or carbohydrate breakdown) to **lactic acid** – the molecule that gives you muscle soreness after unaccustomed anaerobic exercise like chopping wood – yielding only a little energy and reducing power. Note that during anaerobic glycolysis, oxidation (of glyceraldehyde 3-phosphate; pp. 164–6) occurs in the absence of oxygen.

In the presence of O_2 sugars undergo full catabolism to CO_2, thereby fueling energy production via oxidative phosphorylation. The reverse process, in which sugars are synthesized endogenously from small precursor molecules, is termed **gluconeogenesis**; this takes place during periods of low-sugar stress such as starvation or prolonged exercise.

Unlike sun-fueled plants, animals satisfy most of their anabolic needs by scavenging environmental foodstuffs that contribute the carbohydrate (sugar and glycogen) and lipid requirement (Figure 1.11). Most important structural and functional macromolecules, however, are synthesized from scratch using ingredients obtained from the digestive metabolism of dietary molecules. These ingredients include not only the above-mentioned amino acid components of proteins, but also the molecular constituents of **genes**.

Figure 1.11 The major metabolic transitions. Animals primarily metabolize via oxygen (lower panels) whereas plants and some bacteria may not need it (upper panels).

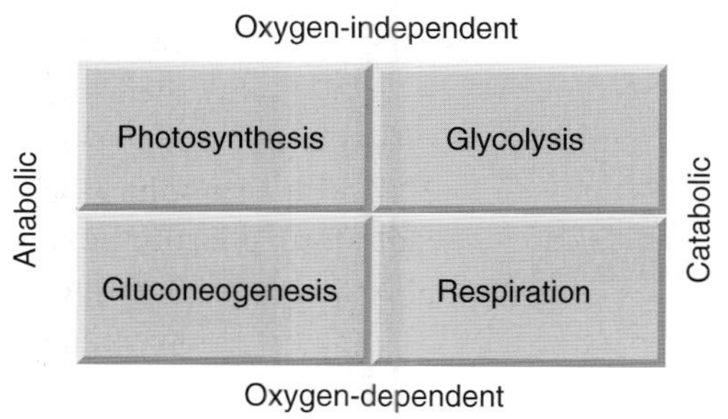

Oxygen-independent

| Anabolic | Photosynthesis | Glycolysis | Catabolic |
| Gluconeogenesis | Respiration |

Oxygen-dependent

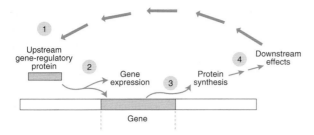

Figure 1.12 Upstream and downstream concomitants of gene expression. As shown, the relationship between gene and protein expression is essentially circular.

Genes are used by proteins to make more proteins

The transition from chemistry to biology – the origin of life – requires molecules to **self-replicate**. Replication is not sufficient for life, however, since inanimate substances such as crystals may also replicate themselves. Two additional features of living systems are:

1. Fidelity of vertical (intergenerational) information transfer – this process is termed **heredity**.
2. Diversification of intergenerational information transfer due to the interplay of random genetic variants and errors with environmental survival threats – this adaptive evolutionary process is termed **selection**.

Life therefore demands a dynamic mode of information storage, **genetics**, which can be passed through successive generations of the same organism. The unit of biological storage, defined as a **gene**, represents the minimum quantum of information able to specify a physical feature. The concept of the gene took almost a century to be elucidated in structural terms; this reflects the fact that most organisms contain at least 100-fold more protein than gene mass, making the average gene as hard to find as a needle in a haystack.

Genes have no intellectual status. They do not reason or conspire; accordingly, no student of biology should feel intimidated by genes. Their defining attribute is that they make faithful (daughter) copies of themselves – a process which, when simulated in the laboratory, is termed **cloning**. The digital quality of genetic information, that is the inheritability of traits on an all-or-none basis rather than as a blend, is designated Mendelian genetics after the pea-breeding monk who first proposed the particulate nature of genes. Mendelian genetics resembles Newtonian physics: a good-enough approximation of genetic reality for day-to-day purposes, but one which falls short of describing the dynamic complexity of the living genetic code.

Genes encode intermediary templates for protein assembly and thus provide the apparatus for their own replication. Far from being inert blueprints, genes are highly interactive molecular loci involved in both sensing and effecting signals (Figure 1.12). Genes respond to **upstream** regulatory interactions which switch the gene on (or off) in response to microenvironmental changes; activated genes orchestrate the **downstream** synthesis and release of protein effectors. Hence, just as proteins cannot transmit information to future generations without genes, so genes cannot influence their environment without proteins.

Hence, genes need proteins just as proteins need genes (Figure 1.13). Both sets of molecules are functionally defined by their structures and, to a lesser extent, are structurally predictable by their functions. Although genes and proteins have a chicken-and-egg relationship in evolutionary terms, it is traditional to ascribe primacy to the gene in view of its role during sexual reproduction – the start point of the biological cycle. This dualistic model can be represented in terms of **genotype** and **phenotype**.

Figure 1.13 The interdependence of protein and gene function. DNA is needed to make RNA, which is needed to make proteins, which are in turn needed to replicate DNA.

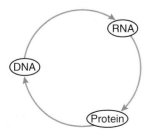

CLINICAL KEYNOTE

Phenotypes and genotypes

Any discernible biological trait that has not been secondarily acquired is a **phenotype**. If transmissible between different generations of the same organism – whether directly or indirectly, predictably or randomly – such a phenotype is **her-**

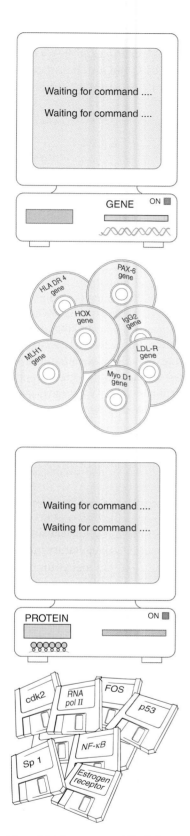

Figure 1.14 "Computer modeling" of genes and proteins. (*Top*) Genes as software. In this model, which is relevant to embryonic development, genes instruct the protein hardware what to do. (*Bottom*) Genes as hardware. In this model, which is relevant to day-to-day genetic functioning, the genome presents a relatively inert face to its immediate environment until instructed by the appropriate protein software how it should respond.

itable and hence likely to have a **genetic** basis. This genetic basis for a hereditary phenotype is termed the **genotype**, irrespective of whether it has been identified in detail; a given phenotype may be associated with a variety of genotypes.

Not all genetic traits are heritable. For example, a deformity that is present at birth (i.e., **congenital**) may result from a genetic abnormality occurring in utero due to, say, inadvertent exposure to rubella virus or ionizing radiation. Since the latter exposures are **genotoxic** (harmful to the genetic material), the congenital phenotype can have a genetic basis even though it may be unlikely to occur in subsequent pregnancies.

Evolution conserves informative gene sequences

Genes are promiscuous. They not only spread vertically, as noted above, but also horizontally – manifesting, for example, as microbial resistance or acute infectious epidemics. Hence, genes are just as capable of wreaking havoc within a biological system as they are of creating and maintaining it. The upside of this genetic promiscuity relates to the capacity for adaptive variation that accompanies it.

Genetic variation underlies the Darwinian notion of survival of the fittest. This translates in molecular terms as genetic **selfishness** – a concept which defines the "selfish gene" as the unit of biological success. The random creation of viable genes is a rare evolutionary event, but one which selects for its own perpetuation. This ability to select for rare events is a central principle not only of evolution but also of molecular biology and human disease.

Structure and function are interdependent in biology. To appreciate this, consider the analogy of computer hardware and software. By convention genes are considered the brains of the outfit, instructing proteins what to do; that is, genes are the system software and proteins are the hardware. This distinction is valid in genetic terms since genes are a stable information repository whereas proteins are not, but in day-to-day metabolic processes genes present a relatively inert interface to the system. Since ambient proteins instruct genes how to respond to microenvironmental changes, proteins may also be viewed as software components that program the output of the genetic hardware (Figure 1.14).

The time-honored Cartesian split between brains and brawn, thought and action, blueprints and building blocks is thus incompatible with the two central axioms of molecular biology:

1. **Function** implies structure.
2. **Conserved structure** implies function.

That structure does not automatically imply function is apparent from the existence of genetic material with little discernible utility (see below). Conversely, gene or protein sequences that are evolutionarily conserved (either across species or within a related family of molecules) strongly suggest functional significance. The survival benefit of a gene to an organism determines the need for the organism to conserve the gene in question; if the survival of different species demands the presence of a given gene, the gene will be conserved across those species. To appreciate the degree of functional conservation implied by this, one need only consider that our biosphere comprises several million species – including over 500 000 higher animals and plants – which share a related genetic make-up despite variations in physical size exceeding 20 orders of magnitude.

The conserved set of genes and related genetic material in an organism is termed the **genome**. Entire gene clusters may be inherited within genomes,

Genetic
material

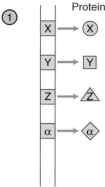

Gene
duplication

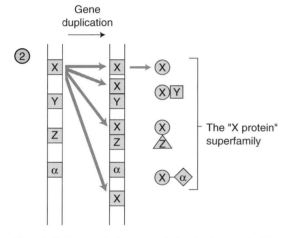

The "X protein"
superfamily

Figure 1.15 The genetic development of molecular superfamilies. Gene X undergoes duplication events throughout the genome, linking up with other genes (Y, Z, α) to form a family of X-containing genes.

across species, and over millions of years; a gene may also proliferate within its own genome, seeding its domains into distant locations and thus cross-fertilizing its way into new applications. Estimates of the number of genes comprising the human genome currently oscillate between 30 000 and 40 000.

MOLECULAR MINIREVIEW

Structural homology and superfamilies

Structural similarity between molecules is termed **homology**, high degrees of which imply a common origin. Homology is quantified by sequence comparison, and ranges from as low as 20% – an arbitrary borderline between homology and random similarity – to as high as 100% (i.e., identity). Homology can extend not only to functionally related molecules in different species, but also to functionally distinct molecules within the same organism. The underlying microevolutionary mechanism, termed **gene duplication**, involves a gene being serially transplanted to other parts of the genome, whether in part or in whole – in practice, only about a third of duplicated genes are successfully transcribed. At the other extreme, intact clusters of genes and regulatory elements may be duplicated. As this process continues, and as gene copies diverge structurally and functionally, **molecular superfamilies** of homologous genes and proteins (paralogs; p. 122) emerge, resembling a genetic patchwork quilt (Figure 1.15). Examples of superfamilies that have arisen via gene duplication include those related to the globin (p. 452) and homeobox genes (p. 401).

Under normal evolutionary circumstances, duplication of a given gene occurs approximately once every 100 million years. The ability of such genes to undergo duplication is balanced by a process whereby redundant genes are silenced. Some such genes may disappear from the genome but others, termed **pseudogenes**, persist as defunct genomic relics of active genes. Note, however, that pseudogenes may also arise prospectively via the genomic insertion of defective sequences. For example, the human olfactory receptor superfamily regulating the sense of smell includes many inactivated gene "ghosts" which reflect the loss of olfactory sensitivity in primates.

We have now refreshed our knowledge as to the basics of chemistry and biochemistry. Amino acids make up proteins; proteins are encoded by genes. In the next section we look more closely at the structure of the gene.

Nucleic acids

Nucleotides are base-sugar-phosphate building blocks

Just as proteins are assembled as linear arrays of amino acids, so are genes synthesized as a primary sequence of informational subunits. These subunits, termed **nucleotides**, link to form consecutive polymeric sequences termed **nucleic acids**, and synthetic molecules of this type are called **oligonucleotides**. Nucleic acids may be either **single-stranded** or **double-stranded**; human genes consist of double-stranded nucleic acids which encode single-stranded nucleic acids. A nucleotide is a tripartite structure which consists of:

1. A nitrogen-containing base
   - A **pyrimidine** (one carbon ring): **cytosine** or **thymine/uracil**.
   - A **purine** (two carbon rings): **adenine** or **guanine**.
2. A pentose (five-carbon) sugar
   - **Ribose** (for single-stranded nucleic acids).
   - **Deoxyribose** (for double-stranded nucleic acids).

Table 1.3. Nucleotide nomenclature and structure. Note that although adenosine and guanosine are (dephosphorylated) nucleosides, the similarly named cytosine is a nucleotide. Note also that incorporation of the nucleotide triphosphate into nucleic acid requires two phosphoanhydride bonds of energy; it is the nucleotide monophosphate which is ultimately incorporated

Abbreviation	Base	Nucleoside	Nucleotide (triphosphate)	Base type	No. of H bonds	Pairs with	Base structure
A	Adenine	Adenosine	ATP	Purine (two rings)	2	T/U	
G	Guanine	Guanosine	GTP	Purine	3	C	
U	Uracil	Uridine	UTP	Pyrimidine (one ring)	2	A	
T	Thymine	Thymidine	TTP	Pyrimidine	2	A	
C	Cytosine	Cytidine	CTP	Pyrimidine	3	G	

3. A phosphate group
   - A **triphosphate** (in newly formed nucleotides).
   - A **monophosphate** (following incorporation into nucleic acids).

The identity of each nucleotide is distinguished by a nitrogenous ring which is termed a **base** because of its ability to accept (acidic) hydrogen ions. All human nucleotides contain a double-ring purine base (adenine, **A**, or guanine, **G**) or a single-ring pyrimidine: either cytosine (**C**), or one of uracil (**U**; in single-stranded nucleic acids) or thymine (**T**; in double-stranded nucleic acids). The ability of these bases to accept hydrogen ions allows them to form stable intermolecular electrostatic linkages via hydrogen bonds.

The informational content of a nucleic acid is specified by the base sequences of its genes, for example A G T T C A A G C, which determine the structures of proteins. Lengths of nucleic acid are usually measured in bases for single-stranded nucleic acids, or **base pairs** (bp) for double-stranded nucleic acids. These units are in turn expressed as multiples of thousands (**kilobases**, kb) or, for genome mapping, millions (**megabases**, Mb). An average gene contains 2–10 kb of coding nucleic acid, but often includes far more noncoding sequence.

A base bound to a five-carbon (pentose) sugar is a **nucleoside** – a pentose bound to adenine represents the nucleoside **adenosine**, for example, whereas a pentose bound to thymine is **thymidine** (Table 1.3). Ribose is linked to phosphate via substitution of a free hydroxyl attached to the 5′ carbon of the sugar;

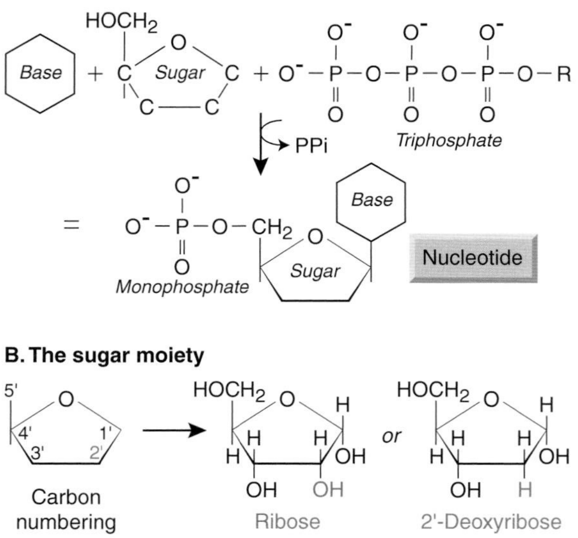

A. Nucleotide synthesis

$$Base + \begin{array}{c} HOCH_2 \\ C \underset{Sugar}{} C \\ C-C \end{array} + O^- - \overset{O^-}{\underset{O}{P}} - O - \overset{O^-}{\underset{O}{P}} - O - \overset{O^-}{\underset{O}{P}} - O - R$$

Triphosphate

↘ PPi

$$= O^- - \overset{O^-}{\underset{O}{P}} - O - CH_2 \quad Base$$

Monophosphate   Sugar

Nucleotide

B. The sugar moiety

5' O
4'   1'
3'   2'

Carbon
numbering

HOCH₂ O H
H   H OH
H   OH
OH   OH
Ribose

or

HOCH₂ O H
H   H OH
H   OH
OH   H
2'-Deoxyribose

Figure 1.16 Structure and synthesis of nucleotides. *A,* Tripartite structure of nucleotides. *B,* Pentose sugar composition: ribose and deoxyribose. PPi, inorganic phosphate.

Figure 1.18 The many guises of adenosine triphosphate (ATP). Not shown is the role of ATP as a purinergic neurotransmitter.

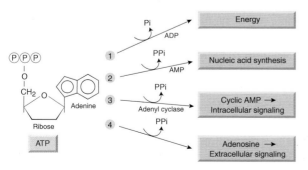

nucleotides are thus **phosphate esters** of nucleosides (Figure 1.16). Nucleosides may arise by dephosphorylation of nucleotides, but nucleotides do not usually arise from nucleoside phosphorylation. Nucleotide formation of **glycosidic bonds** between ribose phosphate and base moieties involves a pyrophosphate-displacing nucleophilic substitution reaction between the attacking nitrogen on the base and the ribose C1. By convention, carbons on the sugar are numbered as primes starting from the carbon joined to the base (1′, one-prime).

The assembly of a nucleic acid strand from unincorporated nucleotides is energy dependent. Hydrolysis of two phosphates (pyrophosphate) from the nucleotide triphosphate yields free energy for the creation of a covalent **phosphodiester linkage** between the remaining hydroxyl group on the 3′ carbon and an oxygen on the monophosphate. Since this leaves a free 5′ phosphate at the origin of the nucleic acid and a free 3′ hydroxyl at the terminus, nucleic acid synthesis is said by convention to occur in a **5′ to 3′ direction**. In this manner the **sugar-phosphate backbone** of the molecule is formed (Figure 1.17).

MOLECULAR MINIREVIEW

Adenosine triphosphate (ATP)

Multi-tasking is nothing new to the nucleotide **adenosine triphosphate (ATP)**, which has been doing it for millions of years (Figure 1.18):

1. ATP is an integral component of nucleic acids
   - The sugar and phosphate moieties link the structure,
   - The base sequence contributes the informational content,
   - Phosphate cleavage provides the energy for nucleotide assembly (as it does for GTP, TTP, and CTP).
2. ATP is the main **energy source** for most living processes. Hydrolysis of the tertiary high-energy phosphate group of the triphosphate moiety yields the free energy of the phosphoanhydride bond; the transferred phosphate confers a negative charge that enables the recipient molecule to oxidize a further molecule. The ATP levels for short-term energy needs are maintained by oxidative phosphorylation, but ATP is too unstable for long-term energy storage (sugars and fat are used for this purpose).
3. ATP may be incorporated into other bioactive molecules. An example is acetyl coenzyme A, or acetyl CoA, which is oxidized (in the citric acid, or tricarboxylic acid, cycle; pp. 151, 165–8) to generate NADH for oxidative phosphorylation.
4. ATP is partly dephosphorylated to a nucleotide monophosphate variously denoted adenosine monophosphate, AMP, or **adenylate**. An enzyme termed **adenyl cyclase** can then cause the single remaining phosphate group to bind two sites on the pentose, yielding the signaling molecule **cyclic adenosine monophosphate** or **cAMP**.
5. ATP is fully dephosphorylated to the purine nucleoside **adenosine** which binds receptors that mediate:
   - Heart rhythmicity and contractility (adenosine is administered intravenously as therapy for certain rapid heart rhythms),
   - Allergic reactions such as asthma,
   - Inhibition of excitatory neurotransmitter release (pain).

Like ATP, the hydrolysis of **guanosine triphosphate (GTP)** provides the energy for certain molecular activities, such as those related to fluid transport or cell movement. **ATPases** and **GTPases** are enzyme classes that release free energy by hydrolyzing polyphosphate groups in ATP and GTP respectively.

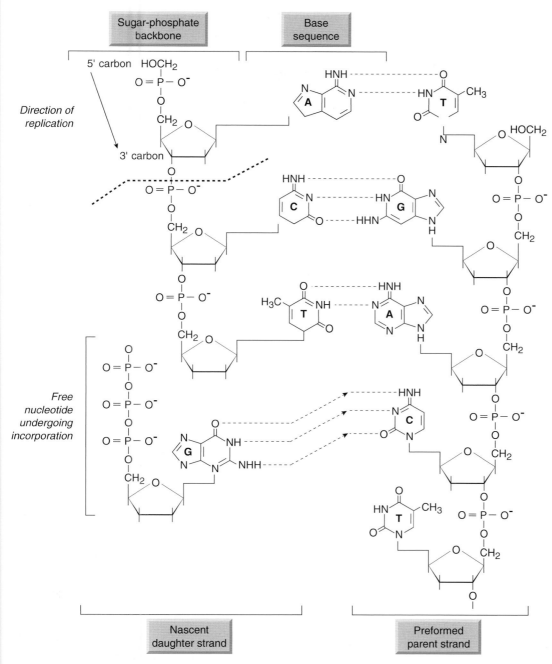

Figure 1.17 Schematic representation of nucleic acid replication. Formation of a complementary (daughter) strand from the original (parental) strand is shown – so-called semiconservative replication. The equivalence of hydrogen bond number, and complementarity of base size, is illustrated.

Efficient nucleoside excretion is needed for nitrogen balance

The digestive breakdown of amino acids in protein-rich food enables us to synthesize nitrogen-containing purine and pyrimidine bases. However, unlike carbon and hydrogen and oxygen – which can be excreted via metabolism to CO_2 or H_2O – nitrogen requires a special excretion mechanism. Fish excrete nitrogenous waste mainly as **ammonia**; birds, as **uric acid** (urate); and mammals as **urea**. Humans excrete most nitrogen in the form of urea, including that from pyrimidine ring breakdown. As in birds, however, human purine excretion occurs exclusively via the uric acid pathway. Being polar and hence water soluble, urea and urate are excreted in the urine; plasma urea levels therefore tend to be inversely proportional to renal function. Abnormally high

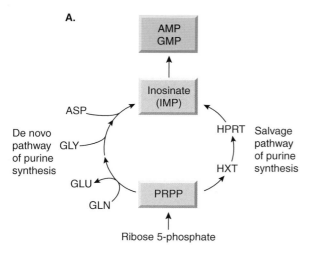

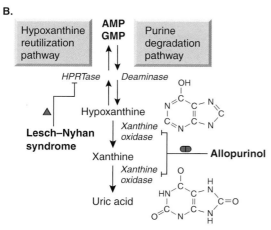

Figure 1.19 Purine synthesis and degradation. *A*, Synthesis of purines (AMP, GMP) via either de novo or salvage pathways. The latter pathway requires the reutilization of hypoxanthine (HXT) via hypoxanthine-guanine phosphoribosyltransferase (HPRT) catalysis to inosinate. *B*, Purine degradation by sequential deamination and oxidation.

urate levels or **hyperuricemia** may result not only from kidney failure but also from metabolic uric acid overproduction.

To understand purine excretion and its associated clinical disorders, one first needs to understand purine biosynthesis. Most nucleotides are synthesized by the interaction of a preformed pentose phosphate with either precursor amino acids (de novo nucleotide biosynthesis; i.e., from scratch) or recycled bases (the salvage – reutilization – pathway). This **5-phosphoribosyl-1-pyrophosphate** (**PRPP**, ribose phosphate) molecule connects the de novo and salvage purine synthesis pathways. In the labor-intensive de novo pathway, PRPP interacts with amino acids to construct a double-ring purine nucleotide. Far more efficient than de novo synthesis, however, is recycling of the partly degraded purine base **hypoxanthine** by recombining it with PRPP via a salvage pathway. This key reaction is catalyzed by **hypoxanthine-guanine phosphoribosyltransferase** (**HPRT**). Lesions damaging the *HPRT* gene may thus prevent the reutilization of PRPP; the resultant PRPP excess triggers constitutive purine biosynthesis leading to hyperuricemia (Figure 1.19*A*).

The purine nucleotide excretion pathway begins with dephosphorylation and subsequent nucleoside deamination. Hydrolytic cleavage of the sugar moiety from a deaminated purine nucleoside produces either xanthine (from guanine) or hypoxanthine (from adenine), just as deamination of the pyrimidine cytosine produces uracil. If any of these deamination events affect nucleosides, they can be repaired by enzymes termed **glycosylases**. Hypoxanthine is in turn oxidized to the nitrogenous waste product **xanthine** by xanthine oxidase – the same enzyme which, when expressed in human breast milk, inhibits bacterial growth through its oxidative activity. A further oxidation by this enzyme yields the end-product of purine metabolism, uric acid (Figure 1.19*B*); mice oxidize urate one step further to allantoin via urate oxidase, but in humans this gene has been silenced. Uric acid may thus function as an endogenous antioxidant, suggesting that hyperuricemia may have benefits.

Dysfunction of the **adenosine deaminase** (*ADA*) gene may lead to a **severe combined immunodeficiency** (**SCID**) syndrome due to defective nucleic acid polymerization in T lymphocytes. Immune cell dysfunction due to ADA deficiency may reflect the accumulation of deoxy-ATP. Rare patients with **purine nucleoside phosphorylase** (**PNP**) **deficiency** incur a milder immunodeficiency due to deoxy-GTP accumulation in immune cells, and this is associated with hypouricemia. In patients with hematologic malignancies, ADA may be inhibited by the anticancer drug **pentostatin**.

CLINICAL KEYNOTE

Uric acid

Impaired function of the *HPRT* gene causes hyperuricemia due to an inability to reutilize hypoxanthine in the salvage pathway, leading to: (1) oxidation of hypoxanthine to urate, and (2) underutilization of PRPP and excess de novo purine biosynthesis. Affected (male) infants with this **Lesch–Nyhan syndrome** exhibit cerebral palsy, writhing movements (chorea), anemia, and self-mutilatory biting of the fingers and lips. These self-destructive features, which occur 10–15 years earlier than the joint manifestations, may reflect dysfunction of dopaminergic neurons due to HPRT deficiency. Detection of uric acid crystals in the urine is a diagnostic pointer. Unlike patients with mutations affecting the **adenine phosphoribosyltransferase** (*APRT*) gene, who are prone to develop 2,8-dihydroxyadenine renal

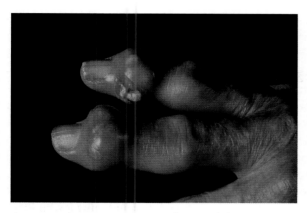

Figure 1.20 Disease as a consequence of purine imbalance: Gouty tophi in a patient with severe hyperuricemia (Wellcome Medical Photographic Library, no. N0010608C).

stones, patients with HPRT deficiency do not derive benefit from the xanthine oxidase inhibitor **allopurinol**.

Childhood malignancies such as **acute lymphoblastic leukemia** are often associated with high rates of growth and turnover as well as high sensitivity to anticancer drug therapy. Such patients are at risk of extremely high plasma and urinary urate levels following induction chemotherapy and consequent cytolysis. If this complication is not treated prophylactically with a xanthine oxidase inhibitor, the resulting **tumor lysis syndrome** can cause renal failure and death. During adult life, crystallization of uric acid out of solution is favored by high concentrations and/or low ambient pH in body fluids. Urate overproducers and underexcretors are thus prone to **acute gouty arthritis** caused by urate crystal formation within joint cavities. Patients who have a chronic metabolic predisposition to hyperuricemia and gout may also develop **tophi** – soft tissue deposits of uric acid – as urate crystals accumulate in cartilage, tendons and other tissues (Figure 1.20). Therapeutic alkalinization of the urine may improve the solubility of urate by maintaining it in the ionized form, thus preventing **kidney stone** formation.

Nucleic acids transmit data via complementary base pairs

Although the capacity for self-replication is fundamental to biology, Nature finds it easier to produce mirror images than exact replicas. A solution to this problem is first to create a mirror image and then to develop a second mirror image of the first. This two-step procedure – in which an initial nonidentical pairing prepares the way for a subsequent pairing which replicates the original – is the basis of nucleic acid function. The structural **complementarity** of base pairing, and hence the complexity of life, is based on only two variables:

1. **Base size**
   - In a double-stranded nucleic acid of constant width, only a pyrimidine (one carbon ring) can pair with a purine (two carbon rings).
2. **Number of hydrogen bonds**
   - Two bonds per base: hence, adenine must pair with thymine/uracil,
   - Three bonds per base: hence, guanine must pair with cytosine.

Steric considerations thus preclude the same nucleotide binding to itself – despite having the right number of hydrogen bonds – whereas bond stoichiometry prevents the wrong purine binding a pyrimidine. These factors explain the specificity of base pairing which in turn determines how nucleic acids transmit information. The Velcro™-like process by which two complementary nucleic acids zip together to form a hydrogen-bonded duplex is termed **annealing**. Guanine and cytosine stick more tightly to each other than do adenine and thymine, paralleling the number of hydrogen bonds. Hence, AT-rich and GC-rich sequences may serve slightly different genetic functions.

Human genes consist of two nucleic acid strands which are interwoven via the knit of hydrogen bonds forming ladder-like rungs. This double-stranded nucleic acid replicates itself as two complementary **daughter** strands, each one of which remains bound to a **parental** nucleic acid strand. Ingeniously, this so-called **semiconservative** replication of double-stranded nucleic acids is completed in a single step since both strands are replicated at once. The term **hybridization** denotes the experimental use of a synthetic complementary nucleic acid (the "probe" – usually radioactive; pp. 557–8) to identify a nucleic acid sequence of interest on a filter.

The two nucleic acid strands that comprise a human gene are termed the **template strand** and the **sense strand**. Importantly, it is the template rather than the sense strand which is physically copied. The sense strand is so-called

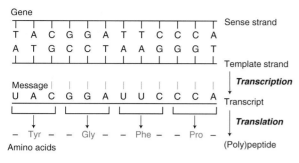

Figure 1.21 Simplified model of (gene) transcription and (transcript) translation. Trinucleotide sequences provide a code for specifying each one of the 20 amino acids.

because it mimics the (complementary) sequence of the template-encoded gene copy or **message** – albeit with substitution of T for U – and thus provides the official gene sequence. Hence, the uncopied sense strand gives rise to the template or **antisense** strand during replication, and vice versa (Figure 1.21).

The template strand prescribes the assembly of its complementary message in the form of a ribbon-like single-stranded **messenger** nucleic acid in a process termed **transcription**. The transcription machinery recognizes the correct binding site on the template strand via complex interactions with conserved sequences upstream of the gene (pp. 85–9). Single-stranded nucleic acid **transcripts** in turn provide docking sites for complementary trinucleotide-based nucleic acid adaptor molecules which align amino acids to form linear polypeptide chains – a process termed **translation** of the messenger nucleic acid. These two reactions, transcription and translation, are the central events of molecular biology (Figure 1.21).

PHARMACOLOGIC FOOTNOTE

Nucleotide-targeted anticancer drug therapy

Certain toxic drugs impersonate nucleotides or their precursors and thus become spuriously incorporated into actively replicating nucleic acids; these drugs are termed **antimetabolites**. Such agents include the purine mimics **azathioprine** – often used as an immunosuppressive agent to treat **autoimmune diseases** – and the anticancer drugs **6-mercaptopurine** (6-MP) and **6-thioguanine** (6-TG). Azathioprine is a pro-drug which is converted in vivo to 6-MP. However, azathioprine is also partly metabolised to thioguanine which is then methylated by endogenous repair enzymes, leading to misincorporation of thymine on the complementary strand during DNA replication; this mutagenicity may explain the high frequency of second malignancies following the use of azathioprine in organ transplantation.

These cytotoxic purine analogues are metabolized via the uric acid degradation pathway. Inadvertent co-administration of azathioprine or 6-MP to an allopurinol-treated patient may therefore result in severe antimetabolite toxicity unless the dose is reduced fourfold. Conversely, interindividual variations in purine metabolism are correlated with differential clinical responses to such drugs.

Antimetabolites based on pyrimidine mimicry include the cytotoxic drug **5-fluorouracil** (5-FU) which inhibits **thymidylate synthase**, and the antileukemic agent **cytosine arabinoside**. A genetic defect of pyrimidine catabolism, familial deficiency of the enzyme **dihydropyrimidine dehydrogenase** (DPD), results in pyrimidinemia and hypersensitivity to 5-FU that manifests clinically as mucositis and cerebellar syndrome. **DPD inhibitors** are now being investigated for their ability to enhance the efficacy of oral fluoropyrimidines.

Here let us pause to retrace the narrative of human molecular biology. About five billion years ago our planet was formed, at which time the Earth's surface was an asteroid-battered boiling soup cloaked in a reducing haze of carbon, hydrogen, and nitrogen. These elements reacted to form compounds such as formaldehyde and hydrogen cyanide. As the Earth's crust cooled over the next billion years, these precursor compounds gave rise to organic molecules capable of fermentation – an energy-producing reaction that drove other intermolecular interactions such as polymerization and phosphodiester bond formation. This transition from inorganic to organic chemistry was accelerated by terrestrial energy catalysts such as meteorite bombardment, ultraviolet light, and lightning. As a result the molecular pea-soup came to incorporate the fundamental ingredients of biology as we know it – amino acids and nucleotides.

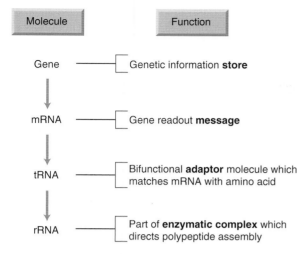

Figure 1.22 Functions of different nucleic acid subspecies during transcription and translation.

Ribonucleic acid can act as a template, adaptor or enzyme

Four billion years ago a random strip of nucleotides may have formed a primitive gene which directed the assembly of a short peptide. Although such a peptide would have lacked any complex structural attributes, it may have contained residues, such as cysteine or histidine, that could bond with metal cations (such as Zn^{2+}, Mg^{2+}, and Ca^{2+}) and thus acquire chemical reactivity. Such metal-dependent peptide motifs have been preserved in the active sites of enzymes and the nucleic acid-binding sites of gene-regulatory proteins.

This first gene was probably made of single-stranded **ribonucleic acid** (**RNA**). Aqueous RNA was an ideal candidate for the first self-replicator since it encapsulates structure and function in a single molecule: in addition to the information contained within its nucleotide sequence (genotype), primeval RNA molecules possessed catalytic activity (phenotype). The remnants of such catalytic or **enzyme** activity persist in some human RNAs, and autocatalytic RNAs or **ribozymes** can be generated in vitro ("in glass", i.e., in the lab) using selective constraints to mimic evolution. RNA may also exist complexed with proteins, in which form it is termed **ribonucleoprotein**. The properties of human RNA include the following (Figure 1.22):

1. Template function (nucleotide sequence recognition and/or transmission)
   • **Messenger RNA** (**mRNA**, or "the message").
2. Adaptor function (the matching of an mRNA sequence to amino acids)
   • **Transfer RNA** (**tRNA**).
3. Enzyme function (protein transesterification)
   • **Ribosomal RNA** (**rRNA**).

RNA is a highly successful nucleic acid by any standards, being present in human tissues in approximately fourfold greater abundance than double-stranded nucleic acids. Nonetheless, there remain objections to the credibility of "RNA world" origin-of-life scenarios (which, even if valid, may only have persisted for one hundred million years or so). As it happens, life on Earth has all but given up using RNA as genetic material over the last billion years – a change that reflects both the structural instability of the single-stranded molecule, and the appearance on the scene of a major nucleic acid upgrade. •

MOLECULAR MINIREVIEW

RNA instability

The evolutionary failure of single-stranded RNA to monopolize biology relates to its unstable structure – an undesirable feature in a molecule designed to cascade down the generations. The reasons for this instability include:

1. RNA is exquisitely vulnerable to enzymatic digestion by ubiquitous proteases termed **ribonucleases**. In contrast, double-stranded nucleic acids are far less sensitive to nuclease digestion.
2. The hydroxyl group at the 2′-carbon position of **ribose** exacerbates the susceptibility of RNA phosphodiester bonds to hydrolysis, especially in the presence of divalent cations. Substitution of a hydrogen for the hydroxyl, as seen in **deoxyribose**, reduces this tendency. Similarly, the RNA-specific pyrimidine base **uracil** is said to be less stable than its methylated form, thymine (see below).
3. The single-stranded structure of RNA lacks the **proof-reading** capabilities of a double-stranded nucleic acid – that is, it cannot check the sequence of a freshly replicated strand against a pre-existing complementary sequence. RNA is therefore prone to accumulating errors over successive generations.

The consequent **error-proneness** of RNA provides a survival advantage for some microorganisms which, by dint of their changing genome, avoid host immune surveillance via selectable alterations in protein expression. A notorious example is that of the **human immunodeficiency virus** (**HIV**) which has thus far evaded attempts to produce a reliable vaccine.

Genes use double-stranded nucleic acids to store information

A key priority for any molecule entrusted with genetic information is to maintain the fidelity of that information through successive generations. This demands the selection of a carrier able to cope with informational complexity and yet resist structural derangement. Such a description fits the master genetic molecule on our planet, **deoxyribonucleic acid** (**DNA**). The main structural differences between DNA and RNA are:

1. DNA is **double-stranded** whereas RNA is single-stranded.
2. DNA forms a **double-helix** whereas RNA assumes linear conformations.
3. DNA contains the reduced sugar **deoxyribose**; RNA contains ribose.
4. DNA contains the pyrimidine base **thymine** whereas RNA contains **uracil**.

Genetic information is better transmitted by DNA than by RNA. Double-stranded nucleic acids lack the instability of RNA, with phosphodiester bonds in DNA having a half-life of 200 million years in the absence of degrading nucleases or oxidant damage. In practice, intact kilobase-length DNA sequences have been retrieved from Egyptian mummies, and broken DNA from bony fragments of 100 000-year-old Neanderthals (note, however, that intact proteins have been extracted from fossils 100 million years old). In addition to its superior sequence fidelity, the double-stranded structure of DNA improves its speed of replication over that of RNA: instead of having to replicate a complementary sequence twice in succession, a two-strand nucleic acid only replicates once to produce an identical molecule.

Even before the structure of DNA was elucidated using crystallography, certain considerations favored a helix for storing genetic material:

1. Any multisubunit structure in which adjacent subunits bear a fixed asymmetric relationship to each other will form a helix – rather like rowing a boat with one oar (Figure 1.23). Hence, a polymeric dinucleotide is likely to assume this conformation, as will many repetitive polypeptides.
2. The compact interdigitated structure of the helix permits massive condensation of the molecule, thus maximizing information storage potential.
3. Helical twist, or **supercoiling**, provides a mechanism for storing and releasing free energy (for example, to drive transcription).

This is not to say that helices lack their drawbacks. Perhaps the most obvious of these relates to the need to disentangle replicating DNA. Fortunately, by the time double-stranded DNA appeared, molecular solutions to such problems had already evolved to cope with the circular genomes of microorganisms.

Removal of the 2′-hydroxy group of ribose also has the disadvantage of making the *N*-glycosyl bonds of DNA more readily hydrolyzable. Since a milliliter of aqueous DNA can store 10^{19} bits of information, even a minor degree of genetic instability might be expected to have significant ramifications. Hence, there are many things that can (and do) go wrong during the maintenance and replication of human genomes. This problem has necessitated the evolution of watchdog proteins termed **DNA repair enzymes**.

Figure 1.23 Helix formation from asymmetric subunits. *A,* Asymmetric rowing (one oar) causes the boat to assume a curved path. *B,* Two rowing boats fastened to each other can form a fixed asymmetric structure. *C,* A succession of asymmetric structures builds an ascending helix.

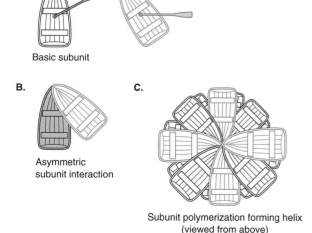

A.

Basic subunit

B.

Asymmetric subunit interaction

C.

Subunit polymerization forming helix (viewed from above)

Circular DNA

Unlike the linear genomes of higher organisms, genomes of simple microorganisms – **bacteria** – are circular, and measure about 0.5 mm in diameter if fully unwound. A circular genome is easier to develop and maintain since there are no specialized structures or endpoints to be negotiated. However, the advantages of a circular genome decline as the size of the genome increases, since it becomes difficult to access specific regions of the genome in a systematic manner.

Nucleic acids can also form circles termed **plasmids** which vary in size between 1 and 100 kb. RNA plasmids may have first evolved from coatless algal viroids, but more complex DNA plasmids have since developed genes with which to modify bacteria. If the plasmid enhances survival of the bacterium it will be replicated in tandem with the host genome; such plasmids may insert themselves into the circular bacterial genome. These plasmids represent **mobile genetic elements** which are passed from one bacterium to another as well as between unrelated bacterial strains. Bacterial plasmids carry two types of survival-enhancing genes:

1. **Virulence genes**, for example:
   - Host recognition proteins such as **adhesins** and **invasins**,
   - Host evasion proteins such as **hemolysins** and **toxins**.
2. **Resistance genes**
   - Biosynthetic enzymes to enhance bacterial survival,
   - Antibiotic resistance enzymes, e.g., for inactivating **penicillin**.

Plasmids thus represent a mechanism of horizontal gene transfer, and are used for this purpose as tools of genetic engineering in laboratories (p. 535).

Circular DNA also occurs in plant structures termed chloroplasts which mediate photosynthesis. The chloroplast genome is believed to have evolved from cyanobacteria, and is related to circular genomic structures in humans that are also involved in energy transfer reactions (see below).

DNA repair and recombination

DNA repair enzymes maintain genetic integrity

Sloppy DNA maintenance can be a boon for bacteria. Rapid rates of genome replication are tolerated without time-consuming interference from extra enzymes, whereas the high error rate yields numerous genetic variants capable of adapting to selective pressures. An example is the stomach ulcer microorganism *Helicobacter pylori* which exhibits remarkable genetic diversity leading to multi-strain colonization of the gastric contents; since the bug often recurs following antibiotic therapy, this represents a significant clinical problem. Similar hypermutability occurs in food-borne pathogens such as *Salmonella enteritidis*, *Campylobacter jejuni* and *Escherichia coli* O157:H7.

In contrast, a high level of genomic integrity is essential for higher organisms. Gene sequences in the human genome most often occur as single copies, whereas everything else in the vicinity (e.g., RNA, proteins, fats) is produced in multiple copies. Despite this, unforced replicative errors are detectable in human DNA at approximately one every 10^4 bp per cycle; after repair, however, net error rates drop to approximately 10^{-10}. This contrasts with net error rates of 10^{-5} and 10^{-4} per residue in RNA and protein respectively, making DNA replication by far the most faithful mode of information transfer. This million-fold enhancement of DNA repair fidelity is due to a battery of enzymes including **exonucleases, endonucleases, ligases, insertases, polymerases, helicases, topoisomerases, glycosylases,** and **flippases** (Figure 1.24).

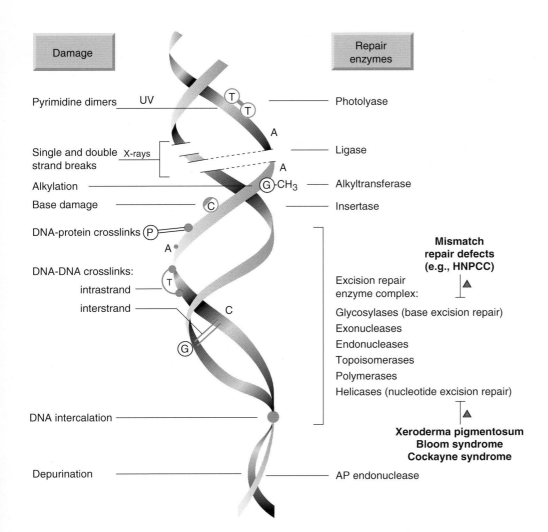

Damage		Repair enzymes
Pyrimidine dimers — UV	(T)(T)	Photolyase
	A	
Single and double strand breaks — X-rays		Ligase
	A	
Alkylation	(G)-CH₃	Alkyltransferase
Base damage	(C)	Insertase
DNA-protein crosslinks (P)	A	
DNA-DNA crosslinks:		
intrastrand	(T)	Excision repair enzyme complex:
interstrand	C	Glycosylases (base excision repair)
	(G)	Exonucleases
		Endonucleases
		Topoisomerases
		Polymerases
		Helicases (nucleotide excision repair)
DNA intercalation		
Depurination		AP endonuclease

Mismatch repair defects (e.g., HNPCC)

Xeroderma pigmentosum Bloom syndrome Cockayne syndrome

Figure 1.24 Types of DNA damage, and enzymes which repair them. Note that excision repair enzymes probably repair all types of damage (e.g., ultraviolet, UV) as well as those indicated. HNPCC, hereditary nonpolyposis colorectal cancer. AP, apurinic/apyrimidinic (site).

Thermal damage causes thousands of depurination and deamination events every day, and additional damage is caused by hydrolysis and nonenzymatic methylation (alkylation). The chemical groups added to DNA by such events are termed **adducts**. Ultraviolet radiation in sunlight induces bulky covalent intrastrand adducts known as **thymine** (or pyrimidine) **dimers**, the removal of which requires **nucleotide excision repair** – a process involving about 30 proteins. The oxidative damage induced by **reactive oxygen species** may be repaired either by nucleotide excision repair or else by **base excision repair** initiated by **DNA glycosylases**. Nontranscribed genes undergo enzymatic methylation, leading to the subsequent deamination of methylcytosine and thus C→T base switching (or G→A if the deamination occurs on the opposite strand). This methylation-dependent modification preferentially affects CG dinucleotides.

DNA damage may cause **nucleotide mismatching**. Cytosine may be deaminated to form uracil, for example, triggering a mismatch with adenine instead of guanine. Hence, excision repair and mismatch repair are two major pathways of DNA repair. Heritable defects of **DNA mismatch repair** (**MMR**) genes may cause **mutator** phenotypes which predispose carriers to genetic instability and cancer (p. 80).

Unrepaired damage may overwhelm DNA proofreading, but most unrepaired lesions prove harmless for one of the following reasons:

1. The lesion is located in a **noncritical** part of the genome
   - Most genetic lesions fall into this category.

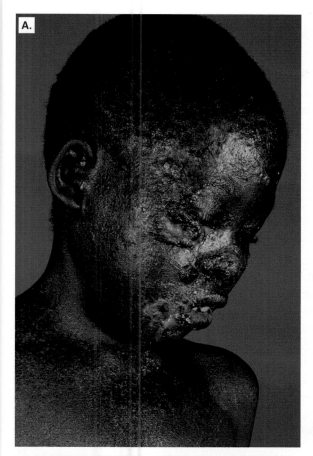

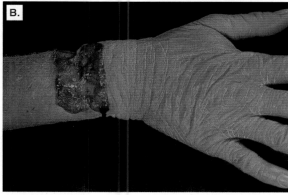

Figure 1.25 Carcinogenesis due to DNA damage. *A*, DNA repair deficiency in a xeroderma pigmentosum patient, showing skin damaged by multiple cancers (Wellcome Medical Photographic Library, no. N0011096C). *B*, An advanced squamous cell skin cancer in an albino patient lacking melanin for UV protection (Wellcome Medical Photographic Library, no. N0010989C).

2. The lesion causes a **conservative** change in amino acid sequence
   • For example, replacement of glutamic acid by aspartic acid.
3. The lesion knocks out gene function but is compensated by other genes
   • This is termed **redundancy**.

Note that gene redundancy may not imply uselessness. From a survival viewpoint it may be useful to have extra genes on tap – rather like firemen, just in case they are needed. Duplicated genes may thus add elasticity and durability to the system. Another model is that of a **parliament of genes** in which the crackpot initiatives of rogue genes may be outvoted by a quorum of uncorrupted genes.

DNA-damaging lesions may be caused by **oxidant damage** due to free radicals induced, for example, by the radiolysis of water. Oxidative injury is responsible for 10^4 to 10^5 lesions (single- and double-strand DNA breaks, base loss or demethylation events) per genome per day. Further oxidant damage is inducible by infection, reperfusion of ischemic tissue, and smoking. While most of these lesions are repaired, a small number accumulate and thus increase the risk of cancer. It is remarkable, however, that germline genomes incur as few as ten unrepaired (i.e., heritable) base changes each year. Such cumulative damage may contribute to the heightened incidence of congenital disorders such as **Down syndrome** with increasing maternal age.

CLINICAL KEYNOTE

Repair enzyme deficiencies

DNA repair disorders are autosomal recessive which often predispose to malignancy conditions, and include:

1. **Ataxia telangiectasia (AT)**. AT individuals are handicapped by their reduced ability to repair DNA strand-breaks. Homozygotes are thus prone to developing **leukemias** and **lymphomas**. Other clinical features include cerebellar degeneration (giving rise to ataxia), abnormal blood vessels in the skin and conjunctivae (telangiectasia), and recurrent chest infections (p. 379).
2. **Excision repair defects**
   • **Xeroderma pigmentosum (XP)**. These patients are hypersensitive to ultraviolet light (UV) because of their inability to repair UV-induced bulky intrastrand DNA adducts (i.e., defective nucleotide excision repair) termed **pyrimidine dimers**. Seven different genes (*XP-A* to *XP-G*) are involved. Affected individuals are at 1000-fold increased risk of skin cancers, usually from the age of eight; neurologic dysfunction may also be seen. Of note, XP affects dark-skinned races as well as Caucasians (Figure 1.25*A*).
   • **Cockayne syndrome**. Sensitivity to both X-radiation and UV radiation, but no increase in skin cancers. Mutations in any one of the five genes controlling **transcription-coupled repair** of UV and oxidative damage are responsible, but the *CSA* and *CSB* genes account for 90% of cases. The resultant excessive cell death may protect against cancer development.
   • **Trichothiodystrophy**. Brittle hair, neurologic damage, sun sensitivity, but no skin cancers.
3. **Bloom syndrome**. A helicase mutation (*BLM*) that causes genetic instability, small stature, immune defects, diabetes and cancers.
4. **Fanconi anemia**. A DNA crosslink repair defect that manifests as bone marrow failure (aplastic anemia), retardation, and acute myeloid leukemia. Most cases are caused by one of two genes.

Genetic complementation groups

Xeroderma pigmentosum (XP), Cockayne and Fanconi syndromes have been linked to heterogeneous gene defects via a process termed **complementation**. This involves mixing experiments that abolish the phenotype of one affected cell line by combining it with genetic material from a cell line isolated from a second patient with the disease, thereby implying the existence of different disease genes.

These genetic varieties of a single syndrome are termed **complementation groups**. For example, of the seven known XP complementation groups (XP-A to XP-G), the XP-A protein binds DNA damage – and thus prevents UVB-induced **skin cancers** – whereas XP-F and XP-G are DNases involved in 5′ and 3′ repair respectively. Hence, one possibility is that the different gene products act together in a multiprotein DNA repair complex, or perhaps sequentially.

Mutations differ in their phenotypic consequences

Genetic variation is intrinsic to life. Organisms that are both genotypic and phenotypic variants are termed **mutants**, and the underlying genetic sequence aberration is a **mutation**. The normal genetic material is termed the **wild-type** (**wt**). A variety of structural and phenotypic criteria are used to classify mutations. In the most conservative case, only a single "letter" of the genetic code is changed – these variants are termed **point mutations**. Such mutations may be structurally conservative, occurring between two purines (A and G) or two pyrimidines (T and C): these mutations are termed **transitions**. More serious (and less common) are **transversions**, purine-pyrimidine base switches that imply more severe functional consequences for proteins.

Larger losses of genetic material – corresponding to the omission of entire "words" or "sentences" – are termed **deletions**, whereas additions of new (inappropriate) sequence are termed **insertions**. A **nonsense mutation** causes transcription to arrest prematurely, thus leading to the production of a truncated protein. In contrast, a **missense mutation** encodes an abnormal amino acid, with the phenotypic consequences depending upon the structural consequences of the substitution. A **loss-of-function** mutation reduces the normal gene effect; a severe version is termed a **null mutation**. Conversely, a mutation that constitutively activates or otherwise augments the normal function of a gene is termed a **gain-of-function** mutation.

Distinction is also made between **germline mutations**, which are responsible for inherited disorders, and **somatic mutations** which are acquired during life and cause adult-onset diseases such as cancer. The extent to which inherited diseases arise because of new germline mutations varies, in part reflecting the reproductive prospects of those affected. **Congenital achondroplastic dwarfism** usually involves new mutations, for example, whereas only 25% of cases of the connective tissue disorder **Marfan syndrome** (arachnodactyly) occur by new mutation – the remaining 75% are associated with a family history. Similarly, the hereditary neurologic disorder **Huntington disease** is seldom seen in the absence of a family history.

In contrast to mutations, phenotypically subtle DNA alterations are readily passed on to successive generations. These sequence variants, termed **genetic polymorphisms**, are usually single-base changes, and are distinguished from mutations by their lack of apparent effect. Variations of this kind may spread widely within a population, and are traceable to specific genetic lineages. This can be helpful when investigating problems relating to forensic medicine (e.g., the identification of bloodstains), or when undertaking family gene mapping.

Mutations are a vital mechanism of genetic variation in bacteria since they trigger the emergence of durable strains in response to selection pressures. Bacteria have a short generation time, permitting the sacrifice of billions of defective mutants in return for one superior strain. For more genetically elaborate higher organisms, however, this "blind watchmaker" strategy is expensive. In humans, most germline mutations reduce survival and are therefore promptly eliminated, usually by spontaneous abortion. It is only with exceptional rarity that a mutation confers a survival advantage on a human cohort.

CLINICAL KEYNOTE

Balanced polymorphisms

Occasional homozygous disorders affecting individuals may be the evolutionary price to pay for less obvious benefits to the species. For example, it is plausible that lethal environmental hazards could select for heterozygote mutations in the gene pool, even though these same mutations confer no benefit in the absence of the hazard. Possible illustrations of this phenomenon include:

1. **Sickle cell anemia** (**hemoglobin S, HbS**) in heterozygous gene dosage (designated **sickle trait, or HbAS**) reduces mortality from blood parasitization by **malaria**, though HbSS homozygosity is fatal. Sickling may reduce parasite entry, prevent replication, and/or enhance the elimination of parasites.
2. Other common hemoglobinopathies such as **thalassemias** and **glucose-6-phosphate dehydrogenase deficiency** may have a similar cause. **Alpha-thalassemia**, for example, may be characterized by increased susceptibility to the less virulent malarial parasite *Plasmodium vivax*, but by reduced lethality following infection with the more fulminant *P. falciparum*.
3. **Cystic fibrosis** – a defect in transmembrane chloride transport – may (in its heterozygous asymptomatic form) confer resistance to lethal epidemic and endemic infections such as **typhoid fever, cholera** or **tuberculosis**.
4. Inherited predisposition to the metabolic disorder **diabetes mellitus** is another condition for which possible survival benefits have been proposed – presumably for mild or subclinical disease – in some stress situations (e.g., reduced infant mortality could be a benefit during famine).

The population frequency of some deleterious recessive mutations may thus be maintained via a heterozygote survival benefit related to an environmental hazard. Such "good-bad" mutations have been termed **balanced polymorphisms**.

Sex promotes allelic variation via DNA recombination

Contrary to popular belief, mutation is not the prime mechanism of human genetic change. Sex evolved not because it was fun but because it was a powerful way of introducing genetic variation (and hence adaptability) into a species. Sexual reproduction is only possible when genomes contain two copies or **alleles** of most genes; that is, the genome is **diploid**. A crucial advantage of this spare-copy arrangement is that **gametes** (sperms and eggs) can shed the spare copy, making these germline genomes **haploid** and hence capable of combining their genetic goods during fertilization. Moreover, if one allele becomes a dysfunctional mutant – that is, if a **heterozygous** mutation occurs – the remaining (wild-type) allele may be able to cover for it. The trait encoded by such a mutation is termed **recessive**, in which case expression of the mutant phenotype requires two copies of the defective gene (a **homozygous** mutation). A variation on this theme relates to individuals who accumulate a different mutation in each allele, thus rendering themselves **compound heterozygotes**; such individuals are often less severely affected than homozygotes.

If the mutant phenotype is apparent even in the heterozygous state, the mutation is termed **dominant**. Loss-of-function mutations thus tend to be recessive, whereas gain-of-function mutations are usually dominant. On occasion, however, heterozygous (allelic) deletions or other loss-of-function mutations may indeed induce a clinical phenotype, indicating that a single wild-type allele cannot provide normal gene function. In this context, autosomal dominant transmission is said to denote **haploinsufficiency** of gene expression.

A mutation that abolishes the normal function of a wild-type allele (e.g., by encoding a defective protein that binds and interferes with the normal protein) is termed a **dominant negative** (p. 586). **Penetrance** of a genetic trait is a measure of phenotype severity in the offspring. If unpredictable, the putative gene is described as **variably penetrant** (perhaps implying functional variation of the other allele). The term **hemizygous** usually refers to a sex-linked gene expressed in males, who have no second allele (pp. 409–10).

Human tumors often undergo aberrant recombinational events leading to allelic deletion or **loss of heterozygosity** (**LOH**), resulting in the eventual loss of growth control. One enzyme group critical for normal recombination is the **RECQ helicase** family: mutations affecting these key proteins are responsible for **Bloom syndrome**, **Werner syndrome**, and **Rothmund-Thompson syndrome** (p. 387). LOH induced by this mechanism renders the affected cell vulnerable to a "second hit" that can wipe out gene function and thus initiate cancer growth.

The ability of sex to inject variation into a species reflects not only the combination of genes from two unrelated organisms, but also the modification of such genes by **genetic recombination** or **crossing over**. This process occurs mainly during gamete formation from a parental diploid genome. Two cognate double-stranded DNA molecules are aligned then nicked, allowing the free single strands to contact complementary sequences on the intact strand of the heterologous DNA molecule (Figure 1.26). This process, termed **homologous recombination**, is exploited in genetic engineering where it is used to create novel organisms in which the expression of a functional gene is blocked or "knocked out" (p. 585). By virtue of its ability to introduce structural variety, genetic recombination underlies the evolutionary ascendancy of sexual (two-parent) over asexual reproduction.

Recombination is not always homologous. Nonhomologous DNA crossing-over sometimes occurs during sexual reproduction, where it is responsible for the important evolutionary processes of gene duplication and "jumping genes" (see below). **Site-directed recombination** events are also nonhomologous, and are relevant to development of the immune system (pp. 475–6).

Figure 1.26 Homologous recombination. DNA strands "cross over" to exchange homologous (but not necessarily identical) nucleotide sequences.

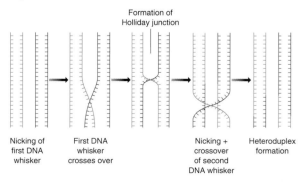

Nicking of first DNA whisker / First DNA whisker crosses over / Formation of Holliday junction / Nicking + crossover of second DNA whisker / Heteroduplex formation

MOLECULAR MINIREVIEW

Recombinational frequency and genomic distance

The huge size of the human genome makes it difficult to locate a gene of interest. Distances within the genome can be measured in a variety of ways: one way of expressing distances between genes involves calculating their **recombinational frequency** within germline tissues. This is a functional measure based on the observation that two genes situated close together will cross over more often during meiosis than will two genes situated further apart.

The eponymous **centimorgan** (cM) is defined as the genetic distance between two loci with a 1% probability of recombination. This approximates one megabase if homogeneous crossing-over is assumed. The total genetic length of the human genome is thus around 3000 cM.

We have learned in this section about the structure of genes – their components, their degradation, their interactions, their maintenance and their alterations. In the next section we consider how genes are packaged within cells, and how the evolution of more complex cells has driven such cells to develop new sources of genetic variation.

Cells and genomes

Bacteria are the genetic ancestors of human cells

The most prevalent life-form on Earth is the humble **bacterium**. RNA-based bacteria appeared around four billion years ago but were vanquished in due course by DNA-based organisms. The most primitive organisms now alive are **mycoplasmas**, tiny nonbacterial parasites familiar in both the laboratory (as contaminants of tissue culture) and the clinic (as causes of pneumonia and/or hemolysis). Since these organisms contain a genome that reproduces itself independently of other genomes, mycoplasmas represent the simplest existing form of **cell**.

Bacteria and mycoplasmas are distinguished from most other cellular species in that they lack a separate membranous compartment to house the genome; in the jargon of phylogeny, bacteria are **prokaryotic**. Prokaryotes are distinguished by their rapid reproductive rate (as often as once every 20 minutes), relative paucity of DNA (less than a megabase), and tough carbonaceous cell wall (a popular antibiotic target). Most prokaryotes contain about a thousand genes – about 2-3% of the number in humans.

The rapid reproductive rate of primitive bacteria provides ample opportunity for genetic selection. This property has led to the evolution of multistep metabolic pathways for processes such as the anaerobic utilization of glucose (glycolysis). Indeed, since bacteria initially evolved during a period when oxygen was scarce on Earth, many have remained obligate anaerobes for which oxygen is toxic. Glycolysis pathway genes (such as those encoding glucose-6-phosphate isomerase and glyceraldehyde-3-phosphate dehydrogenase; pp. 164–6) are conserved all the way from bacteria to Man – so the next time you take an **antibiotic**, be aware that you are killing a distant relative. Primitive yeast-like cells containing a **nucleus** first appeared on the Earth one to two billion years ago.

MOLECULAR MINIREVIEW

The linearization of DNA

How did the first nucleated organelle-free cell evolve? One theory proposes that ancestral archebacteria developed nuclei by invaginating the plasma membrane (the protist or **karyogenic** hypothesis). An alternative theory is that nuclei evolved via an endosymbiotic or phagocytic event between a host (an anaerobic hydrogen-dependent archebacterium) and a wall-deficient eubacterial prey or symbiont (which excretes hydrogen as a respiratory waste product) – the **endokaryotic** or serial endosymbiosis hypothesis.

In the latter model, intranuclear DNA attachment sites may have evolved to enable genome segregation during cell division. Such motile partitioning of the cell was a major breakthrough, since it permitted the linearization of circular bacterial DNA. This allowed replication to occur at many sites simultaneously, in turn facilitating evolution of a larger genome and, hence, embryo-derived multicellular organisms.

A cell is a self-replicating gene machine

To prokaryotic cells the acquisition of a nucleus must have seemed like the early years of computer technology, when the sudden acquisition of hard drives with ample megabyte capacity paved the way for software development on a scale undreamed of in the floppy disk era. These high-storage nucleated cells or **eukaryotes** evolved to be much bigger than prokaryotes, measuring approximately ten-fold greater in diameter ($\sim$10 μm instead of $\sim$1 μm) and containing about 1000-fold more DNA. There remain still millions of different eukaryotic species on the Earth, 75% of which are terrestrial animals living within tropical rainforests.

Eukaryotic cell evolution was a high-water mark in the evolutionary packaging of genes and proteins. The cell nucleus acts as a reference library for the genetic archives. In contrast, most of the cell's engine-rooms or **organelles** reside in the **cytoplasm** between the nucleus and the outer cell membrane. Such organelles include the **endoplasmic reticulum** where proteins are synthesized on **ribosomes** (which in bacteria account for over 30% of dry mass); the **Golgi apparatus**, which modifies proteins following translation; **peroxisomes**, which participate in the oxidative detoxification of free radicals; and **lysosomes**, which destroy time-expired proteins. All such organelles require duplication during cell division, and may be destroyed in certain cell types (e.g., anucleate red blood cell reticulocytes). The evolution of these membrane-enclosed organelles is a key phylogenetic advantage of eukaryotic cells.

In addition to their capacity for replication, eukaryotic cells contain molecular machines and motors which make them metabolize and move. Being obligate aerobes, larger eukaryotic species need to satisfy their formidable metabolic appetites by burning oxygen in another class of cytoplasmic organelles – electron-transfer power plants termed **mitochondria** which produce over 90% of cellular ATP requirements and also contain their own genomic DNA.

MOLECULAR MINIREVIEW

Mitochondrial genomes

The advent of an aerobic atmosphere suddenly made it a competitive priority to develop cellular organelles capable of converting oxygen to energy. These animal analogs of plant chloroplasts are termed mitochondria, 10–1000 of which inhabit every human cell (up to 10^5/oocyte), with each one measuring less than 1 μm in diameter. Mitochondria are the evolutionary fossils of primeval single-cell organisms which wheedled their way inside eukaryotic cells following the fall of the cell wall. Indeed, traces of mycoplasma-like genomes in human mitochondria have been detected. This hypothesis receives further support from the structurally similar genomes of mitochondria and bacteria, most notably *Rickettsia prowazekii* – the causative organism of **epidemic typhus** – which contains an identical set of genes for ATP generation.

In human cells **mitochondrial DNA (mtDNA)** is the only endogenous source of extranuclear genetic material. Individual mtDNA genomes are small – containing only 13 genes, all encoding respiratory-chain enzymes, within 16.5 kb – but recall that there may be up to 1000 mitochondria in each cell.

Features distinguishing the bacteria-like mtDNA from nuclear DNA include:
1. Bacterial and mitochondrial genomes are circular.
2. Bacterial and mitochondrial genomes are not held together by a proteinaceous scaffolding (pp. 52, 62–3).
3. Bacterial and mitochondrial genes are not interrupted (pp. 40–1).
4. Mitochondria do not add caps and tails to their mRNA transcripts (p. 99).
5. Some mtDNA codons represents amino acids distinct from those found in genomic DNA (pp. 78–9).

Mitochondria therefore have triple significance in human biology: first, as evidence of our bacterial ancestry; second, as membranous interfaces for ATP-generating electron transfer reactions; and third, as a repository for genes encoding products involved in cell respiration and cell death.

Mitochondrial DNA is maternally transmitted

Mitochondria replicate their own DNA, which accounts for about 0.5% of haploid cellular DNA. The 16,569 bp of the human mitochondrial genome encode 22 tRNAs, 2 rRNAs (12S and 16S) and 13 proteins from the respiratory (OXPHOS; p. 166) pathway. Each mitochondrion contains 2–12 genomes; the small size of the mtDNA genome enhances its replication rate. Since each cell contains many mitochondria, numerous mtDNA gene copies (up to thousands) may be expressed per cell. Normal and mutant mtDNAs may coexist in the same cell, a condition termed **heteroplasmy**. Deletions of *OXPHOS* genes (e.g., **Kearns–Sayre syndrome**, Figure 1.27) tend to be heteroplasmic if viable, whereas missense mutations (e.g., **Leber syndrome**) are often **homoplasmic**.

Analysis of mtDNA sequences can provide unique information about the ancestry of a cell or organism. This reflects two factors:
1. mtDNA, like the bacterial DNA from which it probably evolved, is poorly repaired and hence has a high mutation rate – at least ten times higher than that of nuclear DNA. This underlies the use of mtDNA as a "clock" for timing cellular evolutionary events, studies of which have spawned the out-of-Africa hypothesis that a sub-Saharan Eve mothered us all (see p. 47). Ageing may also be associated with the accumulation of mtDNA mutations, leading to reduced cell energy production.
2. Unlike nuclear DNA, mtDNA does not have sex. A sperm cell contributes only one ten-thousandth the quantity of mtDNA to the mammalian zygote compared to the oocyte. For practical purposes this means that human mtDNA is maternally inherited via the oocyte cytoplasm. Recombination of mtDNA – either with nuclear DNA or within the ovum – could account for rare instances of paternal mtDNA inheritance. Of note, spermatocytes also fail to pass on any other cytoplasmic organelles.

mtDNA can find its way into cell nuclei where it inserts into nuclear genes to produce chimeric fusion sequences. Many mitochondrial genes may have been lost to the nucleus over the course of evolution, as supported by the far

Figure 1.27 Patient with the mitochondrial DNA defect Kearns–Sayre syndrome, showing muscular weakness due to defective mitochondrial energy metabolism (Wellcome Medical Photographic Library, no. N0009348C).

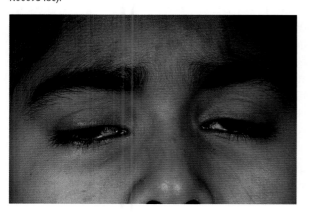

Table 1.4. Diseases of mitochondrial DNA

Primary mtDNA abnormalities
1. **Leber hereditary optic neuropathy** (LHON)
   - Adult-onset blindness; low penetrance,
   - mtDNA-encoded retinal electron-transport chain missense mutations affecting NADH dehydrogenase or cytochromes.
2. Mitochondrial tRNA mutations (usually cause inefficient translation)
   - **MERRF** (myoclonic epilepsy and ragged-red fiber disease),
   - Mutation: tRNA$^{Lys8344/8356}$; causes "horse collar" distribution of fatty tumors,
   - **MELAS** (mitochondrial encephalomyopathy and stroke-like episodes),
   - Mutation: tRNA$^{Leu(UUR)3243}$, i.e., A3243G,
   - Concomitant A12308G polymorphism may be linked to stroke risk,
   - **MMC** (maternally inherited myopathy and hypertrophic cardiomyopathy),
   - Mutation: tRNA$^{Leu(UUR)3260}$ (rarely causes diabetes mellitus).
3. **Kearns–Sayre syndrome** (Figure 1.27)
   - Progressive external ophthalmoplegia, retinopathy, ataxia, and heart conduction defects due to mtDNA deletions.
4. **Pearson marrow-pancreas syndrome**
   - Neonatal pancytopenia, pancreatic/hepatic insufficiency, lactic acidosis.
5. **Cyclic vomiting**
   - Associated with recurrent lactic acidosis, migraine, and sudden death
6. **Leigh syndrome**
   - Mutation of ATPase 6, or nuclear complex II.

higher mitochondrial-to-nuclear DNA ratio of plants and frogs compared to mammals. On the other hand, the mitochondrial genome is not autonomous: proteins encoded by nuclear DNA are essential for mtDNA replication and transcription, making nonmitochondrial genes necessary for normal mitochondrial function. Hence, mutations in genomic DNA may still cause so-called mitochondrial diseases even though cell respiration is regulated by the mtDNA genome.

CLINICAL KEYNOTE

Mitochondrial inheritance

Certain tissues are highly dependent upon mitochondrial energy production. These include the heart, skeletal muscle, central nervous system, and kidneys. Age-related declines in mitochondrial respiration efficiency may contribute to the failure of these organ systems as may nuclear or mtDNA mutations (Table 1.4). One disease that illustrates this pathogenesis is the syndrome of exercise intolerance caused by mutations that affect the mitochondrial *cytochrome b* gene. Another such disorder is **hereditary spastic paraplegia** – a disorder caused by mutation of the somatic *Paraplegin* gene which encodes a protein involved in mitochondrial assembly. Measurements of plasma **lactate** and **pyruvate**, and of muscle **cytochrome oxidase** and **succinic dehydrogenase**, may be helpful in identifying such syndromes.

Not all mitochondrial disorders reflect primary abnormalities of mtDNA. For example, the anti-AIDS drug **zidovudine** (azidothymidine: AZT) may cause muscle weakness in HIV patients because of inhibition of mitochondrial γ-DNA polymerase – in effect, an acquired mtDNA disorder. Similarly, the cardiotoxic effects of the anticancer drug **doxorubicin** (which generates free radicals) may relate in part to mtDNA damage. All such mitochondrial myopathies reflect impaired acidification of muscle fibrils associated with reduced oxygen delivery, with correspondingly sluggish phosphocreatine accumulation and compensatory increases in proton efflux.

Repetition and variation

Introns accelerate evolution by splitting genes

Two bacteria – one for the nucleus and another for the mitochondria – may thus have been the lead architects for human life as we know it. The development of the nucleus was a biological breakthrough which suddenly enabled cells to amass huge genomes. There was still a problem, however, since no mechanism for expanding the number of genes was in place.

A radical solution was forthcoming. Gene subunits were mobilized within the genome, allowing them to generate new genes via a mix-and-match process. This mobilization strategy involved the creation of **split genes**. But what do we mean by this terminology?

The **coding sequence** of a human gene is that part of the gene which ultimately encodes protein. This may not be identical to the full-length gene since eukaryotic RNA transcripts are usually processed prior to translation (p. 100). Hence, human genes are often interrupted by intervening DNA sequences termed **introns** that encode transcripts marked for excision prior to translation.

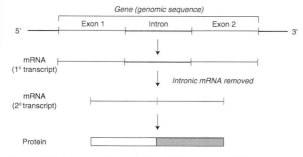

Figure 1.28 Introns and exons. A hypothetical gene split by a single intron is shown. Removal of the intron from the primary transcript leads to formation of the mature (translated) mRNA.

The vast majority of human genes are split by introns, usually 2–20 per gene. Unlike bacteria, only a minority of our genes (e.g., those encoding histone proteins; p. 52) remain intron-free. Whether introns evolved early and were discarded by bacteria (the exon theory) or evolved late and were added to pre-existing genes (the insertional hypothesis) remains a matter for debate.

Gene fragments that encode mature RNA and protein structures are termed expressing sequences or **exons** (Figure 1.28). An alternative way of thinking about this arrangement is to consider exons as **microgenes**. Introns facilitate transgenomic recombination of these integral microgene units – a process termed **exon shuffling** – and thus promote the creation of novel multidomain proteins. According to one theory, the exon universe encoding all polypeptides may comprise as few as 1000 basic DNA motifs, with each of these motifs specifying amino acids as short as 40 residues. This emphasizes both the modular simplicity and the combinatorial complexity of the human genome. An "average" gene consists of:

1. **Genomic DNA** (coding plus noncoding DNA)
   • About 30 kb (range 1–2500 kb),
   • Most of this DNA is contributed by introns.
2. **Coding DNA** (transcribed DNA translated into protein; exons)
   • About 2 kb (range: 0.5–20 kb); this is the length of the mRNA transcript.

Of course, some of the more interesting genes in human biology are far larger than this. The genomic **factor VIII** gene (mutated in the coagulopathy **hemophilia A**) is 186 kb in length, 177 kb of which is accounted for by 25 introns. An even larger gene is that which encodes **dystrophin** – the gene mutated in **Duchenne muscular dystrophy** – which measures over 2 Mb in length and contains over 100 exons. The size and structural complexity of these latter "disease genes" is not coincidental, but rather reflects the abundant room for error during their replication and recombination.

Introns pose technical problems for the mapping of coding sequences within a morass of noncoding DNA. The length of such a gene including introns – that is, the size of the genomic DNA sequence – may be over 100-fold greater than the coding sequence. Homologous genes in different species usually contain introns in similar positions, though the size of such introns varies.

Although variability of intron size suggests a lack of selection pressure on intron structure, it is not accurate to equate introns with genetic junk. Introns may contain regulatory DNA sequences that cause cell dysregulation and human disease when damaged, and intronic mutations may also cause genetic disease by interfering with RNA processing. For example, familial and sporadic tumors of the nervous system including **neurofibromatosis** and **meningiomas** have been linked to intron mutations of certain genes (the *NF1* and *Sis* genes, respectively). Moreover, since genomic DNA sequences tend to be more potently expressed than coding sequences when expressed in animals (pp. 583–4), introns may contribute in unidentified ways to gene regulation.

MOLECULAR MINIREVIEW

Exon shuffling and protein dimer evolution
Enhanced genetic mobility due to exon shuffling may cause structurally homologous domains to appear within functionally divergent proteins. For example, the 45-kb, 18-exon **low-density-lipoprotein** (LDL) **receptor** gene contains domains

A.

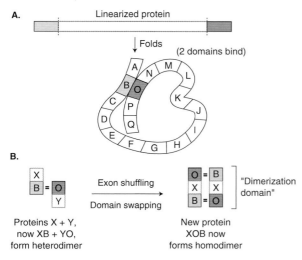

B.

Figure 1.29 Hypothetical evolution of dimers by exon shuffling and domain swapping. *A*, Following translation, the original protein folds, revealing a binding interaction between two domains B and O. *B*, If the exons encoding B and O shuffle and reinsert adjacent to genes encoding proteins X and Y respectively, two new proteins (XB and OY) will be formed. These proteins may thus bind to each other, or heterodimerize, via B and O. If exon shuffling results in protein X being surrounded by new domains B and O, homodimerization may result as shown.

Figure 1.30 Approximate spatial composition of the human genome, showing the proportion of coding to junk DNA.

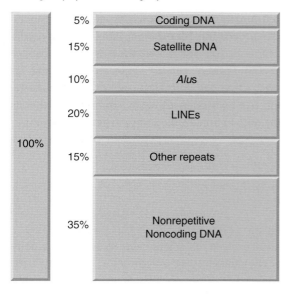

similar to those found in the **C9 complement component** as well as in the **epidermal growth factor** (EGF) precursor. At first glance these molecules do not appear functionally similar, suggesting that the significance of domain swapping events may be at a broader level.

Proteins fold up into three-dimensional structures. The chemistry of the molecular subunits defines a preferred conformation based in part on the relative atomic hydropathy of those subunits. Hence, the folding of a solitary or **monomeric** protein may spontaneously identify subdomains with mutual binding affinity. Imagine, then, that these binding subdomains (let's call them A and B) happen to be encoded by separate exons. Following a few rounds of exon shuffling, we may find that the encoded domains are swapped into different proteins, with protein X containing A and protein Y containing B. As occurred at close quarters within the original folded protein, random juxtaposition of A and B may lead to the stable binding of X and Y. Such protein–protein binding is termed **dimerization**, **oligomerization** or **polymerization**, depending on how many proteins comprise the complex. Some dimers may consist of two identical proteins containing both dimerization subdomains, A and B; such a dimer is termed a **homodimer**. In contrast, the isolated binding of protein X to protein Y is termed a **heterodimer** (Figure 1.29). **Tetramers**, both homo- and hetero-, are particularly stable structures; **trimers** may also occur.

The development of protein dimers was a stroke of evolutionary genius. By introducing the combinatorial complexity of multiprotein interactions, the regulatory capacity of ordinary monomeric proteins was at one stroke hugely enhanced.

Genomes accumulate destabilizing repeat sequences

Less than 5% of human DNA encodes proteins – the other 95% replicates but does not transcribe. This seems grossly inefficient compared to the no-frills genomes of our bacterial cousins, which consist wholly of coding DNA. Strictly speaking, introns and gene-regulatory sequences belong to this class of noncoding DNA. However, the largest subset of noncoding genetic material is the ocean of **junk DNA** which separates islands of functional genes.

Approximately 50% of all noncoding DNA consists of **repetitive DNA sequences** – that is, sequences repeated more than 20 times per genome (Figure 1.30). The widespread infiltration of genomes with such sequences makes repetitive DNA an excellent fossil record of evolution over the last 800 million years. In the human genome, these sequences can be subclassified as:

1. Highly repetitive **tandem repeats** or **satellite DNAs**, e.g.,:
   - $(ACAAACT)_n$ make up 5–10% of the human genome,
   - **Microsatellite** (1-5 bp) **repeats** (e.g., two to four nucleotides: $(CA)_n$, $(CG)_n$, $(GT)_n$, $(AT)_n$ or $(GATA)_n$ / ~100 000/haploid genome),
   - **Hypervariable minisatellite** (14–100 bp) **repeats**, or **VNTRs** (variable number of tandem repeats).
2. Moderately repetitive **interspersed repeats** (**transposable elements**)
   - Make up 35% of the human genome,
   - Short (100–400 bp) interspersed elements (**SINEs**: 14% of the genome); e.g., *Alu* **sequences**: ~1 250 000/haploid genome (10% of the genome),
   - Long (5–7 kb) interspersed elements (**LINEs**: 21% of the genome), e.g., **L1 elements**: ~550 000/haploid genome (17% of the genome) or *Kpn*1 sequences: ~100 000/haploid genome.

This tendency of genomes to accumulate **selfish DNA** should not be confused with the abovementioned concept of selfish genes, an evolutionary paradigm relating to competition within the gene pool.

The number of times a DNA sequence recurs within the genome is termed the **copy number**, with over 50% of all human genes being present in single copy. High copy numbers of repeat sequences destabilize the surrounding DNA, presumably because the recombinational and proofreading machinery becomes confused by vast swathes of identical sequence. Of note, not all repeat sequences are noncoding: functional genes encoding **ribosomal RNA** and DNA-associated **histone proteins**, for example, are also present as tandem repeats.

Junk is not the same as trash. We hoard junk in our attics in the hope that one day it may be useful; trash, on the other hand, we chuck out. Sadly, most of our junk remains useless despite such optimism. Nonetheless, explanations for the survival value of junk DNA (such as the possibility that it compartmentalizes the genome or, more plausibly, introduces variation) may well prove valid. Adaptability will always win out over size or beauty in evolution – newts have six times as much DNA per cell as humans, for example, and are well adapted yet no more intelligent. The need for longlived complex organisms such as humans to resist premature cancer and senescence may also be related in some way to our genome's appetite for scavenging GC-rich junk.

To appreciate the genome's problem, one need only acquire the latest computer megastorage device: against all expectations, the thing fills up with useless information at a pace you can scarcely credit. So it may prove to be with genomic DNA, a storage device which is great for sucking up genetic variation, but in the process appears to have fallen victim of its own success.

CLINICAL KEYNOTE

Junk DNA in human disease

Repetitive sequences such as *Alu*s and L1 elements are not entirely benign in their effects. One way in which these noncoding sequences can cause trouble is by **insertional mutagenesis**, that is, disruption of normal gene function by putting themselves in the wrong place. Examples of these rare mutational events include:

- Insertional mutagenesis of the **factor VIII** and **IX** genes by truncated L1 elements leading to **hemophilia A** and **B** respectively,
- Similar insertional mutagenesis of the *Spectrin* gene to cause **hereditary elliptocytosis**, the *Rhodopsin* gene to cause **retinitis pigmentosa**, the *β-globin* gene locus to cause **β-thalassemia**, or the *LDL receptor* gene to cause **familial hypercholesterolemia**,
- Defective recombination between two nonallelic *Alu* sequences, leading to deletions of the *Hexosaminidase B* gene and, thus, the lysosomal storage disorder **Sandhoff disease**,
- Insertional mutagenesis of the *Dystrophin* gene by L1 elements in **Duchenne muscular dystrophy**,
- *Alu* insertions in the pathogenesis of **Huntington disease**,
- Insertions of L1 sequences disabling the *APC* (**adenomatous polyposis coli**) gene and leading to **colorectal cancer**.

A distinct illustration of the effects of repetitive DNA sequences is provided by neurologic disorders associated with the hereditary accumulation of **trinucleotide repeats** (p. 82).

MOLECULAR MINIREVIEW

Alus

The commonest interspersed repeats are the *Alu* sequences, high-copy-number 300-bp SINEs that contain regions cleavable by a DNA-cutting enzyme called *Alu*1. These sequences account for around 10% of total human DNA. *Alu* sequences originated about 50 million years ago from the inactivation of a primate-specific gene encoding a 7SL RNA species involved in protein synthesis. This process of *Alu* insertion appears to have terminated prior to the phylogenetic divergence of chimps (whose genome has very few *Alu*s) and humans (whose genome is chock-full of *Alu*s), suggesting an evolutionary predisposition for this massive insertional event.

Relevant to this, certain *Alu* subclasses appear able to regulate gene responses in a stress-responsive manner – arguing against a "junk" status for these genetic elements, and away from the paradigm of *Alu*s as inert (albeit mobile) pseudogenes. The latter view is also consistent with the preferential insertion of *Alu*s in gene-rich chromosomal regions, unlike LINEs which (after piggybacking onto *Alu*s; see below) tend to insert into AT-rich heterochromatin. Note that the latter preference explains why LINE-induced genetic diseases are mainly encoded on the X chromosome (pp. 409–10).

Transposons proliferate by jumping through genomes

The commonest long interspersed element, the 6.4-kb **L1 element**, accounts for 80% of LINEs and 17% of the human genome. Both *Alu* sequences and L1 elements insert themselves into the genome by site-specific recombination or **transposition**, that is, they are **transposable elements** or **transposons**. Such sequences spread through the genome as germline mutagens via the same sort of cut-and-paste recombination events that lead to gene duplication.

Unlike *Alu*s, full-length L1 elements can transcribe RNA backwards into DNA, reflecting expression of a catalytic activity termed **reverse transcriptase**. This property allows L1 elements to direct the genomic insertion of RNA species, including those transcribed from other repetitive DNA elements such as *Alu*s (Figure 1.31). This process, termed **retrotransposition**, by definition produces only intronless genes, and the responsible sequences are designated **retro(trans)posons**. The essence of retrotransposition is that what starts out as one sequence ends up as two. Remarkably, as much as 40% of the current version of the human genome (L1 elements + *Alu*s + endogenous retrovirus-like sequences) may have originated in this manner.

LINEs are master retrotransposons. The functional activity of L1 elements underlies their status as **jumping genes**, even though they do not themselves encode proteins. In contrast, since *Alu* sequences do not possess reverse transcriptase activity, they do not qualify as retroposons. Over 95% of LINEs are truncated (averaging 1 kb instead of their full 6 kb length) and hence functionally inactive. Indeed, the human genome may contain as few as 60 full-length active LINEs, representing only 2% of the number active in the mouse genome. Unlike the other main evolutionary family of retroposons – retroviruses – L1 elements do not contain **long terminal repeats** which are stretches of nucleic acid often found in the 3′ region of viral genes. However, their promoters are often contained within the 5′ untranslated region.

Retroposons insert themselves following the nonhomologous repair of double-strand DNA breaks, raising the possibility that endogenous retroelements evolved as part of a DNA repair mechanism. Conversely, bacteria such as *Vibrio cholerae* have developed a mechanism for picking up stray bits of

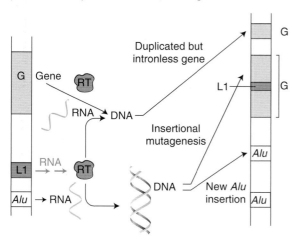

Figure 1.31 Consequences of transposition events. Reverse transcriptase (RT) activity of L1 elements may predispose to gene duplication events, insertional mutagenesis or "jumping gene" proliferation of repetitive DNA motifs, including *Alu*.

DNA that might provide a survival advantage. The molecular basis for this process, referred to as an **integron**, involves a genome-inserting enzyme or **integrase**.

Despite their inability to encode proteins, transposons and retroposons introduce genetic variation by promoting unequal DNA crossing-over and insertional mutagenesis. Sequences (such as exons or promoters) lying 3′ to the retroposon are preferentially inserted into transcribed genes, leading to the expansion and diversification of new genes. Diseases may thus be triggered, with one example being **Fukuyama muscular dystrophy** in which the memorable *fukutin* gene has undergone mutagenesis by retroposon insertion. In addition, retroposons may modulate gene function by insertion into gene-regulatory DNA flanking sequences.

Biologists may also exploit transposons for experimental tasks such as tagging DNA sequences, mapping genes or creating transgenic animals. Perhaps the prime significance of these endogenous human retroelements, however, lies in their close resemblance to another key nucleic acid species – **viruses**.

Cells resemble computers in the sense that both have a physical structure – the hardware – as well as instructions or programs – software – which may be transferred. This design has its problems since undesirable software can also be transferred as rogue programs which inhibit normal function. Such computer viruses bear a strong resemblance to viruses that infect human organisms

MOLECULAR MINIREVIEW

Viruses

Viruses aren't alive, they just feel like they are. Unlike cells, viruses are unable to reproduce independently. Rather, viruses are molecular mimics that hijack the transcriptional and reproductive apparatus of cells. Hence, as with transposons, cellular evolution preceded that of viruses; as with computer viruses, if they didn't exist they would have to be invented.

A virus is a gene machine – *sans* enzymes, *sans* organelles, *sans* everything – which may be single- or double-stranded, RNA or DNA, small (1 kb) or relatively large (300 kb). Viruses remain functionless until they gain cell entry, at which point their genome may integrate into host DNA by mimicking site-specific recombination events. At this point the viral genes become activated and start to control key components of the cell's genetic machinery. Intracellular proliferation of viral particles ensues, causing cell lysis and enabling the liberated viral particles to infect other cells in an exponential manner (Figure 1.32). Of note, some DNA viruses contain prepackaged viral transcripts that can be released into the infected cell even in the absence of transcription.

The **human immunodeficiency virus** (**HIV**) is an example of a **retrovirus** – an RNA virus coexpressing reverse transcriptase, which expedites the integration of a double-stranded DNA copy of the viral genome (the provirus) into host cell DNA. Certain benign retroviruses may have inserted themselves into the human genome where they now function as **human endogenous retroviruses** or **HERVs**. There are 450 000 HERVs which comprise 8% of the human genome: such HERV sequences have been implicated in physiologic functions such as placental morphogenesis, whereas others (HERV-W-like sequences) have been linked to the pathogenesis of diseases such as **schizophrenia**. Porcine endogenous retroviruses or **PERVs** are transmissible by pig islet cell transplantation into immune-deficient mice, casting doubt on the safety of organ xenotransplantation in humans.

Figure 1.32 Viral entry into a naive cell via specific recognition of normal cell surface receptors, followed by ❶ integration, ❷ replication, and ❸ proliferation. Bursting of the infected cell leads to dissemination of virions to neighboring cells.

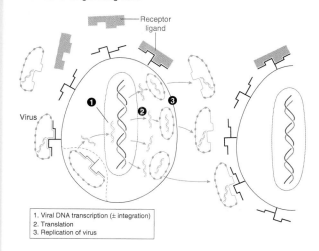

1. Viral DNA transcription (± integration)
2. Translation
3. Replication of virus

Viruses are neither cunning nor evil. Rather, they illustrate how genes and proteins evolve selfishly within a biological system to develop a proliferative advantage, whether in evolution or disease. The positive side of this is that viruses may in time become therapeutically useful as vectors for gene therapy.

Genetic lineages are identifiable by satellite DNA

The human genome is a biological fossil. Genetic analyses of repeat sequences have generated unique conclusions: humans are evolutionarily closer to fungi than plants, Native Americans are closer to Finns than to Chinese, and whales are closer to hippopotamuses than to pigs. These conclusions are based on **molecular clock** paradigms of genetic variability in which mtDNA ticks faster than nuclear DNA, while junk DNA ticks faster than coding DNA. Of note, different clocks – including those based on protein rather than nucleic acid – do not always agree on the time.

Recent clock studies have calculated that humans are now evolving more slowly than other mammals. The human DNA clock turns over at the rate of once every billion years – that is, every nucleotide in the genome will have averaged one mutagenic alteration by that time, though conserved genes such as that for β-globin will vary far less than, say, histone genes or repetitive DNA. In contrast, the rat genome may turn over five times more rapidly than the human genome on a per-nucleotide basis.

Satellite DNA is so-called because its GC-rich nucleotide structure allows it to be separated from other genomic DNA by density gradient centrifugation. This genomic subfraction, which is transcriptionally silent, contains highly repetitive sequences. Any DNA region containing tandem arrays of such repetitive sequences may be termed a **minisatellite**, analysis of which is useful for long-term genotyping; it is the relative speed of minisatellite evolution that is the basis of its utility as a genomic marker. Minisatellite DNA often occurs within introns or within regions immediately upstream or downstream of genes. The variable number of tandem repeats (VNTRs) in such sequences makes them ideal for identifying unique heterozygous pattern. This variability reflects mutational instability, which is often localized to one end of the tandem array. **Microsatellite instability** (MSI) is associated with the pathogenesis of certain familial and sporadic **colorectal cancers**. DNA repeat sequence instability may be induced by mutagens, as documented in survivors of the Chernobyl meltdown; conversely, repeat insertions may also predispose to disease.

Repetitive DNA sequences may thus represent both a cause and an effect of genetic instability, and are therefore useful for analyzing genome identity and ancestry. Such analyses have indicated that the basic body plan of animals has scarcely altered in the last 600 million years; evolution may thus occur in a punctuated fashion. Moreover, much of genetic evolution proceeds in a convergent manner, with the same gene classes evolving in separated species (a memorable example is the puffer fish which has two genes for cannabinoid receptors – and yet, despite its name, does not smoke). Uncertainty as to whether DNA repeats represent genomic hitchhikers or bioterrorists is therefore likely to persist, mirroring Nature's symbiotic balance between parasitism and predation.

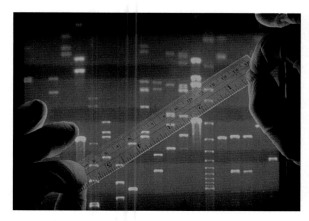

Figure 1.33 DNA fingerprints (Wellcome Medical Photographic Library, no. N0013789C).

DNA fingerprinting

Analysis of DNA sequence variation allows the monitoring of DNA across either time (paleogenetic studies) or space (forensic studies). For example, paleogenetic evidence indicates that human and ape lineages diverged about five million years ago on the African Savannah. The trigger for this divergence appears to have been climatic: replacement of the warm and humid Miocene era by the sunny, dry Pliocene period was accompanied by drying of the ground – making the rapid evolution of bipedalism over the next million years advantageous for locomotion, and thereby encouraging the migration and isolation of selectable population groups (see the movie *2001 A Space Odyssey* if you don't believe this). In true Darwinian style, most of the early bipedal hominids – e.g., *Australopithecus*, four million years ago – duly became extinct, but our own *Homo* genus arose approximately three million years ago and has so far lived to tell the tale. *Homo sapiens* diverged from our Neanderthal cousins a quarter million years ago or so, and is now the sole survivor of about 20 *Homo* species to have walked the Earth. It is only within the last 100 000 years that the exodus of modern humans from sub-Saharan Africa to what we now call the Middle East and Europe occurred, and only in the last 50 000 years that these latter ancestors developed creativity, philosophy and abstract thought. This whole saga has been brought to you courtesy of DNA (mitochondrial and nuclear) clock studies.

Other paleogenetic analyses have placed humans closer to gorillas than to orang-utans and, thankfully, have confirmed only the most distant relationship between ourselves and bats. By the same token, the DNA of cows has been shown to resemble that of dolphins more closely than that of pigs, whereas papaya is closer to cauliflower than to passionfruit (not many people know this).

Forensic studies of repetitive DNA mainly center on minisatellite analysis. Substantial variation exists between individuals as to the number of times a core VNTR sequence is repeated. This observation forms the basis of the **DNA fingerprinting** test now routinely used for identification of tissues (e.g., hair, blood, semen; Figure 1.33) in criminal cases. Other polymorphic DNA variations may be useful for disease detection or gene mapping (pp. 567–8, 573–5).

Enrichment reading

Bedtime reading

Asimov I. *The world of carbon.* Abelard-Schuman, London, 1958

Monod J. *Chance and necessity.* Knopf, New York, 1971

Dawkins R. *The blind watchmaker.* Longman, London, 1988

Cheap'n'cheerful

Atkins PW. *The periodic kingdom.* Basic Books, New York, 1995

Page R, Holmes EC. *Molecular evolution: a phylogenetic approach.* Blackwell, Oxford, 1998

Library reference

Ball P. *Designing the molecular world: chemistry at the frontier.* Princeton University Press, Princeton, NJ, 1994

Summary

Sunlight supplies energy for life on Earth. Molecules are formed by covalent bonding of atoms. Animals use oxygen to burn ingested nutrients. Oxygen pulls electrons off hydrogen donors. Carbon confers structural complexity on living molecules.

Proteins are functional amino acid chains. Phosphate groups transfer energy between proteins. Genes are used by proteins to make more proteins. Evolution conserves informative gene sequences.

Nucleotides are base-sugar-phosphate building blocks. Efficient nucleoside excretion is needed for nitrogen balance. Nucleic acids transmit data via complementary base pairs. Ribonucleic acid can act as a template, adaptor or enzyme. Genes use double-strained nucleic acids to store information.

DNA repair enzymes maintain genetic integrity. Mutations differ in their phenotypic consequences. Sex promotes allelic variation via DNA recombination.

Bacteria are the genetic ancestors of human cells. A cell is a self-replicating gene machine. Mitochondrial DNA is maternally transmitted.

Introns accelerate evolution by splitting genes. Genomes accumulate destabilizing repeat sequences. Transposons proliferate by jumping through genomes. Genetic lineages are identifiable by satellite DNA.

The human genome has been likened to a textbook that an editor has been correcting for millions of years. In this chapter we have reviewed the way in which this genetic narrative has been written; in the next section we take a more detailed look at the higher structures and functions of the human genome.

QUIZ QUESTIONS

1. Describe how an atom is structured, and how covalent bonds form between two atoms.
2. Explain what happens in molecular terms when paper is burnt in air.
3. Discuss the different metabolic processes by which plants and animals derive energy.
4. Name some structural features of a protein that influence its physical behavior.
5. How does gene duplication occur? What use is it?
6. List some of the functions of ATP.
7. What is meant by the term "salvage pathway" in relation to purine biosynthesis?
8. Explain how the specificity of complementary base pairing in DNA is generated.
9. For what evolutionary reasons did sexual reproduction evolve?
10. Explain why the appearance of cell nuclei is regarded as a major evolutionary event.
11. What is an intron? Why do you think we have them?
12. Name some ways the human genome might accumulate repetitive sequences.

2 | **Chromatin and chromosomes**

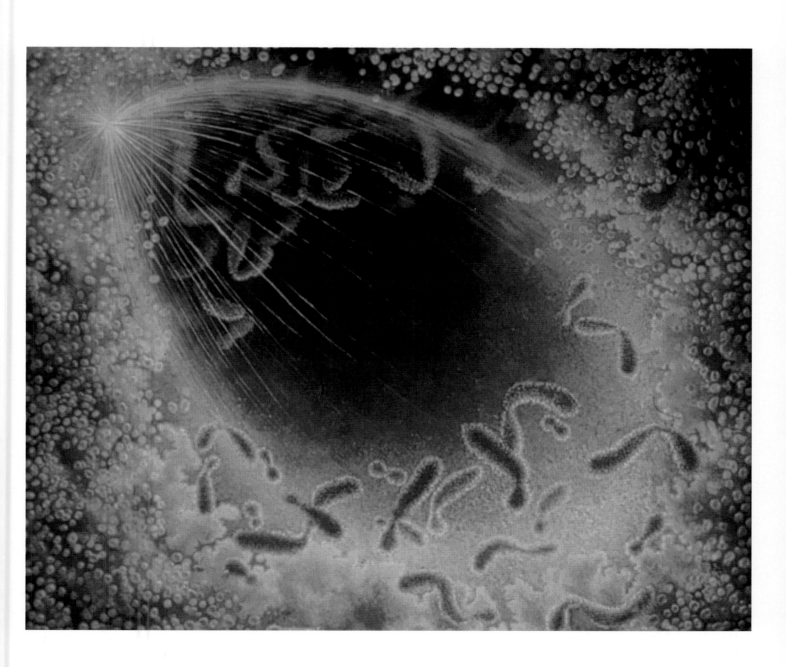

Figure 2.1 (*previous page*) Condensed, newly replicated chromosomes separating during cell division (Wellcome Medical Photographic Library, no. N0012752C).

The informational capacity of the human genome reflects the extraordinary length and compressibility of the DNA molecule. The size of the genome poses special problems for the mapping and cloning of genes implicated in human disease. Here we consider the higher structure of this long and winding molecule.

Chromatin structure

Genomes are characterized by a multilayer architecture

Your body has grown from a single diploid cell to a biological mass of $5 \cdot 10^{13}$ cells. This is an impressive organizational feat for a parental cell measuring 10 μm in diameter with only ten picograms (10 pg) of DNA in its (haploid) genome of $3 \cdot 10^9$ bp. How does DNA do it?

Each one of your cells contains 1000-fold more DNA than a bacterium; if stretched, this DNA would measure about two meters. However, cells of certain flowers (e.g., lilies) contain 100-fold more DNA than human cells. Hence, although genomic structural complexity is a prerequisite for biological complexity, no linear relationship between genome size and biological complexity can be assumed. Put another way, a small genome implies a simple (small and short-lived) organism, but a large genome does not necessarily encode a complex (or large, or long-lived) organism.

The fact that the sum total of DNA in your body could stretch to the Moon and back a certain number of times is of more than Sunday-newspaper significance. The key to this statistic is that DNA exists in a highly condensed state within cell nuclei, several thousand-fold more tightly packed than naked DNA. This condensation is to be expected given the sheer length of DNA – the dystrophin gene alone, for example, measures almost a millimeter when unwound – but also reflects a series of structural transitions embedded within the genetic material (Figure 2.2):

1. **Primary structure**
   • The linear sequence of nucleotides.
2. **Secondary structure**
   • The twisted conformation of the extended double helix.
3. **Tertiary structure**
   • The three-dimensional arrangement assumed by the double helix in the absence of protein binding.
4. **Quaternary structure**
   • The folded and interleaved conformation of protein-complexed DNA.

The information-carrying properties of DNA are inseparable from its ability to compress and decompress itself in a short space of time. Like a huge library archive, the genome has its opening and closing hours during which cellular proteins undertake such responsibilities as quality assurance, cross-referencing, copying, proofreading, repairs and rest. All of these activities occur within defined conformational states of DNA that modulate its ability to accommodate protein visitors.

Figure 2.2 Levels of DNA structure: *A*, primary, *B*, secondary, *C*, tertiary, *D*, quaternary. The latter image depicts the winding of the DNA double helix around histone protein complexes termed nucleosomes.

A.

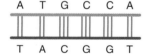

B.

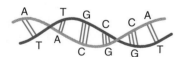

C.

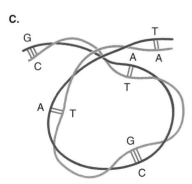

D.

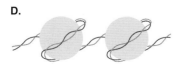

MOLECULAR MINIREVIEW

DNA crystal structures
Solving the structure of the sphinx-like DNA molecule is one of the great stories of scientific history (see Enrichment Reading). The critical data were a set of X-ray coordinates obtained from a DNA crystal. However, we now know that the DNA

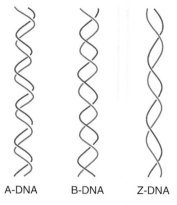

A-DNA   B-DNA   Z-DNA

Figure 2.3 Schematic representation of B-form (right-handed) versus A-form (dehydrated) and (left-handed) Z-DNA.

double helix can exhibit different crystallographic appearances (Figure 2.3) under different in vitro conditions:

1. **B-DNA**
   - Is the usual **right-handed** (Watson-Crick) double-helix.
   - Has a phosphate–phosphate distance of 7 Å (0.7 nm).
   - Predominates in vivo.
2. **A-DNA**
   - Is the right-handed helix seen in **dehydrated** DNA.
   - Is a shorter and fatter helix than B-DNA, with a phosphate–phosphate distance of 6 Å (0.6 nm).
   - Is structurally similar to double-stranded RNA and may participate in RNA–DNA binding.
3. **Z-DNA**
   - Is a **left-handed helix** with a zigzag sugar-phosphate backbone.
   - Is thinner and longer than B-form DNA.
   - Can be induced in vitro by creating stretches of alternating purines and pyrimidines (GCGC . . .) in vivo.

The terms B- and Z-DNA are not simply synonyms for right- and left-handed DNA respectively. Rather, they specify distinct crystallographic structures.

The in vivo role of Z-DNA (if any) remains controversial. Alternating GC-rich sequences often occur upstream of genes; this raises the possibility that the Z-DNA conformation can affect the efficiency of gene transcription. Other evidence points to the formation of Z-DNA in genomic areas with high recombination frequencies, suggesting a possible evolutionary significance.

Another structural DNA variant detected in viruses, **P-DNA**, has its phosphate backbone on the inside and is 75% longer than B-DNA (just 2.6 bp per turn).

Figure 2.4 Secondary structure of B-DNA, showing the position of the major and minor grooves, and the helical coordinates.

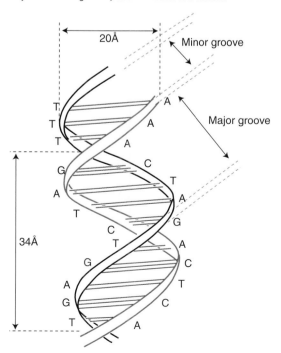

MOLECULAR MINIREVIEW

The grooves of DNA

DNA is a flexible molecule in which certain structural characteristics are constant. The width of the double helix is 20 Å (2 nm), and a full turn of the helix occurs every 10.2 bp (i.e., every 34 Å or 3.4 nm) in solution, or every 10.6 bp in intact coiled DNA. This periodicity of double-helical twist gives rise to the grooves of DNA (Figure 2.4).

The **minor groove** lies between complementary base pairs, whereas the **major groove** lies between noncomplementary base pairs. Despite its name, the minor groove is three to four times as wide as the major groove; the minor groove is broad and shallow, unlike the major groove which is a deep but narrow cleft. Hence, the minor groove measures about 10 Å (1 nm) in breadth – the same width as the phosphate backbone – whereas the major groove is only 3 Å (0.3 nm) across.

The grooves of DNA are important landmarks for DNA-binding molecules. AT-rich sequences favor minor groove binding of the transcriptional machinery in the 5′ flanking region of genes; since complementary AT nucleotides are joined by only two hydrogen bonds, the ability of such sequences to dock protein complexes may be enhanced by this interstrand laxity (p. 59).

Hence, just as an alternating GC nucleotide structure may influence gene transcription via Z-DNA formation (see above), so may the presence of upstream AT-rich sequences affect gene activity. Of note, Z-DNA has a minor groove like B-DNA, but has no major groove; when converting B- to Z-DNA, the base pairs flip upside down so that they lie on the outer convex surface.

Most gene-regulatory proteins bind in the major groove, particularly those binding GC-rich B-DNA sequences upstream of the gene control site (p. 86). On the other hand, small-molecule DNA-interactive drugs – such as those used to poison cancer cells – are usually minor groove ligands.

Eukaryotic DNA is organized by chromatin proteins

The three-dimensional structure of proteins is dictated mainly by the amino acid sequence. In contrast, the nucleotide sequence has little effect on the higher structure of DNA: the spatial conformation of the genome depends primarily upon **protein–DNA interactions**. The language of the gene thus resembles a form of molecular Braille between DNA and proteins – a language based on intermolecular contacts, chemical energy transfers, and steric interchanges.

Much of the higher-order structure of DNA is specified during embryonic development. These long-lived genomic organization events take place in human (but not bacterial) cells via the ordering of **chromatin**, which is a shorthand notation for the structural proteins that bind to DNA and thus form a proteinaceous coat ("Nature's filing system") around the genetic material. Chromatin consists of two classes of DNA-binding proteins:

1. **Histone** proteins
   - Core histones (H2A, H2B, H3, and H4).
   - Linker histone (H1).
2. **Nonhistone** chromatin proteins
   - e.g., High-mobility-group (HMG) proteins.

Histones are 11–13 kDa proteins which are encoded by a family of multicopy genes. A conserved helical **histone fold** at the histone carboxy terminus is responsible for dimerization; mutations affecting this region are responsible for the rare inherited disorder **Coffin-Lowry syndrome**. Amino-terminal **histone tails** may bind heterologous protein sequences termed **bromodomains** and **chromodomains** (see below), permitting interaction of chromatin proteins with the nuclear microenvironment.

The histone **core** – which is composed of two molecules each (hence eight protein subunits in all) of histones 2A, 2B, 3 and 4 – is the centerpiece of a disc-like 206-kilodalton-nucleoprotein chromatin structure termed the **nucleosome**. Nucleosomal DNA spools 146 bp of itself 1.65 times around each histone protein core (Figure 2.5), generating an ultrastructural appearance similar to knots on a string. Nucleosomal beads are spaced about 200 bp apart throughout the genome, localizing preferentially in AT-rich sequences. They are not fixed in position on a sequence-specific basis, however, since locoregional variations in gene activity may be accompanied by ATP-dependent nucleosomal sliding. Nucleosomes compress DNA by about fivefold over the nucleosome-free molecule.

In contrast to the core histones, **histone H1** binds mainly at the core entry and exit sites to internucleosomal or **linker** DNA which stretches between adjacent histone octamers. H1 stabilizes the beads-on-a-string into a solenoid-like structure comprising six nucleosomes, thereby compressing the genetic material a further 40-fold. In so doing histone H1 restricts access of gene-activating proteins to nucleosomal DNA. Hence, histone proteins perform the dual roles of: (1) compacting DNA into nucleosomes, and (2) regulating gene accessibility to heterologous proteins.

Figure 2.5 Nucleosome structure, showing DNA winding around the core histone (H2A, H2B, H3, H4) octamer.

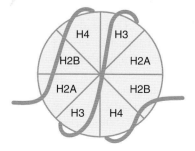

MOLECULAR MINIREVIEW

High-mobility-group nonhistone chromatin proteins

High-mobility nonhistone chromatin proteins are a group (termed HMG) of low molecular weight (<30 kDa) acidic proteins that migrate rapidly on electrophoresis (hence the name) and bind DNA in a non-sequence-specific manner. There are three major subgroups within the HMG family:

1. One structural subgroup, which includes **HMG-14** and **-17**, binds preferentially to nucleosomal DNA in heavily transcribed (active) chromatin.
2. A second subgroup binds AT-rich DNA sequences via a 9-amino-acid motif termed an **AT hook**. A mutation affecting one such gene (*HMGI-C*) has been associated with the development of benign fatty tumors termed **lipomas** and uterine leiomyomata (**fibroids**) in humans. Another AT-hook protein, AKNA, regulates lymphocyte cell death.
3. A third subgroup binds bent DNA sequences via a motif termed an **HMG box**. The latter proteins – which include the important sex-determining gene product SRY (pp. 412–13) – distort and angulate DNA on binding, facilitating access to gene-regulatory proteins. Mutations affecting SRY cause certain intersex syndromes (**hermaphroditism**; pp. 315–18, 413). Like SRY, the histone-mimetic transcription factor **NF-Y** binds proteins containing motifs termed Y-boxes, and this protein is inducible by cellular stresses such as heat shock.

Because HMG nonhistone chromatin proteins indirectly modify gene activity by bending DNA, they are sometimes designated **architectural transcription factors**.

Chromatin controls DNA accessibility

DNA–protein interactions might be easier to understand if the double helix was stripped of its histone and nonhistone chromatin protein coats. But gene expression does not depend upon interactions between naked DNA and diffusible proteins; chromatin-encrusted DNA remains available for regulatory protein interactions, with both DNA synthesis and gene transcription capable of proceeding through intact nucleosomal DNA. Changes in chromatin structure affect the efficiency of such processes by modulating the regional genomic accessibility of specific DNA-interactive proteins. Chromatin confers one of two broad configurations on large regions of DNA:

1. **Euchromatin**
   - Contains most of the potentially active (inducible) genes of a given cell.
   - Becomes decondensed between successive rounds of DNA replication.
2. **Heterochromatin**
   - Is transcriptionally silent.
   - Contains few genes and many repetitive DNA sequences.
   - Remains condensed at all times.
   - Localizes to the nuclear periphery.
   - Undergoes replication only after euchromatin replication is complete.

Heterochromatin, which accounts for about 15% of the human genome, is a gene-silencing invention of recent evolutionary origin. Two subtypes are recognized: **α-heterochromatin** (also termed **constitutive** or **deep heterochromatin**), which affects identical genomic regions in all cells of a given organism, is rich in GC nucleotides and satellite (highly repetitive) DNA sequences, but contains no genes (Figure 2.6); and **β-heterochromatin**, which is activable and contains both genes and mid-repetitive sequences. Heterochromatin can fan out from an **inactivation center** along a double-stranded DNA region, thus protecting local genes from heterologous protein binding. Heterochromatic condensation of the X chromosome (pp. 409–10) may be accelerated by L1 retrotransposons acting as seed crystals for gene inactivation via homologous pairing or mRNA binding.

In contrast, euchromatin maintains DNA in a decondensed configuration open to promiscuous molecular visitations. The 5′ flanking regions of active genes tend to be euchromatic and thus more accessible to DNA-binding

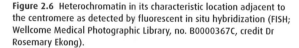

Figure 2.6 Heterochromatin in its characteristic location adjacent to the centromere as detected by fluorescent in situ hybridization (FISH; Wellcome Medical Photographic Library, no. B0000367C, credit Dr Rosemary Ekong).

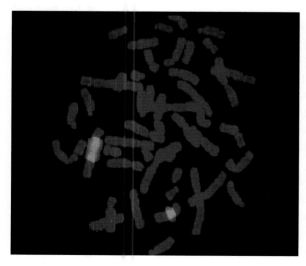

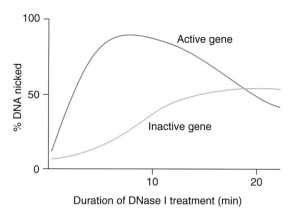

Figure 2.7 Graph of the time-course of nuclease digestion of DNA in transcriptionally active and inactive chromatin, showing the rate of DNA nicking per minute expressed as a percentage of the maximum rate.

Table 2.1. Contrasting features of transcriptionally active and inactive chromatin

Structural feature	Active chromatin	Inactive chromatin
Ultrastructural appearance	Euchromatin	Heterochromatin
Chromatin condensation	Decreased	Increased
Cytosine methylation	Decreased	Increased
Histone acetylation	Increased	Decreased
Histone H1 binding	Decreased	Increased

proteins, leading to faster replication, repair and transcription of these sequences; if euchromatic genes are experimentally reinserted within heterochromatin, however, the efficiency of these processes declines. The congenital neuromuscular syndrome **facioscapulohumeral (FSH) muscular dystrophy** is associated with chromatin rearrangement near an enlarged polymorphic *Kpn*1 tandem array, leading to widespread dysregulation of regional mRNA expression in the vicinity of the FSH gene.

CLINICAL KEYNOTE

Nuclease digestion of DNA in health and disease

Chromatin accessibility can be quantified experimentally by measuring the efficiency with which DNA-cleaving enzymes or **nucleases** degrade genomic DNA in vitro. This involves the use of **DNase I digestion** to demonstrate the presence of **hypersensitive** (i.e., to nuclease scission of DNA) **sites** in active genes. Hypersensitive sites tend to be nucleosome-free, and often correspond to the upstream control regions of active genes; nuclease digestion rapidly cleaves the target DNA into many small nicked fragments. In erythroid (red blood) cells, for example, the gene encoding embryonic **β-globin** becomes DNase-hypersensitive earlier in development than does that encoding adult β-globin, whereas the non-transcribed ovalbumin gene remains resistant to nuclease digestion throughout. This indicates the temporal sequence of gene activation (Figure 2.7).

DNase I may play a role in the pathogenesis of **systemic lupus erythematosus** (SLE) in which autoantibodies to DNA and chromatin proteins occur: mice that have been engineered not to express DNase I are susceptible to this disease. Under normal circumstances DNase I acts as a clean-up enzyme in body fluids containing dead cells, so the abnormal persistence of nucleic acid debris could trigger autoantibody production. The DNase I deficiency in SLE appears to be secondary rather than primary, however, with other clearance-protein defects (e.g., of complement components; pp. 306–8) being recognized.

DNases are used therapeutically to reduce the viscosity of sputum in patients with **cystic fibrosis**, who are prone to recurrent respiratory infections. DNA extruded from cells is intensely viscous, reflecting its length and compressibility; heavy bacterial colonization in these patients leads to viscous secretions partly due to the presence of DNA from lyzed bacterial and immune cells. In contrast, the food-contaminating bacterium *Campylobacter jejuni* expresses a DNase I-like toxin which induces host epithelial cell chromatin disruption and death.

Acetylation of histone proteins permits gene activation

Persistent changes in gene expression can be induced by mutations – that is, via direct alteration of the genetic sequence – or by **epigenetic** modifications of DNA or chromatin (Table 2.1). These epigenetic modifications are themselves heritable, meaning that they can survive both DNA replication and cell division. In functional terms such modifications have been compared to reformatting text words in bold or italics: the digital sequence of information is not altered, but the impact on the reader is. Key epigenetic changes include:

1. Chromatin modification, e.g.,
   - Histone H1 binding to nucleosomes.
   - **Acetylation** of lysine and arginine residues in core histones.
2. DNA modification, e.g.,
   - **Methylation** of cytosine nucleotides.

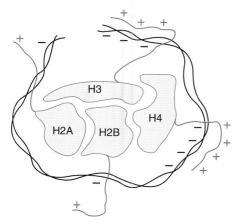

Figure 2.8 Relief diagram of (half) a histone octamer, showing the positions of the amino-terminal lysine tail acetylation sites. In the absence of acetylation, these positive (+) lysine charges bind tightly to the negative (−) charges of the acidic phosphate groups on the DNA backbone.

Core histones consist of a carboxy-terminal histone fold (the business end of the molecule which interacts with the other histones and wraps up DNA) and an amino-terminal tail domain. Histone tails contain basic (positively charged) lysine residues, which, being polar, protrude outwards from the nucleosomal core and into the minor groove, where they appear every 20 bp or so (Figure 2.8). These basic residues exhibit ionic affinity for the phosphate backbone of nucleosomal DNA – which, being acidic, is negatively charged – thus condensing chromatin and reducing the accessibility of heterologous proteins. Loss of the positive histone charge (particularly that of H4) enables loosening of the otherwise tight binding between histones and DNA, allowing chromatin to assume an active conformation that permits the binding of gene-activating molecules. The mechanism by which histones are so modified involves the addition of a greasy **acetyl** group to amino terminal lysines by nuclear enzymes called **histone acetyltransferases** (**HATs**) which are directed to nucleosomes by transactivators; hence, HATs relate to acetyl groups as do kinases to phosphate groups. The gene-activating effect of HATs derives from the nonpolar nature of acetyl groups, which normally participate in fatty acid biosynthesis (pp. 167–8). Heterologous protein bromodomains selectively bind lysine-acetylated histone tails (unlike chromodomains which selectively bind lysine-methylated histones) as part of the chromatin-activating mechanism.

This process of **histone acetylation** is a lubrication mechanism whereby large areas of genomic DNA are prepared for heterologous protein binding and thus for transcriptional activity. An important effect of core histone acetylation is to reduce the nucleosomal binding of **histone H1** by increasing the dynamic on-off rate. This linker-loosening effect makes nucleosome entry and exit sites more accessible to gene-regulating proteins. Different genes require different HAT activities for transcription inducibility, consistent with the presence of multiple coactivating proteins within the HAT complex. Moreover, certain HATs vary their activity in response to phosphorylation. Drug-induced **acute myeloid leukemias** may be triggered by juxtaposition of a HAT and a mitogenic protein.

Genes are repressed by the deacetylation of core histones. Intranuclear **histone deacetylases** (**HDACs**) can silence gene transcription by maintaining a condensed nucleosomal structure that impairs the access of diffusible proteins to DNA sequences involved in gene activation, thus making HDACs potent control genes (Figure 2.9). For example, the **papillomavirus** protein **E7** can induce either warts or cancers by releasing HDAC1 from the growth control protein pRb, and thus reversing pRb-dependent chromatin condensation. Certain HDACs in yeast (silent information regulator or **SIR** proteins) are associated with longevity which is extendable by caloric restriction, suggesting that energy-dependent chromatin activation contributes to cellular ageing.

Figure 2.9 Schema of the interrelationship between histone acetyltransferases (HATs), histone deacetylases (HDACs), and cell growth.

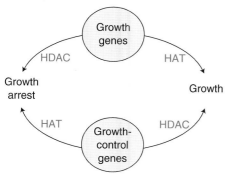

CLINICAL KEYNOTE

Acute promyelocytic leukemia

The consequences of histone acetylation depend on which genes are modified: in particular, mitogenic (growth) or anti-mitogenic (growth control) genes. This is illustrated by the pathogenesis of **acute promyelocytic leukemia** (APL), which usually arises via a pathologic chromosomal fusion (15:17 or 11:17; p. 69) event. The latter gives rise to chimeric genes for **retinoic acid receptor-α** (RARA) downstream of

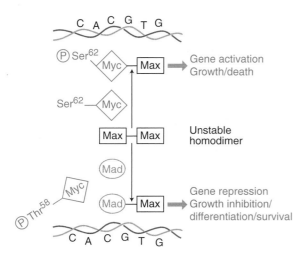

Figure 2.10 Regulation of Myc function by heterodimer formation with Max and Mad. Unstable Max homodimers are replaced by either Myc–Max or Mad–Max heterodimers; this choice is critical in influencing the decision between cell growth and death. Transforming mutations of the critical threonine-58 site (which undergoes reciprocal glycosylation when not phosphorylated) occur in Burkitt and AIDS-related lymphomas.

Figure 2.11 Endemic Burkitt lymphoma (Wellcome Medical Photographic Library, no. N0011143C).

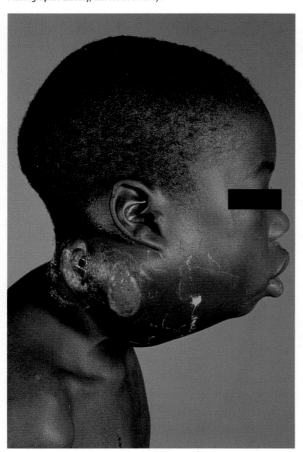

either *PML* (promyelocytic leukemia) or *PLZF* (promyelocytic leukemia zinc finger) control sequences respectively. The growth-suppressive **PML** protein is normally located in the nucleus, whereas the **PML-RARA** fusion protein is both cytoplasmic and nuclear: inhibition of wild-type PML activity by the fusion protein contributes to its leukemogenicity.

Under normal circumstances, the unliganded RARA heterodimerizes with **retinoid X receptors** (RXRs; p. 320) to form a transcriptional repressor complex which includes HDAC1; this complex represses the activity of growth-control genes such as PML. Binding of RA triggers substitution of a HAT activity for HDAC1 in the RARA-bound complex, thereby activating growth-control genes and inducing differentiation.

The PML-RARA fusion protein disrupts RA signaling via competitive inhibition of RARA binding and transactivation of novel target genes. The transcriptional repressor complex bound by PML-RARA is less responsive than wild-type RARA to endogenous RA, but responds to treatment with pharmacologic doses of *all*-trans-retinoic acid (ATRA). PML-RARA is degraded by caspase cleavage in response to ATRA; expression and nuclear localization of PML is thus restored, leading to differentiation and death of APL cells.

The **PLZF-RARA** fusion protein has two repressor binding sites: the additional PLZF-bound repressor complex is ATRA-resistant, explaining the refractory natural history of this molecular disease subtype. Clinical responses may be seen if ATRA therapy is combined with an HDAC inhibitor.

Both ATRA and **arsenic trioxide** (another active treatment) downregulate PML-RARA. Arsenic is detoxified by enzymatic methylation, depleting stores of the methyl donor *S*-adenosylmethionine (SAM; p. 154). Chronic arsenic exposure may thus activate RA-dependent target genes in APL via DNA hypomethylation, while at the same time predisposing to further carcinogenetic events.

MOLECULAR MINIREVIEW

Myc, Max, Mad, and Mad-Max

Myc is a key DNA-binding protein regulating cell growth and death. Transcription is normally activated by a heterodimer of Myc and **Max**, a structurally related protein. This gene-inducing propensity of **Myc–Max** heterodimers is competitively inhibited by the HDAC **Mad** which forms **Mad–Max** heterodimers binding similar **E-box** DNA consensus sequences (Figure 2.10). Part of the inhibitory activity of Mad–Max heterodimers may thus arise from the local HDAC activity of Mad, leading to chromatin condensation.

Chromosomal fusion events that upregulate *Myc* expression in lymphoid tissue are responsible for the pathogenesis of **Burkitt lymphoma** (Figure 2.11). Constitutive transcription in this context reflects the recruitment of immunoglobulin (antibody) genes into the *Myc* translocation breakpoint, thus ensuring lymphoid-specific transactivation.

Epigenetic gene repression is transmitted by DNA methylation

In addition to chromatin modification, cells can vary the behavior of DNA by directly modifying the nucleotide sequence. Such epigenetic modification is carried out by enzymes termed methylases or **methyltransferases** which catalyze **DNA methylation** (alkylation). This process is believed to have been originally invented by bacterial genomes to protect them from their own DNA-cutting enzymes (p. 536).

Certain methyltransferases have prescribed specificities in the same way that other enzymes have consensus substrates. One example is the human

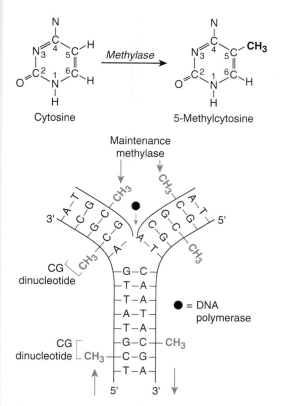

Figure 2.12 Generation of methylcytosine from cytosine via the action of a methylase. A methyl (CH$_3$) group is added to the 5' carbon of the pyrimidine ring; this is initiated by a maintenance methylase and replicated by a DNA polymerase.

histone H3-specific methyltransferase which methylates lysine at position 9 in the histone tail, thus creating a methyl-lysine binding site for the chromodomain of the gene-silencing molecule **heterochromatin protein 1** (HP1).

Similarly, there are at least four human **cytosine methyltransferases** which give rise to the little-known fifth base of DNA, **5-methylcytosine**: just as uracil and its aminated product thymine both bind adenine, so do cytosine and methylcytosine bind guanine. **Maintenance methylases** bind to replicating DNA, which is already hemimethylated (Figure 2.12), thereby ensuring the clonal continuity of the methylated phenotype in replicated DNA (Figure 2.13). Reversal of methylation is likewise inducible via **demethylases**, but little is known as yet about the frequency of this event. The retention of methylcytosine through repeated rounds of daughter DNA hemimethylation is implicated in the following processes:

1. Transcriptional repression
   - Inhibition of transcriptional initiation.
   - Arrest of transcriptional elongation.
2. Suppression of homologous recombination.
3. Developmental modulation of transcription.
   - Differential parental allele expression (genomic imprinting (pp. 406–9)).
   - X-chromosome inactivation (pp. 409–10).

Methylation may occur dynamically during processes such as cell differentiation. Tissue-specific genes that maintain expression despite such differentiation may first require local demethylation of upstream control sequences.

The extent of cytosine methylation varies across species in rough proportion to the size of the genome: humans have 3–5% of their cytosines methylated whereas plants may have up to 25% and insects none. Much of the methylcytosine in human genomes is associated with repetitive transposon and endogenous retrovirus sequences. Methylation may minimize the sequelae of such genomic parasitization (the so-called host defense hypothesis for the evolution of methylation) initially by causing transcriptional repression, and ultimately by predisposing to mutations caused by methylcytosine deamination. Since methylation preferentially affects CG dinucleotides, the latter sequences are mutational hotspots in human diseases.

The dynamic range of gene transcription between full repression and full activation is about 25 000-fold. Cytosine methylation represses gene activity, whereas cytosine hypomethylation facilitates local gene activation. This may be exploited therapeutically by using the hypomethylating agent **5-azacytidine** to enhance the transcription of fetal hemoglobin in patients with blood dyscrasias such as **thalassemia**.

Figure 2.13 Diagrammatic representation of the heritable behavior of a DNA hemimethylase. 5MC, 5-methylcytosine; MT, methyltransferase.

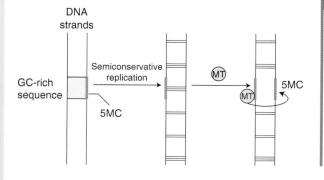

Rett syndrome and ICF syndrome

In addition to the HP1-dependent gene silencing mechanism noted above, methylation-induced gene repression is mediated by **methylcytosine-binding proteins**, of which at least five are known. One such protein, **MeCP$_2$** (methyl-CpG-binding protein 2), recruits a histone deacetylase which causes chromatin condensation by allowing the acidic DNA phosphate backbone to pack tightly to the basic tails of the core histones. This is how cytosine methylation promotes DNA helix stabilization and chromatin inactivation (Figure 2.14). The X-linked dominant neurodevelopmental disorder **Rett syndrome** arises because of defective gene silencing sec-

Figure 2.14 Role of methylcytosine-binding proteins (MeCP$_2$) and HDACs in mediating chromatin condensation. MT, methyltransferase; 5MC, 5-methylcytosine; HDAC, histone deacetylase.

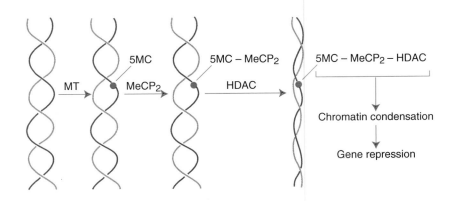

ondary to loss-of-function mutations affecting MeCP$_2$ expression. Patients with the rare **ICF syndrome** (immunodeficiency, centromere instability and facial anomalies) have mutations of the **DNA methyltransferase 3β** (DNMT3β) gene, leading to impaired satellite DNA methylation and heterochromatin formation. Note that the phenotypes of these disorders differ despite a common defect in methylation-dependent chromatin compaction. Other diseases of chromatin organization include **ATR-X syndrome** (α-thalassemia/retardation, X-linked) in which a mutant helicase causes hypomethylation of ribosomal DNA repeats; and **Rubinstein-Taybi syndrome**, in which a histone acetyltransferase activity is deficient.

Gene methylation predisposes to CG→TA mutations

Gene methylation patterns vary with cell lineage and function. Immune cells such as lymphocytes may incur demethylation and hence activation of antibody genes, for example, whereas expression of the **fetal (γ-) hemoglobin** gene (which is used to make blood during embryonic life) is developmentally silenced in adult life by methylation. Similarly, the gene encoding the red blood cell growth factor **erythropoietin** is normally methylated and histone deacetylated, but this inhibition is removed by hypoxia (pp. 450–1). The task of mapping all gene methylation patterns in all human tissues is thus an important one, comparable in scope to the human genome sequencing project.

Genes that need to remain switched on in a given tissue are often demarcated within 5′ flanking regions by hypomethylated 1- to 2-kb GC-rich sequences termed **CpG islands** which comprise more than 55% **cytosine-phosphate-guanine** repeats; about 50 000 CpG islands occur in each human genome. Such islands surround the transcription start sites of 60% of human genes and maintain these genes in a ready-to-transcribe chromatin conformation. Methylation of CpG islands is unusual, but may occur in association with repetitive DNA, as a polymorphic trait, or in tumors.

Methylation can be imagined as the underwear of DNA. Waves of methylation and demethylation define **methylomes** – that is, the usual location of methylation within a given genome. Such methylation is a two-edged sword: it protects chromosomes from deletions and genes from insertional mutagenesis (and perhaps also from oxidant damage), but at the cost of predisposing to conservative point mutations. The genome is normally subject to spontaneous base deamination damage which is efficiently repaired, but the deamination of 5-methylcytosine is unique in that it yields thymine. These transient GT mismatches are poorly recognized by the excision and mismatch repair systems, leaving the C→T transition to be heritably propagated in the next round of DNA replication. Since methylation may also occur on the antisense strand, G→A transitions are an equally frequent methylation-dependent mutation. Such methylation-dependent base transitions are a major force in human genome evolution.

GC-rich versus AT-rich DNA

DNA regions can be characterized in terms of their relative proportions of GC and AT base pairs. The genomes of many bacteria, fruit-flies, and human mitochondria are AT rich; in contrast, human genes tend to be GC-rich. Why? The answer cannot relate only to differences in methylation-dependent DNA damage, since some AT-rich genomes (such as that of *Drosophila* fruit-flies) lack methylases.

GC base pairs are joined by triple hydrogen bonds whereas AT base pairs are joined by double bonds (see Figure 1.17). The idea that "looser" AT-rich nucleic acids may engage more readily in heterologous binding interactions is consistent with certain observations: (1) the multiprotein transcription apparatus binds specifically to a **TATA** upstream gene sequence (p. 86); (2) DNA replication origins are **AT-rich**; and (3) an **AUUUA** sequence in mRNA tails targets transcripts for degradation via protein binding (p. 106), suggesting that substitution of a GC-rich sequence could prevent protein binding via tight annealing to unoccupied GC sites in the same molecule. GC-rich motifs such as CG or CAG, on the other hand, are common in repetitive DNA, suggesting a GC propensity to accumulate. Of note, areas of GC richness are difficult to sequence using conventional DNA analytic technologies.

AT richness often characterizes mutation-prone genomes, such as those of bacteria or mitochondria. This is presumably advantageous to bacteria as it permits rapid genetic selection in response to survival threats. It may also help accelerate the evolution of higher organisms such as humans, since transcriptionally inert (useless) genomic regions will tend to become AT rich via waves of methylation-dependent CG→TA transitions; this can either enhance the possibility of mutation towards more transcriptionally useful DNA, or else predispose to deletion events. On the other hand, the overall GC richness of human genomes may favor the retention of DNA sequence fidelity, thereby militating against maladies such as senescence and carcinogenesis which are of little concern to bacteria (Figure 2.15).

Figure 2.15 Functional interactions between methylation and gene activity. Methylation predisposes to transcriptional repression and AT-rich nucleotide composition, whereas hypomethylation favors transactivation and a GC-rich genome.

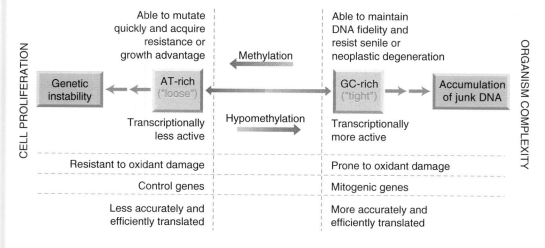

Methylation in cancer

Cancer progression selects for clonally selectable growth advantages. With respect to gene methylation, however, cancer cells may vary the phenotype in either direction:

1. **Hypomethylation**
   - Tends to be global.
   - Activates growth-proliferative genes.
2. **Hypermethylation**
   - Tends to be local.
   - Represses growth-control genes, *and*
   - Predisposes growth-control genes to mutations.

Gene hypermethylation thus represents a selectable tumor strategy for **marking** genomic regions for deletion events that lead to an irreversible loss of growth control, resulting not only in cell growth acceleration but also (more critically) acquisition of genetic instability. Growth-control gene promoters that are often hypermethylated in human cancers include those of:

- The growth-regulatory *Rb* (**retinoblastoma susceptibility**) gene.
- The *CDH1* gene encoding the cell adhesion protein **E-cadherin**.
- The lipid phosphatase *PTEN* gene.
- The *VHL* (**von Hippel–Lindau disease**) gene.
- The *p15* and *p16^INK4A* growth-control genes.

Cells transformed by certain growth-promoting genes exhibit increased levels of 5-methylcytosine. Since similar transformation can be either induced by the 5-methylcytosine transferase gene alone or else abolished by inhibiting histone deacetylase, such transforming genes may act in part by increasing the methylation of growth-control genes.

Figure 2.16 DNA synthesis. *A–C*, Mechanics of bidirectional DNA replication at a replication fork. A, The helicase docks downstream of the replication origin; B, The replication bubble is formed by the forward movement of the DNA polymerase; C, Discontinuous replication of the lagging strand is undertaken by DNA pol α.

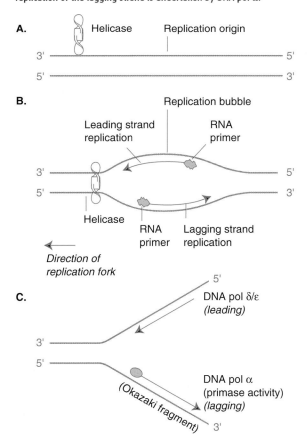

DNA synthesis

Nucleic acids are synthesized by polymerases

The functions of nucleic acids are dependent upon interactions with multiprotein enzyme complexes. Such complexes may include remodeling enzymes termed **polymerases** which catalyze the formation of nucleotide polymers: **RNA polymerases** catalyze DNA transcription (into RNA) whereas **DNA polymerases** catalyze DNA replication (into more DNA). During DNA replication each chain of the helix is separately replicated in the 5′–3′ direction (Figure 2.16). Since the paired strands of the double helix point in different directions, DNA replication is a **bidirectional** process which involves **leading** and **lagging strands** – the latter being replicated discontinuously as a series of so-called Okazaki fragments (Figure 2.16*C*).

The replication of each strand is initiated by a six-protein complex termed a **replisome**, giving rise to a **replication bubble** that propels a zipper-like **replication fork** along the helix (Figure 2.16*B*). As many as 20 000 of these multienzyme complexes are operative in a replicating genome at one time: each 50- to 300-kb domain served by a single replisome constitutes a **replicon**, and clusters of about 100 replicons undergo simultaneous duplication. Despite this military-scale assault, each cell takes between four and eight hours to complete the replication and proofreading of its DNA. At least nine subtypes of DNA polymerase contribute to DNA replication, including:

1. DNA **polymerases-α, -δ**, and **-ε** – replicate nuclear DNA.
2. DNA **polymerase-β**
   - Repairs, recombines and replicates nuclear DNA.
   - Is the smallest and most primitive of the polymerases.
   - Cooperates with glycosidases, endonucleases, and ligases in base excision repair of oxidized or alkylated bases.
3. DNA **polymerase-γ**
   - Replicates mitochondrial DNA.
4. DNA **polymerase-η**
   - Undertakes low-fidelity (error-prone) DNA replication in bacteria.
   - May be mutated in the skin cancer disorder **xeroderma pigmentosum V**.
5. DNA **polymerases-ι,-ζ**
   - Cooperate in the error-prone bypass of DNA lesions: ι initially incorporates nucleotides opposite lesions, whereas ζ is a mispair extender.
6. DNA **polymerase-κ**
   - Mediates sister chromatid cohesion during DNA synthesis.

DNA polymerases-δ and -ε cooperate with an auxiliary molecule termed **proliferating cell nuclear antigen** (PCNA) which enhances the **processivity** of the enzyme – that is, the speed at which the multiprotein complex proceeds along the DNA without pausing. Of note, these polymerases not only replicate but also proofread replicated DNA. In bacteria such as *Escherichia coli* this proofreading activity is due to a 3′–5′ exonuclease activity in the catalytic subunit of DNA polymerase I – termed **Klenow fragment** – which is used in vitro.

Remarkably, polymerases can pass each other when both are working on the same DNA strand. An RNA polymerase can transcribe a gene being replicated, and a DNA polymerase can replicate a gene being transcribed. By judicious use of the complementary strand, these passing maneuvers occur even when polymerases meet head-on. To initiate its replicative function in mid-strand, DNA polymerase-α requires **primers** – short (4–6 bp) RNA sequences encoded by a specialized RNA polymerase called a **primase**. The use of synthetic primers is central to many laboratory DNA techniques including the polymerase chain reaction (p. 550).

PHARMACOLOGIC FOOTNOTE

Aciclovir: an inhibitor of viral DNA polymerase

Viruses resemble splinter-like fragments of genomic DNA which fool the host cell genome into activating viral gene transcription and replication. The structural similarities between viral and human genomes thus represent a challenge for designers of antiviral chemotherapy – namely, that of identifying virus-specific therapeutic targets.

Aciclovir is an antiviral 2′-deoxyguanosine analog with activity against herpesviruses – especially **herpes simplex** (HSV), but also **varicella-zoster** (VZ). Following ingestion, aciclovir is metabolized in herpes-infected cells (HSV, VZ) by viral **thymidine kinase** (TK) to aciclovir monophosphate, and thence by host cell enzymes to aciclovir triphosphate which inhibits viral DNA polymerase. Aciclovir triphosphate then competes with 2′-deoxyguanosine for viral DNA polymerase, causing irreversible inhibition of viral DNA synthesis.

Although humans also express TK in growing tissues, the herpes virus TK selectively phosphorylates aciclovir, thereby inhibiting herpes nucleic acid replication in the relative absence of (human) side-effects; the drug is 50 times more potent with respect to viral than human DNA polymerase. Hence, like other antiviral drugs – including **ganciclovir** (anti-cytomegalovirus; differs from aciclovir by having a 3′ hydroxymethyl group in the acyclic side chain) and **zidovudine** (anti-HIV) – aciclovir functions as an antiviral nucleoside analog. Resistance to aciclovir occurs in herpes viruses that express deficient or defective viral thymidine kinase. **Foscarnet** and **lamivudine** are unrelated drugs that inhibit both viral DNA polymerase and reverse transcriptase.

Replicated DNA is packaged within chromosomes

The replication of human DNA occurs at high speed – about 50 nucleotides per replication fork per second, or about one-tenth the speed of bacterial DNA synthesis. Given that an entire human genome is replicated within a few hours, the accuracy of the process is impressive. As few as a half-dozen genetic errors may be left uncorrected per replicated diploid genome – equivalent to one error per billion base pairs, or less. Replicated DNA does not simply trail around the cell, however, but rather is packaged into microscopically visible nuclear structures termed **chromosomes** (literally, colored bodies; Figure 2.17). Each haploid human genome contains:

1. Twenty-two **autosomes**
   - Numbered 1–22 in order of decreasing size.
2. One **sex chromosome**
   - X or Y.

Each somatic cell contains 23 chromosome pairs, making 46 chromosomes in all; half of these are contributed by each of two haploid parental genomes. Since the X and Y chromosomes are structurally distinct, there are in fact 24 nonhomologous chromosomes in the human genetic universe.

When a diploid cell divides, each chromosome divides into two identical **sister chromatids** to form a close-knit complex termed a **bivalent** which comprises four chromatids. Chromosomes are divided by a structure termed the centromere (see below) into a **short arm (p)** and a **long arm (q)**.

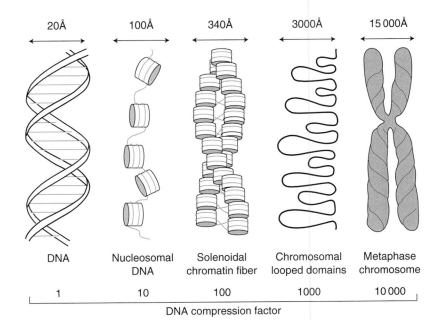

Figure 2.17 Multiple levels of DNA compaction occurring during chromosome condensation, showing the structure of looped domains. The scale in Angstroms is shown at the top.

Male somatic cells contain 44 autosomes, one X and one Y chromosome, whereas female somatic cells contain two X chromosomes – one of which is randomly inactivated by condensation. This latter phenomenon of X chromosome inactivation involves cytosine hypermethylation, histone H4 hypoacetylation, expression of an H2A histone subtype (macroH2A1), and selective transcription of an RNA transcript (XIST; p. 410).

About 70% of chromosomal mass is made up of chromatin proteins, leaving less than one-third composed of DNA. The length of unwound DNA per chromosome averages about 5 cm, ranging from 2 cm (in chromosome 22) to almost 15 cm (in chromosome 1). To put this in perspective, the euchromatic region of chromosome 2 spans 33 Mb and contains 545 genes plus 134 pseudogenes. Each chromosome consists of about 3000 **looped domains** of DNA anchored to an insoluble **nuclear matrix**. Mammoth genes like those encoding factor VIII or dystrophin are not confined within a single chromosomal DNA loop (typically 20–100 kb in size) but rather spill over to contiguous looped domains.

MOLECULAR MINIREVIEW

X-linked inheritance

The Y chromosome is shorter than the X, with the result that some genes on the X chromosome lack alleles on the Y (pp. 409–11. Recessive mutations affecting these X chromosomal genes may thus be apparent in boys but not girls. Such phenotypic **sex-linked** disorders are genotypically described as **X-linked**. Examples include:

1. **Hemophilia.**
2. **Duchenne muscular dystrophy.**
3. **Lesch–Nyhan syndrome.**
4. **Glucose-6-phosphate dehydrogenase deficiency.**
5. **Alport syndrome** (renal failure and deafness).
6. **Testicular feminization syndrome.**

Females with one X chromosome containing the mutant allele are termed carriers. On average, 50% of their sons will be affected whereas the other 50% will be normal; in contrast, few if any of their daughters will be affected but 100% will be carriers. Rare females with mutant alleles on both X chromosomes – usually a result of consanguinity (gene identity due to cousin marriages) – may be affected as severely as males. However, males cannot transmit such diseases to male offspring.

A few diseases exhibit **X-linked dominant** transmission, in which (hemizygous) males are more severely affected, but only half as often as (heterozygous) females. Examples include **ornithine transcarbamylase deficiency** and certain forms of **rickets**. Other X-linked dominant disorders may be uniformly fatal in males, and hence only diagnosed in females.

CLINICAL KEYNOTE

Congenital karyotypic abnormalities

Microscopic recognition of abnormalities in chromosome structure constitutes a branch of ultrastructural analysis termed **cytogenetics** in which the aim is to determine the **karyotype** or chromosomal pattern of the individual in question. Regional differences in chromatin organization may be associated with changes

Meiosis

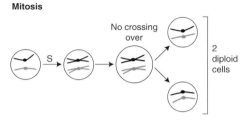

First meiotic division · Second meiotic division · Crossing over · 4 haploid cells

Mitosis

No crossing over · 2 diploid cells

Figure 2.19 Schematic comparison of mitosis and meiosis. Meiosis comprises a reductional division followed by an equational division, whereas mitosis consists of only a single equational division (see text).

2. **Mitosis**
   - Division of one somatic cell with diploid DNA content to form two daughter somatic cells also with diploid DNA content.

Though ethicists may argue, for our purposes human life begins following the fusion of two haploid germ cells – an ovum with abundant cytoplasm, and a sperm consisting of little but nuclear DNA. Each haploid chromosome arises during meiosis of a diploid progenitor. Meiosis is a specialized process unique to the germ cell lineage, and involves two successive cell division events. It takes place continually between adolescence and senescence in males, whereas female meiosis is launched during fetal life and completed on an oocyte-by-oocyte basis prior to ovulation.

Cell commitment to meiosis is made in early G_1 phase. The first meiotic division involves formation of a chromosomal **bivalent** which – by virtue of the tight association (synapsing) between nonsister chromatids – is uniquely susceptible to crossing-over. Because the centromeres remain together and point in the same direction, this division is termed **reductional**. The correct alignment of homologous meiotic chromosomes may be assisted by regions of heterochromatin and invariant repeat sequences, suggesting that these putative junk DNA regions play a key replicative role.

The onset of DNA replication precedes that of meiotic recombination by about two hours. Double-strand DNA breaks induced for the purpose of DNA replication are directly linked to the subsequent onset of recombination within any given chromosomal region. On average, three recombination events occur per chromosomal meiosis, leading to the exchange of large genetic regions. This is one of the chief differences between meiosis and mitosis: genetic recombination is high in the former and very low in the latter.

Failure of correct chromosomal segregation during either the first or second meiotic divisions is termed **nondisjunction**. The risk of nondisjunction rises with maternal age, explaining the concomitant increased incidence of chromosomal disorders such as Down and Turner syndromes. Nondisjunction may also occur during mitotic divisions following conception, in which case milder **mosaic** chromosomal abnormalities (abnormal karyotype in some but not all cells) may be apparent.

The second meiotic division results in diminution of the diploid genome to haploidy (Figure 2.19). Like mitosis, this is an **equational** (cf. reductional) division in which centromeric splitting and segregation occur. Meiosis thus donates one allele of each parental gene to the fertilized cell, with the transmission of a given trait being determined by the net phenotypic effects of both alleles. This random process of **allelic shuffling** contributes further to the genetic variation of meiosis, augmenting the variation induced by chromosomal crossing-over.

Figure 2.20 Fragile X chromosome visualized by atomic force microscopy (AFM). The arrow indicates the fragile site. (Wellcome Medical Photographic Library, no. B0000244C10, credit Dr Ben Oostra).

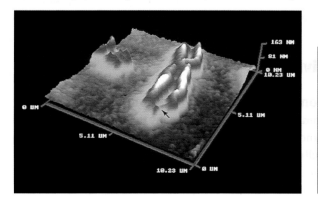

CLINICAL KEYNOTE

Chromosomal fragile sites

Analysis of condensed (mitotic) chromosomes in vitro may reveal weak points susceptible to breakage in a minority of individuals. Depriving cultured cells of the carbon-transfer vitamin folic acid can reveal these **fragile sites**; that is, they are **folate-sensitive** sites. Human diseases associated with fragile sites include:

1. **Fragile X syndrome**: mental retardation in boys (Figure 2.20)
   - The *FRAXA* fragile site on the X chromosome is associated with an accumu-

lation of CG-rich trinucleotide repeat sequences, causing methylation of a nearby CpG island and transcriptional repression of the *FMR-1* gene.
- A distinct *FRAXE* fragile site is associated with a rarer syndrome of mild mental retardation.
2. **Jacobsen syndrome** (mental retardation)
   - The *FRA11B* fragile site on chromosome 11q is associated with a similar repeat expansion affecting the growth-control gene, *Cbl2* (pp. 260–1).
3. Cancers
   - The *FRA3B* fragile site is situated on the short arm of chromosome 3 in a region (3p14.2) that is often damaged or deleted (3p-) in **cervix cancer** or **lung cancer**. This region contains the *Fragile histidine triad* (*FHIT*) gene which encodes a dinucleotide triphosphate hydrolase.

Hypermethylation of CpG islands is also seen in other inherited neurologic disorders involving accumulation of trinucleotide repeats (p. 82).

Massive chromosomal compaction occurs during mitosis

A newly divided human cell takes 18–24 hours to resynthesize its nuclear and cytoplasmic contents and divide again – a repetitive process termed the cell cycle (p. 357). This period of cell division includes three to six hours for DNA synthesis and just one hour for the denouement of somatic cell division, mitosis. For the rest of the time the cell is either resting or doing essential lead-up work for the above two cell division phases. Extracellular molecules that trigger cells to commit to DNA synthesis or mitosis are termed **mitogens**.

Nongermline human cells divide exclusively by mitosis, during which identical genomic copies are passed on to the cell progeny. Unlike meiosis, there are no prizes for introducing variation during mitosis – only cancer – and any reduction of chromosome number is likely to kill the cell.

Mitosis involves the partitioning of the cytoplasm and membranes (cytokinesis) when DNA replication is complete (Figure 2.19). Different phases of chromosomal division are identifiable by light microscopy during mitosis: prophase (the initial separation of replicated chromosomes), metaphase (the alignment of separated chromosomes), anaphase (the early polarization of chromatids), and telophase (the re-formation of daughter nuclei during cytokinesis; Figure 2.21). Most of the cell's life, including DNA synthesis, is spent during the decondensed (pre-mitotic) chromosomal nondividing phase, or interphase.

Mitotic chromosome compaction is mediated by ATP-dependent multienzyme complexes termed **condensins** which compress chromatin-bound DNA tenfold more densely than interphase DNA (that is, 10 000-fold more compact than naked DNA). Being maximally condensed, the metaphase chromosome is used for most cytogenetic studies. Banding may be undertaken following preparation of metaphase chromosomes by cell incubation with the mitotic spindle inhibitor **colchicine**, but finer chromosomal mapping is sometimes undertaken using prophase preparations. Such investigation is undertaken as part of the evaluation of an abnormal neonatal phenotype or else in the characterization of uncommon malignancies.

Figure 2.21 Mitotic phases discernible by light microscopy.

1. Prophase 2. Metaphase

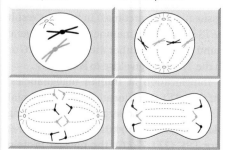

3. Anaphase 4. Telophase

Translocations in leukemias and lymphomas
Diseases of autonomous growth are collectively termed **neoplasia**. Most malignant neoplasms can be subdivided into three groups:

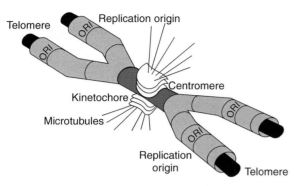

Figure 2.23 The anatomy of a human chromosome. Note that each chromosome in fact contains hundreds of replication origins (ORI).

organizing center (MTOC) in nondividing cells. This solitary centrosome is associated with two **centrioles**: the wayward "daughter" centriole marauds around the cell independently of the "mother" centriole until the time of DNA synthesis and centriole replication. Abnormalities of centrosome number and/or stability are often induced in tumors by transforming proteins such as the human papillomavirus E7 protein (p. 376).

As the time for division draws near, the centrosome duplicates itself, and the two centrosomes then ensure symmetric cell division by migrating to opposite cytoplasmic poles. Centrosome-based nucleation of microtubules leads to alignment of their plus and minus ends: the minus ends are the slow-growing ends pointed towards the cellular poles, whereas the plus ends are the fast-growing ends pointing towards a midchromosomal region termed the **centromere** (Figure 2.23).

The centromere is an active participant in chromosomal segregation, particularly in the initiation of anaphase. Conserved pericentromeric $(GGAAT)_n$ repeats exhibit high thermostability and protein affinity: these satellite repeats contain a 17-bp motif, which is a binding site for the essential mitotic protein **CENP-B**. Other centromere-associated proteins include **CENP-A** (a histone H3 variant specific for centromeric DNA), **CENP-C** (a kinetochore protein) and **CENP-E** (a cell movement protein).

As the chromosomal array aligns itself in mid-cell during late prophase, a protein complex termed the **kinetochore** attaches itself to the centromere. The kinetochore serves as a conduit between this chromosomal region and certain proteins in the spindle apparatus, thus linking the fate of the chromosomes to that of the polarizing spindle (Figure 2.24). Separation of sister chromatids is prevented by hinged α-helical multisubunit complexes termed **cohesins** (homologous to condensins; see above) which stick chromatids together; some instances of congenital abnormality caused by chromosomal nondisjunction may arise through cohesin malfunction. The arrival of anaphase triggers the proteolysis of a cohesin subunit, triggering chromosomal polarization. Another protein destroyed at this time is the endopeptidase **separin** which – by disengaging from its interaction with the anaphase-inhibitory protein **securin** (in turn encoded by a homolog of the *Drosophila* gene, *pimples*) – helps to initiate chromosomal separation.

Figure 2.24 Functional interrelationship between chromosomes and the mitotic spindle. In the nondividing cell, a solitary centrosome acts as the cytoplasmic organizing center for microtubules.

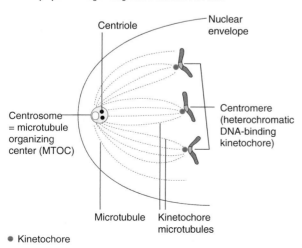

● Kinetochore

Nuclear autoantigens in connective tissue disease
The human body normally produces antibodies that defend it against foreign substances (antigens; p. 198). If this process goes wrong and the body starts making antibodies against normal (self) molecules, the result is **autoimmune disease**. There are two prominent groupings of autoimmune disease: endocrine (hormonal) disorders, and connective tissue (collagen-vascular) diseases.

In autoimmune connective tissue diseases (which affect mainly skin and joints) circulating autoantibodies are often raised against targets in the nucleus. This gives rise to characteristic patterns of antinuclear antibody localization:
1. Rim (peripheral nuclear) pattern
   • Antibodies against double-stranded DNA.
2. Homogeneous (diffuse nuclear) pattern
   • Antibodies against single-stranded DNA or histone proteins.

3. Speckled pattern
   - Antibodies against nonhistone proteins.

All of the above immunolocalization patterns occur in the rheumatic disorder **systemic lupus erythematosus** (SLE). Of note, some SLE patients have antibodies to Z-DNA, which is more immunogenic than B-DNA. Certain related disorders are associated with specific intranuclear autoantibody targets:

1. **CREST syndrome**
   - Calcinosis, Raynaud's, esophageal disease, sclerodactyly, telangiectasia.
   - Associated with **anti-centromere antibodies**.
2. **Mixed connective tissue disease** (MCTD)
   - An overlap syndrome with features of SLE, scleroderma, and polymyositis.
   - Associated with **anti-ribonucleoprotein antibodies** (e.g., to U1; p. 102).
3. Neonatal SLE with **congenital heart block**
   - Associated with **anti-Ro** (SS-A; DNA-binding ribonucleoprotein) **antibodies**.

The extent to which such antibodies influence the course of the disease (i.e., whether they are pathogenic or not) remains unresolved.

MOLECULAR MINIREVIEW

Ku

On the basis of autoantibody studies, the telomeric protein **Ku** was first identified as a DNA-binding autoantigen associated with sclerodactyly. Ku is an end-joining response protein which participates in telomeric capping. It consists of two subunits, **Ku70** and **Ku80**, which combine with a third (catalytic) subunit to form **DNA-dependent protein kinase** (DNA-PK; p. 378). This is a critical nuclear enzyme required for the repair of double-stranded DNA breaks (including telomere uncapping), and also for site-specific antibody gene recombination. Hence, like DNA-PK, Ku is a caretaker protein (pp. 366–7) that binds to telomeres and maintains chromosome stability.

Of note, the sterility phenotype induced by mutation of the **Bloom syndrome** (*BLM*) helicase gene is rescued (complemented) by *Ku70*.

Chromosomal maintenance

Chromosome tips are capped by telomeric nucleoproteins

Being linear rather than circular, human chromosomes contain special end-chromosomal overhanging DNA sequences complexed to proteins. These noncoding protein–DNA caps or **telomeres** (literally, the things at the end) are the only readily accessible chromosomal replication elements in humans. Telomeres contain between 150 and 2000 TTAGGG sequences, which protrude from the 3′ ends of chromosomal DNA strands as 12- to 15-bp terminal overhangs detectable by in situ labeling. These repetitive GT-rich DNA sequences contribute approximately 10 kb to each telomere in human cells; of note, mouse telomeres are over 100 kb. Telomeres stabilize chromosomes via the following means:

1. By protecting chromosome tips from exonucleolytic degradation.
2. By preventing end-to-end chromosomal fusion.
3. By silencing end-chromosomal DNA regions prone to genetic damage.

Terminal chromosome deletions with telomeric loss result in chromosomal instability – that is, such lesions are highly **recombinogenic**. This explains why the treatment-resistant malarial parasite *Plasmodium falciparum* locates its virulence genes within subtelomeric clusters, thus enhancing recombination and (hence) antigenic variation. The recombinogenic nature of telomeres also makes these regions vulnerable to insertional events such as interchromosomal gene duplications. Protection is provided by telomeric induction of heterochromatic transcriptional repression via histone deacetylases.

The evolution of linear DNA is favored by natural selection since it permits rapid replication and recombination and thus enhances genetic diversification. But chromosome ends are difficult to replicate, as the lack of a replication fork means they cannot be initiated using RNA primers. Hence, when you get to the end of the line, there is nothing more to extend. Many viruses deal with this **end-replication problem** by priming with circular DNA, whereas others (such as polio and adenoviruses) use protein primers. Human telomere length, on the other hand, is regulated by DNA-binding ribonucleoproteins termed **telomerases**.

MOLECULAR MINIREVIEW

Human artificial chromosomes (HACs)

The development of **human artificial chromosomes (HAC)** has been made possible by the successful cloning of telomeres, centromeres, and DNA replication origins – in yeast, that is, since human chromosomal origins of replication have only recently been mapped. Yeast artificial chromosomes or **YACs** have long been used as cloning vectors for DNA mapping studies, but the quest to make a HAC has proven much more difficult. The ideal HAC would be a minichromosome 10–20% the size of a normal human chromosome. Such mini-/microchromosomes could be used for gene therapy – that is, for recreating normal function in individuals with specific gene defects such as **Duchenne muscular dystrophy** (p. 244) or **cystic fibrosis** (p. 190).

The technical difficulties that have hindered the creation of a functional HAC illustrate the complexity of normal human chromosomes. A good HAC must have operational centromeres and telomeres, and replication origins (until recently, only telomeres have been available). An advance has been to incorporate pericentromeric α-satellite DNA into HACs – several megabases of 171-bp tandem repeats – thus improving centromere function (and again suggesting that "junk" DNA may be unfairly labeled) and permitting stable gene expression for up to six months in vitro. But optimizing HACs will be only one step in a long path to human gene therapy: delivering HACs to tissues, gaining tissue-specific expression, regulating expression levels of the desired gene product, and avoiding immune reactions against the encoded gene products are all daunting hurdles to be overcome.

Telomerases maintain ageing chromosomes

Telomerases (or telomere terminal transferases) are endogenous ribonucleoprotein enzyme complexes that are inactivated by removing the RNA component. This latter part of the molecule – a AAUCCC RNA template complementary to the TTAGGG telomeric DNA repeat – is distinct from the catalytic **human telomerase reverse transcriptase** subunit, encoded by the *hTERT* gene, that enables telomerases to replicate unprimed DNA at the ends of chromosomes. This structural feature suggests that telomerases evolved via the recruitment of reverse transcriptase activity from L1 retrotransposons.

Telomerases maintain DNA integrity by adding one base at a time to the chromosomal tip, resulting in the addition of numerous TTAGGG repeats to telomeres (Figure 2.25). Cells monitor telomere length by counting the

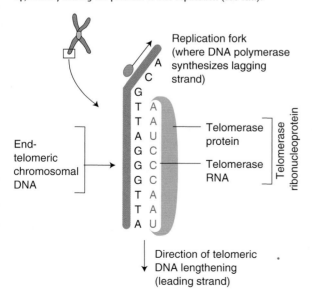

Figure 2.25 Telomeres and telomerase. The telomerase ribonucleoprotein binds complementary sequence at the chromosome tip, cleverly solving the problem of end-replication (see text).

number of copies of a telomere-binding protein. Despite this maintenance, somatic cells lose a little end-chromosomal length each time they divide – perhaps as part of a programmed mechanism to ensure normal ageing and protection from cancer (see below). Human germline cells such as embryonic blastocysts have longer telomeres than do somatic cells. Telomerase-expressing germ cells maintain the length of their telomeres despite numerous cell divisions, whereas the chromosomes of somatic cells shorten with ageing; of note, however, mature sperm cells have low telomerase levels. Similarly, memory T lymphocytes (which confer lifelong immunity) have shorter telomeres and a reduced cell replication capacity relative to naive (unprimed) immune cells. Telomere shortening may thus act as a **mitotic clock** that signals cell growth arrest once a critical size reduction takes place. In this way reductions of telomerase activity may predispose cells to replicative senescence – permanent growth arrest associated with cellular ageing. One rare (1:8 000 000) inherited syndrome of accelerated ageing, **Hutchinson–Gilford progeria**, is associated with accelerated telomeric shortening. In contrast, telomerase gene expression prolongs the life-span of normal human cells.

Age-related replicative arrest may thus occur in response to chromosomal length reaching a critical minimum. Note that not all tissue ageing is due to cellular senescence. Skin ageing, for example, is largely an expression of cumulative photodamage. Indeed, photoinducible mutations of growth-control genes are associated with enhanced telomerase levels in sun-damaged skin, a fetal-like phenotype similar to early cancers. Growth arrest may also occur for physiologic reasons, including a differentiation response in which cells switch off genes that are not relevant to their tissue-specific needs; such differentiation is also associated with a reduction of telomerase activity. Conversely, telomerase levels are at their highest during DNA synthesis and drop to undetectable levels during mitosis. Mice in which the telomerase gene is knocked out exhibit defective spermatogenesis and increased cell death.

Telomerases are sensors of chromosomal damage, and telomerase-dependent healing of chromosomal breaks requires an initial DNA-incisional event. Both the genetic and health consequences of telomerase dysfunction are clear: knockout of telomerase activity in mice leads to aneuploidy and end-to-end chromosomal fusion events, whereas defective telomerase recognition of chromosomal translocation breakpoints is implicated in the development of **thalassemias** (pp. 453–4).

Figure 2.26 Natural history of telomeres. *A*, Telomere length through the life cycle. *B*, M1 and M2 crises in normal and tumor cell senescence. Activation of telomerase following M2 may lead to telomere elongation and (hence) tumor formation.

A.

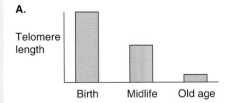

B.

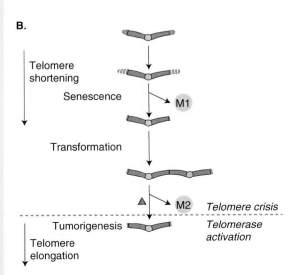

Telomerase activity in cell transformation

Just as cell differentiation is accompanied by reduced telomerase activity, so may cell transformation be accompanied by a rise in telomerase activity. Normal cells senesce and cease replication at a barrier termed **M1** which is activated by telomere shortening. If these cells become transformed (e.g., because of the acquisition of nonreciprocal translocations secondary to telomere attrition), a second growth checkpoint termed **M2** will be reached after approximately 50 more divisions. Attainment of this second checkpoint may trigger a **telomere crisis**: most of the neoplastic subclones will involute, but a few genetically unstable clones may select a survival pathway involving telomerase activation – leading to telomere elongation, cell immortalization and tumor development (Figure 2.26).

Eighty to ninety percent of human tumors are characterized by increased telomerase levels due to transcriptional upregulation. Telomerase detection has thus been used for screening diagnostic biopsy samples and aspirates, and may be overexpressed even in early (in situ) tumors. Hence, telomerase may be regarded as a tumor marker. Rare neonatal **neuroblastomas** that undergo spontaneous regression (so-called stage IV S) are distinguished by a relative lack of telomerase activity, whereas aggressive tumors have high telomerase levels associated with amplification of **N-Myc** which promotes cell immortalization.

The *hTERT* gene undergoes methylation in some tumors, whereas somatic deletions affecting the short arm of chromosome 3 may inactivate a telomerase suppressor gene. The rare X-linked disease **dyskeratosis congenita** – which causes skin and bone degeneration, chromosomal instability, and cancers – is caused by *DKC1* mutations affecting the pseudouridine synthase gene product **dyskerin**, which normally impairs telomerase activity. Telomerase inhibition by telomerase antagonists thus seems an attractive strategy for anticancer drug development. Consistent with this, the antileukemic efficacy of the ancient poison **arsenic** is associated with inhibition of *hTERT* transcription; note, however, that arsenic exposure also causes chromosomal end-to-end fusions and genomic instability. Telomerase may thus benefit cancer cells in two distinct ways: its absence may help promote tumor formation by accelerating nonreciprocal translocations during premalignant growth, and its overexpression may select for immortalized cells during tumor progression.

Cell division demands a cast of characters far in excess of the polymerases and telomerases already discussed. Completion of DNA synthesis requires replication of the entire chromosomal and nuclear structure, which includes not only DNA but also chromatin proteins and the mitotic apparatus. A prerequisite for chromosomal segregation is the untangling (decatenation) of interlinked helices of mitotic DNA. The twisted structure of the double helix thus poses special problems for DNA maintenance – not only during replication but also during recombination, repair, and transcription – which mandate the existence of specialized untangling enzymes termed topoisomerases.

Topoisomerases are DNA-nicking enzymatic swivels

The double helix does not exist as an infinite structure floating in space, but rather as a molecule with ends that are periodically constrained – for example, at the base of chromosomal loops. These constraints convert the twist of the double helix into a form of potential energy (Figure 2.27A) called **superhelicity**. The helix is thus said to be **supercoiled**, representing conservation of potential energy within the molecule. Supercoils within DNA may be **positive** or **negative**, depending on the direction of **writhe**. Z-DNA is stabilized by negative supercoils, which are readily introduced by the passage of an enzyme such as RNA polymerase. Hence, the removal of positive supercoils by such a processive mechanism could trigger the local formation of Z-DNA.

Without enzymes to untangle supercoiled DNA, chaos would soon set in. Synthesis of a 5-kb mRNA would involve the transcript being wrapped 500 times around the helix; while progression of DNA replication forks would necessitate the propeller-like spinning of each replicon, making mitotic decatenation of daughter DNA strands impossible (Figure 2.27B). Enzymes required to maintain DNA during its multiple functions include:

1. **Helicases** (DNA-unzipping enzymes)
   - Open the helix (i.e., transiently split the bases) to permit replisome entry.
2. **Helix-destabilizing enzymes** (single-strand-binding, or SSB, proteins)
   - Prevent nucleic acids forming hairpin structures (p. 97).

Figure 2.27 Topoisomerase actions and effects. *A*, DNA structures disentangled by topoisomerases. *B*, Mechanical requirement for DNA topoisomerases at replication forks, showing how DNA helix rotation may be prevented by topo-induced DNA nicking and unwinding.

A.

Supercoils   Knots   Catenanes

B.

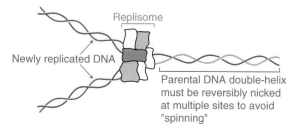

Replisome

Newly replicated DNA

Parental DNA double-helix must be reversibly nicked at multiple sites to avoid "spinning"

3. **Topoisomerases** (DNA-untangling enzymes)
   • Allow the helix to swivel and untwist.

Topoisomerases catalyze the interconversion of supercoiled DNA topoisomers by strand scission and rejoining. Though at least four classes of topoisomerases have been described, two main classes are of interest to human biology:

1. **Type I topoisomerases** (topo I) clamps itself around B-DNA, then introduces transient single-stranded breaks, or nicks, to relax it.

2. **Type II topoisomerases** (topo II) are homodimeric (heart-shaped) protein clamps that trap and then nick DNA in an ATP-dependent manner, thereby causing transient double-stranded breaks which permit DNA strand-passage and supercoil relaxation. Cleavage of the DNA phosphodiester bond powers the formation of a covalent bond between the phosphate and a tyrosine on the enzyme, which in turn stores the energy needed for strand passage. Topo II can also unknot linear DNA and decatenate circular DNA.

Topo I is important for DNA transcription. The type II enzyme modulates DNA replication, recombination, transcription, and repair, and is a marker for cell proliferation; in addition, topo II is a structural constituent of the insoluble nuclear matrix which anchors chromosomal looped domains. Topoisomerases are also autoantibody targets: topo I is the target of the **Scl-70** autoantibody in the disorder **scleroderma**, whereas topo II antibodies are detectable in 15% of patients with **pauciarticular juvenile chronic arthritis**.

Type III topoisomerases selectively relax negative supercoils by transiently cleaving one DNA strand. Genetic stability depends in part upon normal type III topoisomerase function. Diseases of genetic instability such as **ataxia telangiectasia** and **Bloom syndrome** may be associated with abnormal topoisomerase III function.

PHARMACOLOGIC FOOTNOTE

Topoisomerases as drug targets

In addition to their structural and functional roles within human cells, topoisomerases provide highly specific targets for therapeutic drugs:

1. As antibiotic targets, including:
   • Bacterial topoisomerase II (DNA gyrase: target of quinolone antibiotics **ciprofloxacin**, **nalidixic acid**).
   • Gyrase, which introduces positive supercoils into bacterial DNA; eukaryotes do not express gyrase.

2. As antitumor targets, including:
   • Topo II: target of cytotoxic drugs such as **etoposide** (a **podophyllotoxin** derivative) and **doxorubicin**.
   • Topo I: target of the cytotoxic drug **camptothecin**.

These drugs are topoisomerase poisons – as distinct from inhibitors (see below) – which exert their antitumor effects by converting the nicked enzyme–DNA complex into a stable cytotoxic lesion.

Increases in cell topoisomerase content (as may be induced by mitogens) thus enhance the cytotoxicity of these agents, but reduce the effects of true enzyme inhibitors such as the bacterial topoisomerase inhibitor **novobiocin**.

Enrichment reading

Bedtime reading

Jacob F. *The logic of life: a history of heredity.* Pantheon, Beaverton, OR, 1973

Watson JD. *The double helix.* Atheneum, Barcelona, 1968

Cheap'n'cheerful

Goodsell DS. *The machinery of life.* Springer-Verlag, Berlin, 1993

Library reference

Wolffe AP. *Chromatin: structure and function.* Academic Press, New York, 1998

Brown TA. *Genomes.* Wiley-Liss, New York, 1999

Summary

Genomes are characterized by a multilayer architecture. Eukaryotic DNA is organized by chromatin proteins, which control DNA accessibility. Acetylation of histone proteins permits gene activation, whereas epigenetic gene repression is transmissible by DNA methylation which predisposes to mutations.

Nucleic acids are synthesized by polymerases. Replicated DNA is packaged within chromosomes. DNA synthesis is initiated at multiple chromosomal sites.

Meiotic cell division converts diploidy to haploidy. Massive chromosomal compaction occurs during mitosis. Mitotic spindles bind centromeric DNA via kinetochores.

Chromosome tips are capped by telomeric nucleoproteins. Telomerases maintain ageing chromosomes. Topoisomerases are DNA-nicking enzymatic swivels.

QUIZ QUESTIONS

1. Describe the secondary structure and approximate coordinates of a piece of double-stranded DNA. Which is wider, the major or minor groove?
2. Summarize the different levels of compression that cellular DNA may undergo.
3. What are the functional differences between histone H1 and the core histones?
4. Explain the distinction between euchromatin and heterochromatin. Why do you think heterochromatin evolved?
5. What is meant by the term epigenetic inheritance? What mechanisms of epigenetic inheritance are there, and how do they work?
6. Describe how DNA synthesis occurs.
7. Name some structural features that distinguish a human chromosome from a bacterial plasmid.
8. What is meant by the terms (a) aneuploidy, (b) gene amplification, (c) genetic mosaic?
9. How does meiosis differ from mitosis? Why do you think meiosis evolved?
10. Describe the different phases of mitosis as distinguished by microscopic chromosome morphology and localization.
11. Name the phases of the human cell cycle, and explain the main events of each one.
12. Why do you think leukemias are more often curable than cancers?
13. What are the differences between a centriole, a centrosome, a centromere, and a kinetochore?
14. Explain why DNA polymerase cannot replicate chromosome tips.
15. Describe the structure and function of (a) a telomere, (b) telomerase.
16. Why do humans need type II topoisomerases?

3 | Gene expression

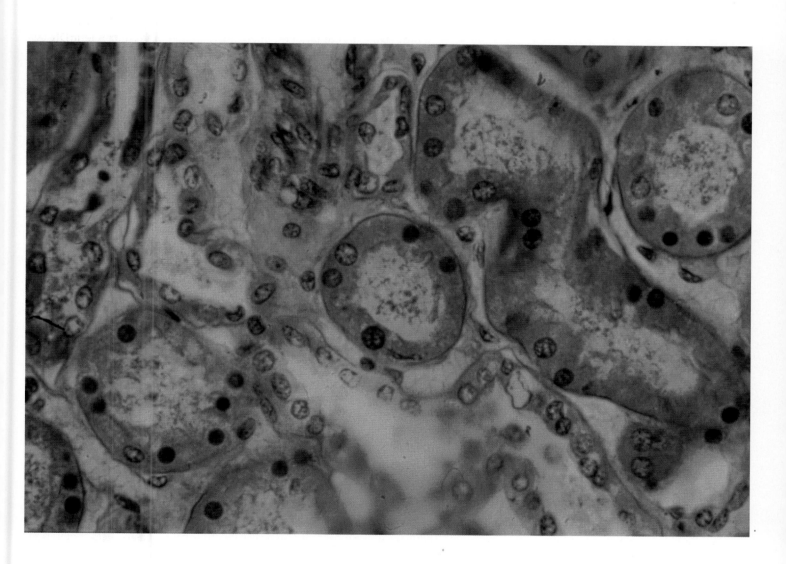

Figure 3.1 (*previous page*) Tissue-specific gene expression generating the morphology of renal tubular epithelium (Wellcome Medical Photographic Library, no. N0009024C).

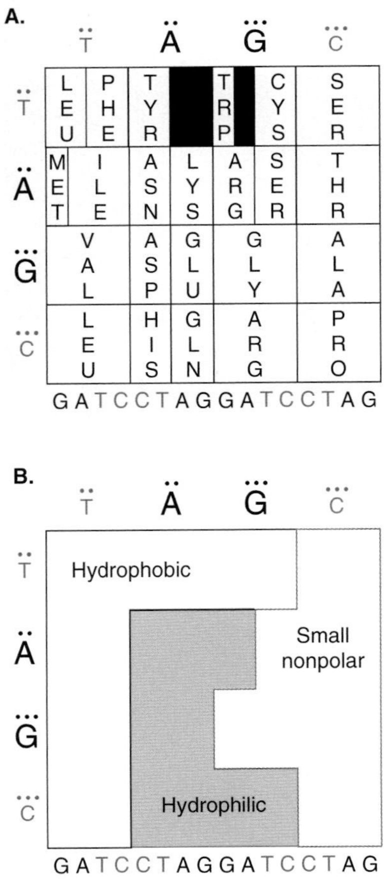

The genetic code

Nucleic and amino acids share a structure–function continuum

The genetic code has traditionally been regarded as an arbitrary encryption device for polypeptide synthesis. This creates a problem for origin-of-life theories: a pure encryption device should require preformed molecular machinery for interpreting and implementing the code, and would thus not exist in prebiotic environments. In fact, amino and nucleic acids exhibit significant structural and functional correspondences that seem likely to have been relevant to the evolution of primordial biomolecules.

With respect to the function of encoded amino acids, the most important codon component is the second base and the least critical the third, with the first occupying an intermediate position. The physical properties of amino acids are linked to the nucleotide sequence of codons: if the second nucleotide is A the encoded residue is hydrophilic (tending to sit on the outside of proteins), whereas if the second nucleotide is U/T, it is hydrophobic (tending to embed itself within the protein core). The survival of simple microorganisms such as bacteria depends more on the rapid mutability of their genomes rather than on conservation of functions: the strain will survive provided at least one organism resistant to environmental threats is available at any one time. Conversely, highly evolved multicellular organisms such as humans require stricter genomic conservation to maintain function.

These diverging paradigms of genetic evolution may be designated neutralist (primarily driven by random mutation) or selectionist (primarily driven by functional conservation). A periodic table for the genetic code can be constructed according to either model by juxtaposing purine and pyrimidine pairs, one version of which is presented in Figure 3.2A. This shows that both acidic and basic amino acids cluster within a common hydrophilic (polar; Figure 3.2B) region, between the hydrophobic region and the small nonpolar residues, supporting the notion of a structure–function continuum between amino and nucleic acids.

Two mutational patterns dominate mammalian genome evolution. First, most nonlethal mutations are transitions rather than transversions; that is, purines tend to substitute for purines and pyrimidines for pyrimidines, thereby minimizing the functional consequences of mutation. Second, base transitions most often occur in a GC→AT direction, reflecting the propensity of CpG dinucleotides to undergo methylation followed by deamination (p. 58). When represented as a nucleic-amino acid map, the minimal **mutational distance** separates functionally similar amino acids (Figure 3.3) – an evolutionary consequence of the most frequent base substitutions causing the least deleterious consequences for protein function. In other words, the genetic code is itself a product of natural selection, with each codon possessing its own selectable phenotype based on mutational stability in the face of adaptive pressures.

Figure 3.2 Nucleic versus amino acid table. *A*, "Periodic table" of the genetic code, showing correlation between codon sequence and amino acids. *B*, Functional amino acid correlation with codon structure, suggesting minimization of mutational distance between related codons.

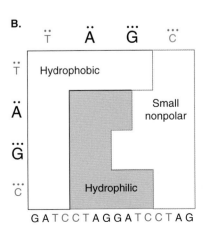

MOLECULAR MINIREVIEW

The genetic code: frozen or fluid?
The language of triplet codons varies between nuclear and mitochondrial DNA – within the mitochondrion, TGA encodes tryptophan rather than "stop" (as in the nucleus); mitochondrial ATA encodes methionine rather than isoleucine; whereas

the (nuclear) arginine-encoding AGA/AGG codons encode "stop" in the mitochondrion. Similar coding divergences occur between the nuclear DNA of humans, fruitflies, and bacteria. Moreover, three amino acids (serine, leucine and arginine) are specified by different first bases, and serine can even be encoded by two second bases. Hence, some of this redundancy in the existing human code may well have evolved from an earlier code(s). We know that this is plausible since other organisms encode ornithine or phosphoserine using codons that mammals use for serine. By the same token, certain human cells can encode the modified amino acid selenocysteine using the TGA "stop codon".

Mutation is a directional process involving the complementary loss and creation of codons. Knowledge of prevailing mutational patterns could therefore permit deduction of the evolutionary (and hence functional) pedigree of a codon. Progressive replacement of complementary GC base pairs by AT is common in transcriptionally inactive DNA, which is typically methylated; conversely, genes that are heavily transcribed should incur less GC→AT switching due to both demethylation and enhanced DNA repair in transcribed sequences, consistent with the hypomethylation of CpG islands adjacent to housekeeping genes. What these patterns of mutational drift are telling us is that the genetic code is not an iceberg but a river: currents of mutation ferry codons around the genome, sometimes being pushed upstream by selective pressures, while at other times being swept downstream by transcriptional neglect and evolutionary irrelevance.

The letters of the DNA alphabet make up three-letter words corresponding to amino acids; changes in even a single letter of this code can cause human disease. Here we consider the mechanics of how these letters are aligned to create a message.

Triplet nucleotide codons are read in frame

The letters of the alphabet that we read on a page make sense because they are grouped into clusters spaced apart from each other. Such spaces create **reading frames** that demarcate sets of letters into words. The digital language of a coding DNA sequence likewise depends upon the words of the sequence being read with the correct punctuation – read, that is, **in frame**. Bacterial genes may sometimes be read in more than one frame, resulting in different proteins. Remarkably, alternate reading frames are also deployed in the human *CDKN2* gene locus, which encodes two distinct proteins (pp. 362–3).

Genes and their transcripts are arranged in consecutive runs of three nucleotides termed **codons** that denote either an amino acid or a (nonsense) stop signal. Depending upon which nucleotide is chosen as the start site, there are three possible reading frames. In human cells (unlike bacteria) only one of these reading frames makes sense; an out-of-frame sequence will sooner or later be punctuated by **stop codons** UAA, UAG or UGA (Figure 3.3). The incorporation of premature stop codons leads to **protein truncation**, which may be readily detectable using standard electrophoretic assays (pp. 547–8).

This **triplet code** specifies the linear sequence of amino acids within a protein. Template DNA sequences such as ACG specify complementary RNA codons such as UGC, which in turn pair with complementary transfer RNA **anticodons** (ACG again). The correct amino acid (in this case cysteine) is thus incorporated into the growing polypeptide chain. Remember that the template DNA sequence is complementary to the nominal gene sequence on the sense strand, and that the mRNA codon is therefore identical (rather than complementary) to the codon of the gene sequence – except that uracil appears in place of thymine. Amino acid specificity is conventionally ascribed to the mRNA codon, with methionine thus being encoded by AUG.

Figure 3.3 Reading frames of a nucleotide DNA sequence. Two of the three triplet reading frames shown are untranscribable due to stop codons.

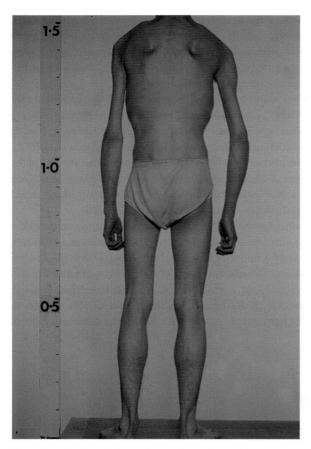

Figure 3.5 Infantile spinal muscular atrophy, a trinucleotide repeat (growing gene) neurologic disorder. Note the winging of the scapulae and the wasting of triceps and biceps (Wellcome Medical Photographic Library, no. N0005393C).

minor groove accessible to the multienzyme complex. The transcribing enzyme then separates from the preinitiation complex and heads off downstream through the open reading frame.

The ensuing phase of **transcription elongation** involves $5' \rightarrow 3'$ movement of the bubble at approximately 50 nucleotides per second. During this process RNA–DNA hybridization prevents backslippage of the attached enzyme. RNA elongation may be interrupted by **pauses** due to the sequence-specific formation of bent RNA regions termed **hairpin** configurations. Following transcription termination, the mRNA is released, processed, recognized by nuclear membrane receptors, and then actively transported to the cytoplasm. On reaching the endoplasmic reticulum, the $5'$ end of the transcript enters the ribosome where it directs translation (pp. 108–10).

CLINICAL KEYNOTE

Growing genes

Insertions of **trinucleotide repeats** that do not alter the reading frame may have transcriptional and clinical consequences. The pathologic effect of these repeat insertions is a dominant gain-of-function phenotype, with only one allele needing to be affected for disease expression. Illustrative of this, heterozygotes for **Huntington disease** (pp. 521–2) are as severely affected as homozygotes.

The accumulation of trinucleotide repeats occurs in hereditary neurologic disorders wherein a defective gene is passed from generation to generation and lengthens with each meiotic division (Figure 3.5). This progressive gene lengthening reflects the replicative instability of GC-rich trinucleotide repeats (e.g., CAG, CGG, CTG) that accumulate either within or adjacent to the gene sequence – some of which are associated with chromosomal fragile sites. These long repetitive sequences may cause DNA to adopt a non-B conformation, or even a hairpin formation, which is difficult for DNA polymerase to negotiate – perhaps causing replication slippage (stuttering) and further sequence expansion.

As many as eight hereditary neurologic disorders arise because of the insertion of CAG repeats encoding **polyglutamine** which, by binding and inhibiting the activity of the neuronal enzyme glyceraldehyde-3-phosphate dehydrogenase (GAPDH), could predispose to neuronal death (though other mechanisms are possible; pp. 522–3). In general, if there are fewer than 40 CAG trinucleotide repeats the phenotype is not apparent, whereas more than 40 repeats causes a phenotype.

Repeats involving untranslated gene regions are another story. For example, in the case of **myotonic dystrophy** the **myotonin** mRNA may be lengthened by over 6 kb by the growing CUG insert, perhaps interfering with the function of CUG-binding splicing proteins or else preventing nuclear export of the enlarged transcript. In the case of **Friedreich ataxia** – which is a recessive loss-of-function disorder, unlike the polyglutaminopathies – the poly-GAA expansion is intronic and should not affect **frataxin** protein synthesis. In the CGG repeat disorder **fragile X syndrome** transcriptional silencing is induced by gene methylation.

The increasing size of trinucleotide repeats between generations accounts for the non-Mendelian phenomenon of **anticipation**, in which an inherited disease becomes more severe with successive generations. This phenomenon parallels the growth in size of the gene. Note that both the length and the position of the repeat sequence vary considerably between disorders (Table 3.1).

Table 3.1. Trinucleotide repeat disorders. The major hereditary neurologic diseases associated with repeat expansions are shown. XR, X-linked recessive; AD, autosomal dominant; AR, autosomal recessive; UTR, untranslated region

Syndrome	Mode of inheritance	Affected gene	Chromosome locus	Insertion site	Repeat sequence	Repeat size (normal)	Repeat size (disease)	Effect on function
Huntington	AD	*Huntingtin*	4p16.3	coding region	CAG	10–35	40–150	gain
Spinocerebellar ataxia (SCA) type 1 (2,3,7)	AD	*Ataxin-1 (2,3,7)*	6p22-23	coding region	CAG	25–35	40–80	gain
Machado–Joseph	AD		14q24.3-q32	coding region	CAG		50–100	gain
Dentatorubral and pallido-luysian atrophy (DRPLA)	AD	*Atrophin-1*	12p12-ter	coding region	CAG			gain
Kennedy	XR	*Androgen receptor*	Xq21.3	coding region	CAG	15–30	40–80	loss
Fragile X	XR	*FMR-1 (FRAXA)*	Xq27.3	5'-UTR	CGG	5–50	100–4000	loss
Myotonic dystrophy	AD	*Myotonin*	19q13.2	3'-UTR	CTG	5–40	50–3000	loss
Friedreich ataxia	AR	*Frataxin*	9q13-q21.1	intron	GAA		100–2000	loss
(Fragile) XE	XR		Xq28		GCC			loss

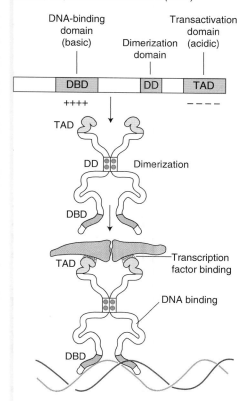

Figure 3.6 Multiple domains within a transcription factor. Following dimerization the complex binds to DNA and then directs activation of the relevant gene. DBD, DNA-binding domain; DD, dimerization domain; TAD, transactivation domain (acidic).

Transactivators consist of functionally distinct modular domains

Everything in biology sticks to everything else; the degree to which two molecules stick is just a question of affinity. In practice this means that the most interesting interactions are those exhibiting high affinity. Consistent with this, major changes in gene-transcribing activity are induced by changes in high-affinity protein–DNA binding. However, not all gene-binding proteins directly affect gene transcription; for example, histones do not. Similarly, not all gene-regulatory molecules are DNA-binding proteins.

DNA-binding proteins that directly affect gene expression are variously termed **transcription factors**, ***trans*-acting factors**, or **transactivators**. These are multifunctional proteins composed of separate domains, such as those for (Figure 3.6):

1. Sequence-specific **DNA binding**.
2. Protein **dimerization**.
3. Gene **transactivation**.

Since the phosphate backbone of DNA renders the molecule acidic (negatively charged), the **DNA-binding domains** of transcription factors are often basic (positively charged; e.g., basic helix-loop-helix domains). Since phosphate groups tend to be acidic, the phosphorylation of DNA-binding domains may inhibit protein–DNA binding, though transactivation may also be inducible by phosphorylation elsewhere on the molecule (e.g., the phosphorylation-dependent activation of the Myc transcription factor; p. 56). Similarly, phosphorylation of STAT-family proteins may induce their nuclear translocation and hence, indirectly, target gene transactivation (p. 305). Of note, the DNA binding of transcription factors may be reduced by 3-5 orders of magnitude due to changes in chromatin structure (i.e., the number of available DNA-binding sites may be reduced to <0.1%).

In contrast, the **transactivation domains** of transcription factors tend to be rich in glutamine and/or proline, and hence acidic. These **acidic activators** bind heterologous proteins in the transcription complex, recruiting them to the gene. One such activator motif is termed an **acid blob**, a negatively charged

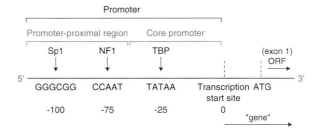

Figure 3.9 Fine structure of the promoter, distinguishing the core promoter from the promoter-proximal region. NF1, general transcription factor; ORF, open reading frame; Sp1, monomeric general transcription factor; TBP, TATA-binding protein.

General transcription factors are invariant components of the transcription machinery that initiate binding to 5′ gene-flanking regions. The target DNA sequence which melts to accommodate the transcription complex generally lies about 25 bp 5′ to the transcription start site, i.e., at −25. This signature sequence, termed the **TATA box** on account of its AT-rich nucleotide sequence, is one of several cis-acting DNA sequences called **upstream elements** which comprise the protein-binding sites of the promoter.

MOLECULAR MINIREVIEW

Upstream elements

The transcription preinitiation complex – which typically includes TATA-binding protein and RNA polymerase II among other molecules – attaches itself to the ~60-bp 5′ gene-flanking region centered on the TATA box. Further 5′ to this binding site, i.e., 40–150 bp 5′ to the transcription start site, lie additional protein-binding DNA regulatory sequences referred to as **accessory sequences**. Upstream elements thus include both the TATA box in the core promoter and accessory sequences in the promoter-proximal region (Figure 3.9):

1. **TATA box**
   - Contains the AT-rich TATAA sequence near −25.
   - Binds the general transcription factor **TATA-binding protein**.
2. **CAAT box** (pronounced "cat box")
   - Contains a GGCCAATCT-containing sequence near −75.
   - Binds the general transcription factor **NF1**.
3. **GC box**
   - Contains the GC-rich GGGCGG-containing sequence near −100.
   - Binds the monomeric general transcription factor **Sp1**.

TATA boxes, CAAT boxes and GC boxes are sometimes termed **constitutive regulatory elements**.

Preinitiation transcription complexes assemble on promoters

The DNA sequence that lies 5′ to the gene and melts to accommodate the transcription complex is termed the promoter. Distinction is made between the **core promoter** and the DNA sequence 100–200 bp 5′ to this, which is termed the **promoter-proximal region**; the latter contains the CAAT box and GC box (Figure 3.9). Most core promoters contain TATA boxes, but exceptions include housekeeping genes such as the general transcription factors themselves.

The TATA box forms a landing site for the saddle-shaped **TATA-binding protein (TBP)**. The unusual symmetry of TBP suggests that it evolved via gene-fusion events affecting a homodimeric trans-activator. Once bound to DNA, TBP radically distorts the conformation of the core promoter. TBP is bound by 8–12 additional **TBP-associated factors (TAFs)**, three of which resemble histones and associate with histone deacetylase complexes. Certain TAF domains termed **bromodomains** consist of polar four-helix bundles which bind amino-terminal histone acetyl groups, perhaps helping to explain how transcription may occur despite the persistence of nucleosomal DNA. The TAF–TBP complex forms an evolutionarily conserved trans-activating apparatus termed **TFIID**, which directs preinitiation complex assembly. Other general transcription complexes (TFIIA, B, E, F, H) can also prime RNA polymerase II activity, however, and neither TFIID nor even TBP itself appears indispensable for transcriptional initiation. TBP is a binding target for the 154-amino-acid hepatitis B transactivating protein X (see below) which is essential for viral replication and hepatitis-associated liver carcinogenesis.

In addition to the TATA box, core promoters may contain an **initiator element** that retains binding of the basal transcription complex following the downstream release of RNA polymerase II, allowing rapid recharging of the transcription complex. Some genes have promoters that favor continual transcription whereas others only initiate transcription in certain tissues. The potency and inducibility of a promoter depends not only on its sequence but also on its chromatin structure and genomic context. Such considerations become important when creating indicator cell lines or transgenic animals (in which context **reporter gene** technology may be of predictive value; p. 565).

MOLECULAR MINIREVIEW

Promoters and enhancers

Promoters and enhancers are both gene-regulatory cis-acting sequences, but enhancers differ from promoters in certain respects:

1. Enhancers are not essential for transcriptional initiation.
2. Enhancers may be positioned at a considerable distance from the transcription start site; for example, the immunoglobulin heavy chain enhancer is positioned over 17 kb from the gene promoter. Hence, these elements are usually situated 5′ to the upstream elements (which in turn lie within ~100 bp of the transcription start site).
3. Enhancers may be positioned downstream from the transcription start site – sometimes lying 3′ to the gene, within introns, or (rarely) within the open reading frame (again, all seen in the immunoglobulin genes).
4. Changing the orientation (5′→3′ or 3′→5′) of the enhancer sequence with respect to the gene does not alter the degree of transcription augmentation. However, some promoters (notably those of certain housekeeping genes) can also support bidirectional transcription.

These criteria can be tested by experimentally cutting and pasting a putative enhancer in different positions and demonstrating equivalent transcription – something that would not be seen with a promoter sequence. Since the effect of enhancers is orientation independent, they may help localize RNA polymerase to the neighborhood of a particular gene without actually aligning it for binding.

Enhancers recruit transcription factors to active genes

Enhancers increase transcription by using sequence-specific DNA-binding proteins to lasso the transcription complex (i.e., the RNA polymerase II holoenzyme) and thus recruit it to an appropriate gene. The transactivator thus binds to the specific **response element** of the enhancer via its basic DNA-binding domain, and also to the transcription complex via its acidic transactivation domain. Interaction of the promoter-bound complex with enhancer-bound transcription factors may occur via DNA looping (Figure 3.8).

Developmental enhancers arranged in tandem over several kilobases upstream of a gene cluster are termed a **locus control region** (**LCR**). The competence of the LCR to be activated depends on chromatin conformation, but the expression of each gene in the cluster depends in addition on transactivator or repressor binding. A well-known LCR is that controlling hemoglobin switching during embryogenesis (p. 453). By recruiting the RNA polymerase into the vicinity of the gene in this manner, enhancer-bound transcription factors increase the probability of transcription initiation. Examples of transcription factors and their DNA-binding sites include:

1. **Jun**
   - Binds to **AP1 sites** (TGACTCA).
   - Mediates responsiveness to mitogenic stimuli.
2. **CREB**
   - Binds to **cAMP response elements** (CREs).
   - Mediates olfaction, circadian rhythm, and pituitary development.
3. **Estrogen receptors**
   - Bind to **estrogen-response elements** (EREs).
   - Mediate effects of estrogens on the breast, uterus, and brain.
4. **STAT**-family transactivators
   - Bind to **GAS elements**.
   - Mediate cytokine and hemopoietic receptor signaling.

The attributes of such proteins may be transferred between polypeptides by mixing-and-matching individual domains. The existence of related motifs thus favors combinatorial interactions between protein superfamilies (Table 3.2); the structural basis of this flexibility is heterodimerization.

Insulator (boundary) **elements** are DNA sequences that demarcate the 5′ and 3′ margins of the gene and its flanking sequences. These elements, which may be affected by regulatory transcription factors or chromatin alterations, prevent enhancers from activating inappropriate genes (Figure 3.10). The

Table 3.2. Recurring motifs in transcription factors

Transcription factor domain	Motif structure	Binding target(s)	Binding mechanism	Examples
Zinc fingers	Metal-based 30-amino-acid recognition bumps in which a 4-amino acid stretch binds a zinc ion	3-bp consensus sequences (which may be palindromic) in the major groove of GC-rich DNA (Figure 3.11*A*)	Dimeric half-sites bind to target DNA-response elements (Figure 3.12)	Steroid hormone receptors: two fingers per molecule, with zinc bound to four cysteine residues (Cys–Cys fingers)
				General transcription factors (e.g., Sp1): fingers of two cysteine and two histidine residues (Cys–His fingers)
				GATA-1 (p. 454), WT1 (p. 408) Hairless*
Copper fist	Knuckles	Metallothionein gene promoter	Knuckles activate promoter	Heavy-metal-binding proteins
Leucine zipper	Helices containing four to five leucine residues each separated by 17 amino acids	Dimeric partner (zipper domain)	The two helices zip to create a clothespeg-like dimeric attachment to DNA	Jun Fos
Basic helix-loop-helix (bHLH)	Two α-helices separated by a loop, adjacent to basic region	E box (CA*XX*TG) DNA site	Dimerization of the two helices yields a basic four-helix bundle binding the major groove	MyoD Myogenin
Helix-turn-helix	Two α-helices separated by a turn		Dimerization permits DNA binding	Homeobox proteins POU-domain proteins
bZIP	Adjacent bHLH and leucine zipper domains		Dimerization by zipper domain; DNA-binding by basic domain (Figure 3.11*B*)	Jun Myc, Max, Mad CREB

Notes:
* Mutated in **alopecia universalis**

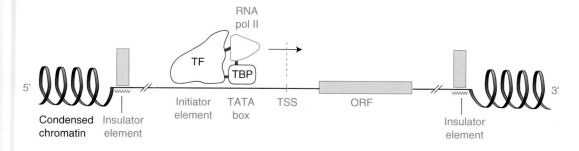

Figure 3.10 Simplified representation of a preinitiation transcription complex, and its relationship to chromatin conformation and gene transcription. Insulator (boundary) elements are shown at the 5′ and 3′ extremes of the active gene region. ORF, open reading frame; TBP, TATA-binding protein; TF, general transcription factor; TSS, transcription start site.

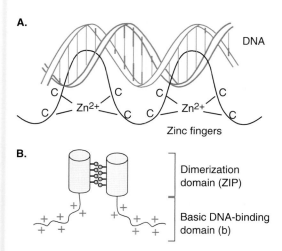

Figure 3.11 Transcription factor motifs. *A*, Cysteine–cysteine zinc finger in steroid hormone receptor binding to its response element in DNA; *B*, bZIP domain, showing the different structural characteristics of the "b" and the "ZIP".

Figure 3.12 Hormone response elements. *A*, Estrogen response element (ERE); *B*, retinoic acid response element (RARE). HRE, hormone response element; N, unspecified nucleotide; TR, thyroid hormone receptor; TRE, thyroid response element; RAR, retinoic acid receptor.

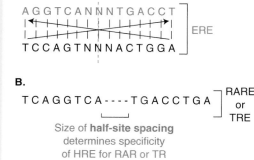

differential expression of parental IGF2 genes (imprinting; pp. 407–8), for example, relates to uniallelic methylation-dependent CpG binding of an enhancer-blocking protein, thereby creating an enhancer boundary or insulator.

Differential dimerization fine-tunes transcription factor activity

The structural motifs that characterize transcription factors (e.g., leucine zippers, helix-loop-helix domains, zinc fingers; Table 3.2) may be responsible not only for DNA binding but also for dimerization. In both leucine zippers and helix-loop-helix proteins, the dimerization interface brings together basic arginine- and lysine-rich peptides which bind the major groove of DNA; this resembles the DNA-binding mechanism of bacterial restriction enzymes (p. 536). Any transcription factor containing a dimerization motif (e.g., leucine zipper) can form dimers with other proteins containing the same motif.

Having the ability to homodimerize or heterodimerize expands the regulatory spectrum of transcription factors. Transcriptional inhibition in human cells often occurs through the differential formation of hetero- or homo-dimeric DNA-binding proteins: homodimeric binding may bend DNA in a manner conducive to gene activation, whereas heterodimers may prevent homodimer binding. Heterodimers are not always inhibitory, however – examples of agonists include **Jun/Fos** (AP1; see below). Examples of important heterodimeric interactions apply to the following transcription factor families:

1. **Myc** and **Max** and **Mad**.
2. **NFκB** and **IκB** (see below).
3. **Retinoic acid receptor** (RAR) and **retinoid X receptor** (RXR; p. 320).

Some transcription factors are activated by binding to a ligand that permits either nuclear translocation or DNA binding. These **nuclear receptors** include the steroid hormone receptor superfamily and the related thyroid hormone receptor family (which includes the RAR/RXR and vitamin D receptors; pp. 313, 317). Each member of the steroid receptor superfamily contains a single domain of two zinc fingers, which binds with high specificity to a **palindromic** DNA sequence called a **hormone response element** (HRE). If bound by homodimeric transcription factors, such sequences exhibit **dyad symmetry**. In such cases the nucleotide sequence itself is recognized by the first zinc finger, whereas the spacing between the symmetric **half-sites** is sensed by the second finger.

In contrast, receptor heterodimers of the thyroid hormone receptor family bind HREs consisting of nonsymmetric tandem half-sites. These hexameric AGGTCA **direct repeat** sequences differ for different hormone receptors of this family only in terms of their half-site spacing (Figure 3.12). Homologs of these receptors may lack known ligands, but such **orphan receptors** may still dimerize and thus affect cell behavior.

Transcription factors in human disease

Mutations of transcription factors in human disease include the following few examples:

1. The zinc-finger-containing **WT1 (Wilms tumor: nephroblastoma)** transcription factor normally inhibits the expression of insulin-like growth factor-2 (p. 408). Germline *WT1* mutations that prevent DNA binding may thus induce kidney tumor growth and/or embryonic malformation (**Denys–Drash syndrome**).

2. Abnormal dimerization of transcription factors may cause end-organ hormone resistance. Examples include a point mutation affecting the **vitamin D receptor** in **hereditary vitamin D-resistant rickets**, and similar disorders affecting the **androgen receptor** and **thyroid hormone receptors**. Similarly, mutation of the POU-family transcription factor **Pit1** can cause pituitary hormone deficiency (**panhypopituitarism**) due to dominant-negative inhibition of pituitary gland gene expression.

3. The **PAX** family of developmental transcription factors is mutated in **Waardenburg syndrome** (*PAX3*; white forelock, deafness, iris heterochromia), **optic nerve colobomas** (*PAX2*) and **aniridia** (*PAX6*).

4. The congenital heart condition **Holt–Oram syndrome** (atrial septal defect plus polydactyly; p. 406) is caused by a null mutation of the **TBX5** transcription factor. Another transcription factor, **NKX2-5**, is mutated in **atrial septal defect with heart block**.

In some diseases transcription factor mutations may affect cellular events outside the nucleus. Oncogenic activation of the cell-surface **Met** receptor tyrosine kinase occurs following the chromosomal translocation of a leucine zipper-containing motif (**Tpr**); this leads to the expression of a fusion protein (**Met-Tpr**), which dimerizes in the absence of growth factor, leading to uncontrolled growth.

Gene regulation

Inhibitory transcription factors silence gene activity

Synergistic and antagonistic interactions between transcription factors are common. The inducing properties of a transactivator may be abolished by the following mechanisms:

1. **Quenching**
   - i.e., Binding of a protein to a functional domain of the transactivator.
2. **Squelching**
   - i.e., Mopping up transcription factors by binding to a strong transactivator.
3. **Phosphorylation**
   - e.g., Of the transactivator's DNA-binding domain.
4. **Heterodimerization**
   - e.g., By reducing DNA affinity or dimer stability.

Prokaryotic repressor proteins inhibit gene activation by binding to DNA-recognition half-sites. For example, the bacterial recognition of tetracycline triggers dissociation of a repressor (**TetR**), thus permitting the expression of a tetracycline efflux/resistance protein (**TetA**). This tetracycline-inducible system is exploited in transgenically engineered animal models (pp. 583–4).

RING finger (C_3HC_4) proteins contain 60-amino-acid motifs that bind Zn^{2+} ions and interact with zinc-finger-containing steroid hormone receptors.

Examples include the **PML** protein (which is fused to RARα in **acute promyelo-cytic leukemia**), the **breast cancer** susceptibility protein **BRCA1**, and the cysteine-rich **Parkinson disease** gene product **parkin** – all of which inhibit gene activity or growth.

Transactivators may become inhibitors because of minor sequence alterations or post-transcriptional modifications. In other words, the same gene can encode both an activator and a repressor. The best-known example is the bacterial **lambda** (λ) repressor gene, but the human **ErbA** (thyroid hormone receptor) and **FosB** genes may also be processed to yield antagonistic protein isoforms (germline FosB inactivation causes a hypothalamic defect that prevents the parental nurturing of offspring).

Some enhancer-like domains may function as transcriptional **silencers**. Gene regions repressed by silencers are termed **silent domains**; whether a gene is active or repressed may thus depend on the net activity of locus control regions and gene silencers. Neuron-specific expression of type II voltage-gated sodium channels reflects the ubiquitous non-neuronal expression of a silencer-binding protein termed REST, for example.

MOLECULAR MINIREVIEW

NFκB and IκB

NFκB (pronounced "enn-eff-capper-bee") is an enhancer-binding nuclear factor originally discovered as a transactivator of the intronic immunoglobulin κ light chain gene enhancer in B lymphocytes. NFκB is a DNA-binding heterodimer of 50- and 65-kDa subunits: the 50-kDa subunit (**p50**) arises from a 105-kDa inactive precursor and binds DNA, whereas the 65-kDa subunit (**p65**) mediates transcriptional activation. Alternatively, p65 may be bound by an inhibitory cytoplasmic protein family collectively termed **IκB**, which prevents nuclear translocation and (hence) the DNA binding of NFκB. Inflammatory cytokine-induced phosphorylation of a degradative motif in IκB triggers IκB proteolysis, liberating NFκB from the inactive heterodimer and permitting NFκB transcription (which in turn prevents cytokine-induced death of inflammatory cells).

Viral double-stranded RNA activates two enzymes that phosphorylate IκB (IκB kinases: **IKKα/β**). Another IκB kinase, IKKγ (a.k.a. **NEMO**, or **NFκB** essential modulator), is mutated in the X-linked dominant genodermatosis **incontinentia pigmenti**. Note that IKKs can induce differentiation via pathways distinct from those involving NFκB, indicating the existence of alternative IKK substrates.

The p65 subunit of NFκB is homologous to the **Rel** gene product (its cancer-causing variant, v-Rel, induces leukemia in turkeys), which activates target genes by binding TATA-binding protein. In contrast, the **Bcl3** protein resembles IκB but transforms cells by associating with DNA-binding NFκB p50 homodimers, leading to potent transactivation. Knockout of p50 increases the susceptibility of experimental animals to infections with pneumococci and *Listeria* spp.

NFκB binds GGGACTTTCC motifs in promoters and enhancers of nonlymphoid as well as lymphoid cells. These NFκB-binding sites occur within many genes encoding putative stress proteins including inflammatory cytokines (such as **tumor necrosis factor**, **interleukins** and **interferons**) and the immediate-early gene product **Myc**.

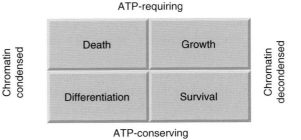

Figure 3.13 Schematic representation of the interrelationship between gene activity and cell outcomes.

NFκB in human disease

Catabolic states induced by cytokines may be accompanied by muscle loss – e.g. in chronic sepsis or **cancer cachexia** – due in part to NFκB-dependent transcriptional repression of muscle-forming proteins (e.g., **myosin**) and differentiating factors (e.g., **MyoD**; pp. 404–5). Muscle loss caused by **glucocorticoid** treatment, on the other hand, may reflect increased muscle proteolysis despite reduced NFκB-dependent inhibition of myofibril growth.

An NFκB-binding site is located in the long terminal repeat (enhancer) of the **HIV1** and **HIV2** viruses. Activation of infected immunocytes may thus be a way in which the human reticuloendothelial system is duped by HIV – as soon as the cell synthesizes NFκB, stimulation of HIV transcription and replication ensues. This is accompanied by induction of the HIV1 **p100 protease** which proteolyzes IκB, thus antagonizing host cell control of NFκB activity and creating a positive-feedback loop driving viral replication. A comparable enhancer containing NFκB sites is found in **cytomegalovirus** (CMV), another virus associated with lifelong infection.

Certain bacteria have worked out how to deal with NFκB: commensal (nonpathogenic, symbiotic) gut *Salmonella* inhibit IκB degradation, for example, thus eliminating any NFκB-dependent inflammatory response. Similarly, the anti-inflammatory drug **aspirin** prevents IκB proteolysis, thus inhibiting NFκB activation. Induction of NFκB expression by **asbestos** is implicated in the epigenetic carcinogenicity of this substance. NFκB is also central to the pathogenesis of the allergic disorder **asthma**.

Changes in gene expression regulate growth and metabolism

Gene activity determines how a cell behaves at any one time. Just as humans vary their behavior during the course of a day, so do cells alternate between different metabolic states depending upon their circumstances (Figure 3.13):

1. Growth
   - Active DNA and protein synthesis.
   - Involves DNA synthesis.
2. Survival
   - Basal gene expression levels.
   - Ready to grow if stimulated; no DNA synthesis.
3. Differentiation
   - Non-tissue-specific genes switched off.
   - May be unable to grow; no DNA synthesis.
4. Death
   - Suicide pathways activated (pp. 377–84).
   - DNA fragmentation.

A fundamental cellular decision is when (or whether) to grow. Cell growth involves much more than DNA replication: it also involves protein synthesis, reduplication of nongenomic nuclear and cytoplasmic organelles, cytoskeletal movement, and maintenance of the cell cycle machinery. Such growth may be continuous during embryonic and fetal life, but requires concomitant cell death to sculpt the shape of limbs and neural circuits. In contrast, tumors may exhibit high net growth rates that are partly due to defects in cell attrition.

The decision to initiate a fresh round of cell growth can be triggered by extrinsic stimuli such as hormones or cell contact. Such triggers unleash a cascade of signaling interactions that culminate in pro-mitogenic gene expression. The first genes induced in a mitogenic cascade of this kind are termed **immediate-early genes**.

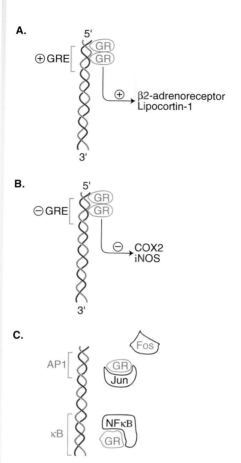

Figure 3.14 Glucocorticoid receptor (GR) actions. *A*, Induction of gene expression via a positive glucocorticoid response element (GRE). *B*, Inhibition of gene expression via a negative GRE. *C*, Inhibition of AP1 and NFκB gene expression via putative dimer-disrupting effects of GR. AP1, activator protein-1; COX2, cyclooxygenase-2; iNOS, inducible nitric oxide synthase; NFκB, nuclear factor transactivating the intronic immunoglobulin κ light chain gene enhancer in B lymphocytes.

MOLECULAR MINIREVIEW

Immediate-early genes

Genes that are rapidly induced (i.e., within an hour) from low basal expression levels by growth stimuli (mitogens) are designated immediate-early genes. These genes include **c-Fos**, **c-Jun**, and **c-Myc**.

Immediate-early genes often encode transcription factors that tend to have a short half-life. In the case of Fos, the latter reflects negative feedback mediated by the binding of the gene product to its own promoter; Fos expression typically peaks ~15 minutes after stimulation and disappears within 60 minutes. Like Myc, Jun and Fos contain heptad leucine repeats (leucine zippers); noncovalent Jun–Fos heterodimerization via these domains generates the so-called **AP1** (activator protein-1) composite transcription factor.

There are at least four Fos (c-Fos, FosB, Fra1, Fra2) and three Jun (c-Jun, JunB, JunD) protein isoforms. The most stable dimer is the AP1 Fos/Jun heterodimer, which binds DNA at either AP1 sites or cAMP response elements (CREs). Like CREB – the CRE-binding transactivator – AP1 binds DNA in a scissors-grip mode. Although Jun–Jun homodimers are also moderately stable (though 500-fold less so than Jun–Fos heterodimers), Fos does not form stable homodimers (and hence does not bind DNA in the absence of a partner) due to destabilizing acidic residues in opposed leucine zipper domains. The differential transcriptional effects of homo- and heterodimer binding may relate to differences in DNA bending induced by the regulatory complex.

Leucine zipper proteins such as Jun/AP1 may liaise promiscuously with zinc finger (e.g., the glucocorticoid receptor) or helix-loop-helix proteins (e.g., MyoD). For example, AP1-inducible collagenase gene expression – a prerequisite for tumor invasion in some systems – is abolished by AP1 binding of activated glucocorticoid receptors or retinoic acid receptors (Figure 3.14), perhaps accounting in part for the antitumor effects of drugs such as **dexamethasone**.

CLINICAL KEYNOTE

Tax in T cell leukemias

Adult T cell leukemia is caused by a retrovirus family, the prototype of which is the human T cell leukemia virus 1 (**HTLV1**), which encodes a 40-kDa transcription factor called **Tax**. Tax stimulates transcription from the long terminal repeat (LTR) of the HTLV1 genome, and strongly drives viral replication. This replicative activity requires Tax to bind to the bZIP domain of **CREB** – thus triggering CREB dimerization, stabilizing CREB–DNA binding, and co-activating three imperfect CREs within the promoter of the HTLV1 genome (Figure 3.15). This Tax–CREB interaction is central to the leukemogenic potency of HTLV1. Another viral transactivator that activates CREB by binding its bZIP domain is the **hepatitis B virus X protein**, which also interacts with TATA-binding protein.

Tax indirectly activates NFκB by inducing phosphorylation of IκB, leading in turn to the induction of Fos, Jun and other immediate-early genes. Tax also induces expression of **interleukin-2** (IL-2) and its receptor, **parathyroid hormone-related protein**, **granulocyte-macrophage colony-stimulating factor** and **platelet-derived growth factor**.

T cell leukemias arising from HTLV1 infection are typically IL-2-dependent for growth in vitro, suggesting that the interaction of Tax with IL-2 receptors has a direct leukemogenic role. Interestingly, transgenic mice that overexpress Tax develop **neurofibromas** and other mesenchymal tumors.

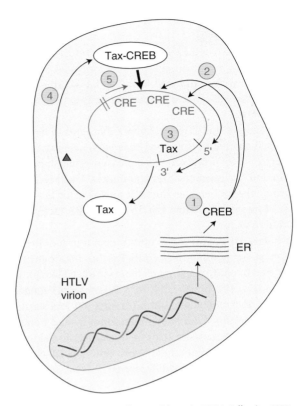

Figure 3.15 Dimerization of CREB with Tax in HTLV1. Following CREB synthesis (1) and binding to CREB-response elements (CRE) (2), *Tax* transcription is activated (3), leading in turn to formation of Tax-CREB heterodimers (4) and acceleration of HTLV1 proliferation (5). CRE, cAMP response element; ER, endoplasmic reticulum.

Differentiated cells express tissue-specific gene subsets

Although the haploid human genome contains over 30 000 genes, as few as 10 000 are expressed in an average cell. **Differentiation** is a property of tissues that demand only a limited number of cell functions, and is induced in large part by switching off unnecessary genes (e.g., those responsible for growth, motility, or secretion of specific proteins). The stability of the differentiated phenotype is critically dependent upon regional chromatin condensation and methylation. Of note, a small number of growth-arrest genes appear to be induced by cell quiescence.

The tissue-specificity of gene expression is illustrated by the large proportion of genes expressed solely in the central nervous system. How do kidney tubular cells know which genes to express and which to silence? Methylation is one mechanism, but many tissue-specific genes remain unmethylated. Transcription factors may be tissue restricted in their expression:

1. **Oct-2** (an octamer-binding activator of immunoglobulin genes)
   - Expressed only in lymphoid tissue.
2. **MyoD1** (pp. 404–5) and **myogenin**
   - Expression mainly restricted to developing muscle.
3. **CAAT enhancer-binding protein** (**CEBP**)
   - Expressed mainly in liver.
4. **Pit-1/GHF-1** (a regulator of pituitary hormone gene expression)
   - Expression restricted to the pituitary gland.
5. **GATA** factors (p. 454) and **Myb**
   - Expressed mainly in hemopoietic tissues.

Tissue-specific phenotypes may depend not only on the transcriptional regulation of new protein synthesis, but also on post-transcriptional mRNA processing and post-translational protein activation. Hence, functional specificity may be maintained despite a degree of transcriptional **leakiness** from putative tissue-specific promoters.

> **MOLECULAR MINIREVIEW**
>
> **Tissue-specific gene expression**
>
> All human cells contain the same gene sequences, yet cell types in different organs express different genes and gene products. In pregnancy, for example, the placenta synthesizes 11 pregnancy-specific glycoproteins, all of which are encoded on chromosome 19. Despite this, tissue-specific gene expression remains a relative rather than an absolute concept. Low-level ectopic (non-tissue-specific) transcription has been documented for many 'tissue-specific' genes, including the anti-hemophilic blood clotting protein **factor VIII**, the red cell oxygen-binding protein **β-globin**, and the embryonic sex-differentiating peptide **antimüllerian hormone.**
>
> Analysis of mutant gene function in human disease may require biopsy of the affected organ (e.g., liver, brain, heart) for documentation of reduced expression and mutation characterization. However, the detection of **illegitimate transcripts** from accessible tissues such as peripheral blood lymphocytes may permit the detection of coding sequence deletions identical to those in the diseased organ. Successful application of this strategy to diseases such as **Duchenne muscular dystrophy** has permitted the noninvasive recognition of known dystrophin gene defects using peripheral blood analysis. This approach may prove applicable to family screening for patients with characterized deletions.

Enrichment reading

Bedtime reading
Kauffman S. *At home in the universe*. Oxford University Press, Oxford, 1995

Cheap'n'cheerful
Latchman DS. *Eukaryotic transcription factors*. Academic Press, New York, 1999

Library reference
Barrow, JD. *Theories of everything*. Oxford University Press, Oxford, 1991

Summary

Nucleic and amino acids share a structure–function continuum. Triplet nucleotide codons are read in frame.

A multienzyme complex transcribes DNA into RNA. Transactivators consist of functionally distinct modular domains. Cis-acting DNA sequences are bound by transacting proteins.

Preinitiation transcription complexes assemble on promoters. Enhancers recruit transcription factors to active genes. Differential dimerization fine-tunes transcription factor activity.

Inhibitory transcription factors silence genes. Changes in gene expression regulate growth and metabolism. Differentiated cells express tissue-specific gene subsets.

QUIZ QUESTIONS

1. Imagine you have a gene X, which makes a protein Y. If X is constitutively transcribed, how may the cellular effects of Y be varied?
2. Explain the physical relationship between the sense strand of DNA and the encoded mRNA transcript.
3. How many different nucleotide triplet codons are there? How does this compare with the number of amino acids, and why?
4. In general, which is worse for gene function: a point mutation, a frameshift mutation, or an inversion?
5. What is the genetic phenomenon of anticipation? Give an example of a disease in which anticipation occurs.
6. Explain the distinction between the promoter and the transcription start site.
7. What is the difference between (i) a DNA-dependent DNA polymerase, (ii) a DNA-dependent RNA polymerase, and (iii) an RNA-dependent DNA polymerase?
8. What do TATA boxes, CAAT boxes, and GC boxes have in common?
9. Name three differences between promoter and enhancer sequences.
10. What is the difference between a cis-acting sequence and a trans-acting sequence?
11. Which of the following transcription factor motifs may be capable of dimerization as well as DNA binding: (i) zinc finger, (ii) basic helix-loop-helix domain, and (iii) leucine zipper?
12. Explain how homodimeric transcription factors bind to DNA. How might gene expression so induced be affected by heterodimer formation?
13. What does the transcription factor NFκB do, and how?
14. Explain what is meant by the terms cell survival and cell differentiation. How does differentiation occur?
15. Name three immediate-early genes. What types of stimuli might induce them?

4

RNA processing and translation

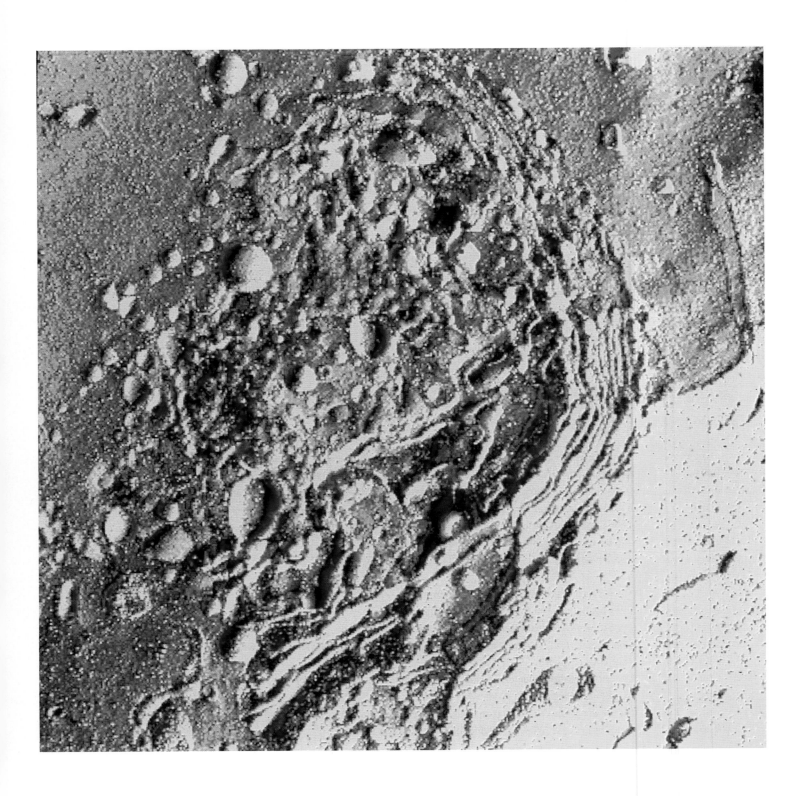

Figure 4.1 (*previous page*) Freeze-fracture cell preparation, showing the microanatomy of cytoplasmic organelles abutting the nucleus. Following nuclear export of mature messenger RNAs to the endoplasmic reticulum, mRNA translation gives rise to polypeptides which are then modified in the Golgi apparatus (Wellcome Medical Photographic Library, no. N0013286C).

RNA function

RNA has different forms and functions

The three-dimensional structure of single-stranded RNA differs from that of a linear polypeptide strip. First, RNAs contain only four inward-facing side-chains, whereas proteins contain 20 outward-facing side-chains. Second, RNA packs loosely and with low cooperativity, unlike the tight binding seen in proteins; this makes it more difficult for RNAs to specify a unique shape. Third, the structural stability of RNA is high, unlike that of most proteins. For example, long GC-rich sequences that are folded back upon themselves may have dissociation half-times of years, unlike a protein α-helix which dissociates within microseconds.

In contrast, the higher structures of RNA and DNA exhibit strong similarities. The formation of double-stranded regions occurs in short nucleic acid sequences termed **inverted repeats** or palindromes, the nucleotides of which snap back upon themselves to form in vitro structures called **cruciforms** in DNA and **hairpins** in RNA (Figure 4.2). Formation of these hairpins affects the transit of the transcription machinery along the elongating mRNA; hence, transcription may be punctuated by **pauses** involving additional protein–RNA and RNA–DNA interactions. The **stem-loop** hairpin is the principal secondary structure of RNA, with such structures providing targets for regulatory protein interactions in defined systems such as the HIV virus. The initial formation of RNA secondary structures can occur within 10^{-5} seconds, but the search for a stable folded tertiary structure may take seconds, or even minutes.

Unlike DNA, RNA may exist as an intermediary message or as a functional end-molecule. The composition of RNA subtypes in human cells is as follows:
1. 75% is **ribosomal RNA (rRNA)**, which translates mRNA to protein.
2. 15% is **transfer RNA (tRNA)**, which matches mRNAs and amino acids.
3. 9% is **heterogeneous nuclear RNA (hnRNA)**, which comprises several RNAs:
   - **Small nuclear RNAs (snRNA, e.g., U2; 4%)** process mRNAs,
   - **Small nucleolar RNAs (snoRNA, e.g., U22; 1%)** process rRNAs,
   - **Messenger RNA (mRNA; 4%)** transfers DNA sequence to ribosomes.
4. 1% is **guide RNA (gRNA)**, which edits mature mRNA transcripts (pp. 104–6). Cells generally contain about twice as much RNA as DNA, with the two nucleic acids together comprising about 1% of dry body mass. When people talk about RNA, however, they are usually talking about mRNA. It should be clear from the above, however, that mRNA represents only a minor proportion of total RNA – just as genes represent only a minor proportion of total DNA.

The variety of RNA structures is a reflection of the many functions of this molecule. As noted earlier, RNA has the remarkable ability to act both as an information-carrying nucleic acid and as an enzyme that can assist its own replication. The latter phenotype, which accounts for less than 1% of total cellular RNA, is referred to as **catalytic RNA**.

Figure 4.2 Primary and secondary structures of RNA. *A*, Linear strip of RNA. *B*, Creation of a stem-loop motif within an RNA molecule by complementary nucleotide binding.

A. Linear RNA

B. Stem-loop RNA

MOLECULAR MINIREVIEW

Catalytic RNA
The first RNA molecules on Earth may have functioned not merely as templates but also as catalytic molecules – **ribozymes** or gene shears – which can cut, splice, and form bonds between carbons, nucleotides or peptides. These reactions include the cleavage of phosphodiester bonds and esterase reactions. Hence, the first RNA

polymerase may not have been a protein but rather an RNA molecule itself. Single-cell microorganisms contain the evolutionary skeletons of RNA's catalytic function:

1. **Ribonuclease P**, a tRNA-processing endonuclease found in *Escherichia coli*, consists of a 375 bp RNA sequence coupled to a 20 kDa enzyme.
2. **Self-splicing (class I) introns** are noncoding intervening sequences in yeast mitochondria that interrupt genes and encode endonucleases which function as RNA maturases (splicing enzymes) or DNA recombinases. The human **delta (δ) virus** – a defective virus composed of circular RNA, and implicated in exacerbations of human **hepatitis B** infections – may have originated as an escaped self-splicing intron.

Modern human cells retain vestiges of catalytic RNA in two catalytic structures, spliceosomes and ribosomes (described in detail later), which contain respectively:

1. **Snurps** – small nuclear ribonucleoproteins (snRNPs) with names like U2 – that consist of proteins complexed with snRNAs which contribute to spliceosome formation (p. 102). Since snurps splice nuclear RNAs; snRNAs are suspected to have evolved from self-splicing introns.
2. Ribosomal RNA (**rRNA**) – which catalyzes **peptide bond formation** via peptidyl-tRNA translocation within ribosomes (pp. 108–9).

Ribosomal subunits lose their peptidyl transferase (enzymatic) activity following exposure to RNase but not proteinase, confirming the ability of rRNA to catalyze protein synthesis. In addition, rRNA has a functional role in mRNA decoding.

    Ribozymes are metalloenzymes that are being evaluated as possible therapeutic reagents (p. 592). Clinical trials of ribozymes have been undertaken in diseases as diverse as **HIV infection, hepatitis, cancer, psoriasis,** and **vascular disorders**.

Messenger RNA is regulated at multiple levels

Genes are expressed in the nucleus but proteins are synthesized in the cytoplasm, implying the existence of a molecular go-between. Messenger RNAs are described as abundant (or **superprevalent**) if there are more than 10000 transcripts per cell. Perhaps as few as a dozen mRNA species per cell (e.g., actin, albumin) would qualify as abundant by this definition, with these messages comprising about 10% of total cellular mRNA mass. Approximately 500 genes are expressed at around 1000 transcripts per cell at any one time, with such **active gene** transcripts making up about 50% of total cellular mRNA. In contrast, messages from a further 10000 regulatory genes may be present in fewer than 50 copies per cell, and these **low-level mRNA** transcripts comprise about 40% of total cellular mRNA. Note that expression level does not correlate particularly well with importance, since many low-expression transcripts are critical for cell regulation.

    RNA is more than a passive intermediary in information transfer. Messenger RNA fine-tunes gene expression via a number of mechanisms:

1. Alternative **mRNA splicing**.
2. Variations in nuclear **mRNA stability**.
3. Regulation of **nucleocytoplasmic mRNA transport**.
4. Modulation of cytoplasmic **mRNA translational efficiency**.
5. Messenger RNA **editing**.

As detailed below, these RNA-based regulatory mechanisms may alter protein expression in different developmental stages, tissues, and metabolic states. An additional RNA-dependent regulatory mechanism in bacteria and viruses is that of **antisense mRNA transcription**, in which transcripts produced from the noncoding DNA strand hybridize with (and thus prevent the translation of) complementary mRNAs. Antisense transcription occasionally modulates mRNA stability or RNA splicing in eukaryotic cells, but it is viruses that more often use this mechanism for usurping control of host cells (Figure 4.3).

Figure 4.3 Sense and antisense mRNAs, illustrating the effect of antisense oligonucleotide annealing on mRNA translation. *A*, Normal mRNA molecule ready for translation into protein. *B*, Hybridization of an antisense oligonucleotide to the above, preventing interaction with the translational machinery.

A.

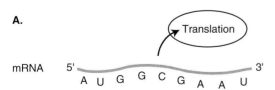

B. Add antisense oligodeoxynucleotide

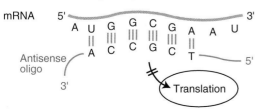

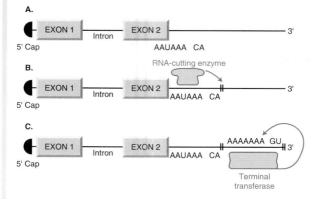

Figure 4.4 Conversion of a primary mRNA transcript to a mature polyadenylated mRNA. *A,* Capped primary transcript with 3′ AAUAAA and CA motifs. *B,* Proposed interaction of an RNA cleavage enzyme with the AAUAAA motif, leading to scission of the primary transcript 20–30 nucleotides downstream. *C,* Addition of a poly(A) sequence to the 3′ free end of the cleaved primary transcript.

This strategy has been experimentally exploited by synthesizing complementary sequences that are either microinjected into target cells or else expressed via gene therapy. Such reagents are termed **antisense oligonucleotides** and are usually cDNAs, since endogenous RNase degrades RNAs too rapidly. The name given to this therapeutic approach is **antisense therapy**. Complementary DNAs can also be designed to bind target gene sequences along the double helix, forming a **triple helix** that impairs gene transcription (p. 593).

Primary transcripts are capped and tailed

A newly transcribed mRNA molecule is termed a primary transcript. By the time its synthesis is complete, the primary transcript has undergone two structural alterations:

1. **5′ capping**
   - Addition of a positively charged 7-methylguanosine **cap** to the 5′ triphosphate moiety of the message. This motif signals ribosome binding and thus the **translation start site** of the transcript by marking the relevant mRNA translation codon.
2. **3′ polyadenylation**
   - Endonucleolytic cleavage followed by the addition of a ~200-adenine tail to the 3′ end of most mRNAs (but not all; Figure 4.4); histone mRNA is one exception. This modification regulates **mRNA stability**.

3′ polyadenylation and 5′ capping may be catalyzed by the same protein in some viral transcripts, consistent with a common function in enhancing translational efficiency.

Translational initiation is signaled by an **AUG** motif in the transcript corresponding to an ATG trinucleotide at the 5′ of the open reading frame of the gene. For this reason, the amino terminus of a protein almost always begins with a methionine residue; the relevant AUG codon is recognized by its proximity to the 5′ cap. In addition to localizing the translation start site, 5′ capping may trigger the **nuclear export** of mRNA to the cytoplasm.

Primary transcripts undergo another series of enzymatic modifications prior to nuclear export, perhaps contributing to that event. This refers to the removal of noncoding intervening mRNA sequences or **introns** from mRNA molecules. These enzyme-dependent transcript excisions are collectively designated **RNA processing**.

MOLECULAR MINIREVIEW

Elongin

Gene function is not determined exclusively by transcription initiation. Following initiation, transcripts undergo **elongation**, a process that is interrupted by RNA polymerase II at various sites in the gene sequence. In human cells transcript elongation is accelerated by a protein called **elongin**, which reduces RNA polymerase II pausing. Elongin is a heterotrimeric transcription factor with subunits termed A, B (which has a ubiquitin-like structure), and C: its functional activation results from binding of the A subunit to the B–C complex, resulting in inhibition of RNA polymerase II pausing and a high mRNA production rate. The absence of elongin is accompanied by frequent and prolonged transcriptional pauses, leading to low or undetectable expression of certain target genes such as the immediate-early mitogenic genes *Myc* and *Fos* (p. 93). Defective transcript elongation may contribute to the "poisoned dwarf" phenotype of the DNA-repair deficiency **Cockayne syndrome**.

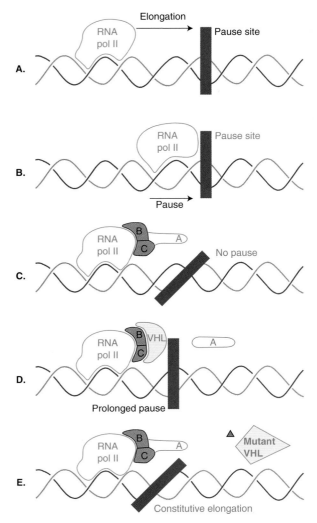

Figure 4.5 Transcription elongation. *A*, Normal transcript elongation by RNA polymerase II (RNA pol II). *B*, Transient pausing of RNA pol II following arrival at a transcriptional pause site within the gene. *C*, Binding of the heterotrimeric protein elongin to RNA pol II, enabling the enzyme to traverse the pause site. *D*, Restoration of the pause site by substitution of VHL protein for subunit A of elongin. *E*, Constitutive mRNA elongation due to a loss-of-function mutation affecting VHL, leading to unopposed elongin action.

von Hippel–Lindau disease

The function of elongin depends critically on its interaction with another protein – the product of a chromosome 3p25.5 gene, which is mutated in the autosomal dominant disorder **von Hippel–Lindau disease**. The 30-kDa wild-type **VHL** protein normally sequesters the elongin B–C complex, thereby preventing interaction with elongin A and so predisposing to a low transcription frequency. In other words, the higher the ratio of elongin A to VHL, the more rapidly transcribed is the gene. This equilibrium breaks down in von Hippel–Lindau disease due to mutation of the *VHL* gene and the consequent failure to sequester elongin B–C subunits, such that the unopposed action of elongin A suppresses RNA polymerase II pausing in target genes (Figure 4.5). The result is a clinical syndrome of **cerebelloretinal hemangioblastomatosis** consisting mainly of angiomas (blood vessel tumors) in the retina, cerebellum and/or spinal cord; in these tumors the second *VHL* allele is also mutated. The profuse vascularization of these tumors reflects inhibition by normal VHL of **hypoxia-inducible factors** (**HIFs**) which in turn induce the expression of blood vessel mitogens such as vascular endothelial growth factor (p. 343). Relevant to this, some VHL patients also develop **pheochromocytomas** (epinephrine-secreting tumors), **hypertension** (high blood pressure) or **polycythemia** (excess red blood cells), and are thus prone to **subarachnoid hemorrhage**.

VHL disease is also associated with **familial renal cell carcinoma**; both of these syndromes can be caused by deletions affecting chromosome 3p. Indeed, 80% of patients with **sporadic nonpapillary renal cell** (**clear cell**) **carcinomas** have somatic *VHL* mutations within the tumor. Such tumors express a hypoxia-inducible endogenous antisense transcript to **HIF1α** mRNA which arises from the 3′ untranslated region of HIF1α mRNA. The proliferation of such tumors is generally dependent upon the **insulin-like growth factor-1** (IGF1; pp. 325–8) pathway. Other genes implicated in the pathogenesis of renal cell cancers are the growth-inhibitory **tuberous sclerosis** (*Tsc*; p. 286) genes, and the *Met* growth factor receptor gene (mutated in **hereditary papillary renal cell cancers** with normal VHL function).

Mature transcripts are derived by intron excision

A **polycistronic gene** can encode more than one protein by making use of multiple translation start sites. Such genes occur in bacteria, reflecting the lack of 5′ cap sites in bacterial mRNAs. So-called **polyproteins** are sometimes produced in human cells: a single transcription event gives rise to a precursor protein, which is subsequently cleaved to form multiple polypeptides. A well-known example of polyprotein production is that of the **pro-opiomelanocortin** (**POMC**) gene product, which is overproduced by some cancers and cleaved to form several bioactive signaling molecules: **met-enkephalin, adrenocorticotrophic hormone** (**ACTH**), **β-lipotropin** and **α-melanotropin** (**α-MSH**). These cleavage products mediate the phenotype of certain **paraneoplastic syndromes**.

A more common mechanism whereby human cells enhance the flexibility of gene expression is RNA processing. Most primary human mRNA transcripts contain introns, reflecting the split gene structure that favors more complex gene evolution. **RNA splicing** is the process whereby introns are removed by an enzyme complex, leaving only the coding **exons**. The borders of introns are usually marked by GT-AG dinucleotide branch-points, but splice-site recognition involves an **exon scanning** mechanism triggered by 3′ sequences that identify codon wobble sites. Export of processed RNAs to the cytoplasm may be initiated by intron removal.

An interesting structural variation concerns glucose-6-phosphate dehydro-

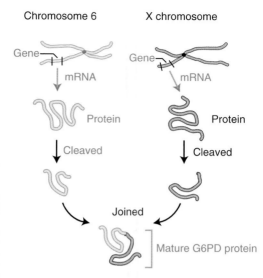

Chromosome 6   X chromosome

Gene   Gene
   ↓ mRNA   ↓ mRNA
      Protein   Protein
   ↓ Cleaved   ↓ Cleaved

                Joined

                   Mature G6PD protein

Figure 4.6 Biosynthesis of the glucose-6-phosphate dehydrogenase (G6PD) protein. Two genes, one located on chromosome 6 and the other on the X chromosome, are transcribed to yield full-length mRNAs, which are in turn translated to full-length proteins. Proteolytic cleavage of these two proteins yields two truncated isoforms, which in due course combine to form a single chimeric G6PD protein.

genase (G6PD), an enzyme involved in generating the nucleotide component ribose-5-phosphate. An X chromosomal gene encodes the minor subunit of this enzyme as well as part of the major subunit; the amino terminal segment of the major subunit, however, is encoded by G6PD exons 1 and 2 on chromosome 6, indicating that the mature protein is chimeric (Figure 4.6). No fusion mRNA molecule has been isolated, suggesting that the hybrid subunit arises via **post-translational transpeptidation** or **ribosome hopping**.

The ability of RNA to be processed to different transcripts complicates the one-gene-one-polypeptide model of eukaryotic gene regulation: one-polypeptide-one-gene seems a more accurate rule of thumb. Translated proteins are responsible for DNA and RNA synthesis, and information flow in human cells thus tends to be unidirectional. This is not the case in **retroviruses** which, as the name suggests, have a penchant for doing things backwards.

RNA processing

Snurps catalyze messenger RNA splicing
RNA splicing is executed by **small nuclear RNAs** (snRNAs), which have the following characteristics:

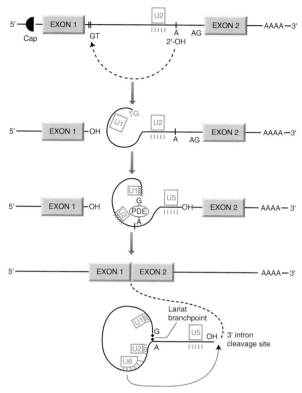

Figure 4.7 Spliceosomal excision of an intronic lariat from a primary mRNA transcript. A pre-mRNA intron is bound by the U2 snurp near an adenosine residue which puts the 5′ donor splice site under nucleophilic attack, cleaving it from exon 1 adjacent to the U1 snurp binding site. A phosphodiester bond (PDE) then forms between the free guanine base and the aforementioned adenosine residue, creating a lariat branchpoint at the adenosine. The U5 snurp situated at the 3′ acceptor splice site interacts with the spliceosomal U6 snurp to cleave the 3′ site, discharging the intron and permitting exon ligation.

1. Small (<250 nucleotides).
2. Nuclear (not cytoplasmic).
3. Complexed with protein to form **ribonucleoproteins** (RNPs).
4. **U-rich** composition; hence, designated **U1, U2, U4, U5, U6.**
5. Form ribosome-like catalytic RNP complexes (see below).

Some of these small nuclear ribonucleoproteins – snRNPs, or **snurps** – such as U2 and U6 play a catalytic role, whereas others such as U4 can repress U6 activity. All bind complementary sequences within the intron (Figure 4.7).

Unlike mRNAs, which are exported from the nucleus to the cytoplasm, snurps are imported into the nucleus where they assemble themselves into a **spliceosome** that catalyzes esterification reactions. Briefly, the cap-binding snurp U1 binds the 5′ end of the intron (the **donor splice site**), cleaves it, and transforms it to a **lariat** structure by coupling to the 3′ **acceptor splice site**. This lariat of noncoding DNA contains a nucleotide region termed the **branchpoint** 10–50 nucleotides 5′ to the acceptor splice site. Initiation of lariat formation occurs following the complementary binding of U2 to the branchpoint, followed by nucleophilic attack on the 5′ splice site by an adenosine within the branchpoint (intronic mutations within the branchpoint cause the genetic human disorder **fish-eye disease**). The lariat is discarded as the two exons are joined. Meanwhile, the 5′ splice site pairs to U6, which directs it to the spliceosomal catalytic center; U6 duplexes with U4 which is in turn sequentially displaced from the spliceosome in an ATP-dependent manner, allowing U6 snRNA to refold and thus re-engage in splicing. An average 6-kb primary transcript might be reduced to a length of 1500 bp by such processing.

Accuracy of RNA processing is essential. **Cryptic splice sites** need to be identified, whereas **exon skipping** due to defective branchpoint recognition must be avoided. This is no mean feat when processing a gene with 50 exons in which some of the introns are as long as 200 kb. Splice site selectivity is distorted by mutations, including those affecting exons, snurps, and the splice sites themselves. Such derangements may lead to disorders as diverse as cancer, blood dyscrasias and autoimmune disease.

CLINICAL KEYNOTE

Snurps as autoantibody targets

Snurps are diagnostically (and perhaps pathogenetically) relevant to human autoimmune connective tissue diseases:

1. **RNP antibodies** (anti-RNP) are anti-snurps present in high titre (>1:1000) in **mixed connective tissue disease**, an overlap syndrome mimicking **scleroderma, polymyositis** and **systemic lupus erythematosus**.
2. **Sm antibodies**, frequently present in systemic lupus erythematosus with renal involvement, are anti-snurps that inhibit RNA splicing. Sm proteins are general snRNP proteins that bind to U1 RNA and thus expose a cap-binding site necessary for the formation of the nuclear localization signal.
3. The speckled pattern of **antinuclear antibody** staining (pp. 70–1) commonly seen in systemic lupus erythematosus corresponds to the distribution of U1 and U2 immunoreactivity, implicating these molecules as autoantigens.

Alternative splicing diversifies cell behavior

Despite being translationally silent, introns can modify gene expression. For example, the tumorigenic activity of the Ras gene may be enhanced by a point mutation within an intron. Rarely, one gene's intron may be another gene's exon. Introns may even be concealed within other introns, suggesting that such "twintrons" may be spliced in separate reactions. However, a more common mechanism of varying human gene transcription involves modifying the positional recognition of transcription start and termination sites, thus altering the sequence of exons within an mRNA. Mechanisms underlying such **alternative mRNA splicing**, which in some cases may generate dozens of different transcripts from the same gene, include:

1. Use of alternative 5′ promoters to provide variable transcriptional start sites, thus varying the relative expression of:
   - Erythroid-specific versus housekeeping forms of the heme-metabolizing enzyme **porphobilinogen deaminase** (pp. 457–8).
   - Pancreatic versus salivary forms of the digestive enzyme **α-amylase**.
2. Use of alternative 3′ polyadenylation signals to vary transcription termination sites, thus varying the relative expression of:
   - Membrane-bound versus secreted immunoglobulin isoforms.

These variant reactions may be regulated by variables such as tissue, gender, or developmental stage. Examples of the differential effects of alternative splicing include:

1. Alternatively spliced extracellular molecules termed **fibronectins** (pp. 226–7) may exert different functions in thrombus formation, secretion or cell adhesion.
2. The affinity of some growth factor receptors for ligands may vary if alternative splicing affects the extracellular domain. Similarly, differential synthesis of soluble and membrane-bound growth factors may be determined by alternative splicing.
3. The normal and neoplastic cell expression of certain peptide hormones (e.g., **parathyroid hormone-related peptide**; p. 418) may be regulated by alternative splicing.
4. In the **calcitonin/calcitonin gene-related peptide** (**CGRP**) gene, a combination of proteolytic cleavage and alternative splicing results in the expression of calcitonin in thyroid tissue but CGRP in the brain (p. 419).

Viruses exploit alternative splicing to maximize their ability to replicate. For example, the E1A gene of **adenovirus** encodes a protein that interferes with the human replication control apparatus (p. 371); this critical mRNA is spliced to yield five different transcripts.

CLINICAL KEYNOTE

RNA processing defects in β-thalassemia

The hemoglobinopathy **β-thalassemia** often results from alterations in donor or acceptor splice sites that abolish normal β-globin mRNA splicing (p. 453). Complete ablation of the donor (GT) or acceptor (AG) splice junctions wipes out mature β-globin production, leading to **thalassemia major** (**β⁰-thalassemia**). Less drastic mutations in the vicinity of normal splice sites cause reduced but still detectable β-globin (**β⁺-thalassemia, thalassemia minor**).

A common β-thalassemia variant in South-East Asia is **HbE disease** – a clinically mild disorder unless crossed with β-thalassemia heterozygotes. HbE results from a single mutation affecting codon 26 of the β-globin chain; this base mutation converts a cryptic RNA splice site into an active GT donor splice site, leading to abnormal alternative splicing (and hence abnormal β-chain production) in approximately 50% of transcripts. HbE heterozygotes and homozygotes tend to be asymptomatic and may be protected from **malaria**. Hence, this phenotype may not necessarily represent a disease as such yet still requires genetic counseling to avoid severe hemoglobinopathies relating to HbE-β-thalassemia heterozygosity.

Mutations affecting tissue-specific RNA splicing have also been implicated in the pathogenesis of **acute intermittent porphyria**, whereas exon skipping is implicated in the pathogenesis of **neurofibromatosis** and **hereditary elliptocytosis**. Phenotypic rescue of a metabolic myopathy has been associated with alternative splicing of a mutant exon, leading to the continued expression of a functional (truncated but still correctly translated) protein with remission of the disease.

MOLECULAR MINIREVIEW

Alternatively spliced dystrophin isoforms

A common variety of infantile muscular dystrophy, the X-linked disorder **Duchenne muscular dystrophy** (**DMD**), occurs because of mutations affecting a large protein in skeletal muscle termed **dystrophin**. Neurons express a 14-kb dystrophin mRNA, which differs from the muscle-specific transcript in the position of its transcriptional start site and 5′ splice junctions. The finding of this brain-specific dystrophin isoform may help explain the clinical observation that 30% of DMD patients are mentally retarded – a difficult phenomenon to reconcile with mutation of a muscle-specific protein. Of note, tissue-specific variability in muscle dystrophin expression also occurs, as seen in **X-linked dilated cardiomyopathy** which arises because of dysregulated cardiac-specific dystrophin gene expression.

Yet another dystrophin isoform, encoded by a 6.5-kb mRNA and having a molecular weight of 71 kDa, is highly expressed in nonmuscle tissues such as liver and brain and is the first dystrophin isoform to be expressed in fetal life. This molecule consists of the cysteine-rich carboxy-terminal dystrophin domains, but lacks the actin-binding amino-terminal domain and most of the spectrin repeat domain. Variably present in muscle, this liver dystrophin is actually more abundant in glial and neuronal cells than are the putative muscle and brain dystrophin isoforms respectively. However, since DMD deletions are not recognized to cause liver pathology, the function of this dystrophin species remains unclear.

Processed messenger RNA sequences may undergo editing

Up to 50% of mature mRNA transcripts in tropical parasites such as *Trypanosoma brucei* (responsible for **sleeping sickness**) and *Leishmania* spp. (responsible for **kala-azar**) do not correspond to the encoding nucleic acid sequence. Fully processed mRNA transcripts may thus continue to be post-transcriptionally modified in vivo. This phenomenon, termed **RNA editing**, involves the following steps (Figure 4.8):

1. Splitting of mRNA transcripts by **guide RNA** (gRNA) molecules containing long tails of uridine nucleotides.
2. **Uridine addition** to cytoplasmic mRNA transcripts by formation of mRNA–gRNA chimeras – a process termed **transesterification**.
3. **Uridine deletion** from transcripts via a reverse process.

The main distinction between RNA editing and RNA splicing is that the intron-like sequences removed by editing are very small. Recognition of mRNA editing sites is not sequence-dependent as in splicing, but rather is based on regional alterations of mRNA secondary structure associated with low thermodynamic stability.

A. Insertional editing (e.g., mitochondrial genes in *T. cruzi*)

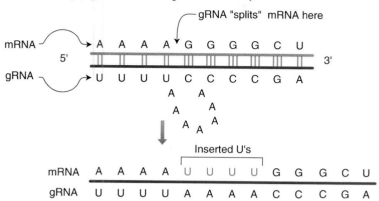

B. Substitutional editing (e.g., apoB)

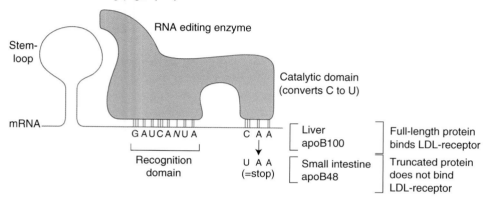

Figure 4.8 mRNA editing. *A*, Insertional editing as seen in trypanosomal genes. The mRNA transcript is split by guide RNA (gRNA), permitting the insertion of poly(U). *B*, Substitutional editing as seen in human apoB transcripts. The putative RNA editing enzyme contains one domain that recognizes an appropriate mRNA-binding site as well as a catalytic domain which modifies an appropriate downstream editing substrate. In the case of apoB, the latter is a CAA codon which, in the small intestine, is converted to a stop; this means that the truncated intestinal transcripts do not encode proteins that bind the LDL-receptor.

Parasite gRNA is encoded by mitochondrial DNA (mtDNA). Deleterious mutations in mtDNA genes can be corrected by gRNAs, suggesting that RNA editing may play a proofreading role. However, editing may occur only at times of demand for the protein of interest, suggesting an additional regulatory role. RNA editing is also a source of genetic variation in **parasites**, representing an important mechanism of antibiotic resistance (Figure 4.9).

A different kind of editing provides a strategy for viruses to increase the coding capacity of their tiny genomes: double-stranded RNA sequences within the human hepatitis delta virus genome are recognized by an **unwindase** which converts adenosine to inosine. Yet another variation on the editing theme is implicated in human lipid metabolism (see below).

Figure 4.9 Trypanosomes editing RNA while circulating in the bloodstream of a patient with sleeping sickness.

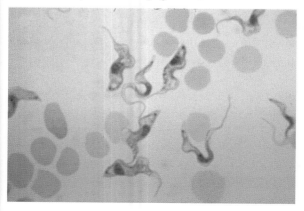

CLINICAL KEYNOTE

RNA editing in human blood and brain

RNA editing in human cells has been well documented in relation to the differential tissue-specific expression of the lipid-binding protein **apolipoprotein B** (apoB):

1. Apolipoprotein B in the liver is translated from the full-length 29-exon 4563-codon mRNA to yield a massive 512-kDa lipid receptor ligand termed **apoB100** which is implicated in **hyperlipidemia** and **cardiovascular disease** (p. 169).
2. In the intestine, however, transcription of the apolipoprotein B gene coding sequence precedes systematic alteration of nucleotide position 6666 by a $C \rightarrow U$ conversion, leading to a premature in-frame UAA stop codon in place of the glutamine-2153-encoding CAA. This results in the production of a smaller 250-kDa

protein, **apoB48** (48% of apoB100 size), an essential component of intestinal fat carrier proteins termed chylomicrons. About 90% of apoB in the human small intestine is of this edited variety.

This type of mammalian RNA editing probably evolved to enable hepatic targeting of dietary lipid; starvation reduces liver editing, while refeeding markedly increases it. Strictly speaking, however, apoB editing – which probably involves cytosine deamination – is distinct from classic protozoal RNA editing.

Mammalian RNA editing is similarly implicated in the production of three brain-specific neurotransmitter receptor (non-NMDA glutamate receptor; where NMDA is *N*-methyl D-aspartate, an artificial glutamate analog; p. 499) subtypes in the central nervous system by alteration of a glutamine-encoding CAG codon to an arginine-encoding CGG.

A number of processes modify RNA messages in the interval between transcription and translation. Two of these processes have just been considered: RNA splicing and RNA editing. A third – RNA degradation – is discussed in the following section.

Poly(A) tails protect transcripts from degradation

Less than 10% of all the RNA transcribed in the nucleus reaches the cytoplasm. Why? The answer relates to a critical variable – **RNA stability**.

Messenger RNAs consist of three key regions: a 5′ untranslated region, a coding region, and a 3′ untranslated region. The latter section of the molecule is modified by a process called **polyadenylation** which occurs when a transcribed AAUAAA sequence (a **polyadenylation site**) signals an endonucleolytic cleavage event 10–30 nucleotides downstream. This cleavage event leads to the addition of a string of adenyl residues (AAAAA . . .) termed the **poly(A) tail** by an enzyme called **poly(A) polymerase** which interacts with the U1 snurp. A practical significance of polyadenylation lies in the ability to identify transcriptionally active genes by purifying mRNAs using **oligo-dT** columns to hybridize poly(A) sequences. These mRNAs can then be eluted and incubated with reverse transcriptase to produce a cDNA library, a key technique of recombinant DNA technology (pp. 569–70).

The poly(A) tail has been implicated in many functions including translation initiation, nuclear mRNA export, and control of RNA processing, but most likely it shields the transcript from exonuclease degradation. This protective effect probably involves formation of RNA secondary structures such as stem-loops and pseudoknots, which protect the 3′ end of the message via interaction with diffusible **poly(A)-binding proteins** (Figure 4.10). Tissue-specific modulation of poly(A)-binding protein expression could thus explain alterations of mRNA stability; for example, the normal half-life of **vitellogenin** mRNA in unstimulated egg cells is 16 hours, whereas a 30-fold prolongation (to 500 hours) occurs in estrogen-stimulated cells. Poly(A) tails are sometimes referred to as **translational enhancers** because of their synergistic interaction with 5′ methylguanosine caps: these structures cooperate to recruit and tether ribosomes to 5′ transcript termini.

Destabilizing sequences can be located in the 5′ or 3′ regions of mRNAs. The best characterized of these is the AU-rich (Shaw–Kamen) sequence **AUUUA** in the proximal 3′ untranslated region. This sequence targets transcripts for rapid mRNA degradation by binding a 32-kDa degradative protein, suggesting that protein lysis pathways may be involved in mRNA degradation. Such sequences are commonly present in cytokine and immediate-early growth gene mRNAs – e.g., *Myc* or *Fos* – enabling these transcripts to disappear within

Figure 4.10 mRNA destabilization by 3′ destabilizing sequences. *A*, Stable mRNA with a poly(A)-binding protein interacting with the poly(A) sequence. *B*, Insertion of an AU-rich sequence either side of the poly(A) sequence permits the formation of a stem-loop structure; this may prevent interaction with the poly(A)-binding protein via the binding of another protein, making the transcript susceptible to ribonuclease digestion.

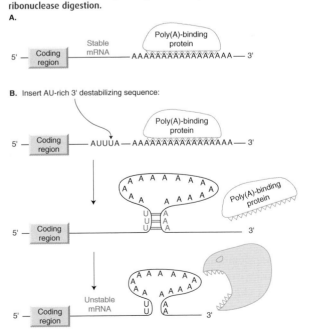

Table 4.1. Comparison of approximate messenger RNA (mRNA) and protein half-lives in a selection of molecules. HMG, hydroxymethylglutaryl; PEPCK, phosphoenolpyruvatecarboxykinase

Gene	Message half-life (hours)	Protein half-life (hours)
Alcohol dehydrogenase	10	50
Dihydrofolate reductase	5	100
Glucokinase	3	10
Glucuronidase	30	100
HMG-CoA reductase	3	3
Ornithine decarboxylase	3	0.5
PEPCK	1	5
Pyruvate kinase	2	24
Thymidine kinase	2	2.4

30–60 minutes of transcription cessation. In contrast, long-lived mRNAs (such as those encoding **albumin**, **β-globin** and the milk protein **casein**) may persist for over 24 hours following cessation of gene expression. Note that the stability of an mRNA does not necessarily correlate with that of its protein, though proteins are usually more long-lived than their mRNAs (Table 4.1).

MOLECULAR MINIREVIEW

RNA silencing

Cells need protection against viruses and mobile genetic elements. Without such protection, genomic integration of viral or transposed DNA sequences may disrupt key genes. Cells may detect the presence of foreign nucleic acid invaders via the recognition of double-stranded RNA (dsRNA). This recognition event activates a sequence-specific post-transcriptional defence mechanism termed **RNA interference** or **RNA silencing**.

The initial step in RNA silencing involves cleavage of the target dsRNA into 21-22 bp duplex fragments by RNase III. These small interfering RNA fragments (**RNAi**) are then used to guide a subsequent attack by a different RNase on single-stranded mRNA transcripts produced by the parent dsRNA.

RNA silencing occurs in worms, flies, parasites, and mammalian cells, and may prove to be important in developmental gene regulation. In mammalian cells, however, dsRNA also activates a nonspecific viral RNA-inactivating mechanism via the activation of two enzymes: **2′,5′-oligoadenylate synthetase** (which activates the mRNA-destroying **RNase** L), and the RNA-dependent protein kinase **PKR** (which phosphorylates and thus inactivates **eIF2a**; pp. 109–10).

CLINICAL KEYNOTE

mRNA stability in human disease

Efficient 3′ mRNA polyadenylation is needed for message stability and protein production, with the choice of polyadenylation signal influencing alternative splicing decisions. Variations in 3′ transcript processing and mRNA stability may also have pathologic consequences, however:

1. Some **herpesviruses** encode snRNAs that bind host spliceosomal proteins to form hybrid snurps. The viral transcripts contain AUUUA sequences at their 5′ ends, and these sequences compete for binding to the host degradative protein. These viruses, which are implicated in some **lymphomas** and **leukemias**, may thus transform host T cells by antagonizing the degradation of AUUUA-containing host mRNAs, which are normally short-lived.
2. Alterations in RNA stability may be associated with human tumors. For example, whereas the normal *Myc* message has a half-life measurable in minutes, the modified *Myc* transcript resulting from the 8:14 chromosomal translocation in **Burkitt lymphoma** has a half-life of around 6 hours.
3. Mutations in the AAUAAA polyadenylation signal are responsible for reduced globin expression in some **β-thalassemia** patients.

Message stability is not exclusively regulated by the poly(A) tail. Expression of mRNA encoding the cytoskeletal protein **β-tubulin**, for example, may be terminated via activation of nonspecific ribonucleases by unpolymerized β-tubulin subunits. Similarly, the 3′ untranslated region of histone mRNA – which lacks a poly(A) tail – may modulate transcript stability by forming a nuclease-resistant stem-loop structure which melts on binding free histone.

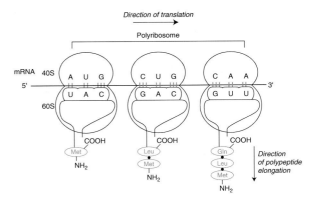

Figure 4.11 Polyribosome translation of mRNA. A series of ribosomes line up along a single mRNA strip; GTP-dependent ribosomal translocation is associated with lengthening of the polypeptide.

Figure 4.12 Secondary and crystal structures of transfer RNA. *A*, Cloverleaf representation of tRNA secondary structure. *B*, L-shaped crystal structure of tRNA.

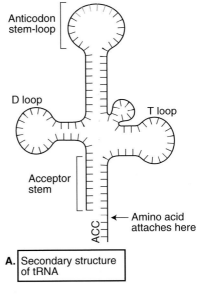

A. Secondary structure of tRNA

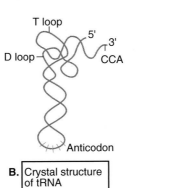

B. Crystal structure of tRNA

Translational control

Ribosomal RNAs link to messenger RNAs via transfer RNAs

Intranuclear organelles termed nucleoli are the sites in which **ribosomal RNAs (rRNA)** are modified by cleavage of pre-rRNAs. **Small nucleolar RNAs (snoRNAs)**, of which there are perhaps 50 different kinds in human cells, specify methylation sites in rRNA precursors. Some of these snoRNAs are encoded within intronic DNA. Mature rRNAs are exported to the cytoplasm.

Approximately 40 different proteins complex with cytoplasmic rRNAs to form protein-synthesizing factories termed ribosomes. These organelles consist of small (40S; 30S in prokaryotes) and large (60S; 50S in prokaryotes) subunits containing light (18S) and heavy (28S) rRNAs respectively (to put this in perspective, over 50% of ribosome mass is composed of rRNA). Ribosomes align themselves along the same mRNA transcript to form a long protein-synthesizing array termed a polyribosome or polysome (Figure 4.11).

Coupling of the mRNA codon with the polysome is initiated via an intermediary RNA species termed **transfer RNA (tRNA)**, which is 76 nucleotides in length. Although its stem-loop structure confers a cloverleaf shape on X-ray crystallography, tRNA folds as an L-shape in vivo. Transfer RNAs are rich in **pseudouridine**, a more versatile molecule than uridine due to a greater hydrogen-bonding capacity: uridine is modified by enzymatic cleavage and rotation of the bond between ribose and uracil, creating a new angle. Two functional domains characterize this family of noncatalytic adaptor molecules:

1. A trinucleotide adaptor or **anticodon**, which binds specific mRNA codons.
2. A helical **acceptor stem**, which binds specific amino acids (Figure 4.12).

Each tRNA acceptor stem is coupled to an amino acid: tRNA^Tyr couples to tyrosine, tRNA^Cys couples to cysteine and so on. Interestingly, the number of anticodons for an amino acid does not equal the number of codons, with glutamine and asparagine having more anticodons than (say) glutamate and aspartate.

Amino acids and transfer RNAs are coupled by aminoacylation

How do tRNAs translate mRNA codon information into specific amino acid binding? Specificity of binding is conferred by a reaction termed **aminoacylation**. Translational fidelity depends upon accurate recognition of a given tRNA by one of 20 phylogenetically ancient enzymes termed **aminoacyl-tRNA synthetases**. Two nucleotide regions within the tRNA molecule specify a binding site for the aminoacyl-tRNA synthetase destined to bind a given tRNA and amino acid. Correct aminoacylation is ensured by a proofreading mechanism prior to nucleocytoplasmic export of processed tRNAs. Curiously, cleavage of certain aminoacyl-tRNA synthetases yields smaller polypeptide fragments which activate inflammatory pathway signaling. **Jo-1 autoantibodies** to aminoacyl-tRNA synthetase are often detectable in patients with the autoimmune disorder **polymyositis** (especially with lung involvement) though the pathogenetic significance of this is uncertain.

During translation, the carbonyl group of the amino acid is first activated by aminoacylation, and then the aminoacyl group is transferred to the ribose moiety of tRNA in an esterification reaction that can be catalytically accelerated by RNA itself. These paired reactions create a covalent **peptidyl-tRNA linkage** which persists following detachment of the enzyme (Figure 4.13). The anticodon of the detached tRNA-amino acid complex binds the mRNA codon and thus becomes aligned. Peptide chain synthesis commences after the 40S ribosomal subunit recognizes and binds the mRNA 5′ cap, an event which is

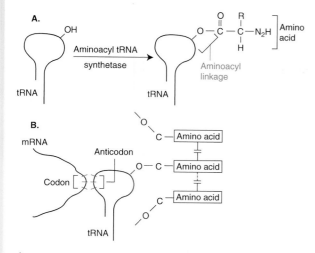

Figure 4.13 Aminoacylation of transfer RNA (tRNA) and amino acid. *A*, Enzymatic activation of the amino acid carbonyl group by aminoacyl-tRNA synthetase. *B*, Secondary alignment of the aminoacylated tRNA-amino acid complex via anticodon binding to mRNA.

followed by downstream migration of the ribosome–tRNA–amino acid complex to the AUG mRNA start codon. Three distinct ribosomal regions bind the aminoacyl–tRNA–amino acid complex:

1. The **A-site** of the 40S ribosomal subunit receives the *a*nticodon stem-loop of the incoming aminoacyl-tRNA-amino acid complex.
2. The **P-site** of the 40S ribosomal subunit binds the *a*nticodon stem-loop of the tRNA-amino acid complex in which the *p*eptidyl-tRNA linkage is first hydrolyzed to provide energy for creating a new peptide bond in the nascent polypeptide chain. This reaction, catalyzed via **peptidyl transferase** activity associated with the ribosome, takes place at a rate of around 100 new bonds per minute. Such peptide bond formation can be catalyzed in vitro using naked ribosomal RNA alone.
3. The **E-site** is where the tRNA *e*xits from the ribosome.

GTP-dependent **translocation** of the tRNA-bound complex from the A-site to the P-site is a fundamental step of protein synthesis, and one which is selectively inhibited by antibiotics.

PHARMACOLOGIC FOOTNOTE

Antibiotic inhibition of bacterial ribosome function

The molecular basis of bacterial protein synthesis is similar but not identical to that of human protein synthesis. These differences permit the development of antibiotics – drugs that are selectively toxic to microorganisms.

Prokaryotic ribosomes are smaller than the human variety: 30S and 50S instead of 40S and 60S. The bacterial RNA–ribosome interaction is a common focus for antibiotic action:

- **Aminoglycosides** prevent mRNA binding to a conserved sequence of 30S ribosomal RNA, which normally mediates the interaction between the codon and the aminoacyl tRNA anticodon; this interaction is sensed by the ribosome under normal circumstances. Hence, classic aminoglycosides such as **streptomycin** prevent initiation of protein synthesis by binding to the ribosome and thus triggering mistranslation. Resistance to aminoglycosides often occurs because the drug is phosphorylated, acetylated or adenylated.
- **Tetracyclines** prevent tRNA binding to 30S ribosomes.
- **Chloramphenicol** blocks peptidyl transferase reactions, thus preventing elongation of nascent polypeptides.
- **Erythromycin** blocks ribosomal tRNA translocation; the antistaphylococcal drug fusidic acid also inhibits translocation. Methylation of the ribosomal binding site is a readily acquired resistance mechanism, however.

Note that there are many other mechanisms of antibiotic action; for example, inhibition of RNA polymerase by **rifampin**, or inhibition of bacterial cell wall synthesis by **penicillins** (p. 177).

Translation involves initiation, elongation, and termination

RNA translation requires a battery of molecules to initiate, synthesize, and terminate the growing polypeptide chain as it is passed along the polysome. Only when the carboxy terminus is added does the mature protein detach from the ribosome-laden (rough) endoplasmic reticulum; the smooth endoplasmic reticulum is mainly involved in lipid metabolism. Protein synthesis is carried out by:

1. **Initiation factors (eIFs)**.
2. **Elongation factors (EFs)**.
3. **Termination factors**.

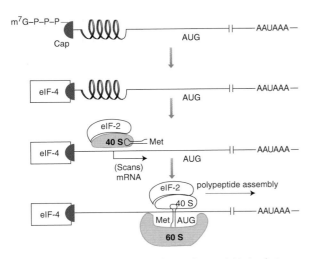

Figure 4.14 Initiation of mRNA translation. The eIF4 initiation factor complex binds to the 5′ methylguanosine cap where it catalyzes ATP-dependent unwinding of RNA secondary structure through its helicase ability. This unwinding permits the binding of the 40S ribosomal subunit, together with that of eIF2 and an initiator methionyl tRNA. This complex then scans the 3′ mRNA sequence for the nearest AUG. When this is located, the 60S ribosomal subunit joins the complex and polypeptide synthesis proper is initiated.

Chain initiation is triggered by a family of **initiating factors** termed **eIFs**. Initiation of protein synthesis involves the formation of a ternary complex with Met-tRNA (involving an initiating protein termed **eIF2**) followed by the joining of mRNA caps to the polyribosome (catalyzed by a 25-kDa mRNA cap recognition protein of the **eIF4** family). This reaction involves the ATP-dependent unwinding of RNA secondary structure by eIF4, permitting the binding of the 40S ribosome. Polyribosome scanning for the mRNA initiation codon is then initiated by a complex of this ribosome subunit, eIF2, and the Met-tRNA, culminating in the addition of the 60S ribosomal subunit to the complex (Figure 4.14).

Translation can be inhibited by the binding of heterologous molecules to eIF4, but such inhibition can be presented by anabolic mitogens such as insulin which cause phosphorylation of eIF4-binding molecules. The immunosuppressant **rapamycin** inhibits such phosphorylation, thereby blocking cell cycle progression. Conversely, cells can be transformed by either eIF4 overexpression or by eIF2 dephosphorylation.

Translation errors occur at a frequency approximating 1 per 100 000 residues synthesized. In mammalian cells this level of accuracy reflects the proofreading capability of aminoacyl-tRNAs. **Elongation factors** (**EFs**) – not to be confused with transcription elongation proteins (pp. 99–100) – are a family of GTP-binding timer molecules that introduce a delay into peptide synthesis and thus optimize the recognition of codons by anticodons. Not until a ternary complex of EF, GTP, and aminoacyl-tRNA is formed does ribosomal binding take place: codon recognition leads to GTP hydrolysis, permitting the delivery of aminoacyl-tRNA to the ribosomal A-site.

The tRNA-EF-GTP complex binds to the appropriate codon with high affinity; at the same time, EF prevents the bound amino acid from detaching. When EF hydrolyzes GTP following codon recognition, tRNA is released as EF detaches from the ribosome, allowing the amino acid to be incorporated into the growing polypeptide chain. This **translocation** of tRNA from its aminoacyl to peptidyl binding site is associated with a ratchet-like rotation of the 30S relative to the 50S ribosomal subunit. Hence, EF-dependent GTP hydrolysis powers the shuttling of tRNA along the ribosome in the same direction as 30S ribosomal subunit rotation. Because EF delays amino acid incorporation, mismatched tRNAs have a greater chance of detaching on account of their weaker codon-anticodon affinity.

Translational termination is signaled by the DNA poly(A) motif, which is transcribed to poly(U), leading to mRNA hairpin formation – in effect, a mechanical stop signal mediated by RNA–protein interaction. These RNA structural interactions are often mediated by RNA helicases termed **DEAD-box proteins** characterized by the conserved motif DEAD (Asp-Glu-Ala-Asp). Such proteins may stabilize mRNAs, but are not exclusively involved in terminating translation; the initiator complex eIF4 also contains such helicases.

Translation elongation, initiation, and disease
The efficiency of protein synthesis is controlled by the phosphorylation status of eIF2a (which inhibits protein synthesis) and of eIF4E (which enhances protein synthesis). **Adenovirus** infection antagonizes the antiviral effects of interferon by promoting eIF2a phosphorylation and eIF4E dephosphorylation; similar mechanisms

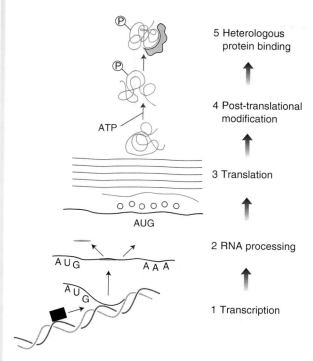

5 Heterologous protein binding

4 Post-translational modification

3 Translation

2 RNA processing

1 Transcription

Figure 4.15 Phases of gene and protein regulation that modulate the effects of mRNA transcription.

may operate in other viral infections such as **Epstein–Barr virus, HIV, polio,** and **influenza**. Transfection and antisense studies have implicated eIF4E in normal and malignant cell growth regulation, and have suggested a role for another elongation factor (**EF-1a**) in cell transformation.

With respect to elongation, **diphtheria toxin** dysregulates the EF needed to translocate the polypeptide-tRNA from the ribosomal acceptor site to the donor site. As little as a single molecule of this toxin can poison an entire cell.

mRNA functionality varies with translational efficiency

Because living organisms need to adapt to environmental changes, human cells have evolved a variety of molecular maneuvers for modifying gene behavior. These include not only transcriptional gene regulation and post-transcriptional mRNA processing, but also a number of translational and post-translational modifications (Figure 4.15):

1. Translational regulation of protein production.
2. Post-translational modification of the mature gene product (p. 127).
3. Heterologous regulation by an interacting gene product; e.g., a ligand binding its receptor or a protein forming a dimer with another protein.

Stem-loop structures within mRNAs may be targets for regulatory protein interactions in defined systems such as the **human immunodeficiency virus**. Such interactions may modulate mRNA translational efficiency through effects on spliceosomal or ribosomal interactions, inhibition of translational initiation via competitive binding to ~100-bp 5′ untranslated leader sequences, or direct inactivation of translation by masking transcripts. Secondary structural changes such as hairpin formation may also slow ribosomal scanning of the mRNA transcript and thus enhance recognition of translation start sites. Leaky ribosomal scanning of this type may result in translation of functionally antagonistic molecules, the balance of which provides an additional level of cell control. Translational efficiency may be further impaired by damage to the 3′ untranslated region, deletions of which have been implicated in **lysosomal storage diseases** such as **aspartylglucosaminuria**.

The effects of translational control on net gene function are illustrated by the example of iron metabolism. Three-quarters of human iron turnover is related to red cell heme biosynthesis: **ferritin** is a large parenchymal iron-storage protein that sequesters (and thus detoxifies) up to 4500 Fe atoms per molecule during iron excess, whereas **transferrin** is a circulating iron-scavenging protein that binds and distributes plasma iron to peripheral tissues. After binding two ferric (Fe^{3+}) atoms, transferrin binds a dimeric transferrin receptor on the surface of iron-requiring cells such as hepatocytes, and iron is endocytosed and released for use in acidic endosomes. Ferritin and the transferrin receptor are thus functional opposites, with one acting as a storage protein and the other as a distributor: changes in microenvironmental iron balance lead to reciprocal effects on the availability of ferritin and transferrin receptor mRNAs. Of note, cell transformation by the immediate-early *Myc* gene (p. 93) requires direct repression of ferritin gene transcription.

MOLECULAR MINIREVIEW

Translational regulation of iron metabolism
Iron abundance activates a stem-loop **iron-response element** (IRE) in the 5′ untranslated region of the ferritin mRNA; this IRE sequence is a potent translational

repressor. Increases in extracellular iron concentration interact with the IRE to cause translational derepression of ferritin mRNA, resulting in 50-fold enhancement of ferritin synthesis. Like other heavy metal response elements (such as those activating the metallothionein gene), IREs are not activated by iron per se but by a regulatory protein (the **IRE-binding protein**) which may be inactivated by inflammatory mediators such as nitric oxide (p. 351). This protein does not bind iron, but rather recognizes the mRNA secondary structure of both the ferritin and transferrin receptor transcripts (i.e., the stem-loop IRE). A molecule playing a reciprocal role in ferritin mRNA translation is **ferritin repressor protein**, which is degraded in the presence of iron.

Iron deficiency converts the IRE-binding protein to a high-affinity RNA-binding state, leading to the repression of ferritin translation. However, absolute concentrations of ferritin mRNA may remain high despite iron flux. The transferrin receptor mRNA also contains IREs – five in all – which are positioned in the 3′ untranslated region of the message. Iron deficiency has no effect on transferrin receptor translation, but potently inhibits receptor mRNA degradation. Hence, unlike ferritin, iron deficiency increases transferrin receptor mRNA concentrations, whereas iron excess reduces mRNA levels. In summary (Figure 4.16):

1. Ferritin and transferrin receptor are functionally opposed molecules which both contain IREs in their untranslated mRNA sequences. The ferritin IRE lies in the 5′ untranslated sequence, whereas the transferrin receptor IREs lie in the 3′ untranslated sequence.

Figure 4.16 Regulation of transferrin receptor and ferritin mRNA translation by iron availability. *A*, In the transferrin receptor mRNA, binding of iron-response elements (IREs) by binding proteins (IRE-BPs) in the 3′ untranslated region leads to increased abundance, reflecting inhibition of mRNA degradation. *B*, In contrast, binding of an IRE-BP to the single IRE in the 5′ untranslated region of ferritin mRNA prevents translation of the coding region. Hence, iron availability differentially modulates the effects of these iron-regulatory molecules on iron availability.

A. Transferrin receptor

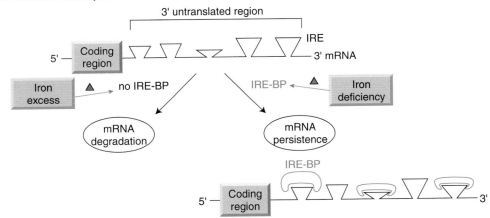

B. Ferritin

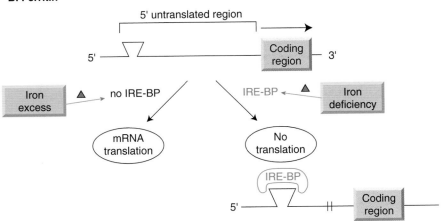

Enrichment reading

Bedtime reading
Judson HF. *The eighth day of creation.* Simon and Schuster, New York, 1979

Library reference:
Richter JD (ed). *mRNA formation and function.* Academic Press, New York, 1997

Gesteland RF, Cech T, Atkins JF (eds). *The RNA world.* Cold Spring Harbor Laboratory Press, Cold Spring Harbor, 1999

QUIZ QUESTIONS

1. Describe some of the possible structures and/or functions of RNA in (a) messenger RNA, (b) transfer RNA, and (c) ribosomal RNA.
2. What are some of the ways in which the function of a messenger RNA transcript can be varied?
3. Explain how an antisense oligonucleotide can influence the effects of gene expression. What problems relate to using this approach as a therapy?
4. How are the 5′ and 3′ ends of messenger RNA modified, and what purpose do these modifications serve?
5. Explain how pharmacologic inhibitors of viral reverse transcriptase work.
6. What is a snurp?
7. Define the term intron, explain how they are recognized, and state whether they are transcribed, translated or replicated.
8. Describe in detail the location and sequence of events in which an intron is spliced out of a primary transcript.
9. What is alternative messenger RNA splicing, and why might it exist? How does RNA editing differ from RNA splicing? Can you describe an example of editing in human cells?
10. What mechanisms regulate the stability of mature messenger RNA transcripts?
11. Describe in detail how messenger RNA, transfer RNA and ribosomal RNA can all interact during the translation of RNA into protein.
12. What does an aminoacyl-tRNA synthetase do?
13. Name some steps of bacterial protein synthesis that are inhibited by antibiotics.
14. Distinguish the role of elongation factors in protein synthesis from that of elongin in transcriptional elongation.
15. Explain how the translational efficiency of ferritin and transferrin messenger RNAs affects iron metabolism.

2. Activation of the 5′ (ferritin) IRE by iron deficiency causes translational repression; ferritin synthesis thus depends on ferritin mRNA translational initiation.
3. Activation of the 3′ (transferrin receptor) IREs by iron deficiency leads to mRNA stabilization. The net rate of transferrin receptor synthesis therefore depends primarily on the transferrin receptor mRNA half-life.

Hence, common regulatory sequences in the 5′ untranslated region of ferritin mRNA and the 3′ untranslated region of transferrin receptor mRNA coordinately regulate opposite net effects on ferritin and transferrin receptor biosynthesis.

CLINICAL KEYNOTE

3′ Untranslated region (3′ UTR) diseases

Drastic abnormalities of evolutionarily conserved genes are usually fatal, perhaps explaining why mutations of gene coding regions and 5′ control sequences are relatively uncommon. The effects of mutations in the 3′ untranslated region (3′ UTR) may be more subtle, however, reflecting the less catastrophic nature of most post-transcriptional modifications. This means that 3′ UTR anomalies may be sufficiently viable to be expressed as diseases. Examples include:

1. Nondeletional **α-thalassemia** of the **α-globin Constant Spring** (α^{CS}) variety. A UAA→CAA antitermination mutation in the α^{CS} allele permits ribosomal translation to continue into the 3′ UTR, but this is associated with reduced mRNA half-life due to an unprotected poly(A) tail, leading to thalassemia (pp. 103, 453).
2. **Myotonic dystrophy**. Accumulation of CTG trinucleotide repeats in the 3′ UTR leads to abnormal nuclear retention of *DMPK* mRNA transcripts due to recognition of CUG codons by a binding protein (**CUG-BP**). The resulting translational deficit of **myotonin** leads to reduced serine-threonine phosphorylation of ion channels in muscle, hence the clinical phenotype (p. 265).
3. **Fukuyama congenital muscular dystrophy**. Retrotransposed insertion of 3 kb junk DNA into the 3′ UTR of *Fukutin* destabilizes the mRNA, leading to a neuronal migration defect.
4. **Neuroblastoma** and **mantle-cell lymphoma**. Amplification of the *N-Myc* gene in neuroblastomas correlate with tumor aggressiveness, and also with the presence of two 3′ UTR cis-acting AU-rich elements (AREs) which bind a 40-kDa RNA-binding protein that stabilizes both *N-Myc* and *Fos* mRNAs. Similarly, the *Bcl1* mRNA produced in cyclin D1-overexpressing mantle-cell lymphomas is stabilized by deletional loss of AREs in the 3′ UTR.

Summary

RNA has different forms and functions. Messenger RNA (mRNA) is regulated at multiple levels. Primary transcripts are capped and tailed. Mature transcripts are derived by intron excision.

Snurps catalyze mRNA splicing. Alternative splicing diversifies cell behavior. Processed mRNA sequences may undergo editing. Poly(A) tails protect transcripts from degradation.

Ribosomal RNAs are linked to mRNAs via transfer RNAs (tRNAs). Amino acids and tRNAs are coupled by aminoacylation. Translation involves initiation, elongation, and termination. Gene functionality varies with the efficiency of mRNA translation.

5

Protein structure and function

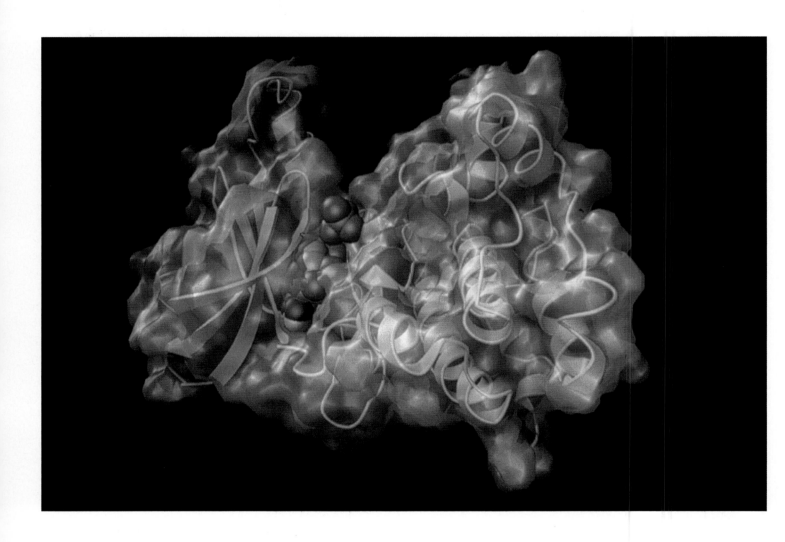

Figure 5.1 (*previous page*) Modeling of the three-dimensional structure of a protein kinase (Wellcome Medical Photographic Library, no. B0000443C02).

Proteins yell stage directions at DNA, and DNA reads its genetic script back to protein; in this way the cytoplasm talks to the nucleus and vice versa. This dialogue is well illustrated by cell fusion experiments in which the nucleus of one cell is added to the cytoplasm of another, redirecting the latter cell's behavior. In the following chapter we discuss how proteins direct the life of cells.

Protein structure

Proteins are amino acid polymers

With the exception of a few genes – such as those encoding ribosomal RNA (rRNA) – human genes are transcribed and translated to form proteins. Perhaps as many as three or four different protein forms are produced in the body by each gene, reflecting the diversifying influence of downstream transcript and protein modifications.

Proteins are conglomerations of amino acids, which originate as linear ribbon-like structures synthesized by ribosomes in response to instructions from transfer RNA (tRNA), messenger RNA (mRNA) and DNA. Each ribosome binds two tRNA molecules and approximately 40 base pairs (bp) of mRNA. Since an average amino acid has a molecular weight of ~120 daltons, a 50-amino-acid polypeptide weighs in at around 6000 daltons (6 kDa). An "average" protein contains about 400 amino acids, corresponding to a molecular weight of around 50 kDa, but the range extends from less than 10 kDa to over 1000 kDa. Up to 20 amino acids per second are incorporated into a growing polypeptide chain, implying that an average protein is synthesized in less than a minute.

At any one time, a typical differentiated human cell synthesizes fewer than 10 000 different proteins, most of which are present at low levels. Proteins are classified according to size as either peptides (implying fewer than about 50 amino acids – that is, smaller than 6 kDa – and hence capable of being artificially synthesized) or polypeptides. Functional protein groupings include:

1. **Structural molecules**
   - e.g., Collagen, keratin, actin, spectrin.
2. **Functional molecules**
   - **Enzymes**, e.g., proteases, glycosylases, helicases (names end in -ase).
   - **Signaling molecules**, e.g., transcription factors (such as Myc, NFκB, and receptors (e.g., the visual pigment rhodopsin).
   - **Transport/storage molecules**, e.g., transferrin, ferritin, and hemoglobin.
   - **Antibodies**, e.g., IgG and IgM.

Structural proteins lack catalytic activity but may nonetheless signal. An example is that of **collagen**, which acts as an extracellular activating ligand for cell-surface adhesion molecules. Fibrous biomaterials such as hair, nails, skin, cartilage, wool, and silk express structural proteins in abundance. When dehydrated, your body consists of approximately 80% protein by mass – about five times greater than the total amount of carbohydrate and ten times greater than total fat content (in lean individuals).

Nonpolypeptide molecules called **prosthetic groups** may be complexed with proteins. These groups participate in electron transfer reactions such as occur in cell respiration and drug metabolism. An example of a prosthetic group is the iron-containing heme moiety of the oxygen-carrying blood protein **hemoglobin**. Proteins that temporarily lack prosthetic groups, e.g., iron-free apolactoferrin, are designated **apoproteins**.

Aminoacidopathies

The process of degrading and excreting old amino acids requires a number of enzymes. Mutations that reduce the function of such enzymes will therefore cause accumulation of amino acid metabolites. Genetic abnormalities of amino acid metabolism include:

1. **Homogentisate oxidase** deficiency (the first single-gene disorder described)
   - Is characterized by an inability to degrade homogentisic acid, a breakdown product of phenylalanine and tyrosine metabolism.
   - May present with the passage of black urine (**alkaptonuria**; the original name for the syndrome) due to homogentisate excretion.
   - Can present with black cartilage (e.g., visible in ear) termed **ochronosis**.
   - Causes joint damage because of impaired **lysyl oxidase** activity.
2. **Phenylalanine hydroxylase** deficiency
   - Is characterized by an inability to convert phenylalanine to tyrosine.
   - Causes central nervous system demyelination and mental retardation.
   - May be detected by urine screening of neonates (Guthrie test).
   - Is termed **phenylketonuria** (PKU) and managed with dietary manipulation.
3. **Maple syrup urine disease**
   - Is due to impaired degradation of (iso)leucine and valine.
   - Reflects a mutation affecting a branched-chain ketoacid dehydrogenase.
4. **Ornithine transcarbamoylase** deficiency
   - Is a deficiency of an X-linked mitochondrial enzyme that drives the synthesis of citrulline from ornithine.
   - Causes hyperammonemia, hyperglutaminemia, and hypocitrullinemia.
   - Is treatable with sodium phenylacetate/phenylbutyrate, which activates nitrogen excretion pathways.
5. **Cystinuria**
   - Impaired renal reabsorption of COAL (cystine, ornithine, arginine, lysine).
   - Absorptive defect also affects the intestine.
   - Is distinct from **cystinosis** (impaired lysosomal destruction of cystine).

Hartnup disease is a rare aminoaciduria affecting neutral amino acids (p. 153). **Tyrosinemia** may respond to treatment with ascorbic acid.

Amino acid solubility influences polypeptide packing

Proteins are polyionic molecules that contain a mixture of charged, neutral, and aromatic amino acids. The side-chains of these molecules are classifiable on the basis of their biochemistry at neutral pH:

1. **Hydrophobic** (water-insoluble, greasy) amino acids include:
   - Valine, leucine, and isoleucine (large nonpolar side-chains).
   - Tryptophan and phenylalanine (nonpolar aromatic side-chains).
2. **Hydrophilic** (water-soluble) amino acids include those with polar side-chains such as:
   - Glutamate, aspartate (acidic).
   - Lysine, arginine (basic).

Cell systems are characterized by high concentrations of macromolecules in close proximity. The interactions between these macromolecules depend on **solvation forces** which vary with the state of the water molecules between them. Such forces may be either attractive or repulsive depending upon the relative hydration states of the macromolecules in question.

The critical influence of hydrophilic–hydrophobic interactions on the tertiary structure of globular proteins is termed the **hydrophobic effect**. Amino acid sequence analysis can predict the hydrophilicity of peptide sequences within a protein (**hydropathy analysis**). One application of hydropathy analysis is the identification of membrane-spanning regions within a protein, since lipid-rich membrane sequences are hydrophobic. Transmembrane regions within proteins consist of 20–25 nonpolar amino acids (the length of a membrane-spanning α-helix) with positively charged basic residues marking the cytoplasmic side. Sequences in which polar and hydrophobic residues are juxtaposed in this way are termed **amphipathic**, and such sequences determine the orientation of membrane-spanning proteins.

Hydrophobic residues embed themselves in the interior of large proteins, providing a clue to three-dimensional protein structure. Mutations that eliminate the hydrophobicity of key amino acids may thus create destabilizing cavities within the protein. Hydrophilic residues, on the other hand, stud themselves around protein exteriors where they may provide interaction sites for heterologous proteins such as those involved in cell signaling. These divergent attributes of hydrophilic and hydrophobic residues mean that mutational interconversion of such sites tends to have major phenotypic sequelae.

CLINICAL KEYNOTE

Missense and nonsense mutations

Replacement of a hydrophobic by a hydrophilic amino acid, or vice versa, is a classic deleterious **missense mutation**. Such substitutions usually affect the second (or, less often, the first) base in the mRNA codon, e.g., exchanging an A for a U (see Figure 3.2). Examples of mutations causing major amino acid alterations are as follows:

1. A valine-for-glutamate (GUG-for-GAG) substitution in the sixth amino acid of β-globin underlies **sickle-cell anemia** (pp. 456–7). This mutation creates a pathologic hydrophobic area on the surface of the hemoglobin molecule, favoring its collapse (and hence red cell sickling) in response to oxidant stress.
2. Deletion of the hydrophobic phenylalanine residue at position 508 (Δ508) of the **cystic fibrosis transmembrane-conductance regulator** (CFTR, a chloride transport channel; p. 190) is responsible for 70% of **cystic fibrosis** cases.

Major deleterious substitutions such as the Arg→Gly substitution at codon 664 of the **c-Kit receptor** may be expressed as mild disorders in heterozygotes (who in this case present with the autosomal dominant human white spotting phenotype **piebaldism**; p. 339) and yet be lethal in double-allele dosage. Conversely, null mutations that eliminate protein expression may be well tolerated if the deficiency can be compensated: an example is the recessive disorder **analbuminemia** in which less than 1% of the normal serum albumin level is present in homozygotes, who may suffer only edema or hyperlipidemia.

Nonsense mutations are frameshifts or stop codons that result in chain termination; their phenotypic severity depends on the extent of protein truncation.

Linear polypeptides form helices and sheets

Like nucleic acids, polypeptides can be characterized in terms of different structural levels: primary, secondary, tertiary, and quaternary. Primary protein structure consists of the linear amino acid sequence – unlike the base sequence of nucleic acids, this sequence largely determines the secondary and tertiary structures. Secondary protein structure arises because amino acids contain polar carboxy and amino termini which, when folded into the protein's hydrophobic core, require neutralization by hydrogen bonding. This

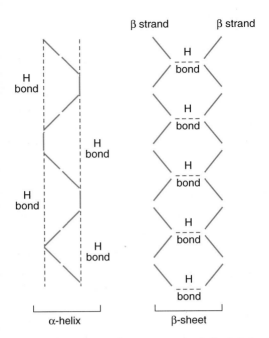

Figure 5.2 Protein secondary structures. *A*, α-helix. *B*, β-sheet. Hydrogen bonds are shown as dotted lines.

Figure 5.3 Progressive folding of a polypeptide from linear to mature tertiary structure.

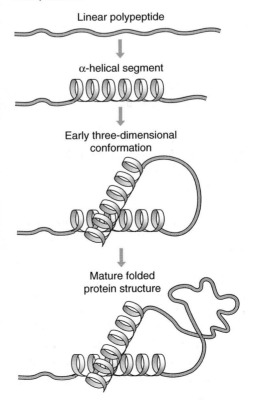

is accomplished by pairing the polar amino- and carboxy-terminals within repeating structures. Hydrogen bonding between such repeating motifs gives rise to one of two common secondary structures: (1) **α-helices** and (2) **β-sheets**. α-Helices most often occur on the exterior of proteins. Hydrophobic residues within such helices tend to embed themselves within the protein core, giving rise to an interdigitating conformation with a periodicity averaging 3.6 residues per turn. A common quaternary arrangement of α-helices in human proteins is the **four-helix bundle**.

β-Sheets are composed of short (6–12 amino acid) β-strands that cross-link horizontally to form a pleated pattern (Figure 5.2). The **β-ribbon** is a double-stranded β-sheet conformation that has been implicated in nucleic acid-binding. Like α-helices, **β-barrels** are often present within lipid-rich hydrophobic regions such as those associated with membranes. In general, secondary structures can be predicted from amino acid sequences with ~75% accuracy (that is to say, with far greater predictive accuracy than tertiary structures).

Secondary structures give rise to tertiary structures, which involve the polypeptide folding back upon itself to form recognition sites for protein–protein and protein–DNA interactions (Figure 5.3). Examples of such tertiary structures include DNA-binding **helix-loop-helix** (HLH) motifs, calcium-binding **EF hands** (a variant of HLH), and **coiled coils**. The latter are intertwined α-helices occurring in keratins, (tropo)myosins, tubulins and some heat-shock proteins. This motif is also the basis for the leucine zipper dimerization seen in transcription factors such as Fos: the coiled coil zipper forms the stem of a Y-shaped dimer which binds DNA via a scissors-grip.

Nature is not ambidextrous. Like the B-form DNA double helix, α-helices in human proteins are invariably right-handed in terms of twist, reflecting the left-handed structure of their constituent amino acids.

PHARMACOLOGIC FOOTNOTE

Enantiomers and drug toxicity

Amino acids are asymmetric molecules that exhibit chirality or handedness, which determines the lock-and-key substrate specificity of their three-dimensional structure. Whereas endogenous sugars are right-handed (e.g., dextro-glucose or dextrose), virtually all natural proteins are left-handed, that is, **S-enantiomers** (formerly called L-enantiomers). The few exceptions include neuropeptides such as dermorphin and the deltorphins (p. 508), bacterial peptidoglycans, and senescent human proteins in lens cataracts (**crystallins**) and in **Alzheimer disease** (**β-amyloid**).

Nonpeptide synthetic drugs such as propranolol, ibuprofen, warfarin, verapamil, and terbutaline often contain mixtures of left- and right-handed (**R-enantiomers**; i.e. the D-isomers, formerly called D-enantiomers) molecules. Such **racemic mixtures** have been implicated in the pathogenesis of therapeutic side-effects – thalidomide being the most notorious example, containing as it does the teratogenic S-enantiomer in addition to the therapeutic (anti-morning sickness) R-enantiomer. The epidural anesthetic bupivacaine is another example, depending for its therapeutic effect on the S-enantiomer; the R-form is four-fold more potent in causing cardiotoxic side-effects. Similarly the S-enantiomer of the oral anticoagulant drug warfarin is five times more potent than the R-enantiomer.

Ibuprofen is a popular anti-inflammatory drug for which the S-enantiomer is three times more potent than the other; similar relative potency is exhibited by the

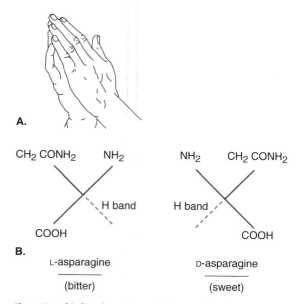

A.

B.

L-asparagine — (bitter) D-asparagine — (sweet)

Figure 5.4 Chirality of enantiomeric drugs. *A,* Figurative representation of opposed chiral configurations. *B,* Mirror-image structures of L- and D-asparagine corresponding to their respective aromas.

Figure 5.5 3D spectrum of higher-order protein structures. *A,* Globin domain. *B,* Immunoglobulin-like domains. *C,* Trefoil-shaped ligands.

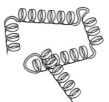

A. Globin conformation

B. Immunoglobulin-type loops

C. Trefoil peptide

S-enantiomers of indomethacin and naproxen, two other nonsteroidal anti-inflammatory drugs (NSAIDs). The antirheumatic drug penicillamine is only used as its *R*-enantiomer (D-penicillamine), since L-penicillamine depletes vitamin B_6 following its incorporation into proteins.

Enantiomers may have markedly different physical characteristics: *S*-limonene smells of lemons and *R*-limonene of oranges, *R*-carvone tastes of spearmint and *S*-carvone of carraway seeds, and asparagine isomers taste either bitter or sweet (Figure 5.4). In general, *R*-enantiomers tend to be more antigenic and toxic than their *S*-enantiomeric counterparts.

Protein folding is stabilized by higher-order interactions

Primary and secondary protein structures possess a biological significance that goes beyond mere chemical curiosity. For example, linearized peptide antigens are presented to T cell receptors for phagocytosis (p. 204), unlike native folded antigens which are only recognized by immunoglobulins. Most protein functions, however, require the molecule to adopt a higher-order conformation that is classifiable as either tertiary (i.e., the three-dimensional structure of a protein as determined by binding between distant residues; Figure 5.5) or quaternary (i.e., the arrangement of subunit contacts within multisubunit proteins).

Higher-order protein folding does not occur randomly. Even when completely unfolded or **denatured** in vitro, many solubilized polypeptides spontaneously reacquire their correct conformation – a process termed **renaturation**. Such proteins fold in the most energetically favorable manner by minimizing the energy cost of conformational transitions. This efficiency also applies to heterologous interactions between different proteins, accounting for the high specificity of enzyme–substrate, antigen–antibody and ligand–receptor interactions. Key determinants of higher-order protein structure include:

1. Covalent amino acid interactions
   - Disulfide bonds.
2. Noncovalent amino acid interactions
   - Hydrophobic stabilization.
   - Steric constraints (space-filling characteristics).
3. Weak interactions affecting protein secondary structure
   - Hydrogen bonding.
4. Weak interactions, often without major structural effect
   - Electrostatic interactions, especially between polar amino acids.
   - Van der Waals forces, especially between nonpolar amino acids.
   - **Cis–trans isomerization** of proline-containing peptides (p. 487).

Three-dimensional protein modeling based on crystal structures can yield elaborate visualizations of protein configuration (Figure 5.6). Structural prediction based on sequence analysis alone, however, is bedeviled by difficulties. In particular, it may be impossible to model which distant parts of the amino acid sequence (e.g., potential cysteine pairings) interact with each other.

Misfolded proteins are detected while still in the endoplasmic reticulum (ER), where they are retained in a complex with calcium-binding and stress proteins. An example is the cystic fibrosis gene product (CFTR; p. 190), which, even in normal individuals, may be correctly folded in a minority of translations. CFTR mutations may cause abnormal processing of sugar-coated (glycosylated) residues, leading to ER retention and protein degradation. Other genetic disorders also cause protein misfolding (see below).

The **sacsin** gene, which encodes the largest single-exon gene product known (12.8 kb), has the features of a heat-shock/chaperone protein. Its mutation gives rise to the early-onset autosomal recessive neurodegenerative syndrome, **spastic ataxia of Charlevoix–Saguenay (SACS)**.

Cellular stress differs from psychologic stress. The latter induces the expression of an entirely different set of "stress" proteins including the noradrenaline metabolite **3-methoxy-4-hydroxyphenylglycol** and the hypothalamic hormone **corticotrophin-releasing hormone**.

Protein function

Different polypeptide domains serve distinct functions

Gene sequences may exhibit regions of homology that suggest a common evolutionary origin. If these genes all resemble each other with (say) more than 50% homology at the nucleotide level, they are said to belong to the same multigene **family**. DNA motifs defining a genetic family may occur in either coding DNA (e.g., the *histone* gene family), noncoding DNA (e.g., the *Alu* family), or both coding and noncoding DNA (e.g., the *β-globin* pseudo/gene family). Larger groups of genes sharing less stringent homology may constitute a looser union called a **superfamily**. Examples of genetic superfamilies include the steroid hormone receptor superfamily of signaling molecules, and the opsin superfamily of photosensitive pigment receptors. Two main evolutionary mechanisms inject variation into genomes:

1. **Gene duplication**.
2. **Single-base nucleotide changes** (mutations and polymorphisms).

Genetic superfamilies arise via recurring cycles of gene duplication (due to transposition or defective recombination) with or without chromosomal translocation. If the (imperfectly) duplicated gene can incorporate sufficient structural divergence to generate a new function, it may be selected for retention within the genome. Nonidentical members of such a genetic superfamily (i.e., evolutionarily conserved variants) are termed **paralogs**, whereas homologs of the same gene expressed in different species are termed **orthologs**. As a rule of thumb, paralogs can be recognized by detection of at least 1 kb of common (>90% identity) sequence.

Approximately 6% of the human genome originated via gene duplication events. This represents a tenfold higher frequency of gene duplication than has occurred in fly and worm genomes, for example. Most of this gene duplication activity seems to have occurred around the evolutionary time of the human-great apes transition.

Functional redundancy creates selective pressure on paralogous genes to mutate towards a new function, meaning that duplicated genes are hotspots for genetic evolution. The GC-rich pericentromeric regions of the human genome adjacent to α-satellite DNA are especially recombinogenic, and it is this location which attracts the insertion of most intrachromosomal gene duplications; in contrast, interchromosomal insertion of duplicated gene sequences takes place mainly within subtelomeric regions. Note, however, that only about a third of gene duplication events are associated with subsequent transcription.

A high degree of cross-species homology (i.e., ortholog identity) suggests an important role for the conserved sequences. For example, there are over 30 000 species of spiders that spin silk from liquid proteins termed fibroins which have been conserved for over 100 million years. Conversely, ancestrally unrelated genes may come to be selected for similar functions, leading to the gradual evolution of structural similarity in the absence of close genetic similarity. This paradigm of genetic selection to fill a common environmental niche is termed **convergent evolution**.

Protein **domains** are polypeptide regions that are able to fold autonomously into functional units. Domains are often encoded by single exons that provide modular genetic subunits capable of being disseminated through the genome. However, the number of distinct protein-folding motifs or **superfolds** within the biological universe appears finite, perhaps numbering somewhere between 500 and 2000.

Exon shuffling and **intron capture** are modes of gene variation that permit structural change within protein domains. Exon shuffling may result in patchwork proteins in which domain homologies reflect functional similarities at the molecular level. Examples of such domain homologies are the immunoglobulin-like, epidermal-growth-factor-like, zinc finger, and kringle-bearing domains.

CLINICAL KEYNOTE

Protein isoforms in human disease

Structural variants of proteins occur in many forms. At the level of atomic structure, for example, the Maui coral extract palyotoxin ($C_{129}H_{223}N_3O_{54}$) has been calculated to have one sextillion (10^{21}) possible **isomers**. By the same token, members of the immunoglobulin superfamily exist as different **isotypes** such as IgG-κ and IgM, which are encoded by separate genes (p. 199). Proteins that bear strong structural and functional similarities to each other are termed **isoforms** or (in the case of enzymes) **isozymes**. Such protein isoforms may be encoded either by the same differentially processed gene or else by two structurally similar genes. Examples include:

1. The MM, MB, and BB isoenzymes of **creatine kinase,** which are used in the diagnosis of cardiac and muscle disorders.
2. **Lactate dehydrogenase** (LDH) isoforms 1–5, which may be used in the diagnosis of cardiac and liver disease.
3. The four isoforms of **alkaline phosphatase**, which are routinely used in the diagnosis of bone, liver, and neoplastic disease. The alkaline phosphatase family comprises non-tissue-specific (released from liver, bone, and kidney), placental, germ cell, and intestinal isoenzymes. Of these, the latter three are more than 90% homologous – their functional differences probably reflect alterations in a surface loop of the molecule.

An occasional mechanism of isoform variation termed **protein splicing** affects the RecA (recombination) gene of *Mycobacterium tuberculosis*. Protein sequence, rather than DNA sequence, determines the site of excision; the excised spacer proteins (**inteins**) represent binding sequences for DNA site-specific homing endonucleases which promote recombination. These inteins, which are typically ~50 kDa in size, are not involved in the protein splicing reaction, which takes several hours. Intein structure is remarkably consistent, beginning with a serine or cysteine and terminating with an asparagine. The surrounding protein sequences, the amino- and carboxy-terminal **exteins**, are also characterized by specific amino acid junctional residues which fuse following splicing.

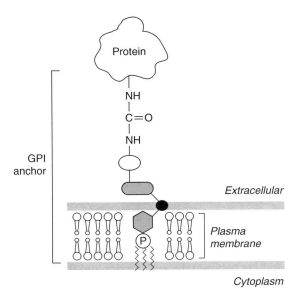

Figure 5.15 Attachment of an extracellular protein to the plasma membrane via a glycosylphosphatidylinositol (GPI) anchor.

molecule in the biosynthesis of cholesterol. Choice of the "X" residue in the target CAA*X* sequence – usually methionine or serine (farnesylation) or leucine (geranylgeranylation) – determines the modification, either of which results in hydrophobic membrane association following terminal tripeptide cleavage. **Farnesylation** generally targets molecules to outer cell membranes, whereas **geranylgeranylation** more often directs proteins to cytosolic membrane surfaces. Isoprenylation of the **hepatitis delta virus antigen** has been implicated as a prerequisite for viral virulence, whereas defective prenylation is associated with the inherited pigmentary retinopathy **choroideremia**.

Another post-translational modification that targets newly synthesized proteins to the membrane is **glypiation;** that is, the addition of a GPI anchor. These lipid-containing anchors are synthesized in the ER and then attached to the carboxy terminus of protein precursors destined for plasma membrane expression (Figure 5.15). Hydrolysis of GPI anchors may occur in response to the sugar-utilization hormone insulin.

CLINICAL KEYNOTE

Paroxysmal nocturnal hemoglobinuria and PIG-A

Carboxy-terminal addition of GPI anchors not only targets newly synthesized proteins in the ER to insert into the plasma membrane, but also helps to determine the polarity of transmembrane protein insertion. In other words, it determines whether the protein's carboxy- or amino-terminal points in or out of the membrane (not to be confused with polarity of charge). Such GPI anchors are expressed in protozoal parasites (e.g., falciparum malaria, *Toxoplasma gondii*, *Giardia lamblia*, *Leishmania* spp., and trypanosomes) in which they mediate virulence.

Paroxysmal nocturnal hemoglobinuria (PNH) is a clonal defect of protein attachment to the cell surface due to defective expression of GPI anchors mainly in hemopoietic tissues. This phenotype arises because of somatic mutations affecting the X-chromosomal *PIG-A* (*phosphatidylinositolglycan A* complementation group) gene – a glycosyltransferase required for the early stages of GPI anchor biosynthesis. *PIG-A* mutations may lead to secondary deficiencies of at least 25 GPI-anchored proteins in hemopoietic stem cells, including complement-regulatory polypeptides such as **DAF** (**decay accelerating factor** or **CD55**) and **CD59**. This causes complement hypersensitivity and chronic hemolysis with anemia (which may be associated with bone marrow aplasia). Note that DAF is the cell-surface attachment site used by **echoviruses** to gain cellular entry.

Platelet activation by complement is responsible for the thrombotic tendency of PNH. *PIG-A* mutations are present in many normal individuals, suggesting that this genotype may be necessary but not sufficient for the PNH phenotype.

Secretion is signaled by a cleavable leader sequence

The most common shared motif in precursors of secretory and transmembrane proteins is a hydrophobic 10- to 25-amino-acid amino-terminal **signal peptide** or **leader sequence**. This leader sequence binds a cytosolic α-helical ribonucleoprotein chaperone called **signal recognition particle** (SRP), which prevents folding of the nascent polypeptide chain. SRP binds to a docking protein (SRP receptor) on the ER membrane before detaching, thus directing polyribosomes to ER membrane receptors. At this point the still-unfolded polypeptide chain commences elongation, while at the same time the leader sequence undergoes cleavage by a **signal peptidase** bound to the ER membrane. This cleaved leader sequence then acts as an activating ligand for a **ribo-**

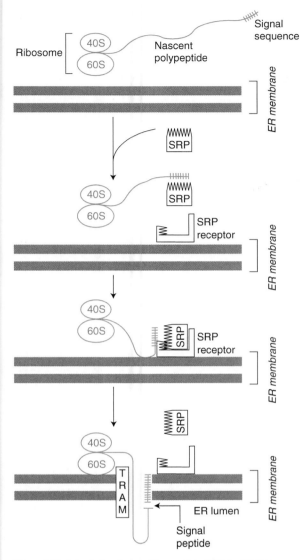

Figure 5.16 Role of signal recognition peptide (SRP) in directing proteins to insert in membranes. Binding of SRP to the signal peptide is followed by membrane localization, and cleavage of the protein–protein complex accompanies transmembrane protein migration. TRAM, translocation-associated membrane protein.

somal tunnel at the ER membrane; similar proteinaceous **channel tunnels** direct polypeptide transport across nuclear and mitochondrial membranes.

Transmembrane protein translocation occurs with the aid of a membrane-bound glycoprotein termed **TRAM** (translocation-associated membrane protein). Proteins destined to be soluble (e.g., secretory factors or lysosomal enzymes) undergo cleavage of a membrane-bound carboxy-terminal peptide and are released into the lumen of the ER. These luminal proteins may then bud off together with their surrounding ER membrane, travel to and fuse with the plasma membrane, and undergo secretion into the extracellular space.

Future integral transmembrane proteins, on the other hand, remain anchored within the lipid bilayer of the ER due to a **signal-anchor sequence**. After further post-translational modification (e.g., disulfide bond formation, N-glycosylation), these polypeptides are processed in the Golgi apparatus before being exported to their cell destinations. Such ER-embedded proteins integrate with the lipid bilayer of the plasma membrane instead of passing to the exterior (Figure 5.16). Mutations affecting any step in this sequence may lead to failure of protein targeting, resulting in protein deficiency phenotypes. Failure of protein addressing may also occur with gene mutations despite conservation of the normal targeting machinery.

CLINICAL KEYNOTE

Sialic acid in health and disease

Bacteria generally do not glycosylate proteins (though there are certain exceptions, e.g., *Chlamydia* spp. and gonococci). This has proven a problem in using *Escherichia coli* to clone proteins destined for human use, since differentially glycosylated proteins tend to be immunogenic. Lower eukaryotes such as yeast add oligosaccharides but often in different patterns (**glycotypes**) to that seen in human cells. Even phylogenetic neighbors such as mice glycosylate proteins differently to humans. This means that an antibody directed to (say) the extracellular domain of a human protein may not recognize the protein when the human gene is expressed in mouse cells.

Blood-borne glycoproteins – such as erythropoietin or tissue plasminogen activator – require additional oligosaccharide masking of terminal N-linked carbohydrate groups to prevent rapid in vivo degradation. The oligosaccharide most often used to mask carbohydrate residues in human cells is **sialic acid**.

Virulent microorganisms such as group B **meningococci** (which cause epidemic meningitis) use sialic acid to mask the recognition of extracellular bacterial antigens by the immune system (Figure 5.17). Sialic acid also functions as a cell-surface receptor for influenza virus **hemagglutinin**; the other major influenza antigen, **neuraminidase**, cleaves terminal sialic acid residues from host cell and viral glycoconjugates, thereby propagating newly synthesized virions from infected cells.

MOLECULAR MINIREVIEW

The asialoglycoprotein receptor

When a glycoprotein loses sialic acid (**desialylation**), the carbohydrate moiety so exposed is recognized by hepatic receptors. Degradation of desialylated glycoproteins occurs as a direct consequence of uptake by these reticuloendothelial **asialoglycoprotein receptors** or ASGRs, which are **galactose lectins** expressed on the sinusoidal surface of the liver cell membrane. The receptor is a hetero-oligomer

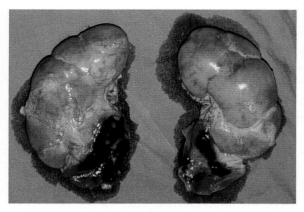

Figure 5.17 Post-mortem evidence of catastrophic adrenal infarction (Waterhouse–Friedrichsen syndrome) following fulminant meningococcemia. Sialic acid modification of extracellular antigens (capsule and lipooligosaccharide represents a key virulence mechanism in these bacteria (Wellcome Medical Photographic Library, no. N0002433C).

Figure 5.18 Nuclear import of proteins. *A*, Nuclear pore of nuclear envelope represented in cross-section. *B*, Protein with nuclear localization sequence (NLS) binds to nucleus-binding protein (NBP), which in turn facilitates protein passage via the nuclear pore into the nucleoplasm.

A.

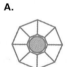

Nuclear
pore
(cross-section)

B.

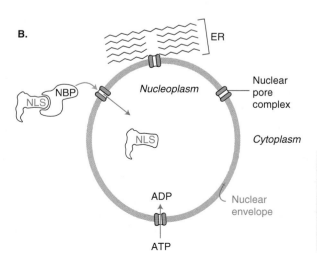

consisting of two structurally related galactose-binding subunits (**GalNAc receptors**) which multimerize to form an antenna-like structure.

A classic clathrin-coated pit receptor (p. 197), the ASGR recognizes penultimate galactose residues, which are revealed in proteins that have shed terminal sialic acid moieties. Recognition of this abnormal *N*-acetylgalactosamine oligosaccharide sequence leads to internalization and endosomal degradation of the target ligand with recycling of the receptor. Hyperimmune rejection of transplants and ABO blood transfusion incompatibility both reflect the immunogenic effects of an α-galactosyl epitope.

Mechanisms other than ASGR binding mediate glycoprotein clearance and degradation. For example, the glycoprotein luteinizing hormone (LH) is cleared via a hepatic endothelial SO_4-GalNAc receptor specific for sulfated *N*-glycosylated oligosaccharides. Other glycoproteins are cleared via mannose receptors (in alveolar macrophages) or mannose-6-phosphate receptors (in lysosomes).

Nuclear entry is specified by acidic localization sequences

Like RNA, proteins may cross the nuclear envelope in either direction. mRNA, tRNA, and rRNA subunits are actively transported from the nucleus into the cytosol, whereas proteins travel mainly in the opposite direction. These passages take place across a nuclear membrane bilayer: the outer membrane of the nuclear envelope is continuous with the ER membrane, and the space between the two leaves of the nuclear envelope is continuous with the lumen of the ER.

Proteins have been identified that migrate back and forth across the membrane – a process termed **nucleocytoplasmic shuttling**. Molecular migrations involving the nucleus occur via a huge octagonal aqueous 125-kDa **nuclear pore complex** consisting of a large central pore – a channel almost 10 nm (100 Å) in diameter – surrounded by eight smaller peripheral channels. This pore complex consists of 30 different proteins, which comprise a basic subunit repeated 16 times: the nuclear side of the pore forms a single **nuclear basket**. Small peptides cross peripheral channels by simple diffusion, whereas larger proteins require active transport via the central pore.

The small GTP-binding protein **Ran** (p. 283) facilitates nuclear import and export in conjunction with proteins termed **importins** (α, β) and **exportin** respectively. Importins bind cytoplasmic proteins containing **nuclear localization sequences** – peptide sequences of strongly basic residues resembling those of the tumor virus SV40 T antigen. A split (bipartite) distribution of such residues has since been suggested as an underlying consensus nuclear import signal. This bipartite basic peptide binds a nuclear import receptor, which is phosphorylated prior to chaperoning the target protein in either direction along tracks between the nucleolus and cytoplasm via the pore complex (Figure 5.18). Examples of nuclear proteins containing such motifs include the NFκB/IκB/Rel heterodimer family, steroid hormone receptors, topoisomerases, the growth control proteins p53 and cdc25, the RNA/DNA polymerases, and the growth signaling genes Jun, Fos and Raf.

MOLECULAR MINIREVIEW

ADP-ribosylation
ADP-ribosylation is a post-translational modification that affects both cytoplasmic and nuclear proteins. ADP-ribosylation of actin filaments is induced by **clostridial toxins** – inhibiting actin polymerization and thus accounting for the toxin-mediated

pathology induced by these bacteria – whereas ADP-ribosylation of G-protein subunits results in the secretory diarrhea of **cholera** (p. 276). **Diphtheria toxin** acts by causing the ADP-ribosylation of an elongation factor involved in ribosomal protein synthesis (p. 111). ADP-ribosylation may be experimentally inhibited either by the antagonist 3-aminobenzamide, or else indirectly by the fungal metabolite **brefeldin A**, which prevents the binding of cytosolic proteins to Golgi membranes.

Poly(ADP-ribosyl)ation of DNA-binding proteins occurs within the nucleus following the induction of DNA strand-breaks by noxious stimuli such as ionizing radiation. This protein modification is catalyzed by the enzyme **poly(ADP-ribosyl) polymerase** or **PARP**, which is itself is a substrate for the intracellular enzymes that trigger cell death in response to cell damage (p. 383). Poly(ADP-ribosyl)ation thus appears to play a protective role in the DNA damage response. Of note, high expression levels of the *PARP1* gene have been linked to longevity.

Protein degradation

Polypeptides targeted to lysosomes are destroyed

Translation is only one determinant of protein availability. An efficient protein degradation system is required for several reasons:

1. To remove damaged (and/or misfolded) proteins from the cell.
2. To enable the rapid flux of intracellular signaling molecules.
3. To recycle constituent amino acids for new protein synthesis.

Unlike the genes by which they are encoded, proteins generally do not survive for the life of the cell but rather are involved in a constant round of synthesis, proteolytic cleavage, covalent modification, and degradation. This turnover is reflected in the wide range of protein half-lives. In general, structural proteins are long-lived whereas signaling molecules are rapidly degraded. Two key degradative routes include:

1. **Lysosomal degradation** – of transmembrane or endocytosed molecules.
2. **Proteasomal degradation** – of ubiquitin-tagged cytosolic proteins.

Lysosomes – literally, dissolution bodies – are intracellular bags of acid surrounded by glycosylated membrane proteins. Lysosomes are responsible for heavy-duty molecular degradation, and derive their constituent detergent enzymes (tagged by mannose-6-phosphate residues; p. 132) from the trans-Golgi. These acid hydrolases are highly active within the pH 5 environment of the lysosome but cause minimal damage on leaking into the pH 7.2 cytosolic milieu; they receive substrates from either endosomes or phagosomes containing extracellular particles, including microorganisms.

Null mutations of the integral lysosomal membrane protein **LAMP-2** cause **Danon disease**, an autophagic impairment manifesting as cardiomyopathy and myopathy. Many other diseases arise due to derangements of lysosomal structure or function, including not only I-cell disease (see above) but also **Hermansky–Pudlak syndrome**, **Chediak–Higashi syndrome** and the **X-linked oculocerebrorenal syndrome**.

MOLECULAR MINIREVIEW

The N-end rule

Protein stability is determined by rates of protein degradation, much of which occurs during rather than after translation. The stability of many such proteins is critically related to two sequence motifs:

1. The protein's amino-terminal residue – the basis of the so-called **N-end rule** for predicting protein degradation in bacteria and higher organisms such as man.
2. The presence of an internal lysine-binding site for **ubiquitin** (see below).

The primary amino-terminal degrading residue (or **N-degron**) is arginine. However, other amino acids (aspartate, glutamate, asparagine, and glutamine) may be metabolized to arginine via conjugation.

By ensuring the loss of partially cleaved protein remnants, this process prevents inadvertent interactions between such remnants and functional proteins. An illustrative example involves the **cohesin** protein complex which regulates sister chromatid cohesion during DNA replication. Cleavage of a cohesin subunit by the protease **separin** yields a 33-kDa carboxy-terminal cohesin fragment with a destabilizing amino-terminal arginine residue, leading to rapid proteasomal degradation of cohesin; this permits the release of sister chromatid binding, triggering the onset of anaphase. Organisms engineered to disobey the N-end rule exhibit a high frequency of chromosomal loss, consistent with failure of sister chromatid release.

Ubiquitin marks proteins for proteasomal destruction

Many cytosolic and membrane proteins are degraded by reversible crosslinkage to an abundant (indeed, ubiquitous) 76-amino-acid polypeptide called **ubiquitin**. Free lysine residues in acceptor proteins attach to ubiquitin side-chains which in turn promote hydrolysis of the modified protein substrate by ATP-dependent proteases. Internalization of transmembrane receptors may also be enhanced by ubiquitination, accelerating their degradation; ubiquitin is then recycled. Ubiquitination requires three enzymes:

1. **E1** (ubiquitin activators).
2. **E2** (small ubiquitin-conjugating enzymes).
3. **E3** (ubiquitin-protein ligases).

Following ubiquitin activation, E3 recruits E2 to the protein of interest. E2-bound polyubiquitin is then transferred by E3 to the target. E3 proteins belong to a sequence-structure superfamily of **RING finger** proteins – including **BRCA1**, **PML**, **HDM2**, and the kinase-extinguishing **Cbl** – all of which are growth-regulatory proteins implicated in human carcinogenesis.

Ubiquitinylated proteins end their days in a heptameric barrel-shaped 20S (750 kDa) 28-subunit catalytic chamber termed a **proteasome** (the 20S proteasome) sited within a still larger 26S (>2000 kDa) structure – which, confusingly, is also called a proteasome (the 26S proteasome). These endosomal protease-containing repositories are strategically located adjacent to the ER where they serve a proofreading role for exported proteins: up to 30% of all newly synthesized proteins are improperly folded (defective ribosomal products, or **DRiPs**) and hence require efficient detection and destruction. Phagocytosed foreign antigens may be ubiquitinylated, processed within proteasomes, and then re-exported to the cell surface for presentation in peptide form to T lymphocytes (Figure 5.19). **Ubiquitin-like domains** in certain DNA repair proteins interact with the 26S proteasome, implying a link between DNA replication and protein degradation.

Ubiquitin may recognize its substrate and signal its degradative intention by binding a so-called **destruction box** consisting of a **PEST** (proline, glutamate, serine, threonine) sequence which is detonated, as it were, by phosphorylation (for example, in the inhibitory transcription factor, IκB; p. 91). The intracellular pathogen *Listeria monocytogenes* maintains host cell (and hence its own) viability by including a PEST sequence within its secreted pore-forming protein **listeriolysin O**. In the absence of this PEST sequence, the internalized cytolytic toxin becomes longlived and kills the cell.

Figure 5.19 Protein degradation pathways. Certain classes of proteins are degraded via the lysosomal route, while others undergo proteolytic destruction within the proteasomal complex.

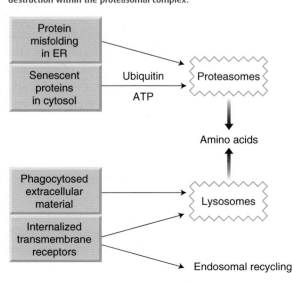

Proteins targeted for ubiquitinylation include damaged polypeptides such as denatured hemoglobin, suggesting that peptide sequence alone is insufficient to explain this recognition. Ubiquitinylation may also modify growth-controlling substrates such as cyclins, p53, Myc, and Fos. For example, the transforming E6 protein of papillomavirus acts by targeting the control protein p53 for ubiquitinylation. The muscle wasting of **cancer cachexia** has been linked to ubiquitinylation of muscle proteins.

CLINICAL KEYNOTE

Protein degradation pathways in disease

Efficient lysosomal degradation of unwanted cellular products is essential for human health. The importance of this cellular garbage disposal system is emphasized by its associated clinical disorders:

1. **Familial hypercholesterolemia** may be caused by a defective amino acid internalization signal within the cytoplasmic domain of the **low-density-lipoprotein (LDL) receptor**, leading to failure of LDL receptor downregulation in response to high plasma cholesterol.
2. Increased lysosomal ubiquitin–protein conjugates are seen in association with senile neuritic plaques and neurofibrillary tangles in patients with **Alzheimer disease**, and also in **Creutzfeldt–Jakob disease**.
3. Neurologic trinucleotide repeat disorders such as **spinocerebellar ataxia** or **Huntington disease** may cause neuronal toxicity due to intracellular accumulation of degraded proteins.

Insoluble amyloid polymers resist degradation

Inherited defects of proteolytic enzymes or protein trafficking can lead to accumulation of noxious proteins in the body. Another group of diseases characterized by protein accumulation are the **amyloidoses**.

Amyloid (starch-like) proteins are waxy fibrillar molecules consisting of β-sheets – hence the name, β-amyloid. Formation of the β-sheet conformation permits abnormal protein aggregation and (thus) amyloid fibril formation. These insoluble fibrils, which appear eosinophilic on histochemistry, are deposited in human tissue as a result of neoplastic disorders, chronic inflammatory conditions, familial syndromes, transmissible infections, **Alzheimer disease**, and **Down syndrome**. The latter two disorders are associated with the cerebral deposition of amyloid fibrils which aggregate to form pathogenetic neuritic plaques. Many amyloid proteins occur in different disease contexts, including **β-amyloid** (see below), **amylin (type 2 diabetes)**, **calcitonin (medullary thyroid cancer)**, β_2**-microglobulin (chronic hemodialysis)** and **immunoglobulin light chains (myeloma)** (pp. 474–5).

Familial mutations affecting the serum thyroxine- (and retinol-) binding protein **transthyretin** cause **senile cardiac and neuropathic amyloidosis** presenting with heart failure and arrhythmias. Transthyretin binds βAP and thus prevents its tissue deposition (rather like **apolipoprotein E2** and α_2-**macroglobulin** which protect against **Alzheimer disease**).

Mutations affecting the **lysozyme** (egg white) gene cause abnormal polymerization of the protein, leading to **autosomal dominant hereditary amyloidosis**. Other molecules implicated in genetic amyloidoses include **gelsolin**,

from the breakdown of ferritin shells. Excessive tissue deposition of hemosiderin is a hallmark of iron-loading anemias, but urinary excretion of hemosiderin is also a diagnostic test for chronic intravascular hemolysis. Usually, however, hemosiderosis occurs secondary to multiple transfusions for conditions of ineffective erythropoiesis such as thalassemia or sideroblastic anemia. Serum iron and ferritin are both elevated, and iron chelation using desferrioxamine is effective prophylaxis.

Idiopathic hemochromatosis (IHC) is the commonest genetic "disease" known. This autosomal recessive disorder of chronic iron hyperabsorption affects up to 1 in 200 Caucasians i.e., the carrier rate is as high as one in seven among Northern Europeans; compare this with the 1:90 and 1:30 000 carrier and homozygote frequencies, respectively, for Wilson disease. Serum ferritin levels may be extremely high in IHC patients, reflecting two- to threefold dietary iron hyperabsorption. Clinical manifestations are similar to those seen in severe hemosiderosis, but may also include pigmentation and pancreatic endocrine failure (bronze diabetes), cirrhosis, arthropathy, and hypogonadism. The phenotype is more severe in males, perhaps reflecting menstrual iron losses in females. However, this parent-of-origin effect could also reflect genomic imprinting (pp. 406–9).

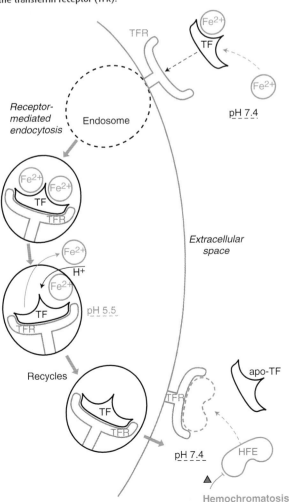

Figure 6.11 Cellular iron metabolism, showing the interplay between the hemochromatosis gene product (HFE), apotransferrin (apo-TF), and the transferrin receptor (TFR).

MOLECULAR MINIREVIEW

Hemochromatosis, HFE and C282Y

Idiopathic hemochromatosis (IHC) arises because the *HFE* gene, which encodes a 348-residue transmembrane glycoprotein, is mutated. The *HFE* gene cosegregates with major histocompatibility complex (MHC or HLA; p. 204) genes on chromosome 6, where it is located 6 Mb telomeric to (and in linkage disequilibrium with) the *HLA-A3* locus. Consistent with this, the HFE gene product is itself an MHC class I α-chain that has lost the ability to bind peptides. Instead, HFE associates with the 90-kDa **transferrin receptor** (TFR), which is bound with high affinity by two HFE molecules. TFR-bound insoluble ferric (III) iron undergoes reduction at the duodenal brush border by a cytochrome-like **ferric reductase** (Dcytb), the activity of which is upregulated by iron deficiency and downregulated by dietary iron repletion. The reduced ferrous (II) iron is unstable (i.e. prone to re-oxidation to ferric iron), but capable of absorption across the duodenal crypt cell membrane via a **divalent cation transporter**, DCT1. Internalization of the tripartite TFR-TF-Fe^{2+} complex into the more acidic cell interior leads to iron release, permitting recycling of the receptor–apotransferrin complex to the cell surface where the basic pH triggers its dissociation. HFE binds avidly to TFR at this pH, however, sterically inhibiting TFR binding of Fe^{3+}-bound transferrin (Figure 6.11).

Approximately 85% of European IHC patients are homozygous for a C282Y HFE substitution derived from a Celtic founder 60–70 generations ago. This substitution, which is now expressed by 5% of the European/Caucasian population, leads to impaired heterodimerization of the HFE protein and β2-microglobulin. The α-chain therefore fails to bind TFR, leading to 200–300% increased dietary iron absorption. About two-thirds of patients with the C282Y mutation also have an H63D mutation affecting the other allele, which worsens the phenotype. Allele for allele, however, H63D is less severe than C282Y (15–20% of the population is heterozygous for H63D). Elevated transferrin saturation appears a reliable screening test for C282Y.

Heterozygotes for C282Y have impaired HFE function, accompanied by higher than normal serum iron and ferritin levels, but rarely associated with complications of IHC (e.g., liver damage) in the absence of other disease such as **alcoholic cirrhosis**. This raises the question as to whether the heterozygous phenotype confers an evolutionary survival advantage. Only about 50% of C282Y homozygotes fully express the sequelae of IHC, and as many as 30% may appear phenotypically normal; conversely, occasional IHC patients have no detectable missense mutation of HFE. Of note, C282Y carriers may be at fourfold increased risk of developing **type II diabetes mellitus**, accounting for as much as 15% of the incidence of this disease.

Transferrin transports extracellular iron to cells

As noted for copper, most minerals circulate in the bloodstream complexed to a carrier protein. Transferrin is a circulating 80-kDa β1-globulin which transports up to 4 mg of body iron at any one time. Each transferrin molecule binds two Fe^{3+} and two bicarbonate molecules. Like intestinal iron absorption, hepatic synthesis of transferrin increases in response to iron deficiency and reduces in response to iron excess. These alterations are accompanied by changes in ferritin and transferrin receptor mRNA availability (pp. 111–13).

Alterations in transferrin expression occur more quickly than those of hemoglobin concentration or serum iron levels. Under normal circumstances transferrin is only about 30% saturated. Following its release from the reticuloendothelial system, transferrin-bound iron is shuttled from the peripheral circulation to the bone marrow where it attaches to **transferrin receptors** on reticulocytes and nucleated red cells. Following reduction at the proximal intestinal membrane, transferrin-bound iron crosses the membrane and is released as soluble, acidified cytosolic Fe^{2+}.

Transferrin availability and transferrin receptor expression correlate with cell growth. Extracellular transferrin-bound iron may act as an electron acceptor, thus stimulating intracellular redox enzymes such as **NADH:ferricyanide oxidoreductase** – a target of cell growth promoters. Conversely, ferritin gene expression may cause cell growth arrest in vitro.

Lactoferrin is a transferrin-like free radical scavenger that is found in tears, breast milk, mucosal cells, and leukocytes. Lactoferrin inhibits bacterial replication by sequestering microenvironmental iron. Consistent with this, the virulence of many bacteria (e.g., *Hemophilus, Neisseria, Yersinia* spp.) correlates with their ability to utilize iron: the sleeping sickness parasite *Trypanosoma brucei* encodes up to 20 different transferrin receptors, allowing it to internalize transferrin-bound iron while circulating in the bloodstream of different species, while the thrush fungus *Candida albicans* expresses two high-affinity iron permeases with multiple transmembrane domains. One microorganism that appears to evade the requirement for iron (thereby side-stepping the antibiotic effects of lactoferrin) is the Lyme disease agent *Borrelia burgdorferi*.

CLINICAL KEYNOTE

Hemopoiesis and iron metabolism
Primary and secondary abnormalities of iron homeostasis occur in many human diseases, as follows:

1. Iron deficiency, usually secondary to blood loss, is characterized by low serum iron, high transferrin and low ferritin. Apart from anemia, long-standing iron deficiency may be characterized by **pica** (a craving to eat unnatural substances, e.g., dirt), glossitis, spooned nails (**koilonychia**), esophageal webs (**Plummer–Vinson–Paterson–Kelly syndrome**), and perhaps immune deficiency or **atrophic gastritis**.
2. Chronic disease (e.g., severe **rheumatoid arthritis**) leads to increased serum ferritin and marrow iron stores despite reduced serum iron and transferrin saturation, absent marrow sideroblasts (red cell precursors), abnormally low

erythropoietin activity, normochromic anemia, and reticulocytopenia. This may reflect a functional iron reutilization defect secondary to impaired reticuloendothelial iron release.

Many other hematologic disorders – such as primary **sideroblastic anemias**, for example – are associated with secondary abnormalities of iron metabolism.

Sugars

Carbohydrate catabolism provides energy

Compounds that can be formulaically rendered as $C_x(H_2O)_y$ are termed **carbohydrates**. These include simple **sugars** and larger starch-like molecules such as **glycogen**. Starches are degraded by salivary and pancreatic **amylases** to oligosaccharides such as **maltose**.

Both sugars and starches avidly bind water. Carbohydrates combine readily with the other main biomolecular species – nucleic acids, proteins, and fats – to form the sugar-phosphate backbone of DNA, proteoglycans, and glycolipids respectively. In these molecules the carbohydrate modification usually plays a structural role. Free carbohydrates, on the other hand, are more often involved in the storage of energy, which can in turn be released by sugar breakdown or **glycolysis**. Digestive proteases in the human small intestine release three main products of dietary polysaccharide breakdown:

1. **Glucose.**
2. **Galactose.**
3. **Fructose.**

Sugars such as **sucrose** and **lactose** are hydrolyzed by intestinal brush-border enzymes to yield these monosaccharides. Starvation, on the other hand, is accompanied by the breakdown of macromolecules to fuel. **Glycogenolysis** (not to be confused with glycolysis) is one such catabolic mechanism, which involves the reverse generation of glucose from glycogen stores in liver and muscle. This occurs for about 24 hours after initiation of fasting, at which time liver glycogen stores are depleted. Glucose may also be synthesized de novo – a process termed **gluconeogenesis**. About two-thirds of hepatic glucose production in the first day of fasting arises via gluconeogenesis, and the rest via glycogenolysis.

Feeding (carbohydrate ingestion) causes transient hyperglycemia and consequent changes in peptide hormone availability: **insulin** secretion, which enhances plasma glucose utilization, and suppression of the insulin antagonist **glucagon**. The liver responds by removing plasma glucose for glycogenesis (glycogen formation) and/or glycolysis (pyruvate/lactate generation from glucose), while at the same time hepatic gluconeogenesis from fatty metabolites such as acetyl CoA declines. Inherited metabolic defects impairing glycogenolysis manifest as **glycogen storage diseases** (Table 6.3).

Carbohydrate absorption normally continues for 1–6 hours after a meal. After this time plasma insulin levels fall whereas levels of glucagon rise: these hormonal changes lead to increased hepatic synthesis of catabolic enzymes while inhibiting the glycolytic pathway. Catabolic hormones such as glucocorticoids (pp. 315–20) enhance transcription and stabilize the mRNA of gluconeogenic enzymes such as **phosphoenolpyruvate carboxykinase** (PEPCK). Plasma and intracerebral glucose levels are maintained by gluconeogenesis from 12–16 hours of fasting until starvation sets in after approximately 72 hours.

Table 6.3. Glycogen storage diseases

Glycogen storage disease type	Clinical manifestations	Enzyme deficiency
0	Hypoglycemia	Glycogen synthase
1	Hypoglycemia, hepatomegaly	Glucose-6-phosphatase
2 (Pompe disease)	Myopathy and heart failure	Lysosomal acid, α-1,4-glucosidase
3	Hypoglycemia, hepatomegaly, myopathy	Debrancher enzyme: amylo-1,6-glucosidase
5 (McArdle syndrome)	Cramps, myoglobinuria	Muscle phosphorylase
7	Weakness, hemolysis	Muscle phosphofructokinase

Table 6.4. Insulin-inducible and -repressible genes

Insulin-inducible genes

1. Glycolytic enzymes: pyruvate kinase, glucokinase, phosphofructokinase, aldolase.
2. Fat-synthesizing enzymes: fatty acid synthase, glucose-6-phosphate dehydrogenase, glycerol-3-phosphate acyltransferase.
3. (Brown adipose) uncoupling protein.
4. Growth hormone receptor.
5. Glucose transporters 1, 2, 4.
6. IGF1.
7. Prolactin.
8. Lipoprotein lipase.
9. Fos, Jun, Myc, Ras.

Insulin-repressible genes

1. PEPCK.
2. Growth hormone.
3. Apolipoprotein B.
4. Insulin-like growth factor binding proteins (IGFBPs).

Notes:
PEPCK, phosphoenolpyruvate carboxykinase.

Alactasia and celiac disease

The commonest metabolic nutritional disorder of the human race affects disaccharide metabolism. **Lactose intolerance** arises because of a primary or secondary deficiency of **lactase**, a hydrolytic enzyme that converts lactose to the absorbable glucose and galactose monosaccharides. When inherited, this condition is termed **alactasia** and is commoner in ethnic Chinese races than in Caucasians. Secondary deficiencies of intestinal lactase can accompany some diarrheal conditions, making it prudent to avoid dairy products during the healing phases of such disorders.

Gluten-induced enteropathy or celiac disease results from dietary exposure to wheat **α-gliadins**. Modification of gliadin by **transglutaminase** appears necessary for a maximal T cell response to the antigen, raising the possibility of using desensitization treatments to the modified epitope.

Insulin drives efficient cellular utilization of plasma nutrients

Rates of dietary protein absorption from the gut vary between "fast" proteins (e.g., whey) and "slow" proteins (e.g., casein): ingestion of fast proteins causes a rapid appearance of amino acids in the bloodstream, whereas slow dietary proteins cause a more gradual rise in plasma amino acids. Sudden availability of free plasma amino acids triggers a major increase in protein synthesis, but more gradual elevations blunt this anabolic response. A homeostatic balance between anabolism and catabolism is thus autoregulated by plasma amino acid availability.

Insulin is an additional anabolic stimulus. When insulin and glucagon are coexpressed, insulin-mediated transcriptional inhibition of the gluconeogenic pathway is dominant. Lack of insulin leads to the human disease **diabetes mellitus**, in which carbohydrates fail to be directed to the anabolic pathway, and organ damage ensues because of the default deposition of glycation products.

In normal individuals carbohydrate ingestion induces hepatic enzymes that convert glucose to short- and long-term energy stores. Enzymes induced by oral carbohydrate loads include glycolytic and fat-synthesizing enzymes (Table 6.4). Ingestion of fat represses these genes, whereas insulin increases their expression. For example, insulin regulation of **glucokinase** is independent of glucose availability; in contrast, **pyruvate kinase** (a downstream glycolytic enzyme) requires glucose for the transcriptional effects of insulin.

Like liver cells, insulin-stimulated muscle cells take up glucose, which undergoes conversion to glycogen. Working muscle splits glucose out of glycogen and converts it to pyruvate, which is in turn either converted to acetyl CoA by **pyruvate dehydrogenase** or else catabolized to lactate (Figure 6.12). ATP is produced by the mitochondrial metabolism of acetyl CoA; if these measures are not sufficient to satisfy muscle energy needs, muscle tissue is broken down to yield **phosphocreatine** as an emergency ATP source. Like muscle and liver cells, adipose tissue takes up glucose in the presence of insulin, but this is destined for long-term energy storage as fat (usually triglyceride).

Aerobic metabolism enhances ATP yield from glucose

On entering the cell, most glucose molecules are tagged for cytosolic retention in an ATP-dependent phosphorylation reaction catalyzed by **hexokinase**. The newly phosphorylated metabolite, **glucose-6-phosphate**, participates in the glycolytic pathway. This anaerobic pathway yields a net gain of two ATP, NADH

Figure 6.12 Glucose metabolism under aerobic and anaerobic conditions. Organic waste is metabolized to lactate under anaerobic conditions, or excreted as CO_2 under aerobic conditions.

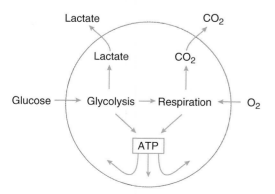

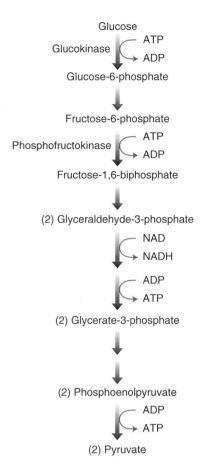

Figure 6.13 The glycolytic pathway. A net gain of 2 ATP molecules per cycle is forthcoming.

Figure 6.14 Oxidative phosphorylation in the mitochondria, showing the transmembrane direction of electron transport.

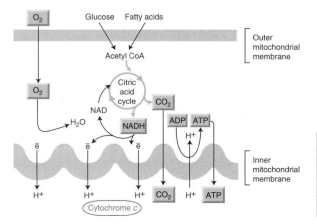

and pyruvate molecules for each glucose (Figure 6.13). Antibiotics such as **metronidazole** inhibit this pathway in anaerobic microorganisms.

The evolution of mitochondria (which ushered in aerobic metabolism) put a new spin on cellular energy management. Mitochondria are responsible for three energy-producing (oxidative) pathways:

1. **β-oxidation**: oxidative conversion of fatty acids to acetyl CoA (see below).
2. **Citric acid cycle**: generation of NADH from acetyl CoA oxidation.
3. **Oxidative phosphorylation**: production of ATP from oxidation of glucose.

Human cells produce most of their ATP by burning reduced carbon compounds. Glucose and other cellular foodstuffs are thus oxidized to produce the electron donor NADH (nicotinamide adenine dinucleotide, reduced). These electrons are in turn combined with oxygen to produce water as an oxidative excretion product (Figure 6.14). The efficiency of these reactions and the associated body heat production is regulated in brown fat by inner mitochondrial membrane **uncoupling proteins** or UCPs, which are implicated in the pathogenesis of obesity (pp. 433–4). Note in this context that mitochondrial maintenance of body temperature (through the oxidative "burning" of glucose) is not a waste of energy, but rather is essential to ensure the efficient catalysis of most biochemical reactions. **Ubiquinone (coenzyme Q)**, a mitochondrial cofactor for UCPs, may be depleted by the **statin** class of hypolipidemic drugs, leading to **myopathy** due to mitochondrial dysfunction.

Complete oxidation of glucose can be achieved by the creation of a positive charge and reduced pH on one side of the mitochondrial membrane. This is effected by carrier molecules termed the **electron transport chain** (ETC), a biochemical storage battery that drives ATP synthesis by a chemiosmotic mechanism. Five respiratory enzyme complexes underpin this series of reactions: complex I, **NADH: ubiquinone oxidoreductase** (a large L-shaped proton-translocating complex); complex II, **succinate:ubiquinone reductase** (an FAD-containing citric acid cycle component which feeds electrons to the ETC); complex III, **cytochrome bc$_1$** (also known as ubiquinone cytochrome *c* reductase; couples electron delivery to the creation of a proton gradient, hence a redox crossroads); complex IV, **cytochrome oxidase** (a proton pump which pulls electrons from cytochrome *c*); and complex V, **ATP synthase**. Mutations of complex I or II enzymes may cause quinone-responsive mitochondrial encephalomyopathies. Clinical improvement may be obtained using oral **ubidecarenone**.

By incorporating NADH and pyruvate into the malate/aspartate shuttle (and thence to the citric acid cycle; Figure 6.15) an additional six ATP molecules can be produced above the yield obtainable from glycolysis. Hence, for each molecule of glucose, one cycle of **oxidative phosphorylation** – if we include mitochondrial decarboxylation of pyruvate to acetyl CoA, metabolism of succinyl CoA to NADH and FADH$_2$, and the consequent production of ATP – adds a whopping 36 ATP molecules to the two yielded by glycolysis.

CLINICAL KEYNOTE

Diseases of oxidative phosphorylation

There are as many as 1000 proteins involved in oxidative phosphorylation, only 13 of which are mitochondrial. Most known oxidative phosphorylation disorders are thus

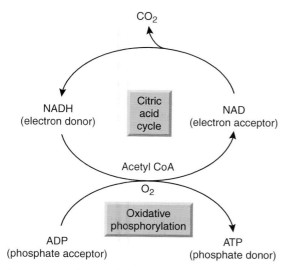

Figure 6.15 Coupling of the citric acid cycle to oxidative phosphorylation, leading to NADH-dependent enhancement of ATP production.

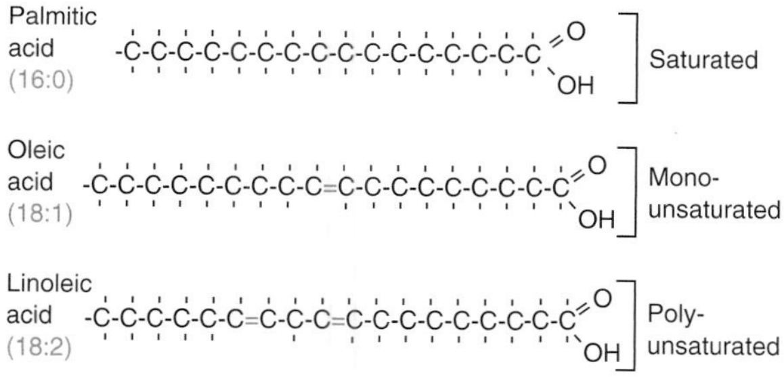

due to nuclear rather than mitochondrial genes; the symptoms of these disorders usually reflect ATP depletion or free radical excess. Typical presentations of such disorders include lactic acidosis (usually neonatal), visual failure (retinal degeneration), optic neuropathy), ophthalmoplegia and ptosis, myopathy with or without cardiomyopathy, and **myoclonic epilepsy**.

Over 50 mutations of mitochondrial DNA (mtDNA) are known. The same mutation can give rise to different phenotypes, whereas similar phenotypes may arise from different mutations. Mutations that impair the function of the electron transport chain will increase the NADH:NAD ratio and reduce α-tocopherol levels, leading to impaired fatty acid β-oxidation (see below) with secondary carnitine deficiency. In a potentially lethal side-effect, the enzyme **carnitine palmitoyltransferase-1** (CPT1, which normally facilitates mitochondrial entry of long-chain fatty acids) is inhibited by a rise in malonylcarnitine levels triggered by the pediatric sedative drug **propofol**, clinically mimicking an acute mitochondrial myopathy. The CPT1 inhibitor **etomoxir** inhibits metabolism of fatty acids while promoting that of glucose, and thus appears especially useful in treating chronic heart failure secondary to **cardiomyopathy**.

Fats

Dietary fatty acids are converted to acetyl CoA by β-oxidation

Fats are critical dietary constituents. Without cholesterol, for example, we would be unable to synthesize cell membranes, myelin sheaths, bile acids, steroid hormones or the visual receptor rhodopsin. Adipose tissue provides an enormous energy store for mobilization during fasting or exercise, but such mobilization is a slow process; since oxidation of muscle glycogen stores releases energy at four times the rate of lipolysis, muscle fatigue usually accompanies glycogen depletion. Mitochondrial enzymes involved in the latter process include **glycogen phosphorylase** and **pyruvate dehydrogenase**.

The varieties of fat include **fatty acids, phospholipids, sphingolipids, isoprenoids**, and **triacylglycerols**. Fatty acids are mainly obtained from the diet, and include the essential fatty acids **linoleic** and **linolenic** acids. Linolenic acid is metabolized by desaturation to arachidonic acid, which in turn gives rise to prostaglandins and other pro-inflammatory molecules (p. 292).

Fatty acids are classified by their cis-alkyl double bond content as either **saturated** (i.e., full of single bonds) or **unsaturated** (i.e., not full of single bonds; hence, containing double or triple bonds; Figure 6.16). The number of double bonds (degree of unsaturation) and the shortness of the fatty acid chain reduce the melting point and thus enhance the fluidity of unsaturated fats: unsaturated fats thus tend to be oils at room temperature, whereas solid fats (e.g., lard) are usually saturated. In chemical notation, the length of the fatty acid chain is represented by one number (e.g., 16), which is followed by a second digit indicating the number of double bonds (e.g., 0 = saturated).

The essential fatty acids are unsaturated and hence represented as linoleic (18:2) and linolenic (18:3) acids; the other unsaturated long-chain fatty acids are **oleic** and **palmitoleic** acid. Saturated fatty acids predisposing to vascular disease (**atherosclerosis**) when consumed in excess include **lauric acid** (12:0), **myristic acid** (14:0), and **palmitic acid** (16:0). These dietary fats may be endogenously elongated or desaturated (e.g., to promote membrane fluidity). Note that neither short-chain saturated fats nor stearic (18:0) acid elevate LDL-cholesterol levels (see below), suggesting that not all saturated fats are atherogenic. Unsaturated fatty acids include:

Figure 6.16 Saturated and unsaturated fatty acids. The more double (or triple) bonds, the more unsaturated the molecule.

Palmitic acid (16:0) -C-C-C-C-C-C-C-C-C-C-C-C-C-C-C-C〈O OH Saturated

Oleic acid (18:1) -C-C-C-C-C-C-C-C-C=C-C-C-C-C-C-C-C-C〈O OH Mono-unsaturated

Linoleic acid (18:2) -C-C-C-C-C-C=C-C-C=C-C-C-C-C-C-C-C-C〈O OH Poly-unsaturated

Table 6.6. Lipoproteins

1. **LDL**
   - Major carrier of endogenous cholesterol and cholesteryl esters
   - ApoB100 is the sole apoprotein.

2. **Chylomicrons**
   - The largest and most triglyceride-rich lipoprotein particle (85% w/w)
   - ApoB48 is the major apoprotein (also apoAI, apoE).

3. **Chylomicron remnants**
   - Major carriers of dietary cholesterol
   - Contain apoB48 and apoE.

4. **VLDL**
   - Another major triglyceride carrier (50% w/w)
   - ApoB100 is the major apoprotein.

5. **β-VLDL**
   - A mix of chylomicron remnants and VLDL remnants (IDLs)
   - Contain chylomicron-derived apoB48 *plus* VLDL-derived apoB100.

6. **HDL**
   - The smallest and most protein-rich lipoprotein
   - Subclassified as larger HDL_2 and smaller HDL_3
   - ApoAI is the major apoprotein.

7. **Pre-beta HDL**
   - Electrophoretic HDL subfraction which binds directly to cells
   - Scavenges cell-associated cholesterol for reverse transport to the liver (p. 437).

8. **IDL**
   - Intermediate-density remnant of VLDL catabolism
   - Cholesterol (40%) and triglyceride (25%) rich
   - ApoE3 is the major apoprotein.

9. **Lp(a)**
   - LDL-like cholesterol-rich (45%) lipoprotein; scarce
   - ApoB100 and apo(a) are the sole apoproteins
   - A ligand for LDL receptors and plasminogen receptors.

disease. The common late-onset form of Alzheimer disease has been linked to the apolipoprotein E allelotype in approximately 50% of cases. The three common apoE alleles (E_2, E_3, and E_4) are encoded on chromosome 19.

1. **Apolipoprotein E_4** increases the risk and reduces the age of onset of dementia, with E_4 homozygotes having a higher risk than heterozygotes who are in turn at higher risk (three-fold) than E_4-null individuals. Hence, E_4 gene dosage increases the risk of Alzheimer disease (tenfold greater risk in E_4 homozygotes compared with E_4-null) just as amyloid precursor protein (APP) does in **Down syndrome**. The vascular effects of E_4 may contribute to neuronal ischemia; consistent with this, the ability of estrogen to protect against cognitive decline are negated in E_4-allele holders. Alternatively, E_4 may sequester β-amyloid peptide (βAP) in senile plaques (predisposing to neuronal death) or inefficiently bind tau (predisposing to neurofibrillary tangles). Of note, this genotype is more useful for predicting when, rather than whether, a given individual develops Alzheimer disease. A positive test is not of diagnostic utility in isolation – fewer than 30% of apoE$_4$ polymorphs will develop Alzheimer disease – but can improve the specificity of the diagnosis. Moreover, the E4 allele is predictive of failure to respond to cholinesterase inhibitor (tacrine) treatment.

2. **Apolipoprotein E_2** exerts a protective effect over and above that seen in E_4-null individuals, presumably by preventing neuronal death.

Functional magnetic resonance imaging (FMRI) studies of brain function have indicated that E_4 carriers exhibit more widespread cerebral activation and more intense hippocampal activity in response to memory tasks than do E_3 homozygotes, a phenomenon that appears predictive of subsequent memory loss. Mutations affecting **α_2-macroglobulin**, another ligand for the apoE$_4$ receptor (LRP), are also linked with disease onset. α_2-macroglobulin is a protease that mediates βAP clearance, suggesting a further pathogenetic mechanism for apoE$_4$.

Plasma lipids are transported by lipoproteins

Lipid profiles are reported in terms of total serum cholesterol and triglycerides. These lipid levels are measures of circulating saturated lipoproteins, the functions of which are presented in Table 6.6.

Long-chain dietary fatty acids are converted within intestinal mucosal cells to triglycerides, which are complexed with apoB48 and apoA prior to chylomicron uptake (Figure 6.19). After entering gut lymphatics, chylomicra are transported to the circulation where they take up apoC and apoE from HDLs. ApoCII activates **lipoprotein lipase** on capillary cell walls, thus hydrolyzing core triglycerides to free fatty acids which enter adipose tissue for storage, or muscle (particularly cardiac muscle) for oxidative fuel generation. The triglyceride-depleted chylomicron detaches from lipoprotein lipase – leaving behind its apoCII moiety – to yield a smaller cholesterol-rich particle recognizable by residual apoB48 and apoE surface markers. Hence, chylomicra and their triglyceride-depleted remnants are the main carrier proteins for dietary triglycerides and cholesterol respectively.

Chylomicron remnants are removed from the circulation by both receptor-dependent and receptor-independent mechanisms, with the latter being mediated by apolipoprotein binding to either intrahepatic LDL receptors or to apoE-binding **LDL receptor-related proteins** (LRP); the family of LDL receptor-like proteins is shown in Table 6.7. The efficiency of remnant clearance depends upon the affinity of apoE isoforms for their receptor, with apoE$_4$ having the highest and apoE$_2$ the lowest affinity; total and LDL-cholesterol levels therefore tend to be higher with apoE$_4$ expression.

VLDLs are catabolized in a fashion similar to chylomicra. Following triglyceride hydrolysis and cleavage of apoCII by lipoprotein lipase, the liberated

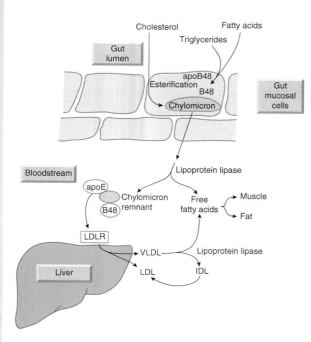

Figure 6.19 Transport of dietary lipid across the gut mucosa and into plasma. Chylomicra and associated apolipoproteins are then routed through the liver, leading to feedback regulation of hepatic lipoprotein synthesis; free fatty acids, on the other hand, are incorporated directly into muscle or fat. apo, apolipoprotein. IDL, intermediate-density lipoprotein; LDL, low-density lipoprotein; LDLR, LDL receptor; VLDL, very low-density lipoprotein.

VLDL remnant particle (i.e., IDL) undergoes endocytosis by hepatic LDL receptors and/or lipase-inducible conversion to LDL. Indeed, LDLs are taken up by LDL receptors far less readily than IDLs, reflecting the 20-fold lower LDL receptor affinity for apoB100 than for apoE. Oxidized LDL is associated with increased atherogenicity, suggesting that the anti-atherogenic action of estrogens may derive from their inhibitory effects on LDL oxidation.

MOLECULAR MINIREVIEW

Lipoprotein (a)

Lipoprotein (a) (Lp(a)) is an LDL-like molecule with non-LDL-like molecular interactions. Lp(a) is an unusual lipoprotein among mammals, being only expressed in humans and East African hedgehogs. Lp(a) – pronounced "ell-pee-little-ay" – resembles LDL in terms of size (about 25 nm across), apoprotein composition (B100), and cholesterol content (around 50% by mass).

Unlike LDL, the 510-kDa apoB100 moiety of Lp(a) is disulfide-linked in the endoplasmic reticulum to an equally massive (300–800 kDa) **plasminogen-like protein** called **apo(a)** – plasminogen being the precursor of an endogenous protease that dissolves blood clots (that is, it is fibrinolytic; pp. 466–8). The apo(a) protein consists of an amino-terminal domain containing up to 37 plasminogen kringle IV repeats, a single kringle V domain, and a plasminogen-like protease domain. Apo(a) structurally resembles a giant variant of plasminogen, and probably arose by duplication of the nearby plasminogen gene on chromosome 6. More than 20 codominantly inherited apo(a) isoforms of different sizes exist. Plasma Lp(a) concentrations tend to be inversely correlated with the apo(a) size polymorphism. Since 80% of the Caucasian population express larger apo(a) variants, the population Lp(a) distribution is heavily skewed to the left.

Lp(a) is cleared from plasma mainly via LDL receptor uptake; the presence of apo(a) impairs the binding of apo B100 to the LDL receptor. Lp(a) also competes for the occupation of plasminogen-binding sites in endothelial cells. Since the apo(a) domain of Lp(a) lacks the arginine residue specifying the cleavage site of plasminogen, Lp(a) is resistant to proteolytic activation. Lp(a) thus antagonizes fibrinolysis by competitively inhibiting plasminogen; hence, high Lp(a) levels predispose not only to atherosclerosis but also to thrombosis.

Individual variations in plasma Lp(a) concentrations have a stronger genetic basis than do those of any other lipoprotein, with 70% of variability being accounted for by the apo(a) locus. Moreover, neither dietary nor therapeutic measures usually succeed in lowering plasma Lp(a). Patients with familial hypercholesterolemia have twice the normal risk of high Lp(a) levels.

Summary

Normal cell function requires exogenous nutrients. Vitamin C is an antioxidant needed for collagen synthesis. B-group vitamins are coenzyme precursors. Single-carbon reactions require water-soluble vitamins. A metal–carbon bond in vitamin B_{12} provides reactivity. Homocysteine causes oxidative damage to endothelial cells.

Dietary trace elements maintain protein function. Copper regulates cellular oxidation and respiration. Tissues store intracellular iron bound to ferritin. Transferrin transports extracellular iron to cells.

Table 6.7. The LDL receptor family

LDL receptor
VLDL receptor
LDL receptor-related protein (LRP)
Apolipoprotein E receptor-2
Megalin

Enrichment reading

Library reference

Brody T. *Nutritional biochemistry.* Academic Press, New York, 1998

Combs GF. *The vitamins: fundamental aspects in nutrition and health.* Academic Press, New York, 1998

Stipanuk MH (ed). *Biochemical and physiological aspects of human nutrition.* WB Saunders, Philadelphia, 1999

Carbohydrate catabolism provides energy. Insulin drives efficient cellular utilization of plasma nutrients. Aerobic metabolism enhances mitochondrial ATP yield from glucose.

Dietary fatty acids are converted to acetyl CoA by β-oxidation. Lipoproteins are circulating apoprotein sandwiches. Plasma lipids are delivered to cells by lipoproteins.

QUIZ QUESTIONS

1. Name some proteins in which covalently modified amino acids are incorporated, and explain the change in function caused by the amino acid modification.
2. Which vitamins have antioxidant properties? How do deficiencies in these vitamins arise, and what clinical syndromes result?
3. Name one clinical condition resulting from an excess of free radical generation, and another resulting from a deficiency thereof. What effects do these free radical imbalances cause?
4. Describe the biochemical functions of the B-group vitamins thiamine, niacin, and pyridoxine. What clinical effects result from their dietary deficiency?
5. How may a person become niacin deficient, other than through dietary insufficiency?
6. How does folic acid affect the function of thymidylate synthase?
7. What are the functional differences between hydroxocobalamin, cyanocobalamin, and methylcobalamin?
8. Describe the function of R-proteins, and their relationship to intrinsic factor.
9. What does selenium do, and how does its deficiency manifest?
10. Name two proteins functionally regulated by copper.
11. Explain the importance of iodine in thyroid hormone metabolism.
12. Briefly describe the different roles of transferrin and ferritin in iron metabolism, and their different alterations in disease.
13. Describe the sequence of biochemical events that occurs in response to starvation.
14. What is gluconeogenesis? When does it occur, and which molecules are involved?
15. Describe in broad outline the glycolytic pathway.
16. Explain the difference between saturated and unsaturated fatty acids, and discuss their relationship to atherogenesis.
17. Describe the structural relationship between cholesterol, triglycerides, and free fatty acids.
18. Explain the difference between a lipoprotein and an apolipoprotein using examples.

7

Membranes and channels

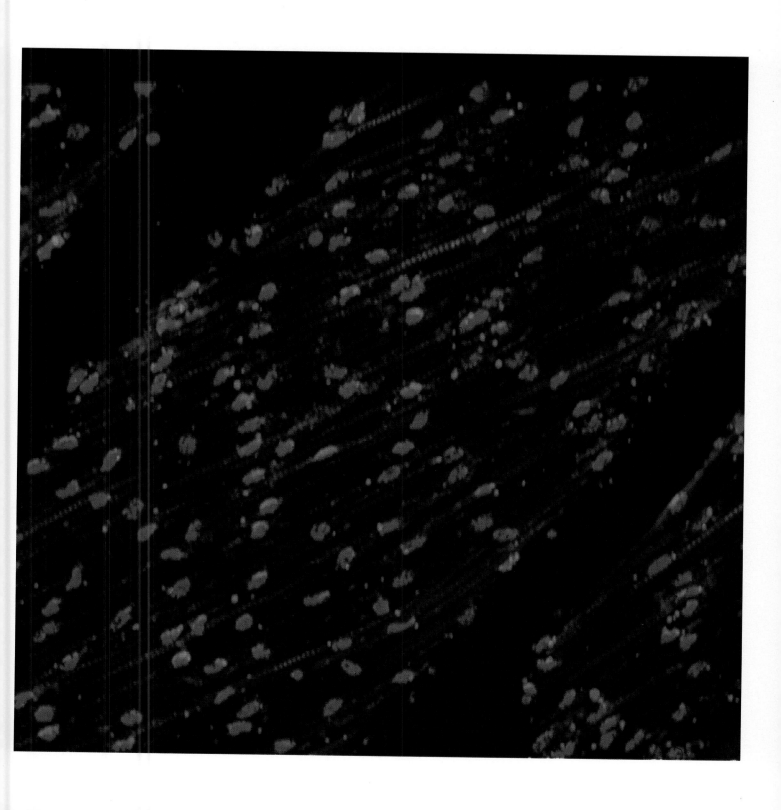

Figure 7.1 (*previous page*) Confocal image of heart muscle cells. The nuclei are red. The green spots indicate gap junctions between the cells, which facilitate the conduction of electrical impulses through the heart, thus coordinating its contraction. (Wellcome Medical Photographic Library, no. B0000108C00, credit Dr David Becker).

Our focus in the previous sections has been restricted to intracellular molecules. Many of the molecules we know most about, however, are associated with the plasma membrane – the outer lining of the cell. In this section we consider the role of membrane-associated molecules in linking extracellular and intracellular events.

Membranes

Hydrophobic membranes divide cells into compartments

Human cells contain over 200 different lipids, many of which are derived from glycerol. When three fatty acids bind glycerol, a triglyceride molecule is formed. One of the three fatty acids in triglycerides can be replaced by a negatively charged phosphate group, which binds choline, serine or ethanolamine to form **phosphatidylcholine** (dipalmitoyl lecithin), **phosphatidylserine** and **phosphatidylethanolamine** respectively. These **phospholipids** comprise most of the lipid content of cell membranes, with the 50% nonlipid portion of the membrane being protein.

The fatty acid tail of the phospholipid is hydrophobic whereas the polar phosphate group is hydrophilic. Membrane phospholipids therefore align themselves with the phosphates pointed out (i.e., extracellularly and into the cytosol) and the fatty acid tails pointed into the membrane core. The resulting film-like bilayer configuration of the protein-phospholipid sandwich (Figure 7.2) – described as **amphipathic** to indicate the charge asymmetry of the constituent phospholipids – is accompanied by a characteristic distribution of phospholipids within the membrane leaflets:

1. The outer membrane monolayer mainly consists of:
   - **Phosphatidylcholine** (lecithin).
   - **Sphingomyelin**.
2. The inner membrane leaflet mainly consists of:
   - **Phosphatidylinositol** (p. 289).
   - **Phosphatidylinositol (4,5)-bisphosphate** (PIP$_2$).

In addition to shielding the cell contents from the extracellular space, membranes line the Golgi cisternae, mitochondrial cristae, endoplasmic reticulum, and nuclear envelope. Unless polymerized by proteins such as spectrin (pp. 242–3), the lipid bilayer is fluid. Membrane fluidity enhances molecular diffusion through the plasma membrane, facilitating cell functions such as budding, adhesion, phagocytosis, and migration.

Figure 7.2 Membrane structure, showing the amphipathic structure of the lipid-protein sandwich.

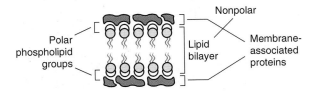

Polar phospholipid groups

Nonpolar

Lipid bilayer

Membrane-associated proteins

MOLECULAR MINIREVIEW

Choline

The essential three-carbon amine nutrient **choline** becomes lipidated to form a variety of signaling molecules. Choline may undergo the following transformations:

1. Phospholipidation to phosphatidylcholine or sphingomyelin.
2. Acetylation to the neurotransmitter **acetylcholine**.
3. Conversion to lipid signaling molecules such as **diacylglycerol** or **platelet-activating factor**.
4. Oxidation to the methyl donor **betaine** (which remethylates homocysteine as part of the methionine synthase pathway; p. 154).

Choline deficiency causes a reduction in membrane lecithin. Enzymes termed **flippases** (phospholipid translocators) flip choline-containing phospholipids from one side of the endoplasmic reticulum membrane to the other – but do not flip inositol-, ethanolamine- or serine-containing phospholipids, hence maintaining the asymmetry of the bilayer.

CLINICAL KEYNOTE

Antiphospholipid syndrome

Phospholipid antibodies occur in autoimmune diatheses of the lupus (**systemic lupus erythematosus**, SLE) cluster. According to one theory, phospholipid antibodies are formed in response to phosphatidylserine exposure on the outside of membranous blebs attached to dying cells (pp. 383–4). Consistent with this, lupus patients often have high concentrations of circulating dead cells associated with antinucleosomal (DNA-histone) antibodies formed in response to cell rupture. Such autoantibodies may belong to one of the following categories:

1. Anti-cardiolipin antibodies.
2. Lupus anticoagulants.
3. False-positive reaginic tests for syphilis.

Cardiolipin (diphosphatidyl glycerol) accounts for ~20% of inner mitochondrial membrane phospholipid. About 30% of patients with systemic lupus erythematosus (SLE) will have one or other of these antiphospholipid antibodies, some of which may be drug-induced.

Clinical hallmarks of the associated **antiphospholipid syndrome** are thrombosis, thrombocytopenia, hypertension, and recurrent miscarriages. Coagulation is accelerated in vivo (especially with IgG antibodies) but inhibited in vitro by the so-called lupus anticoagulant; the latter phenomenon reflects impaired interaction between prothrombin (p. 468) and the phospholipid moiety of the prothrombin activator complex. A putative target autoantigen for antiphospholipid antibodies is **lysobiphosphatidic acid** (LBPA) in the endosomal vesicular membrane. This lipid is a marker of the late endosome (p. 197); that is, LBPA enrichment indicates that the endocytosed endosome is about to fuse with lysosomes. Reduced expression of the anticoagulant hormone **annexin V**, which normally separates coagulant proteins from activating phospholipids, is also implicated in the pathogenesis of the thrombotic tendency.

Surface glycolipids protect and insulate cells

Membrane biosynthesis is initiated by fatty acids combining with serine to form **sphingosine**, an amino alcohol. Addition of a further fatty acid to sphingosine forms **ceramide**. Following export to the Golgi lumen, ceramide is combined with phosphocholine to form **sphingomyelin** or with oligosaccharides to form **glycolipids** (or glycosphingolipids). The latter are sugar-containing membrane lipids in which the glycosyl groups protrude into either the Golgi lumen (i.e., at the time of post-translational modification) or the extracellular space. **Shigatoxins** produced by notorious *Escherichia coli* serotypes such as O157:H7 cause their clinical sequelae (e.g., the **hemolytic-uremic syndrome**) by first attaching to specific glycosphingolipid (globotriaosylceramide: **Gb3**) receptors on capillary endothelial cells.

Sialic-acid-containing glycolipids termed **gangliosides**, of which approximately 50 are identified, are negatively charged molecules that contribute up to 10% of myelin membrane lipids in nerve cells. The charge on these molecules facilitates neurotransmission. Ganglioside G_{M1} stimulates dopaminergic neuron sprouting (and hence is used in the experimental treatment of **parkinsonism**) and represents an autoantibody target in **amyotrophic lateral sclerosis**

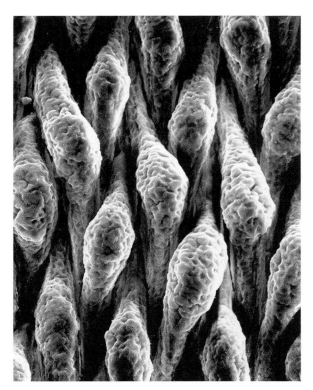

Figure 7.3 The inner surface of the small intestine is covered with millions of tiny folds called intestinal villi. This scanning electron micrograph (SEM) shows part of the ileum in the small intestine and its leaf-shaped villi. This shape allows the villi to lie closely together in an alternating pattern, increasing the surface area and absorption of nutrients. (GAB ref. IV-140 n.3.) (Wellcome Medical Photographic Library, no. B0001113B06 courtesy of Professor Giorgio Gabella).

these DNAs insert into the PBP genes to produce non-penicillin-binding variant proteins. Transposons can mediate similar resistance.

β-Lactam entry into Gram-negative bacteria depends upon hollow membrane proteins termed **porins**. Hence, the resistance of *Pseudomonas* spp. to the antibiotic **imipenem** may be due to null mutations affecting the D2 porin, and similar resistance mechanisms are operative for **aminoglycosides** and **fluoroquinolones**. Increased antibiotic efflux is a well-documented enterobacterial resistance mechanism for **tetracyclines** (p. 109).

Intercellular communication

Intercellular information is exchanged by cell contact

Cell–cell contact is central to intercellular communication. Partly for this reason, cells and tissues may maximize their available surface area by forming corrugated structures such as microvilli and villi respectively (Figure 7.3).

Cells experiencing deformative stress become aware of the external stimulus through a process termed **mechanotransduction**, which involves the conversion of kinetic forces to biochemical signals (Figure 7.4). Stretch-inducible activation of **baroreceptors** (pressure receptors) in the cardiovascular and pulmonary systems provides one example of this mechanism. Other mechanotransduction examples include:

1. Activation of intracellular signaling (e.g., via calcium release) by muscle stretch.
2. Stretch-inducible activation of genes mediating uterine relaxation prior to parturition.
3. Changes in basilar membrane potential due to acoustic mechanotransduction by auditory hair cells in the ear (p. 505).

All cell types sense shear stress to some extent. This is indicated by the variety of genes expressed in response to such stress, including immediate-early genes, chemoattractants, and growth factors. Torsional membrane stresses are transmitted to cells through adhesive surface molecules, whereas the afferent loop of such responses is mediated by proteins responsible for cell shape (pp. 239–40).

Efferent responses to mechanical stimuli may involve the activation of transmembrane ion-permeable **channels**. For example, alterations in cell volume related to changes in extracellular osmolarity may modulate the activity of the transmembrane channels that regulate intracellular ion concentrations. The activation of mechanosensitive ion channels occurs in prokaryotes (e.g., *Mycobacterium tuberculosis*) via a homopentameric channel which resembles the nicotinic acetylcholine receptor (p. 494). Baroreceptor activation may alter the patency of such channels in human cells, activating compensatory shifts in fluid balance.

The in vitro growth of normal cells to confluence results in density-dependent growth inhibition, a homeostatic mechanism that is often abrogated in tumor cells. Density-dependent growth arrest may be associated with the downregulation of mitogen receptors, suggesting that membrane-bound ligands mediate this effect.

Cells communicate via connexins

Intercellular communication occurs not by touch but by molecular exchanges between the cells. These exchanges take place via membrane connections.

Figure 7.4 Mechanisms of mechanotransduction by membranes: activation of transmembrane receptors and/or ion channels by stretch.

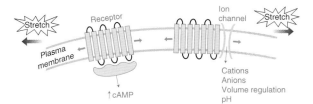

Such connections comprise a variety of structures that are distinguishable by electron microscopy:

1. Gap junctions
   - Gasket-like intercellular channels.
2. Tight junctions
   - Areas of membrane contact or fusion which define cell orientation by distinguishing the apical and basolateral plasma membranes (Figure 7.5).
   - Function as fences or gates.
   - Prevent paracellular loss of large proteins.
   - Are leaky in **celiac disease** (p. 165) due to gut overexpression of **zonulin**, a protein that promotes the disassembly of tight junctions.
   - Contribute to the blood–brain barrier (see below).
3. Adherens junctions
   - Are thickened membrane regions that contain adhesive glycoproteins (**cadherins**; pp. 211–12) which undergo homophilic binding to create transmembrane connections with cytoskeletal microfilaments.
   - Adhesion plaques, also called focal contacts, are a subtype of adhesive junction that occurs between certain cell adhesion molecules (**integrins**; p. 222) and a substratum composed of **extracellular matrix proteins**.

Gap junctions are water-filled spaces that allow the intercellular transit of small (<1 kDa) nutrients and electrolytes which may then migrate intracellularly via carrier/transporter proteins or aqueous channels (Figure 7.6). These hexagonal structures are composed of protein subunits termed **connexins** which are categorized into α and β families and named on the basis of their molecular weight (e.g., connexin46 – **Cx46** – is 46 kDa in size). Epithelial cell communication is critically dependent upon gap junctions: such **gap-junctional intercellular communication** (GJIC, 'metabolic cooperation') can be measured experimentally by dye transfer between cells, and plays a key role in embryonic development, heart muscle contraction, synaptic coupling in the brain, and the function of tissues such as the optic lens, retina, and cochlea. In contrast, normal skeletal muscle cells lack gap junctions.

The efficiency of GJIC depends on cell type and connexin isoform composition. GJIC is implicated in tumorigenesis: certain transforming proteins inhibit GJIC by phosphorylating the gap junction protein **Cx43**, whereas increased Cx43 expression can revert the malignant phenotype of brain tumor cells. Over 100 heritable mutations affect **Cx32** in an X-linked subtype of the polyneuropathy **Charcot-Marie–Tooth disease** (Figure 7.7), reflecting involvement of Cx32 in myelin cross-linking. Similarly, mutations affecting **Cx26** are the commonest single cause of genetic deafness (p. 505), whereas the severe congenital heart malformation **visceroatrial heterotaxia** arises secondary to Cx43 mutations.

Figure 7.5 Insertion of proteins into cell membranes, illustrating cell and protein polarity. Cell polarity is based on the demarcation of basolateral borders between epithelial cells, as indicated here by the presence of a tight junction (*A*). Transmembrane protein polarity (*B*) is determined by the position of the amino- and carboxy-terminal ends with respect to the intracellular and extracellular space; here the hydrophilic (heavily phosphorylated, denoted by the encircled letter P) terminus is intracellular, whereas cysteine residues (C, which are oxidized extracellularly to cystine) predominate in the extracellular region. ER, endoplasmic reticulum.

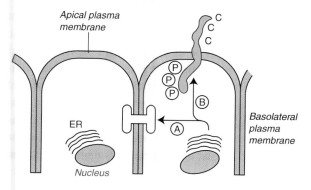

PHARMACOLOGIC FOOTNOTE

Tight junctions, drug delivery, and the blood–brain barrier
Molecules (such as drugs) in the peripheral circulation are presented to the central nervous system – brain, spinal cord, and cerebrospinal fluid or CSF – at a functional tissue interface consisting of several components:
1. Blood–CSF barrier
   - Mainly consists of choroid plexus epithelium.

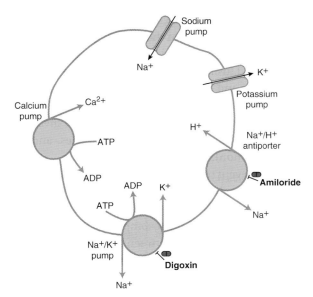

Figure 7.9 Different ion transporters: channels, pumps, exchangers, and their energy requirements.

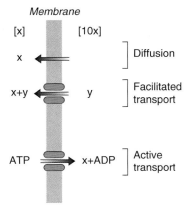

Figure 7.10 Active versus facilitated transport: the former requires ATP to proceed against a concentration gradient, whereas the latter occurs via cooperative interaction with another solute.

that allow the bidirectional passage of molecules smaller than 30 kDa. Because the concentration of molecules such as glucose and electrolytes needs to be tightly controlled in different cell compartments, strict entry and exit mechanisms are required. These are provided by transmembrane molecular transport proteins (Figure 7.9):

1. Pore-forming proteins
   - **Ion channels**.
2. Carrier proteins
   - **Pumps**: ATP-dependent membrane allosteric proteins (ATPases),
   - **Transporters**: e.g., *Mdr* multidrug transporter, copper transporters,
   - **Exchangers** (also known as **antiporters**), for example:
     Na^+/K^+ pump (a ubiquitous ATPase).
     Na^+/H^+ antiporter (pH-dependent).
     H^+/K^+-proton pump (acidifies gastric lumen).
   - **Ion-coupled membrane transporters**: e.g., serotonin transporter.

Ion channels, such as the Na^+ channel responsible for nerve action potentials, are pores of a certain width that permit selective transmembrane molecular migration. Channels that permit more solute to flow into the cell than out are termed **inward rectifiers**, whereas those that favor extracellular solute transport are termed **outward rectifiers**. Potassium channels may thus be divided into three groups: the two-transmembrane domain inward rectifiers, the four-transmembrane domain pore channels, and the six-transmembrane domain voltage-gated channels.

Ion channels rank among the most fundamental transmembrane molecular constituents. The cellular influx of monovalent ions influences cell volume and electrical conductivity, whereas the influx of divalent cations modulates enzyme activity. Since neuromuscular and renal epithelia are key ion-transporting tissues, clinical disorders of channel function (**channelopathies**; Table 7.2) often affect the nervous system or kidneys.

Membrane transit via carrier proteins may be energy-dependent or energy-independent. These mechanisms are respectively termed active transport (involving pumps or exchangers; for example, **glucose–galactose cotransporters**) and facilitated diffusion (e.g., involving **glucose transporters**). The latter process occurs down a concentration gradient by a valve-like mechanism (Figure 7.10). In contrast, active transport involves large pumping movements of the transmembrane domains.

Pumps use the chemical energy of ATP to move ions between cell compartments. Certain pumps undergo autophosphorylation (P) of a conserved aspartate residue in the central catalytic domain, and are thus termed **P-type ATPases**: these include Ca^{2+}-ATPase, Na^+/K^+-ATPase, and gastric H^+/K^+-ATPase. Of note, P-type ATPases lack a structural motif called the **P-loop** that is found in other ATPases and GTPases.

Exchangers or antiporters are bidirectional pumps. Ion-coupled membrane transport proteins (secondary transporters) use energy supplied by pre-existing transmembrane ion gradients to shift solutes or toxins against concentration gradients: examples include the **sodium-glucose cotransporter** (mutated in **glucose-galactose malabsorption**) and a bacterial transporter implicated in antibiotic resistance. The **sodium/hydrogen exchanger** (Na^+/H^+ antiporter), which comes in six isoforms, protects cells from acidosis (e.g., during ischemia) by actively extruding hydrogen ions. Under such circumstances the rise in intracellular sodium triggers reciprocal activation of the Na^+/Ca^{2+} exchanger – leading to a secondary rise in intracellular calcium

Table 7.2. Channelopathies

Clinical disorder	Protein affected	Phenotype	Transmission mode
Episodic ataxia type 2 (acetazolamide-responsive), familial hemiplegic migraine, spinocerebellar atrophy type 6	Calcium channel (cerebral P/Q type, voltage-dependent, α_{1A}-subunit, CACNA 1A)	Episodic or chronic ataxia, epilepsy	AD
Familial hypokalemic periodic paralysis	Calcium channel (muscle, α_1-subunit)		
Cystic fibrosis	Chloride channel (CFTR)	Viscid secretions: pulmonary and pancreatic insufficiency	AR
Bartter syndrome	Chloride channel (renal)	Normotensive, hyper-reninemic, hypokalemic alkalosis	AR
Dent disease, X-linked recessive hypophosphatemic rickets	Chloride channel, (CLC-5, outward-rectifying, renal)	Familial hypercalciuric nephrolithiasis	XR
Episodic ataxia type 1	Potassium channel	Ataxia, myokymia (rippling muscles)	AD
Benign familial neonatal convulsions	Potassium channel (KCNQ2)	Recurrent clonic fits in infancy	AD
Long QT syndrome (type 1)	Potassium channel (cardiac, slow, voltage-gated)	Syncope, sudden death	AD
Long QT syndrome (type 3)	Sodium channel (cardiac; SCN5a)	Syncope, sudden death	AD
Hyperkalemic periodic paralysis, paramyotonia congenita	Sodium channel (muscle, α_1-subunit)	Weakness, myotonia	AD
Pseudohypoaldosteronism type I	Sodium channel (epithelial: α,β and γ subunits)	Hypotension	AR
Liddle syndrome	Sodium channel (epithelial: β and γ subunits)	Low-renin hypertension (pseudohyperaldosteronism)	AD
Gitelman syndrome	Sodium-chloride transporter (renal, thiazide-sensitive)	Bartter-like syndrome	AR
Generalized epilepsy with febrile seizures	Sodium channel, voltage-gated β_1 subunit	Recurrent seizures	AR
Hypophosphatemic rickets, hypercalciuria	Sodium-phosphate transporter	Rickets	AR
Glucose-galactose malabsorption	Sodium-glucose transporter 1	Failure to thrive	AR
Renal glycosuria	Sodium-glucose transporter 2	Positive dipstick test for glycosuria	AD, AR
Cystinuria type I	Dibasic amino acid transporter (apical, renal)	Semi-opaque renal stones	AR
Distal renal tubular acidosis	Anion exchanger (basolateral, renal)	Nephrocalcinosis, renal calculi	AD
Nephrogenic diabetes insipidus, non-X-linked	Aquaporin-2 water channel	Polyuria	AD, AR

which may result in cell death (pp. 383–4). The diuretic **amiloride** inhibits the Na^+/H^+ exchanger, leading to renal sodium (and water) losses unaccompanied by intracellular potassium retention (hypokalemia); i.e., this is a potassium-sparing diuretic. Newer amiloride derivatives such as **cariporide** and **eniporide** are being used prior to ischemia or reperfusion (e.g., before **coronary angioplasty**) in an effort to attenuate the expected rise in intracellular calcium and thus limit infarct size.

PHARMACOLOGIC FOOTNOTE

Anti-influenza chemotherapy

The integral envelope protein **M2** of influenza virus exhibits pH-dependent monovalent proton channel activity. When the virus is endocytosed into the endosomal

Enrichment reading

Bedtime reading

Loewenstein WR. *The touchstone of life: molecular information, cell communication, and the foundations of life*. Penguin, London, 1998

Library reference

Ashcroft FM. *Ion channels and disease: channelopathies*. Academic Press, New York, 1999

Summary

Hydrophobic membranes divide cells into compartments. Surface glycolipids protect and insulate cells. Bacterial cell wall transpeptidases bind β-lactam rings.

Intercellular information is exchanged by cell contact. Cells communicate via connexins. Vesicles shuttle proteins between cell compartments.

Solutes cross membranes via pumps. Ion channels are transmembrane protein pores. Transmembrane ionic flux is gated by voltage or ligands. Transporters use ions to drive macro molecular transit.

QUIZ QUESTIONS

1. Explain the consequences of the lipid-rich structure of membranes.
2. Describe how proteins insert into membranes and assume their correct orientation.
3. What are some possible effects of cell contact? How are these mediated?
4. Name some different kinds of intercellular junctions and their functions.
5. Give examples of diseases caused by the abnormal functioning of ion channels?
6. Describe mechanisms by which channels are extracellularly or intracellularly activated.
7. Summarize the molecular pathophysiology of cystic fibrosis.

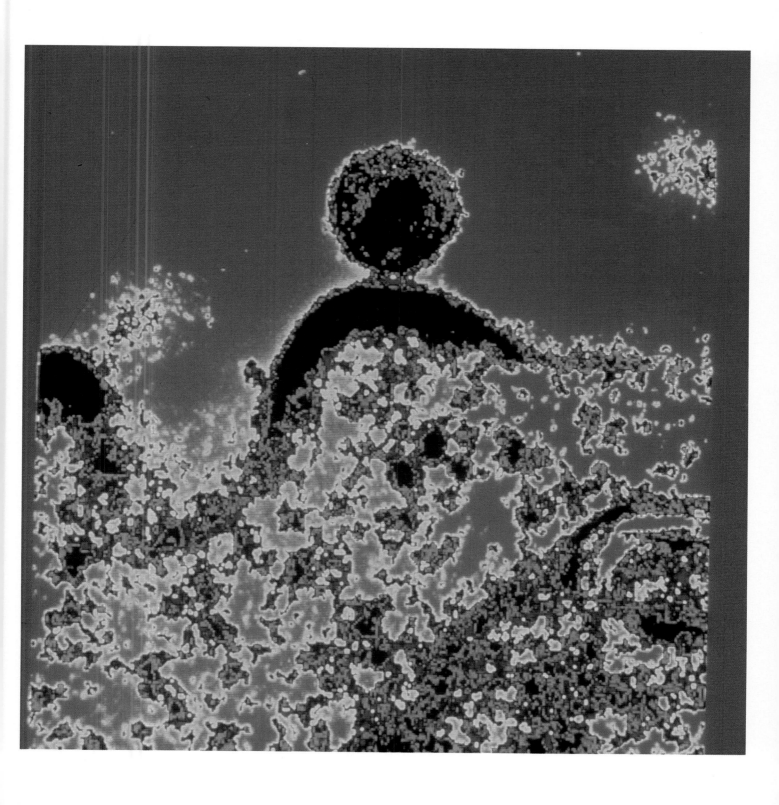

8

Figure 8.1 (*previous page*) Human immunodeficiency virus (HIV). The virus binds to CD4 receptors on the surface of helper T cells, thereby gaining entry to the cell interior via a process of internalization. (National Medical Slide Bank, Wellcome Trust Photographic Library, no. 12260).

To communicate at the cellular level, multicellular organisms must have ways of making intercellular contact. The human body contains about ten trillion (10^{13}) cells (actually, it contains far more than that – but most of those additional cells are bacteria!). All these cells need to talk to each other, and to this end have evolved elaborate networks of cell-surface recognition and signaling molecules as described below.

Cell-surface receptors

Extracellular events trigger intracellular signaling

The surface of the plasma membrane is studded with proteins inserted into the bilayer which connect the extracellular space with the cytoplasm. This network of integral membrane proteins enables cells to sense what happens around them. Transmembrane proteins are stabilized by the insertion of a hydrophobic domain(s) into the amphipathic lipid environment of the membrane bilayer (Figure 8.2): since there are no hydrogen donors or acceptors in the membrane, the hydrogen bonding of transmembrane domains needs to be fully satisfied within the main chain of the peptide itself. Membrane-spanning domains fulfill this requirement for internal hydrogen bonding by adopting repeating main chain secondary structures of bundled α-helices or β-barrels in the presence of apolar side chains. Bacteria have exploited this hydrophobic effect by producing pore-forming toxins such as **α-hemolysin**, which insert tenaciously into human cell membranes via their nonpolar oligomeric β-barrel structures.

Human cells communicate with each other via two specific molecular mechanisms: first, by motility (i.e., by using a membrane-bound molecule to activate a neighboring cell's protein sensor by direct contact); and second, by secretion (i.e., by using a soluble molecule to activate a distant cell's sensor without the necessity for cell contact). In addition, however, cells may sense their environment by mechanisms other than the interaction of preformed biomolecules with specific receptors. Extrinsic stimuli such as heat, electricity, hypoxia, and mechanical force can also initiate adaptive cell responses that include the activation of nonspecific stress response pathways (p. 290). Nonetheless, most cell responses involve transmission of signals by either:

1. Changes in transmembrane ionic transport
   - Affecting the intracellular availability of Na^+, Cl^-, K^+, Ca^{2+}, H^+; or
2. Initiation of intracellular signaling by phosphorylation cascades
   - Usually dependent upon ATP or GTP.

These two modes of signaling are not mutually exclusive. Many phosphorylation events modify intracellular ionic homeostasis; similarly, alterations of ionic balance can enhance or dampen the enzymatic activity of kinases and phosphatases.

Figure 8.2 Simplified microanatomy of a transmembrane cell-surface receptor, showing the extracellular, transmembrane, and intracellular domains.

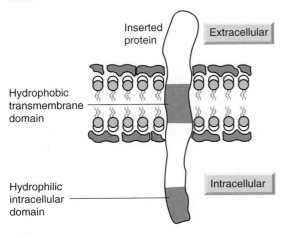

Inserted protein

Extracellular

Hydrophobic transmembrane domain

Intracellular

Hydrophilic intracellular domain

Membrane receptors

Transmembrane receptors are protein sensors that transduce extracellular information to the cell interior. The orientation of such receptors is specified by the charge of amino acid residues flanking the transmembrane domain: basic residues (arginine, lysine) tend to cluster on the cytoplasmic side. Transmembrane proteins can thus be categorized on the basis of whether their amino-terminals poke out into the extracellular space (type I membrane proteins: e.g., epidermal growth factor (EGF) receptor, insulin receptor) or into the cytoplasm (type II membrane proteins: e.g., transferrin receptor, asialoglycoprotein receptor). **Sorting** of proteins to the apical or basolateral end of cells may be signaled by post-translational modifications such as glycosylphosphatidylinositol (GPI) anchors. Cell-surface receptors occur in a variety of configurations, including:

1. **Single-transmembrane-domain receptors**
   • e.g., Most receptor tyrosine kinases.
2. **Seven-transmembrane-domain receptors**
   • G-protein-coupled receptors.
3. **Twelve-transmembrane-domain transporters**
   • e.g., Glucose transporters (the transported ligand represents the transduced signal).

In general, any molecule that protrudes from the plasma membrane into the extra-cellular space is likely to be some sort of receptor. (This may even apply to unligated ion channels, which comprise tetrameric subunits of six transmembrane domains, if the triggering stimulus is regarded as a ligand and the resultant ion flux as a receptor signaling event). Ligated receptors may diffuse laterally through the membrane when activated, leading to receptor aggregation and/or oligomerization. The cytoplasmic portion of such a protein may or may not contain a catalytic domain; if not, the signal may be transduced via a conformational change that tweaks a heterologous catalytic molecule into action.

Ligands induce conformational changes in receptors

The activation status of receptors usually depends upon the local availability of **ligands** (binding molecules). The receptor tends to be the larger molecule in this protein–protein interaction: this makes sense since the ligand tends to be just the messenger (i.e., the upstream transducer) in this pathway, whereas the receptor is the more informative signaling molecule (i.e., the downstream effector). Molecules homologous to known receptors, but for which no endogenous ligand is identified, are termed **orphan receptors**. Ligands modify receptor function in steps (Figure 8.3):

1. Ligand binding may stabilize extracellular receptor domains by causing them to fold and thus assume a high-affinity ligand-binding conformation.
2. By modifying the extracellular domain conformation, ligands may induce:
   • Transmission of an allosteric change to the intracellular domain, or
   • Relief of a negative constraint that permits receptor oligomerization.
3. By activating catalytic activity of either the receptor or a heterologous molecule, ligand binding may initiate a wave of post-translational modifications (usually phosphorylation) of receptor substrates.
4. Substrate modification may induce one of the following:
   • Binding of the substrate to another molecule.
   • Localization of the substrate to a particular cell compartment.
   • Catalytic activation of the substrate, resulting in downstream signaling.

Receptors and ligands are often expressed in low abundance, making their detection difficult. The cell may nonetheless remain sensitive to even small increments in ligand availability. This is because receptor activation triggers a self-amplifying signal transduction cascade within the cell – a transient positive feedback loop that is terminated by negative feedback (pp. 260, 280).

Not all receptors are activated extracellularly. The **steroid hormone (nuclear) receptor** superfamily is a class of receptors activated by circulating ligands that diffuse across the plasma membrane before binding target molecules in the

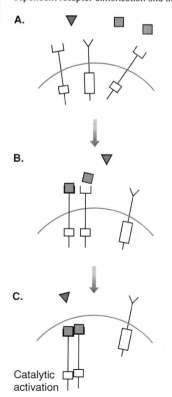

Figure 8.3 Activation of cell-surface receptor molecules by diffusible ligands. *A*, Unliganded receptors; *B*, Receptor-ligand binding; *C*, Ligand-dependent receptor dimerization and internalization.

A.

B.

C.

Catalytic activation

cytoplasm or nucleus. Like membrane-spanning receptors, however, nuclear receptors also undergo ligand-dependent receptor oligomerization.

MOLECULAR MINIREVIEW

Receptor oligomerization

Cell-surface receptors that transduce intracellular signals may do so as oligomers, including homodimers and heterodimers:

1. **Homodimeric** receptors include:
   - Ligand-activated **receptor tyrosine kinases**
     (Note that the insulin receptor subfamily remains dimeric even in the absence of insulin because of an extracellular cystine linkage.)
2. **Hetero-oligomeric** receptors, include:
   - Ligand-gated ion channels.
   - **Antigen receptors** (immunoglobulins, T cell receptors).
   - **Cytokine receptors**.
   - Heterodimeric **receptor serine-threonine kinases**.
   - **Adhesion molecules** (e.g., integrins).

Activation of catalytic receptors – which are most often kinases or phosphatases – usually involves dimerization. For example, ligand-inducible dimerization of receptor tyrosine kinases is required for receptor transphosphorylation and (thus) substrate binding and signal transduction; the process is not unlike rubbing two sticks together to spark a flame (Figure 8.3). Note that this receptor class can also heterodimerize. Although steroid hormone receptors are noncatalytic, their binding to DNA as transactivators likewise depends upon the formation of homo-dimers or heterodimers.

  Why does nature complicate life with receptor oligomers? As discussed earlier in the context of transcription factors, dimerization creates huge combinatorial possibilities – synergistic, antagonistic, and modifying – from a relatively small number of modular protein motifs. It is this enhancement of signal tuning which is the regulatory advantage of receptor oligomerization.

Transmembrane receptors are catalytic or noncatalytic

One fundamental distinction between transmembrane receptor families lies in whether they possess intrinsic catalytic activity or whether they signal by ligand-dependent structural switches (Figure 8.4):

1. Transmembrane receptors containing catalytic domains; for example,
   - Receptor protein kinases (pp. 259, 334).
2. Noncatalytic transmembrane receptors; for example:
   - Receptors activating downstream catalytic molecules
     – Cytokine receptors (pp. 303–4).
     – G-protein-coupled receptors (p. 278).

Additional criteria for subclassifying receptors are presented in Table 8.1.

  Receptors are capable of distinguishing between homologous molecules such as the pituitary octapeptides vasopressin and oxytocin. Receptors for hormones and growth factors usually bind diffusible ligands synthesized by distant or local cell networks respectively. However, the distinction between ligand families such as **peptide hormones** and **polypeptide growth factors** may be blurred. For example, hypothalamic hormones act exclusively within the local (anterior pituitary) environment; the signal-transducing properties of receptors for insulin are identical to those of growth factors; and insulin-like growth factors circulate in peripheral blood bound to carrier proteins.

Figure 8.4 Cell-surface receptors. Ion channels may be activated by voltage, ligands, or heterologous receptors. G-protein-coupled receptors are noncatalytic receptors that signal via second messengers. Cytokine receptors are also noncatalytic, but transduce signals by interaction with catalytic effector molecules. Protein receptor kinases have intrinsic catalytic activity, phosphorylating heterologous signaling molecules on tyrosine or serine/threonine. Ag, antigen; C, cytokine; GF, growth factor; Pk, protein (receptor) kinase; Tk, tyrosine kinase.

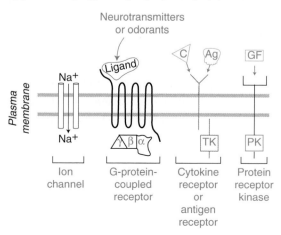

Table 8.1. Classification of receptors

1. **Ligand-binding characteristics**
   - Hormone receptors
     - e.g., Growth hormone receptor, glucagon receptor, estrogen receptor
   - Growth factor receptors
     - e.g., Nerve growth factor receptor, platelet-derived growth factor (PDGF) receptor
   - Extracellular matrix receptors
     - e.g., Hyaluronic acid receptor, integrins (pp. 222–6)
2. **Signal-transducing properties**
   - Receptor tyrosine kinases
     - e.g., PDGF receptor, insulin receptor
   - G-protein-coupled receptors
     - e.g., Vasopressin receptor, glucagon receptor
   - Ligand-gated ion channels
     - e.g., Nicotinic acetylcholine receptor
3. **Structural homology:**
   - Immunoglobulin-like receptor family
     - e.g., PDGF receptor, T cell receptor, CD4
   - Nerve growth factor (NGF) receptor family
     - e.g., Tumor necrosis factor receptor, NGF receptor
   - Steroid hormone receptor superfamily
     - e.g., Vitamin D_3 receptor, thyroid hormone (T_3) receptor
   - Cytokine receptor family
     - e.g., Growth hormone receptor, erythropoietin receptor
4. **Functional similarity:**
   - Adhesive receptors
     - e.g., T cell receptor, hyaluronic acid receptor, CD4
   - Catabolic receptors
     - e.g., Glucagon receptor, T_3 receptor
   - Pressor receptors
     - e.g., Atrial natriuretic peptide receptor, vasopressin receptor

Figure 8.5 Differential intracellular routing of newly synthesized proteins. Following the internalization of transmembrane ligand–receptor complexes by receptor-mediated endocytosis, the endosome enters the vesicular system. The vesicle contents are then routed to the lysosome for degradation, to the trans-Golgi for processing, or back to the plasma membrane (recycling). ER, endoplasmic reticulum.

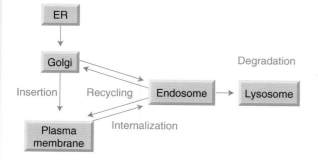

In contrast, **steroid hormones** (such as the sex hormones estrogen and testosterone) are hydrophobic nonpeptide cholesterol-derived molecules which circulate in a protein-bound state before binding and dimerizing intracellular transcription factors (i.e., DNA-binding nuclear steroid hormone receptors) that induce genes for local growth factor release.

Activated receptors may internalize, recycle, or degrade

Extracellular molecules communicate with the cell interior by a variety of mechanisms, including:

1. Small molecule (<1 kDa) uptake via aqueous channels or transporters.
2. Small molecule (e.g., folate) uptake via plasmalemmal vesicles or caveolae (potocytosis; p. 180).
3. Macromolecular uptake via **receptor-mediated endocytosis** involving pinocytosis of membranous endosomal vesicles (e.g., applies to LDL, transferrin, toxins, and polypeptide growth factors).

Receptor-mediated endocytosis is initiated by plasma membrane invaginations termed clathrin-coated pits. These pits contain proteins called **adaptins** which recognize tight-turning oligopeptide motifs in receptor cytoplasmic domains. The receptor–ligand complex becomes internalized within an endocytic (clathrin-coated) vesicle which then becomes uncoated and incorporated into an endosome. The endosome-bound receptor may be either recycled to the plasma membrane, or dispatched for lysosomal degradation (Figure 8.5). This pathway regulates many cell-surface receptors including those for growth factors, transferrin, and LDL.

Cell-surface receptors thus act as sensors for the presence of upstream ligands, and also propagate downstream signals. Hence, a receptor is an informative molecule that **transduces** biochemical information. A typical signal transduction cascade involves a **first messenger** or ligand (e.g., adrenaline), which causes its receptor to activate an **effector** molecule (e.g., adenyl cyclase) that triggers the release of a **second messenger** (e.g., cAMP; pp. 269–70) responsible for a common pathway of cell signaling (Figure 8.6).

This sequence of events gives rise to changes in gene expression, protein interaction and/or cell metabolism. Receptors may bind ligands with high or low affinity, leading to modification of one or more downstream substrates.

Conversations between ligands and receptors are rarely monologues. **Crosstalk** occurs between and within cells: as one molecule speaks, another is silenced. Molecules involved in cell signal transduction often **transmodulate** each other's activity in this way, streamlining communication and fine-tuning cell behavior. Such negative feedback control loops are critical for the prevention of malignant transformation.

PHARMACOLOGIC FOOTNOTE

Drugs acting via receptors

Many drugs act by binding to specific cellular receptors. Such drugs are said to be agonists or antagonists depending upon whether they mimic or block the function of the endogenous ligand. Such drugs include:

1. **Receptor agonists**
   - **Salbutamol:** β_2-adrenergic receptor agonist.
   - **Clonidine:** α-adrenergic receptor agonist (in the brain).

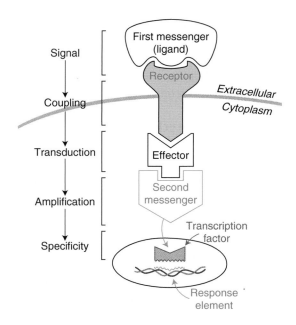

Figure 8.6 Sequence of events following the ligation of cell surface receptors. Activation of the receptor triggers effector activation, leading in turn to signaling by one or more second messengers. Most signaling cascades end at the nucleus (leading to changes in gene expression) or at the cell membrane.

Table 8.2. Proteins containing immunoglobulin-like domains

1. Antigen receptors
   - T cell receptors
   - B cell surface immunoglobulins (IgM, IgD)

2. Major histocompatibility complex (MHC) proteins
   - Formerly called human leukocyte antigens (HLA)

3. Other lymphocyte cell adhesion receptors; for example:
   - CD4, CD8
   - CD2, CD28

4. **Cell adhesion receptors**; for example:
   - N-CAM (on neurons, glia, muscle)
   - ICAM1 (binds leukocyte counter-receptors)
   - DCC (deleted in colonic cancer) and carcinoembryonic antigen (CEA; p. 211)

5. **Growth factor/cytokine receptors**; for example:
   - Platelet-derived growth factor (PDGF) receptor
   - Interleukin-1 receptor

- **Goserelin**: gonadotrophin receptor agonist often used to downregulate receptor function.
- L-**DOPA**: dopamine receptor agonist.

2. **Receptor antagonists**
   - **Tamoxifen**: estrogen receptor antagonist.
   - **Bromocriptine**: dopamine (and prolactin) receptor antagonist.
   - **Ranitidine**: histamine (H$_2$) receptor antagonist.
   - **Metoprolol**: β$_1$-adrenergic receptor antagonist.
   - **Prazosin**: α$_1$-adrenergic receptor antagonist.
   - **Losartan**: angiotensin II receptor antagonist.
   - **Ondansetron**: serotonin (5-HT$_3$) receptor antagonist.

Agonists may have weak antagonist effects, and vice versa. For example, administration of a weak opiate receptor agonist to a narcotic addict may cause acute dysphoria and withdrawal symptoms due to functional antagonism (competitive inhibition) of the stronger agonist.

Antigen recognition

Immunoglobulin-like domains make proteins sticky

A common structural motif in the extracellular portions of cell-surface receptors is the **immunoglobulin-like domain** – so-called because it was first defined in antibody (immunoglobulin) proteins. The stickiness of these domains is useful for microbial defense but exposes a cellular Achilles heel: **rhinovirus** enters cells by first binding to an immunoglobulin-like domain just as **HIV** does (pp. 483–4).

Immunoglobulin-like domains consist of a β-sheet sandwich comprising about 100 amino acids. Examples of cell-surface molecules belonging to this immunoglobulin superfamily are presented in Table 8.2. Immunoglobulins encoded by antibody genes are hypervariable structures that collectively can recognize an indefinite number of foreign **antigens**. These and other **antigen receptors** are expressed on immune cells – principally B lymphocytes (bursal cells) or T lymphocytes (thymic cells) – as follows:

1. Extracellular antigen receptors
   - **Immunoglobulins** (Ig), or antibodies
     - Expressed on the surface of bone-marrow-derived B lymphocytes, or secreted into the circulation by plasma cells.
     - Bind **native** antigens which are diffusible in the extracellular space,
   - Multisubunit **T cell receptors** (TCR)
     - Expressed on the surface of thymus-derived T lymphocytes.
     - Bind processed (linear) antigens presented at the cell membrane.
2. Intracellular antigen receptors
   - **Major histocompatibility complex** (MHC) proteins
     - Are intracellular antigen receptors that transport processed antigens to the cell surface but do not participate in antigen internalization.
3. T cell membrane **coreceptors**
   - **CD4** and **CD8**
     - Bind MHC proteins and thus participate in antigen presentation (Figure 8.7).

The immunoglobulin-like domains in these molecules confer adhesive properties. Such molecules may communicate with neighboring cells by direct contact or by interaction with secreted products in the extracellular space. For example, B cells (which express surface immunoglobulin) that recognize antigenic deter-

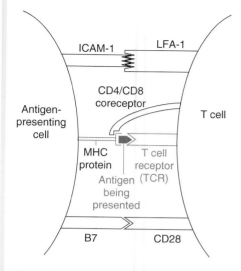

Figure 8.7 Receptor connection between a T cell and an antigen-presenting cell (APC) in response to antigen challenge. The antigen is presented by the APC to the T cell receptor (TCR) and coreceptor (CD4 or CD8, for helper or cytotoxic T cells respectively). The cell–cell interaction is further stabilized by the cell-specific B7-CD28 binding, and also by reciprocal binding of complementary adhesive molecules (p. 216). 1 CAM-1, intercellular cell adhesion molecule 1; LFA-1, leukocyte function-associated antigen; MHC, major histocompatibility complex.

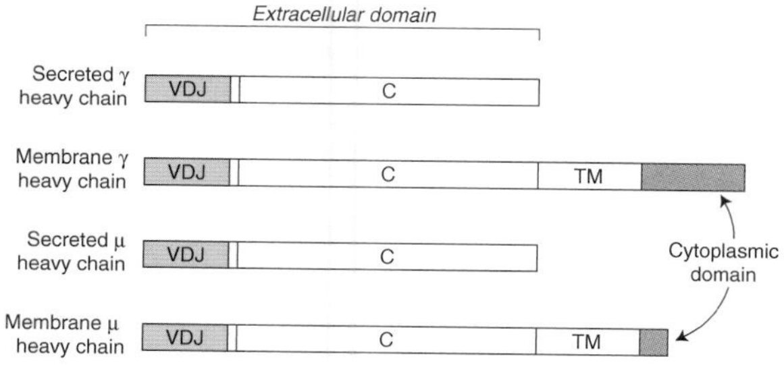

minants on the surface of foreign cells will form an intercellular **synapse** in which clustered antigen receptors efficiently acquire membrane antigens.

MOLECULAR MINIREVIEW

Leukocyte cluster of differentiation (CD) antigens
Leukocyte cell-surface proteins may be identified by raising **monoclonal antibodies** to fractionated plasma membrane components. The isolation of such antibodies enables direct determination of the target protein's molecular weight and pattern of tissue-specific expression. It also permits cloning of the molecule's gene sequence, leading to functional protein characterization.

This approach has identified numerous cell-surface molecules that have been given the designation **CD (cluster of differentiation) antigens**. Different cell types (e.g., functional T cell subgroups) are characterized by surface expression of certain CD antigens, some of which may serve more than one function; for example, CD4 and CD8 act as both adhesion molecules and antigen coreceptors (see below). Characteristics of CD molecules are shown in Table 8.3.

Hypervariable antibody loops bind complementary antigens

An immunoglobulin (Ig) or antibody is a Y-shaped molecule that consists of four disulfide-linked subunits: two 24-kDa **light chains** (κ or λ) and two effector 55- to 70-kDa **heavy chains** (γ, μ, α, δ, ε; or G, M, A, D, E), making ten possible immunoglobulins (e.g., IgG-λ, IgM-κ). These can be further divided into heavy chain subtypes such as IgA_2 (with α2 heavy chain) and IgG_4. IgG makes up 80% of circulating immunoglobulin, while IgA accounts for 12%, IgM 6%, IgD 1%, and IgE less than 1%. These immunoglobulin **classes** have distinct functions (Table 8.4).

Immunoglobulins usually circulate as monomers but some are multimeric (e.g., IgA dimers, IgM pentamers). The expression as either membrane-bound or secreted antibody isoforms may be regulated by alternative mRNA splicing (Figure 8.8). Proteolysis of the immunoglobulin **hinge region** splits the molecule into two portions (Figure 8.9):

1. Amino-terminal variable **antigen-binding fragments** (**Fab**).
2. Carboxy-terminal **crystallizable fragments** (**Fc**).

Fc fragments are bifunctional: they bind and activate **complement**, and also interact with cell-surface receptors that trigger immune effector functions.

The synthesis of a mature antibody requires several genes, each of which specifies a single region of the eventual immunoglobulin. The **variable** (V) **region** of the molecule is separated from the **constant** (C) **region** by a **joining** (J) **segment**. Unlike light chains, heavy chains also contain a **diversity** (D) **region**. Each V region (V_H plus V_L domains) contains three divergent amino acid regions termed **hypervariable loops** or **complementarity-determining regions** (CDRs), which form an antigen-binding site; in contrast, the constant (C) region binds the antibody to the cell surface. A mature antigen receptor gene transcript consists of the recombinant fusion of one V with one J region, with or without a D – that is, via **V(D)J** recombination (Figure 8.10).

The antibody's six CDRs adopt asymmetric configurations to recognize three-dimensional antigenic structure, flexibly rearranging themselves

Figure 8.8 Formation of alternatively spliced membrane-bound (B cell) and secreted (plasma cell) immunoglobulin heavy chain isoforms of IgM and IgG. C, constant region; D, diversity region; J, joining segment; V, variable region; TM, transmembrane domain.

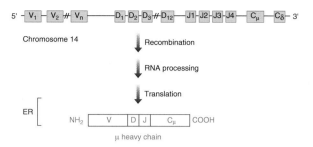

Chromosome 14

Recombination

RNA processing

Translation

ER

NH₂ [V | D | J | Cμ] COOH

μ heavy chain

Figure 8.10 Generation of antibody diversity by V(D)J recombination. ER, endoplasmic reticulum. Note that antibody light chains lack the (D) – diversity-region.

and γ (the subunit responsible for signal transduction, ligand internalization, and antigen presentation). These receptors are integral membrane proteins that belong to the immunoglobulin superfamily – a notable exception being that of the low-affinity IgE receptor **FcεRII**. A ligand for the latter molecule is the heavily glycosylated complement receptor CR2 which is the B cell portal of entry for **Epstein–Barr virus** (EBV).

The different biological activities of immunoglobulin isotypes (e.g., IgG_{1-4}; Figure 8.11) relate to differences in their target FcRs. Even within the same FcR subclass, cell-specific RNA splicing patterns may dictate functional differences. For example, the B cell isoform of FcγRII forms part of the cytoskeleton-associated membrane cap on lymphocyte activation, whereas macrophage FcγRII does not undergo capping. Experimental knockout of the murine FcR γ chain in mice results in immunodeficiency due to defects in phagocytosis and cytotoxicity.

FcRs may be secreted into biological fluids where they circulate as soluble immunoglobulin-binding factors. **High-dose intravenous immunoglobulin** (IVIG) may ameliorate symptoms in certain autoimmune disorders (e.g., **Guillain–Barre syndrome**) partly by FcR blockade and partly by accelerating the catabolism of pathogenic autoantibodies: the latter action is mediated by a β_2-microglobulin-containing transport receptor termed **FcRn**.

CLINICAL KEYNOTE

Fc receptors in human disease

Bacteria have evolved FcR-like antibody-binding proteins, and several herpesviruses also encode nonhuman IgG-binding FcR-like glycoproteins expressed on the membranes of infected cells. Higher microorganisms such as parasites (especially *Schistosoma mansoni*, *Leishmania* spp. and trypanosomes) also express FcR-like molecules on their surfaces. This evolutionary development suggests a role for such proteins in microbial pathogenicity, perhaps involving the proteolytic cleavage of bound antibody.

Bacteria also express cell-surface Fc-binding proteins structurally unrelated to FcRs: **protein A** of *Staphylococcus aureus* (used routinely in laboratory practice for polyclonal immunoglobulin purification), for example, and the IgG-binding **protein G** of *Streptococci* spp. Note that whereas antigen binds immunoglobulin via the variable regions of the antibody, protein A and protein G bind via secondary structure interactions with the constant IgG heavy chain domain.

A number of human diseases involve FcRs:

1. Susceptibility to infections in **paroxysmal nocturnal hemoglobinuria** reflects impaired immune complex clearance as a result of reduced leukocyte FcγRIII
2. The **Ebola virus** secretes a glycoprotein that binds neutrophil FcγR (CD16b), thus inhibiting neutrophil activation. It also expresses a transmembrane glycoprotein that binds endothelial cells. Hence, one virulence factor may promote infection whereas the other is responsible for the hemorrhagic phenotype.
3. Dysfunction of macrophage FcγR is associated with autoimmune diseases such as **systemic lupus erythematosus, Sjögren syndrome**, and **dermatitis herpetiformis**. Knockout of FcγR protects NZB/NZW mice (modeling systemic lupus) from autoimmune nephritis.

Rheumatoid factors are circulating IgG-binding proteins present in rheumatoid arthritis and other autoimmune diseases. These autoantibodies may arise as anti-idiotypes directed against virally induced anti-Fc receptor antibodies.

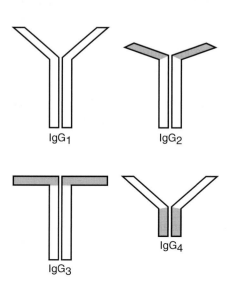

IgG₁ IgG₂ IgG₃ IgG₄

Figure 8.11 Structural variations associated with IgG isotypes 1–4.

T cell receptors

T cell receptors are multisubunit signaling complexes

B cell surface immunoglobulins (IgM, IgD) resemble another antigen-binding member of the immunoglobulin superfamily – the **T cell receptor** (TCR), which mediates nonhumoral cell-mediated immunity. TCRs are not secreted like immunoglobulins, but participate in many of the same processes including antigen binding, clonal selection, and signal transduction. The heterodimerized V_α and V_β chains of TCRs undergo genetic rearrangement similar to that responsible for the generation of antibody diversity (pp. 478–9).

T cell receptors consist of seven proteins. Unlike immunoglobulins, which recognize three-dimensional native (extracellular) antigens, TCRs bind intracellularly processed (linearized, denatured) antigens presented by MHC proteins. TCRs consist of two distinct protein complexes:

1. An antigen-recognition heterodimer composed of disulfide-linked α and β ($\alpha\beta$TCRs) or γ and δ subunits ($\gamma\delta$TCRs). This mainly extracellular complex – designated **Ti** – resembles an immunoglobulin Fab fragment. The TCR antibody-binding surface consists of hypervariable regions of the $V\alpha$ and $V\beta$ domains, which interact with foreign peptides presented by adjacent cells.

2. A subjacent complex composed of **CD3-γ, -δ, -ϵ, -ζ, and -η** (pronounced gamma, delta, epsilon, zeta, and eta respectively) subunits, some of which may be dimerized. This complex is involved in cytoplasmic TCR signaling (p. 258, Figure 11.7).

Unlike Ti, CD3 proteins contain large cytoplasmic domains. CD3 domains are structurally invariant, whereas clonotypic TCR-α and -β subunits contain variable antigen-binding regions similar to those in antibodies. Cross-linking experiments suggest a physical association between Ti-β and CD3-γ which may reflect the presence of oppositely charged amino acid moieties in the transmembrane portions of these molecules. Activated TCRs undergo ζ- and δ-subunit ubiquitination, targeting the receptor for degradation.

The first thing to note about $\gamma\delta$ (gamma-delta) **TCRs** is that they have nothing to do with γ- and δ-CD3 subunits – even though (like $\alpha\beta$TCRs) they are noncovalently associated with the CD3 transmembrane signaling complex. Antigen recognition by $\gamma\delta$TCRs appears fundamentally different from that mediated by $\alpha\beta$ T cells, with no requirement for CD4 or CD8 expression, MHCI/II antigen processing (see below) or peptide specificity. The γ and δ TCR chains are encoded on chromosomes 7 and 14 respectively, with the δ chain positioned within the α TCR chain gene locus. $\gamma\delta$ receptors are the first to be expressed during thymic development, and persist in a small proportion of peripheral T cells that lack the far more common $\alpha\beta$TCRs. Commitment of a T cell to the $\gamma\delta$ lineage is favored by the presence of a heterozygous loss-of-function mutation affecting the developmental transmembrane receptor **Notch1** (p. 404) – suggesting that signaling by the latter receptor normally maintains the predominance of $\alpha\beta$ T cells.

Mutations affecting TCR subunits may be responsible for inherited immunodeficiency states. Chromosomal translocations of both the TCR locus and the immunoglobulin-encoding loci are implicated in the development of **lymphocytic leukemias.** Polymorphisms in the V region of the TCR may also occur in **multiple sclerosis,** consistent with oligoclonal lymphocytic involvement in this disorder.

restoration of TAP expression could be therapeutically useful. However, the scarcity of clinical immunodeficiency syndromes associated with antigen transporter defects suggests complementary processing pathways.

Class II defects may result from transcriptional errors affecting either the trans-activators or promoters of the various (-DP, -DQ or -DR) molecules. Binding of antigenic peptides by MHC II is irreversible in vivo, thereby conferring a molecular memory of past antigen encounters upon the class II complex; vaccines mimic such antigenic peptides to produce a prophylactic immune response.

Experimental knockout of β_2-**microglobulin** (a component of MHC receptors; see above) expression also causes immunodeficiency in animal models. Inappropriate immune responses directed against endogenous peptide epitopes may underlie the association of certain MHC molecular combinations with a predisposition to autoimmune disorders, though this remains speculative.

Summary

Extracellular events trigger intracellular signaling. Ligands induce conformational changes in receptors.

Transmembrane receptors are catalytic or noncatalytic. Activated receptors may internalize, recycle or degrade.

Immunoglobulin-like domains make proteins sticky. Hypervariable antibody loops bind complementary antigens. Immune complexes are cleared by Fc receptors.

T cell receptors are multisubunit signaling complexes. Major histocompatibility complex (MHC) proteins present processed peptides to T cell receptors. T cell coreceptors interact with MHC proteins.

Enrichment reading

Cheap'n'cheerful

Lauffenburger DA, Linderman JJ. *Receptors: models for binding, trafficking, and signaling.* Oxford University Press, Oxford, 1996

QUIZ QUESTIONS

1. Explain some of the different ways in which cell-surface receptors work.
2. Distinguish the different mechanisms of action of the different classes of receptor proteins.
3. Discuss the manner in which named drugs act by modulating receptor function.
4. Name some members of the immunoglobulin superfamily. Do they share any functional attributes?
5. What is meant by the term CD antigen? Name three of these and their functions.
6. Explain the structure and function of a secreted antibody molecule.
7. Define the meanings of the terms idiotope and idiotype.
8. How are circulating antibody–antigen complexes cleared by the circulation?
9. What are MHC proteins? What is the meaning of the term MHC restriction?

9

Adhesion molecules and the extracellular matrix

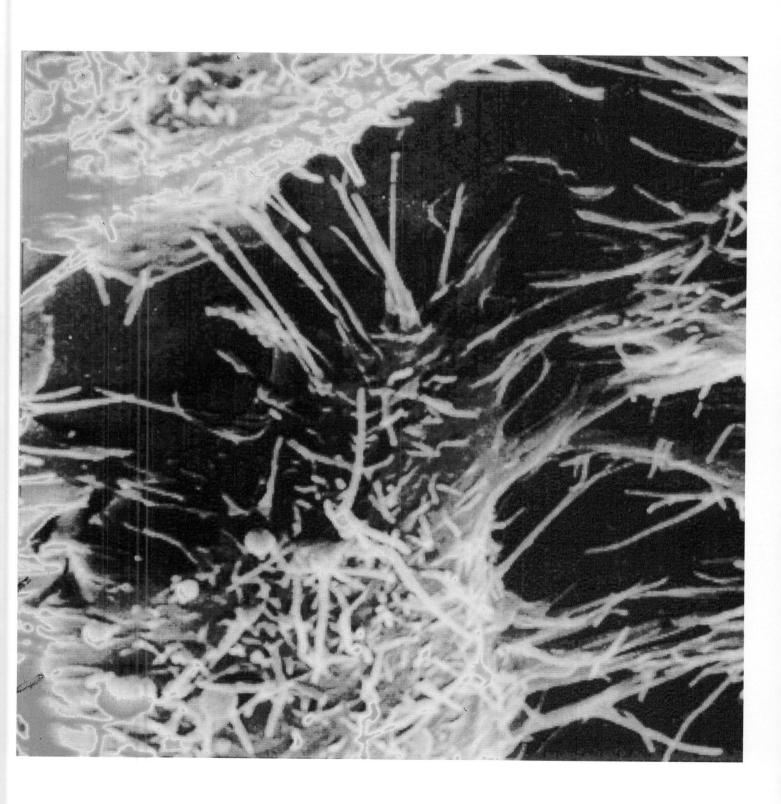

Figure 9.1 (*previous page*) Human tumor cells adhering tightly to each other in monolayer tissue culture. Color-enhanced SEM image (National Medical Slide Bank, no. N0013291C).

Cell adhesion

Cells contact each other via adhesion molecules

Cell adhesion is a mechanical necessity for multicellular organisms. Large groups of adherent cells sharing a common organ-specific function are termed tissues. The behavior of cells and tissues depends on information transfer from surrounding molecules – either those fixed to the surfaces of contiguous cells, or those diffusible within the proteinaceous **extracellular matrix** separating the cells of adherent tissues.

Adhesion to a substratum is a prerequisite for replication of many cell types, a growth requirement termed **anchorage dependence**. Conversely, many cell types will stop proliferating once a certain level of intercellular contact (confluence or crowding) has been reached: this process is termed **density-dependent growth arrest** or **contact inhibition**. Both anchorage dependence and contact inhibition are mediated by plasma membrane **cell adhesion molecules** (CAMs). Dysfunction of adhesion proteins may thus disrupt cell growth control, and contribute to cell transformation.

Cell adhesion molecules participate in **homophilic** or **heterophilic** binding interactions. Homophilic binding occurs when the extracellular domain of one CAM binds to a similar domain of the same CAM expressed by another cell, whereas heterophilic binding denotes interaction between different CAM families. Adhesion reactions between cells of the same type are termed **homotypic**, whereas **heterotypic** adhesion occurs between different lineages. Adhesive interactions that cause cell clumping are termed **aggregation** reactions. Hence, platelets may either adhere (e.g., to endothelium) or aggregate (to each other); in vitro assays distinguish defective platelet adhesion and aggregation in different diseases. Adhesion molecules fall into four major families (Figure 9.2):

1. **Cadherins** – calcium-dependent CAMs which link homotypic adhesion to cell proliferation (via intermediary molecules termed catenins).
2. **Selectins** (LEC-CAMs) – mediators of initial (weak) heterotypic adhesive events between leukocytes, platelets, and activated endothelial cells.
3. **Integrins** – heterodimeric CAMs which link heterophilic cell adhesion with the extracellular matrix and intracellular signaling.
4. **Immunoglobulin-like domain CAMs** – mediators of both homophilic and heterophilic cell adhesion.

Adhesion molecules do more than just stick together. CAMs act as both effectors and sensors of intracellular signaling, enabling adhesive interactions to be modified in response to phosphorylation events within the cell. The variety of adhesion molecules reflects functional differences between these superfamilies in terms of adhesive strength, tissue specificity, and speed of cell binding. In general, the strength of cell adhesion depends more on the number of adhesion molecules than on the affinity of CAM binding (usually weak). The main clinical pathologies involving cell adhesion molecules are: **thrombosis**, **inflammation**, and cancer **metastasis**.

Figure 9.2 The main superfamilies of cell adhesion molecules (CAMs): cadherins, selectins, immunoglobulin-like domain CAMs, and integrins.

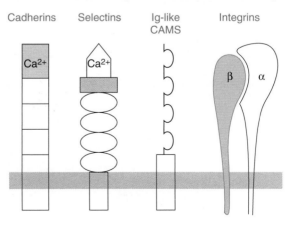

Cadherins   Selectins   Ig-like CAMS   Integrins

Carcinoembryonic antigen (CEA)

The pathologic nature of cancer metastasis implies that nonmalignant cells are constrained from growing inappropriately with respect to neighboring cells and tissues. **Carcinoembryonic antigen** (CEA) is a glycosylated adhesion molecule containing immunoglobulin-like domains. In the clinical context, CEA is often measured in serum as a marker of tumor progression or recurrence, and is sometimes of diagnostic value when measured immunohistochemically.

Normally expressed only during development, CEA mediates homotypic epithelial cell adhesion. During liver metastasis CEA also mediates heterotypic binding interactions between tumor cells and Kupffer cells: CEA exposure induces the release of pro-inflammatory cytokines (p. 300) from Kupffer cells in model systems, leading to adhesion molecule upregulation, tumor cell arrest within the hepatic vasculature, and E-selectin-dependent sinusoidal invasion. The efficiency of the latter step may in turn depend upon the extent of cancer cell surface sialylation, since sialic acid ligands activate E-selectin (p. 218). CEA may thus play a central role in cancer metastasis, particularly in the liver.

Kallmann syndrome

Patients with **Kallmann syndrome** (hypogonadotropic hypogonadism with anosmia) have problems with sex and smell. These patients have anosmia because they do not have olfactory bulbs and/or tracts, whereas their hypogonadotropic hypogonadism is caused by a deficiency of hypothalamic gonadotropin-releasing hormone. On occasion, such patients may have other neurologic abnormalities (nystagmus, mirror movements, sensorineural deafness, and claw-foot), genitourinary tract anomalies or cleft lip/palate (Figure 9.3).

This confusing collection of developmental defects reflect a mutation affecting the *KAL-1* gene on Yq11.21, which encodes a 210-kb adhesion molecule homologous to the immunoglobulin-like neural adhesin N-CAM; the encoded KAL-1 protein is developmentally involved in neuronal migration within the central nervous system. Animal knockout and fetal autopsy studies have confirmed defects in neuronal migration due to null mutations of this gene. Additional defects in neurotransmitter release and calcium channel activity are recognized in Kallman syndrome.

Other congenital neurologic disorders such as **lissencephaly** and **tuberous sclerosis** – a syndrome of mental retardation, seizures, facial rash (adenoma sebaceum), hypomelanic (ash-leaf) skin macules, and tumors of the brain, bowel and heart – may reflect abnormal adhesion molecule function during development.

Cadherins mediate homotypic epithelial cell aggregation

The **cadherin** family of glycoproteins mediates calcium-dependent adhesion. When ambient calcium is removed, the extracellular domains of these proteins bend in such a way as to trigger proteolytic degradation of the molecule. Key members of the cadherin superfamily include:

1. **E-cadherin** – the main cadherin responsible for epithelial cell adhesion; hence, the "glue" or master sculptor for epithelial morphology. It also mediates blastomere compaction in early embryos.
2. **N-cadherin** – the main cadherin responsible for neural cell adhesion; hence, mediates developmental formation of neural ganglia. It is also present in heart and lens cells.

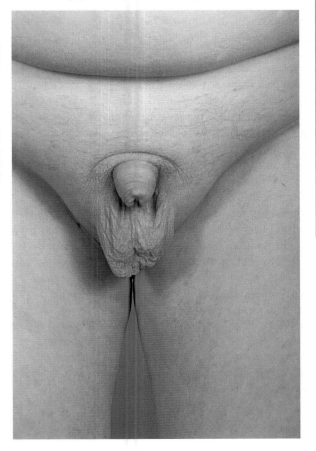

Figure 9.3 Kallmann syndrome, in which all manifestations of the disease (including hypogonadism, as shown here) appear traceable to a single mutation affecting a neural adhesion molecule (Wellcome Medical Photographic Library, no. N0008972C).

3. **P-cadherin** – the main cadherin responsible for placental cell adhesion. Cadherins act by binding other cadherins – that is, homophilic binding via an N-terminal His–Ala–Val (HAV) tripeptide leads to homotypic cell adhesion. E-cadherin is prominently expressed in adherens junctions where it creates tight membranous links between clustered cell-surface CAMs and intracellular cytoskeletal components. A rise in extracellular calcium triggers the formation of cellular projections, termed filopodia, which mediate E-cadherin-dependent membrane zippering at such junctions. Polymerized fibers of the actin cytoskeleton link these membranous puncta, triggering changes in cell shape.

Weaker adhesive forces are mediated in desmosomes by the cadherins **desmoglein** and **desmocollin**. Desmosomes are high-tensile intercellular contact points that abound in cardiac myocytes and the arachnoid layer of the meninges, where they join intermediate filaments (keratin, desmin, and vimentin; p. 238) to membrane attachment points. These cadherin-dependent junctions have little role in cell communication but confer structural integrity on epithelial tissues. **Hemidesmosomes** – which are unrelated to desmosomes – mediate adhesion of epithelia to basement membranes.

MOLECULAR MINIREVIEW

E-cadherin in cancer

During cancer development, cells lose their differentiated phenotype and begin to grow continuously and/or in the wrong place. This process involves either the acquisition of dominant (gain-of-function) mutations or the progressive accumulation of recessive (loss-of-function) mutations. Of the cell-adhesion pathways characterized, genetic abnormalities affecting the cadherin system are most clearly implicated in the pathogenesis of cancer.

The distinctive metastatic phenotype of one human breast cancer subtype that spreads preferentially to serosal surfaces (**infiltrating lobular carcinoma**) is associated with a lack of E-cadherin expression resulting from gene deletions. Prostate cancer, on the other hand, is often associated with the downregulation of E-cadherin and the reciprocal upregulation of (nonepithelial) N-cadherin protein expression. Some kindreds with **familial (diffuse) gastric adenocarcinoma** express an E-cadherin (*CDH1*) donor splice site mutation, resulting in reduced cell adhesion associated with poor tumor differentiation grade. Like infiltrating lobular breast cancer, diffuse gastric cancer is characterised by high rates of peritoneal carcinomatosis, further implicating E-cadherin deficiency in this phenotype.

Progression of **melanoma** from the radial (slow) to the vertical (fast) growth phase is often associated with a switch of expression from E-cadherin to N-cadherin. This switch inhibits interaction between transformed melanocytes and epidermal keratinocytes, but enhances interaction with (and hence invasion of) dermal fibroblasts.

Intercrossing experiments using transgenic mouse models have shown that E-cadherin knockout is accompanied by tumor invasion and metastasis, whereas wild-type E-cadherin expression arrests tumor growth at the adenoma stage. Experimental addition of extracellular E-cadherin domains inhibits homotypic cell binding and promotes tissue invasion, supporting the status of E-cadherin as an invasion suppressor. Still other cadherin knockouts are associated with an inflammatory bowel phenotype resembling **Crohn disease**.

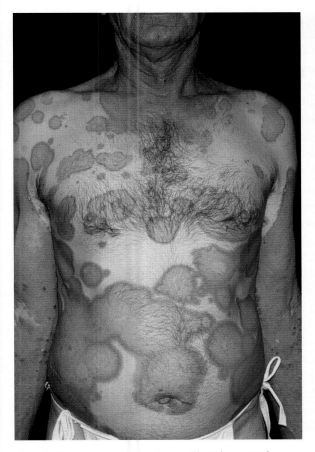

Figure 9.4 Bullous pemphigoid, a disease of hemidesmosomal molecules, shown here as a psoriasiform pattern of involvement. This disorder is sometimes induced as a distant effect of cancer elsewhere in the body (Wellcome Medical Photographic Library, no. N0003119C).

CLINICAL KEYNOTE

Desmosomes and dermatologic diseases

Viewed in cross-section, the stratified squamous epithelium of human skin resembles a brick wall glued together by cement. This wall is composed of a superficial cornified layer composed of dead epidermal cells (the stratum corneum), a basal layer of viable epidermal cells, and the subjacent basement membrane. These layers are held together by desmosomal adhesion; pathologies that disrupt this adhesion cause skin blisters. Such disorders of (hemi)desmosomes include:

1. **Pemphigus vulgaris** – a blistering disorder of old age in which autoantibodies to the desmosomal glycoprotein **desmoglein** (a cadherin) cause loss of adhesion between the basal and superficial epidermal layers (acantholysis).
2. **Pemphigus foliaceous** – another blistering disorder in which autoantibodies to desmoglein cause adhesive loss within the superficial (granular) epidermal layers, leading to fragile (flaccid) blisters. The autoantibodies play a direct role, as indicated by neonatal transmission from affected mothers.
3. **Bullous pemphigoid** – yet another blistering disorder of old age, but caused by autoantibodies to hemidesmosomal antigens (Figure 9.4). These antibodies disrupt adhesion between the basal epidermal layer and the basement membrane (i.e., at the dermo–epidermal junction), resulting in subepidermal blisters that are less fragile than in pemphigus. The disease may be more serious, however, since less normal skin remains following desquamation.

Other blistering skin diseases such as **dermatitis herpetiformis** may affect skin cell adhesion because of autoantibody deposition. The inherited skin disorder **Darier disease** is also associated with loss of desmosomal structures. Hemidesmosomal abnormalities are seen in some varieties of the inherited skin disease **epidermolysis bullosa** (see Figure 10.3). Rarely, the development of bullous dermatoses may herald the presence of an occult malignancy – raising the possibility of a neoplastic origin for autoantibody production.

Adhesion and transcription are linked by β-catenin

Intracellular cadherin domains are anchored to the inner plasma membrane by a belt-like array of proteins termed **catenins** (α, β, γ). These proteins contain motifs termed **arm repeats** which are homologous to sequences in the *armadillo* protein family of fruitflies. **β-catenin** and **γ-catenin** compete for binding to E-cadherin, whereas **α-catenin** bridges β-catenin and the cytoskeletal proteins F-actin and α-actinin (p. 239). Dysfunction or deficiency of catenins inhibits cadherin-dependent adhesion. This is illustrated by **Naxos disease** in which 17q21 deletion of γ-catenin (plakoglobin – a component of desmosomes and adherens junctions) results in woolly hair, palmoplantar keratoderma, and arrhythmogenic right ventricular cardiomyopathy.

Growth-factor-dependent tyrosine phosphorylation of β-catenin has a similar effect on epithelial cell adhesion, suggesting that constitutive growth factor signaling may transform cells not only by accelerating DNA synthesis but also by enhancing cell motility. Null mutations of the E-cadherin gene on chromosome 16q or the β-catenin gene on 3p21 activate the invasive phenotype – as does enzymatic cleavage of the E-cadherin extracellular domain – whereas invasion is suppressed by intact E-cadherin/β-catenin complexes or by cadherin overexpression. In addition to its central role in cadherin-dependent cell adhesion, β-catenin regulates the transcriptional control of cell growth via an outside-in cell signaling pathway (pp. 396–7).

The cytoplasmic abundance of β-catenin is limited in quiescent cells by **glycogen synthase kinase-3-beta** (GSK-3β) which phosphorylates it.

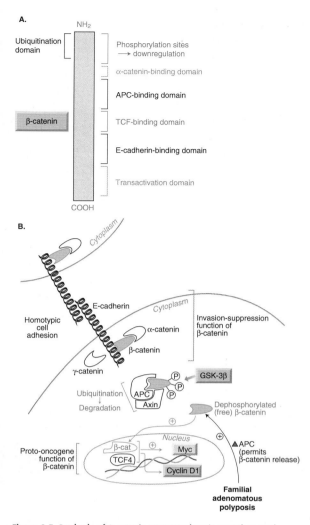

Figure 9.5 Dual role of β-catenin as a cytoplasmic growth control protein (required for the adhesive function of E-cadherin) and a nuclear growth-activating protein (required for the trans-activation of growth genes). *A*, Structure of β-catenin, showing the amino-terminal phosphorylation site responsible for its growth-factor-dependent downregulation. *B*, Invasion-suppressive (cytoplasmic) and proto-oncogene (nuclear) functions of β-catenin. GSK-3β, glycogen synthase kinase-3-beta.

Phosphorylated β-catenin forms a multiprotein complex with another arm-repeat protein – the massive **APC** (adenomatous polyposis coli; see below) gene product – as well as with **axin** (also known as conductin), triggering ubiquitination and proteasomal degradation of the APC–axin–β-catenin complex (Figure 9.5*A*). Inhibition of GSK-3β activity by extracellular ligands termed **Wnts** (pp. 396–7) inhibits β-catenin phosphorylation, permitting its dissociation from the APC complex and redirecting it from ubiquitin-dependent proteolysis to cytoplasmic accumulation and hence to nuclear translocation (Figure 9.5*B*). Some APC-bound β-catenin may also undergo nucleocytoplasmic shuttling, being returned to the cytoplasm by APC nuclear export sequences (see below). Mutations of the *Presenilin-1* gene locus (implicated in Alzheimer disease; p. 142) can likewise destabilize β-catenin, but in neurons this predisposes to cell death.

On entering the nucleus, uncomplexed β-catenin molecules promote cell survival by converting the transcription factor **TCF4** (LEF) from a repressor to an activator. TCF4-inducible gene products include the cell-cycle control proteins **cyclin D1** and **Cdk1**, the immediate-early **Myc** protein, the acid-regulatory hormone **gastrin**, the multidrug transporter **Mdr1**, and the eicosanoid receptor **PPAR-δ** (p. 441). β-catenin thus has the remarkable ability to function as a growth-control protein at the plasma membrane and yet as a transforming protein in the nucleus. In lower organisms these different functions are served by distinct β-catenin isoforms. Interestingly, β-catenin overexpression can cure baldness in mice (at the cost of inducing hair follicle tumors – trichofolliculomas – and giant hindpaws) whereas TCF4 knockout leaves them nude (and with reduced proliferating cells within intestinal crypts).

CLINICAL KEYNOTE

Heritable polyposis syndromes

Multiple steps are involved in the progression of a tumor from a benign to a malignant (invasive/metastatic) phenotype. A common benign precursor lesion is the polyp – a smooth, often pedunculated growth that mainly affects the gut, skin, nasal epithelium or larynx. Up to 75% of sporadic bowel cancers arise from adenomatous polyps; the population prevalence of the latter approaches one in three amongst individuals older than 50, and the lifetime probability of developing one is about 50%. Intestinal polyps have been intensively studied because of their association with colorectal cancer. Several heritable premalignant intestinal polyposis syndromes are recognized:

1. **Familial adenomatous polyposis** (FAP; autosomal dominant)
   - Is usually caused by mutations of the adenomatous polyposis coli (*APC*) gene, resulting in carboxy-terminal APC protein truncation.
   - Is clinically characterized by hundreds or thousands of colonic polyps appearing in early adulthood (Figure 9.6).
   - Generally results in cancer by age 40 unless prior colectomy.
   - May also cause polyps and tumors of other sites (e.g., duodenal or adrenal adenomas, periampullary carcinomas).
   - Is termed **Turcot syndrome** if a brain tumor occurs.
   - Is termed **Gardner syndrome** if mesodermal tumors (e.g., jaw fibromas, desmoids, thyroid tumors) occur.
2. **Juvenile polyposis** (autosomal dominant)
   - May be caused by mutations of either the lipid phosphatase **PTEN** or the growth factor signaling effector **SMAD4**.

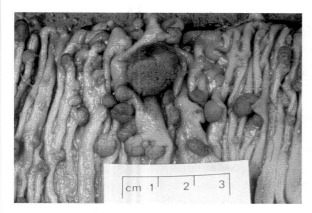

Figure 9.6 Familial polyposis coli, post-colectomy (Wellcome Medical Photographic Library, no. N0009280C).

3. **Peutz–Jeghers syndrome** (autosomal dominant)
   - Is characterized by hamartomatous small bowel polyps,
   - Gives rise to an increased incidence of gastrointestinal and breast cancers,
   - Is associated with pigmentation of lips, mouth, digits, vulva, and eyelids,
   - Is caused by germline truncating mutations of the *LKB1* gene on chromosome 19p13 which inactivate a serine-threonine-kinase regulating cell death; such mutations have not been detected in sporadic gastrointestinal cancer.

A distinct familial colon cancer syndrome, **hereditary nonpolyposis colorectal cancer** (HNPCC or Lynch syndrome, a DNA mismatch repair defect resulting from familial mutations of *MLH1* and similar genes; p. 80), tends not to cause the innumerable pedunculated pancolonic polyps characteristic of FAP. Nonetheless, up to 100 flat or pedunculated tubulovillous adenomatous polyps may occur proximal to the splenic flexure in this disorder.

Classic HNPCC and FAP each account for as few as 1% of all colorectal cancers occurring after the age of 50, but less clearcut genetic predispositions may be operative in a further 10–20% of colorectal cancer cases. *APC* somatic mutation is found in most colorectal cancer cases due to HNPCC, and transgenic knockout of *APC* increases the frequency of *MLH1*-dependent bowel tumors by 50- to 100-fold.

MOLECULAR MINIREVIEW

APC

The *APC* gene on chromosome 5q21 encodes a large (300-kDa) catenin-binding protein spanning 15 exons. A variety of mutations are characterized, many of which encode stop codons leading to protein truncation. Mutations at codon 1309 may be more potent in inducing carcinomas than are other mutations, whereas mutations amino-terminal to codon 157 produce fewer polyps. As many as 95% of FAP mutations occur in a central region 5′ to codon 1500 known as the **mutation cluster region** or MCR. APC nuclear export signals (located 3′ to the MCR) normally enable APC-β-catenin complexes to exit the nucleus, but oncogenic APC mutations delete these signals, thereby inducing nuclear accumulation of β-catenin. Mutation location may also predict whether certain extracolonic disease stigmata occur:

- **Congenital hypertrophy of the retinal pigment epithelium** (CHRPE; in 80% of patients; truncation between codons 463 and 1387).
- Mandibular osteomas or desmoid tumors (**Gardner syndrome**; truncation between codons 1403 and 1578).
- Thyroid cancers, brain tumors, and hepatoblastomas.

APC mutations may have a dominant negative effect (p. 586): single allelic defects inactivate the remaining allele by binding of the truncated protein to the wild-type molecule. Mild FAP syndromes may arise from mutations that render the *APC* allele dysfunctional but unable to bind the wild-type protein, thus abolishing the dominant negative activity and reducing disease severity. In these cases, mutations of the remaining allele may represent a second step in tumorigenesis required for polyp growth and neoplastic progression. This is consistent with the finding that *APC* mutations cause defects in chromosome segregation – presumably reflecting impaired interaction between APC, microtubules and kinetochores. Hence, the oncogenicity of *APC* mutations may derive more from the acquisition of genetic instability than from defects of β-catenin-dependent adhesion.

Up to 85% of sporadic colorectal carcinomas and adenomas harbor acquired *APC* mutations and/or allelic loss, and many of the remaining cases have β-catenin mutations. Codon 1554 is an *APC* mutational hotspot in these sporadic carcinomas. Mutations clustering around codon 1300 tend to be associated with allelic loss, whereas mutations outside this region more often give rise to protein truncation with loss of carboxy-terminal APC function. Of note, *APC* mutations in animal models have been linked to reduced gastric inflammatory responses in chronic *Helicobacter pylori* infection, which is in turn associated with **gastric cancer** development.

Inflammatory adhesins

Inflammation upregulates adhesion molecule function

Leukocytes – lymphocytes, neutrophils, monocytes, basophils, and eosinophils – are programmed to detect and eradicate trouble spots in the human body. To do this they must be able to circulate, adhere, cross endothelial (blood vessel) membranes, and assemble within lymph nodes; this ability to switch between adherent and nonadherent phenotypes requires a repertoire of adhesion molecules. Naive T cells encountering antigen for the first time rapidly express surface CD45R0 and the β_1-integrins, for example, with T cell adhesion to antigen-presenting cells maintained by ongoing expression of LFA1 and CD2. Immunoglobulin-like CAMs bind each other in homophilic or in heterophilic mode.

Cytotoxic T cell function may be inhibited by monoclonal antibodies binding to either CD2 (LFA2) or LFA3 (CD58); these molecules exhibit structural homology and chromosomal linkage, suggesting a common ancestral gene. When LFA3-expressing erythrocytes adhere in vitro to activated CD2-expressing T cells, a **rosette** of adherent erythrocytes forms around the T cell. Rosetting is used clinically as a test of lymphocyte typing and T cell function, and may be absent in immunodeficient states such as **Hodgkin disease**. The mechanism underlying rosetting is not established, though a reduction of sialic-acid-mediated negative surface charge on activated T cells has been proposed.

One of the best-characterized responses to inflammation is the transcriptional induction of the immunoglobulin-like adhesion molecule **ICAM1** in endothelial cells. Heterotypic binding of leukocytes expressing the heterophilic LFA1 integrin mediates the endothelial recruitment of inflammatory cells. The avidity of this interaction is regulated not by ICAM1, which is constitutively receptive, but by LFA1, which is post-translationally converted to a high-affinity state by T cell receptor activation. However, increased ICAM1 expression also occurs because of mRNA induction.

CLINICAL KEYNOTE

Cell adhesion and bacterial virulence

Bacterial adhesion and virulence are intimately related. The virulence of invasive bacteria such as *Shigella* spp. depends upon host cell cadherin expression, permitting adhesion of the microbe to the intestinal cell membrane. The virulence of *Salmonella* spp. likewise depends on strain-specific binding interactions with host tissues, as does that of group A streptococci which bind to extracellular matrix fibronectin (p. 227) on epithelial cells.

Uropathogenic *E. coli* contain composite fibrillar bacterial structures termed **P-pili** composed of structural proteins generically termed **pilins**. P-pili recognize **P blood group antigens** (p. 463) on urothelial cells through the binding of a bacterial adhesin termed PapG at the tip of the pilus. The pilus tip binds to hexagonally arranged urothelial membrane proteins termed **uroplakins**. Urothelial cells contacted in this way self-destruct as part of a nonimmune host defense system, but P-fimbriated bacteria overcome this epithelial shedding by tissue invasion – leading to cystitis and/or pyelonephritis. P-pili binding induces the transcription of an **iron-sensor gene** that drives continued replication of the bacterium in urine. Cranberry and blueberry juices (which contain condensed tannins termed **proanthocyanidins**) inhibit the binding of P-fimbrial adhesins to uroplakins, suggesting a novel prophylactic intervention.

Like enterohemorrhagic *E. coli* (EHEC), enteropathogenic *E. coli* (EPEC) is an attachment and effacing (A/E) pathogen. Central to the A/E virulence of EPEC is the insertion of a nonpilus adhesin designated **Tir** (translocated intimin receptor) into the plasma membrane of human intestinal mucosal cells using a secretion-like mechanism; Tir is tightly bound in turn by the bacterial cell surface protein **intimin**. Activation of inserted Tir by intimin triggers actin nucleation events (p. 240) in the host cell, leading to localized formation of actin-rich pedestals and the associated destruction of the microvillous brush border. *Yersinia pseudotuberculosis* expresses an intimin-like outer membrane protein termed **invasin** which is responsible for virulence.

Leukocytes adhere to inflamed tissues

The classic stigmata of inflammation – rubor, calor, tumor, and dolor (erythema, heat, swelling, and pain) – reflect tissue infiltration by immune cells, and may be absent in individuals with impaired immunity. Tissue inflammation is initiated by cytokines (such as interleukin-1 and tumor necrosis factor) which make vascular endothelial cells sticky by inducing the expression of adhesion molecules. The recruitment of leukocytes to such sites occurs via a series of steps involving different classes of adhesion molecules:

1. **Rolling**
   - Is the initial step in leukocyte recruitment.
   - Involves weak leukocyte adhesion to the endothelial site of inflammation.
   - Is mediated by **selectins** which slow down leukocyte transit.
2. **Adhesion**
   - Is a secondary step in leukocyte recruitment.
   - Involves strong adhesion of leukocytes to the endothelium by activation of integrin binding.
   - Is mediated by β_2-integrins.
3. **Extravasation**
   - Is a late step in leukocyte recruitment.
   - Involves migration of leukocytes through the endothelium, into the extracellular matrix and across the basement membrane.
   - Is mediated by β_1-integrins.

Inflammation can thus be viewed as a multi-step process involving: (1) the initial upregulation of endothelial selectin expression to arrest circulating inflammatory cells via weak endothelial–leukocyte adhesive events, and (2) secondary induction of leukocyte integrin expression to trigger the shear-resistant recruitment of inflammatory cells by activated endothelium. These latter interactions between endothelial immunoglobulin-like CAMs and leukocyte integrins illustrate the adhesive paradigm of CAMs binding to heterophilic **counter-receptors**.

Table 9.1. Selectins: features and functions

1. **E-selectin** (CD62E)
   – Maximally expressed on activated endothelial cells about 4 hours after an endothelial inflammatory insult (cf. E-cadherin, which is epithelial, not endothelial)
   – As with all selectins, **sialyl-Lewis^x-like sugars** (sCD15; p. 462) on neutrophils and monocytes are ligands
   – A second ligand is a **skin-vascular addressin** which localizes E-selectin to cutaneous sites of inflammation

2. **P-selectin** (CD62P)
   – Expressed in α-granules of activated platelets, and endothelial cells
   – Mediates platelet–platelet and platelet–leukocyte aggregation
   – Also mediates rolling of leukocytes in postcapillary venules during the initial inflammatory phase of leukocyte margination
   – Expressed on endothelium within minutes of an inflammatory insult, thus acting as an early warning system
   – The major neutrophil ligand **PSGL-1** is a fucosylated cell-surface glycoprotein that is bound by the parasite responsible for the tick-borne illness **human granulocytic ehrlichiosis**

3. **L-selectin** (CD62L)
   – Expressed on leukocytes
   – Facilitates the emigration of recirculating lymphocytes to peripheral nodal tissue, and recruitment of neutrophils

CLINICAL KEYNOTE

Adhesion molecules in noninfectious disease

The function of adhesion molecules is best characterized in the bloodstream where leukocytes are called upon to mediate inflammatory events. Microbial infection is a major cause of inflammation, but many noninfectious inflammatory diseases may benefit from treatments targeting adhesion molecules:

1. **Rheumatoid arthritis** and other autoimmune disorders.
2. **Adult respiratory distress syndrome** ("shock lung").
3. **Reperfusion injury** following infarction.
4. **Transplant rejection**.

It is important to note that leukocyte recruitment by CAMs occurs not only in overt inflammatory states such as the above, but also in conditions such as **wound healing**, **atherosclerosis** and **degenerative arthritis**. Elevated plasma levels of ICAM1 may be predictive of **myocardial infarction**, for example; this is consistent with both the ability of ICAM1 to recruit leukocytes to vascular endothelium and the model of arteriosclerosis as an inflammatory disease (p. 299).

Mucin-activated selectins tether leukocytes to the endothelium

The selectin family of CAMs (Table 9.1) is characterized by an extracellular domain structure comprising:

1. An amino-terminal lectin-like (**L**) domain.
2. An adjacent epidermal-growth-factor- (EGF-) like (**E**) domain.
3. Two to nine consensus repeats of complement-binding (**C**) proteins.

Selectins are thus alternatively termed LEC-CAMs. **Lectins** are molecules that bind cell-surface carbohydrate/sugar residues, and include ricin, phytohemagglutinin, and concanavalin A. Most lectins are plant-derived but some, such as the galactose-binding lectin domain of the hepatic asialoglycoprotein receptor, are expressed in human tissues. Illustrative of this, human genetic polymorphisms that reduce serum concentrations of the 32-kDa **mannose-binding lectin** predispose cystic fibrosis patients to serious infections with *Burkholderia cepacia*.

Carbohydrate ligands on the surface of such microorganisms provide high binding selectivity since their constituent monosaccharides can be repetitively *O*-glycosylated. One such endogenous *O*-glycosylated moiety, expressed in the zona pellucida of the unfertilized egg cell (p. 392), is the target of a sperm carbohydrate receptor. Many ligands that activate selectin-dependent leukocyte–endothelial adhesion are **mucins**. For example, the endothelial sialomucin **CD34** (a cell-surface marker for hemopoietic stem cells; p. 338) is a ligand for L-selectin. These heavily *O*-glycosylated proteins, of which about a dozen are known, are expressed on the surface of leukocytes and endothelial cells, and may contain immunoglobulin-like domains that further enhance heterotypic cell adhesion.

MUC1 is a hormone-regulated epithelial membrane mucin often expressed in glandular ducts such as the uterine tubes, suggesting that its antiadhesive properties might contribute to the prevention of ectopic (tubal) pregnancy. Consistent with this, low molecular weight variants of the highly polymorphic MUC1 protein are associated with female infertility due to defective embryonic implantation. In contrast, **MUC2** and **MUC7** are secreted mucins in the intestine and salivary glands respectively. Cancer cells are known to alter mucin secretion either by upregulated production, ectopic expression, or aberrant glycosylation; for example, 90% of human carcinomas express abnormally glycosylated MUC1. Moreover, since hepatic sinusoidal endothelium upregulates E-selectin expression in response to tumor cell entry, the liver-metastasizing propensity of certain cancers could relate in part to specific mucin expression phenotypes.

Unlike the sweet-toothed selectins, members of the other heterophilic cell adhesion superfamilies – immunoglobulin-like CAMs and integrins – bind nonglycosylated peptide epitopes. For example, immunoglobulin-like CAMs such as ICAM1 and VCAM1 bind leukocyte integrins such as LFA1 and VLA4 respectively during endothelial inflammation. Integrins and immunoglobulin-like CAMs thus engage in heterologous protein–protein adhesion events that replace weak selectin-dependent interactions with durable leukocyte-endothelial binding.

MOLECULAR MINIREVIEW

H-CAMs and CD44

H-CAMs are structurally unrelated to LEC-CAMs (selectins), and may be expressed on epithelial or glial cells. A key H-CAM is **CD44**, the receptor for the extracellular matrix protein hyaluronic acid (p. 226) that mediates cell aggregation. Activation of CD44 by hyaluronate enhances cell motility and tissue invasion. Of note, CD44 may also bind matrix growth factors such as **basic fibroblast growth factor** and **heparin-binding epidermal growth factor**, and is activated by sulfation induced by **tumor necrosis factor α** (TNFα). Adhesion of group A streptococci to the pharyngeal epithelium is mediated by host CD44 binding to bacterial hyaluronic acid capsular polysaccharide.

Alternative splicing of standard CD44 (**CD44s**) results in a large number of isoforms or splice variants collectively termed **CD44v**; further variation occurs because of differential glycosylation. Abnormalities of CD44 expression are associated with tumor progression, and specific variants such as **CD44v5** and **CD44v6** (which contain the exon products v5 and v6, respectively) are associated with malignant transformation. Normal nonproliferating thyroid cells express only CD44s, for example, whereas malignant thyroid cells express CD44v6 together with the β-galactosil-binding protein **galectin-3**. Such differences in molecular phenotype may facilitate distinction of benign and cancerous thyroid nodules sampled by fine needle aspiration.

Leukocyte chemotaxis is regulated by soluble chemoattractants

Chemotaxins or chemoattractants are polypeptide ligands responsible for directing leukocytes to a specific site. Chemoattractant concentration gradients trigger the extravasation of leukocytes – from either the neutrophil or monocyte lineage – across vessel endothelial basement membranes and into inflammatory tissue. Chemotactic cytokines or **chemokines** (also known as intercrines) are a family of basic 8- to 10-kDa heparin-binding ligands defined by the presence of a four-cysteine (**CXC** or **CC**) motif. Variants on this structural theme include the mucin-like natural killer (NK) cell chemokine **fractalkine**, in which the first two cysteine residues are separated by three intervening residues (**CX$_3$C**), and the two-cysteine **lymphotactin** chemokine.

Approximately 50 chemokines have been identified. **Neutrophil chemokines**, which include **interleukin-8** (IL-8; p. 298), **platelet factor 4** and **GRO** belong to the CXC (cysteine–amino acid–cysteine, or **α**) chemokine family.

Enrichment reading

Cheap'n'cheerful

Ayad S, Boot-Handford R, Humphries M (eds). *The extracellular matrix facts book.* Academic Press, New York, 1998

Library reference

Mousa SA (ed) *Cell adhesion and matrix proteins: role in health and diseases.* Springer-Verlag, Berlin, 1998

Paul LC, Issekutz TB (eds). *Adhesion molecules in health and disease.* Marcel Dekker, New York, 1999

Pearson JD (ed). *Vascular adhesion molecules and inflammation.* Springer-Verlag, Berlin, 1999

Summary

Cells contact each other via adhesion molecules. Cadherins mediate homotypic epithelial cell aggregation. Adhesion and transcription are linked by β-catenin.

Inflammation upregulates adhesion molecule function. Leukocytes adhere to inflamed tissues. Mucin-activated selectins tether leukocytes to the endothelium. Leukocyte chemotaxis is regulated by soluble chemoattractants. Chemokine receptors activate leukocyte motility.

Integrins are integral membrane proteins that integrate signals. Outside-in and inside-out signals are routed via integrins. RGD sequences in matrix proteins activate integrins.

The extracellular matrix is full of glycosaminoglycans (GAGs). Collagens are triple-helical crosslinkers and integrin ligands.

Secreted proteases attack specific substrates. Elastin maintains the tensile strength of connective tissues. Matrix metalloproteinases facilitate tissue remodeling. Cells and tissues alter phenotype via protease inhibition.

QUIZ QUESTIONS

1. Name the main classes of cell adhesion molecule, and describe any functional differences you know of between them.
2. What is a desmosome? How do desmosomal adhesive defects manifest clinically?
3. Explain some of the ways in which dysfunction of the cadherin–catenin adhesion system may contribute to cancer development or progression.
4. What are some of the molecular biologic correlates of the clinical phenomenon of inflammation?
5. Explain the steps involved in white blood cell adhesion to inflamed blood vessel endothelium.
6. Describe the process of chemotaxis, and the molecules implicated in its mediation.
7. What are chemokines, and how are they relevant to the acquired immunodeficiency syndrome (AIDS)?
8. Describe the structure of integrins, the mechanism of their activation, and the potential consequences of such activation in different tissues.
9. Correlate the structure and function of collagen molecules. What are the clinical consequences of collagen mutations?
10. Explain the developmental and pathophysiologic relevance of extracellular proteases.

Cytoskeletal proteins and molecular motors

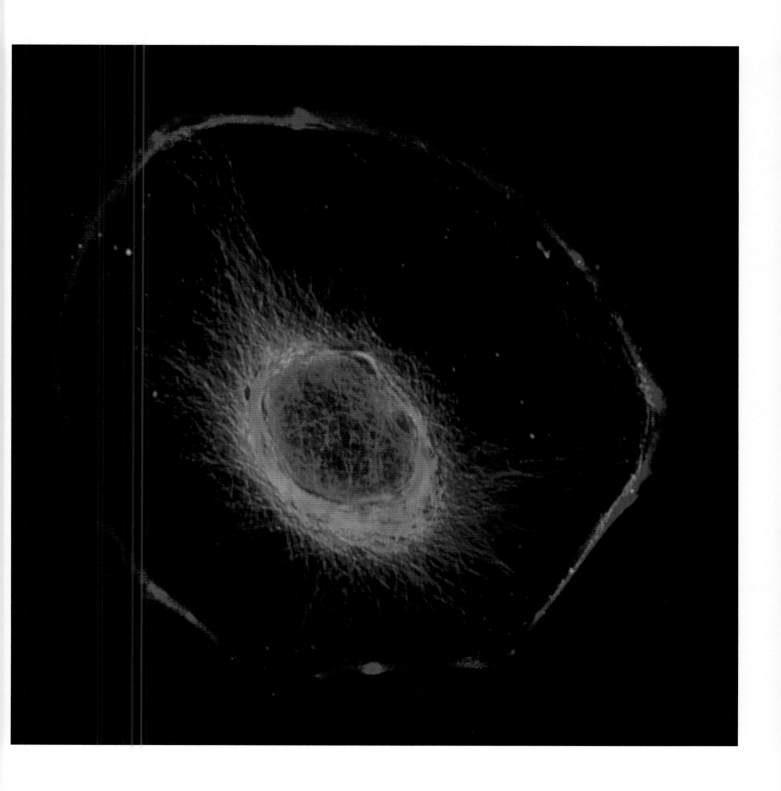

Figure 10.1 (*previous page*) Confocal microscope image of a 3T3 fibroblast cell before it divides in culture. The nucleus has been stained blue, whilst two components of the cytoskeleton, actin myofilaments and neurofilaments, are stained red and green respectively. The cytoskeleton forms the internal framework of the cell, giving it shape (Wellcome Medical Photographic Library, no. B0000103C00, Dr David Becker and K. Whitely).

Human cells express surface molecules that provide channels of communication between and within cells. Communication channels of this kind are needed to coordinate the many functions of a multicellular organism such as Man. Responses to intercellular and intracellular communication include changes in cell shape, movement and proliferation, all of which are mediated by an intracellular network of microfilamentous proteins termed the cytoskeleton; cytoskeletal proteins also mediate the processes of chromosomal condensation and separation in cell division. Here we consider how cell structure and function depend on contractile cytoskeletal proteins.

Cytoskeleton

Cytoskeletal proteins sense extracellular contacts

The cytoplasmic domains of cell adhesion molecules interact with **cytoskeletal proteins** – the filamentous web of molecules governing cell shape, division and movement (Figure 10.2). Extracellular membrane contacts are reversibly created with cytoskeletal proteins via different sets of adhesion molecules:

1. Cadherins
   - Create cell–cell contacts termed desmosomes by interacting with a class of cytoskeletal proteins termed **intermediate filaments**.
   - Create cell–cell contacts termed adherens junctions by interacting with a class of cytoskeletal proteins termed **actin microfilaments**.
2. Integrins
   - Create cell-matrix contacts termed adhesion plaques by interacting with actin microfilaments.

Adherens junctions are multiprotein membrane complexes that consist of cytoskeletal molecules such as the band 4.1 superfamily (**ezrin, talin, merlin, radixin,** and **moesin**) as well as **vinculin, tensin, paxillin,** and **zyxin.** These proteins anchor polymerized actin microfilaments or **stress fibers** to plasma membrane attachment sites. This process may be disrupted during cancer progression, when integrin- and cadherin-dependent tyrosine phosphorylation of cytoskeletal-associated proteins causes adhesion plaque dissolution and impaired intercellular communication. The lack of cytoskeletal proteins in bacterial cells explains why only eukaryotic cells are capable of membrane-dependent morphologic processes such as endocytosis, exocytosis, and cytoplasmic streaming.

Figure 10.2 Schematized interrelationship between cytoskeletal function, intracellular (signaling) and extracellular (adhesive) events.

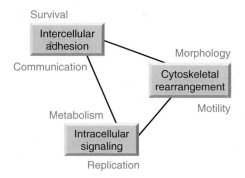

CLINICAL KEYNOTE

Marfan syndrome

Fibrillins are large 350-kDa extracellular matrix proteins that are synthesized by stromal tissues and contribute to adhesive intercellular microfibrils. Whereas normal fibroblasts produce normal microtubular bundles, fibroblasts expressing dysfunctional fibrillins produce fragmented or absent microfibrillar strands.

There are two known fibrillin genes, *FBN1* and *FBN2*. Loss-of-function mutations affecting *FBN1* on chromosome 15 are famous for causing **Marfan syndrome,** which is characterized by a tall thin physique, a high-arched palate, spidery fingers, pectus deformities, kyphoscoliosis, as well as cardiac and aortic defects. These mutations may also cause less global syndromes: ectopia lentis (optic lens dislocation), isolated familial aortic root dilatation and/or dissection, and the MASS (mitral prolapse, aortic dilatation, skeletal abnormality and skin involvement) syndrome. Mutations of *FBN2* on chromosome 5 cause a similar (though not identical) syndrome of **congenital contractual arachnodactyly**.

By virtue of their large size, both *FBN* genes are susceptible to mutation; indeed, most of the 200 or so *FBN1* mutations that have been described in Marfan syndrome have proven unique. *FBN1* exons 23–32 encode numerous epidermal growth factor-like repeats (p. 329), and mutations in this region appear more likely to cause a severe neonatal presentation. Phenotypic severity depends most critically on the net amount of FBN1 protein produced, with mutant FBN1 appearing to exert a dominant negative effect; hence, the mutant:wild-type ratio is important.

Microtubules contain GTP-dependent tubulin polymers

Cytoskeletal molecules participate in contractile events such as locomotion and mitosis. Proteins contributing to the cytoskeleton are classified into three groups based on the morphologic structures to which they contribute:

1. Microtubule (23 nm diameter) proteins
   - **α-** and **β-tubulin**.
2. Intermediate filament (10 nm diameter) proteins
   - **Keratin**,
   - **Lamin**, **desmin**, **involucrin**, **vimentin**, and **synapsin**.
3. Microfilament (6 nm diameter) proteins
   - **Actin**.

Microtubules are cylindrical structures, each one of which is composed of 13 **α-tubulin** and **β-tubulin** heterodimers. These tubular structures exhibit polarity (handedness: + and −) as defined by the perinuclear (−) and peripheral (+) cell regions. Microtubules maintain cell morphology by the GTP-dependent polymerization of monomeric tubulin. However, tubulin also possesses intrinsic **GTPase** activity which permits tubulin depolymerization and hence microtubule relaxation. GTP binds to both α- and β-tubulin, but β-tubulin prevents access of water molecules to the GTP-binding site of α-tubulin, thereby blocking GTP hydrolysis at that site.

The GTP-dependent locomotive properties of microtubules fuel the beating of cilia and flagella, facilitate intracellular transport of membranous organelles and proteins (e.g., between the endoplasmic reticulum and the Golgi apparatus), and enable chromosomal movement during cell division. Cilia are wispy microtubule-rich organelles that beat rhythmically to propel the movement of cochlear hair cells and respiratory tract mucus. Viewed in cross-section, cilia contain an internal structure termed an axoneme, which consists of nine microtubular rods surrounding two central microtubules; each axoneme comprises about 250 proteins. Sperm cells contain motile axoneme-containing organelles termed flagella, which are longer than cilia and may become dysfunctional because of axonemal protein mutations (pp. 248–9, 396).

Cell division requires the destabilization of microtubules, which is induced by the binding of a cytosolic phosphoprotein termed **stathmin** to tubulin. Overexpression of dephosphorylated stathmin blocks cell division, consistent with high stathmin expression levels within neurons. Tubulin polymers may also be stabilized by **microtubule-associated proteins** or MAPs. Smaller (45–65 kDa) MAPs termed **tau** proteins (see below) are expressed in neural tissues within growing axons, whereas larger MAPs localize to dendrites.

Prolonged stabilization of microtubules may be pharmacologically induced by tubulin-binding yew bark derivatives termed **taxanes** (e.g., **paclitaxel**), or else inhibited by antimitotic spindle poisons such as **colchicine** and **vincristine**.

The antihelminthic drug albendazole selectively inhibits tubulin polymerization in parasitic worms such as trichuris, ascaris, strongyloides, and hookworm.

MOLECULAR MINIREVIEW

Tau and tauopathies

Microtubules are normally stabilized by heat-resistant stress-inducible phospho-polypeptides collectively designated **tau** (τ) proteins, these being one subtype of microtubule-associated protein (MAP). Diseases resulting from abnormal tau structure or function may be generically designated **tauopathies**. In **Alzheimer disease**, for example, tau proteins are truncated by alternative mRNA splicing, leading to precipitation within nerve cell bodies to form neurotoxic insoluble **paired helical filaments** that impair axonal transport. Abnormal phosphorylation of tau in this context yields a higher molecular weight species (A68) which is present in the brains of heat-shocked animals as well as in Alzheimer disease. Since tau hyperphosphorylation precedes the development of the neurofibrillary tangles characteristic of Alzheimer pathology, such phosphorylation may prevent tau binding to microtubules and thus trigger its deposition into tangles.

Cytoplasmic aggregation of tau also occurs in the autosomal dominant syndrome of **hereditary frontotemporal dementia** which arises because of tau gene mutations on 17q21. Many of the responsible mutations occur at the 5′ intronic splice site downstream of exon 10; such mutations are believed to disrupt the structure of a primary RNA stem-loop, leading to abnormal tau transcript splicing. Other tauopathies include **Pick disease** and **progressive supranuclear palsy** (Steele–Richardson syndrome).

Tau is normally phosphorylated by **glycogen synthase kinase-3β** (GSK-3β). Inhibition of this kinase by the psychoactive drug lithium allows tau to dephosphorylate and thus re-associate with microtubules.

Intermediate filaments maintain cell integrity

If microtubules are the spokes and inner tubes of the cell, filamentous cytoskeletal proteins contribute the connecting wires and strings. **Intermediate filaments**, of which there exist over 60 different genetic types, are high-tensile fibrous polymers that maintain cell shape and protect plasma membranes. Approximately 1% of total body protein is composed of intermediate filaments, but this rises to 80% in neural and epidermal tissues. All intermediate filament proteins adopt a ropelike structure consisting of two α-helical chains arranged head-to-tail as a coiled-coil dimer: these dimers array themselves to form antiparallel fibrils which in turn intertwine to form the 10-nm filamentous fiber.

Keratins are the largest family of intermediate filaments, comprising more than 30 subtypes. The keratin superfamily can be divided into two subgroups:
1. **α-keratins**
   • The major keratin in skin, hair, and nails.
2. **β-keratins**
   • The β-pleated sheets found in silk.
Keratins reach out to neighboring cells via filament extension to desmosomal cell junctions. Keratin expression is characteristic of epithelial cells: epidermal keratinocyte basal layers express keratins 5 (K5) and 14 (K14), whereas suprabasal layers express K1 and K10. Hair-specific keratins are cysteine-rich

and hence covalently cross-linked to yield a rigid cytoskeleton: having a "perm" to create a new-wave hairstyle involves breaking the disulfhydryl linkages between these keratins. A nonkeratin intermediate filament protein in epidermal cells is the α-helical molecule **involucrin** which acts as a cross-linker in the cornified envelope of keratinocytes.

Keratins are insoluble and hence durable. These properties contrast with the short intracellular half-lives (30 minutes) of other intermediate filaments such as the **lamin** family, which mediates phosphorylation-dependent nuclear envelope formation and dissolution, and **vimentin**, a protein phosphorylated during mitotic reorganization of the cytoskeleton in mesenchymal and brain cells. This tendency to phosphorylation of intermediate filament proteins suggests a nonpolymeric mechanism for protein interaction. Intermediate filaments are also abundant in neurons (neurofilaments) and in astrocytes and Schwann cells where they are composed of a **glial fibrillary acidic protein** (GFAP) network that requires vimentin for assembly. **Synapsins** are cytoskeletal-associated phosphoproteins in nerve terminals that regulate actin polymerization and hence neurotransmitter release (p. 497).

Immunohistochemical detection of vimentin can help to distinguish sarcomas (positive staining) and undifferentiated carcinomas (negative staining). A structurally related molecule in muscle is the intermediate filament protein **desmin**, mutations of which may give rise to myofibrillar fragility associated with skeletal myopathy and cardiomyopathy.

CLINICAL KEYNOTE

Intermediate filament proteins in disease

Mutations of the *K14* and *K5* keratin genes give rise to the blistering skin condition **epidermolysis bullosa simplex** in both humans and mice; this disorder is characterized by basal layer cytolysis (Figure 10.3). Mutations affecting *K9* cause the palmoplantar blistering disorder **epidermolytic palmoplantar keratoderma**, which is characterized by suprabasal cytolysis and clumping of keratin filaments. Other disorders relating to keratin mutations include **pachyonychia congenita** (hair and nail dystrophy; mutations of *K6, K16, K17*); **Meesmann corneal dystrophy** (*K3, K12*), and **white sponge nevus syndrome** (affects esophagus; mutations of *K4, K13*).

Increased expression of K6 and K16 are characteristic of hyperproliferative skin lesions such as chronic blisters or **psoriasis**. Expression of these keratins facilitates the migration of keratinocytes over the skin wound.

Intermediate filament proteins are implicated in the phenotype of certain malignancies. For example, Reed–Sternberg cells (the cytopathologic hallmark of **Hodgkin lymphoma**) over express the protein **restin**, whereas colorectal carcinogenesis is associated with mutations of the cytoskeletal protein **MCC** (mutated in colorectal cancer). Some cases of **amyotrophic lateral sclerosis** (motor neuron disease) may be caused by mutations affecting neurofilaments.

Actin is a microfilamentous protein with ATPase activity

Actin microfilaments – best known for making up the thin filaments of muscle cells, but in fact ubiquitous in human tissues – are polymeric macromolecules that constitute 10–20% of all cell protein. Most of the important architectural molecules in the cell are linked by actin, which is thus a key morphologic determinant (Figure 10.4). A housekeeping gene product, actin is used as a positive control in experimental studies of gene expression.

Figure 10.3 Epidermolysis bullosa, due to a keratin mutation (Wellcome Medical Photographic Library, no. N0004663C)

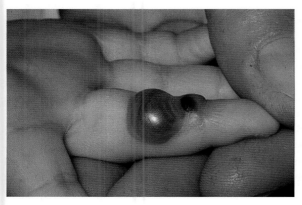

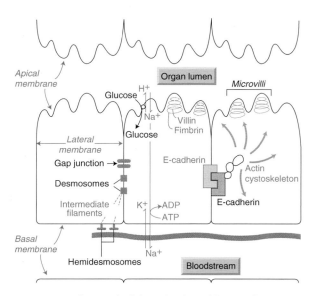

Figure 10.4 Unification of cellular molecules and functions by cytoskeletal molecules (actin microfilaments, intermediate filaments, and microtubules).

Figure 10.5 Transformation of actin via phosphorylation and polymerization. ATPase-dependent hydrolysis of ATP triggers polymerization of monomeric F-actin.

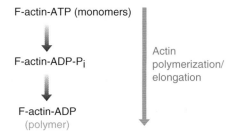

Just as tubulin is a major component of cilia, so is actin a key constituent of intestinal microvilli. However, actin differs from tubulin in two key respects: first, actin filament stability is ATP-dependent rather than GTP-dependent; and second, actin microfilaments exist as a cross-linked meshwork rather than as discrete tubular structures. Polymerization of actin involves two steps – **nucleation** (the rate-limiting step) and **elongation** – which affect different isoforms of the molecule:

1. **Nucleation** begins as a salt-inducible change in configuration affecting **g**lobular (monomeric) **G-actin**, which makes up 50% of cell actin.
2. G-actin is converted to asymmetric filamentous (polymeric) **F-actin**, which then undergoes **elongation**.

There are at least six human actin isoforms (either cytoplasmic or muscle) encoded by separate genes. F-actin is the central cytoskeletal component. Microfilamentous F-actin polymers are stabilized by calcium and ADP, whereas unpolymerized G-actin is stabilized by magnesium and ATP – the extent of interconversion depends on the ATPase properties of the actin molecules involved. Since ATP–actin has a higher affinity for the ends of filaments, the elongation of actin is promoted in an ATP-dependent manner (Figure 10.5). Cellular deformation in some experimental systems is associated with dephosphorylation of tyrosine residues within actin.

The behavior of actin is regulated by **actin-binding proteins**. Monomeric G-actin is bound by a small (15 kDa) actin-binding protein termed **profilin**, which promotes actin polymerization at uncapped barbed ends. Polymerized actin microfilaments are severed by calcium-activated actin-binding proteins such as **gelsolin** or the brush border protein **villin**; the latter molecule can also catalyze polymerization of G-actin, hence maintaining the architecture of microvilli in gut epithelial cells. In nonmuscle cell types, actin severing by gelsolin and villin induces a relaxation of cell shape and thus enhances phagocytosis and cell motility; gelsolin may also terminate actin polymerization by **capping** the barbed (growing) F-actin end. **Thymosin β4** is another actin-binding protein which maintains cellular pools of actin monomers by sterically preventing spontaneous polymerization.

CLINICAL KEYNOTE

Actin in human diseases
Although it is a housekeeping gene product, actin is implicated in a number of human disease states:

1. Massive tissue injury may release large amounts of F- and G-actin into the circulation, leading to microfilament-induced vascular obstruction with life-threatening consequences in conditions such as **septic shock, malaria, adult respiratory distress syndrome**, and **fulminant hepatic necrosis**.
2. The development of circulating pathogenetic autoantibodies in conditions such as **chronic active hepatitis** (smooth muscle antibodies) and **postcardiac injury syndrome** (cardiac muscle antibodies) may reflect intravascular actin release following tissue damage.
3. Failure of actin severing due to a gelsolin point mutation results in **familial amyloidosis** (Finnish type; p. 139).
4. The ability of gelsolin to sever filamentous actin may prove to be significant therapeutically in **cystic fibrosis**, in which high levels of filamentous actin in secretions cause tenacious sputum and pancreatic insufficiency.

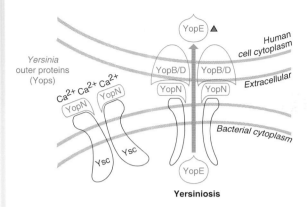

Figure 10.6 Mechanism of damage to the actin cytoskeleton mediated by the *Yersinia* outer protein (Yop) YopE, which is injected into the host target cell. Ysc, a *Yersinia* transmembrane protein.

Actin-dependent cell movement is usually achieved by the formation of spikes (parallel filaments: filopodia) or sheets (orthogonal filaments: lamellipodia). The extension of lamellipodia is accelerated by thymosin β4 (see above), thereby enhancing cell migration; relevant to this, the overexpression of thymosin β4 is associated with the metastatic behavior of certain human cancers.

In *Yersinia* spp. – the vector of **bubonic plague**, among other disorders – immunity to phagocytosis (i.e., virulence) within colonized lymphoid organs is conferred by a battery of secreted *Yersinia* outer protein (**Yop**) molecules including the actin-depolymerizing cytotoxin **YopE** which is upregulated by bacterial contact with host cells (Figure 10.6).

A congenital multigene deletion disorder termed **Williams syndrome** arises in part because of the deficiency of a kinase that phosphorylates and thus activates the actin-depolymerizing protein cofilin (see below): the resulting defect in developmental axonal migration causes a visuospatial cognitive defect and mental retardation.

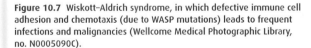

MOLECULAR MINIREVIEW

WASP

The autosomal recessive immunodeficiency disorder **Wiskott–Aldrich syndrome** (WAS; Figure 10.7) is caused by loss-of-function mutations affecting the Wiskott-Aldrich protein or **WASP**, which is selectively expressed in hemopoietic cells. WASP is an actin-binding protein that induces the formation of adhesive contacts by macrophages, neutrophils, platelets, and lymphocytes during the chemotactic response to bacterial infection; this action of WASPs reflects stimulation of the actin-nucleating activity of the actin-related protein 2/3 (**Arp2/3**) complex. WASP-expressing cells normally synthesize podosomes in response to the secretion of bacterial chemoattractants. These adhesive structures are absent in WAS patients, leading to defective chemotaxis and impaired immunity.

In neural cells the combination of phosphatidylinositol (4,5)-bisphosphate (PIP$_2$) and the small GTPase **Cdc42** (p. 284) induces filopodia formation by binding to **N-WASP** – a profilin-binding WASP homolog expressed mainly in the nervous system. On binding to Cdc42, N-WASP induces actin depolymerization – revealing free barbed ends of actin which in turn polymerize to form long actin microspikes. Another actin-depolymerizing phosphoprotein, **cofilin**, mediates the membrane-ruffling and lamellipodium-inducing effects of the small GTPase **Rac** (p. 284); the latter complexes with a WASP-related protein termed **WAVE**.

Figure 10.7 Wiskott–Aldrich syndrome, in which defective immune cell adhesion and chemotaxis (due to WASP mutations) leads to frequent infections and malignancies (Wellcome Medical Photographic Library, no. N0005090C).

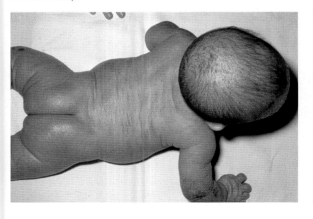

CLINICAL KEYNOTE

VASP and listeriosis

The virulence of the intracellular bacterial pathogen **Listeria monocytogenes** depends on tissue invasion. *Listeria* moves through the host cell cytoplasm at a speed averaging approximately 5 μm (one-half cell diameter) per minute, and is powered by an actin "rocket tail" propelled with the aid of host proteins. When the bug reaches the target cell membrane, filopodia are formed.

How does *Listeria* subvert the host cell machinery? The actin-binding protein profilin is concentrated in those parts of the cell where actin filaments are recruited to a proline-rich profilin-binding protein named **VASP** (vasodilator-stimulated phosphoprotein). The key virulence protein of *Listeria* is a **VASP-binding protein** termed **ActA**, which is expressed at that part of the bacterium's surface where the

A.

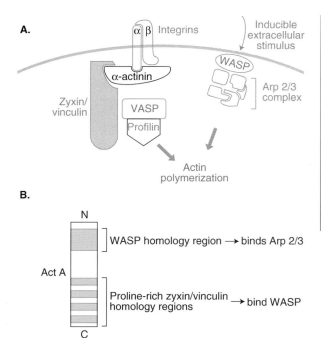

B.

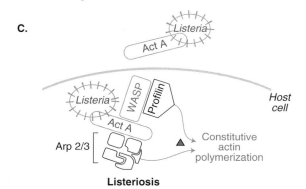

C.

Listeriosis

Figure 10.8 WASP and VASP in health and disease. *A*, Participation of WASP and VASP in normal actin polymerization. *B*, Domain structure of the ActA protein of *Listeria* spp. *C*, Pathogenic mechanism of ActA when released intracellularly by *Listeria*.

actin tail forms. By binding VASP, profilin is recruited to this part of the bacterial cell wall, producing an actin assembly nidus at this site; bacterial migration speed varies in proportion to the length of the actin tail. Distinct ActA domains are homologous to WASP and to the cytoskeletal proteins zyxin and vinculin. This explains why ActA binds to the Arp2/3 signaling complex (which cooperates with cofilin to trigger actin filament disassembly) and VASP (Figure 10.8).

This unique ability of *Listeria* to usurp host cell proteins for its own survival explains its invasive presentations: placental invasion (granulomatosis infantiseptica), gut invasion, and meningitis-meningoencephalitis (often with only a monocytic response in the cerebrospinal fluid). *Shigella dysenteriae*, *Rickettsia* spp., and vaccinia virus also exploit host cell cytoskeletal proteins to travel between cells and proliferate. *Shigella* spp. has developed functionally similar but structurally divergent genes to *Listeria* spp. (i.e., convergent evolution) that permit the polymerization of host cell actin and, thus, the bullet-like propulsion of organisms into adjacent cells.

Ankyrin anchors actin to spectrin

Cell shape, motility, and contractility are regulated by the tugging of actin on tightly bundled actin-crosslinking proteins within focal adhesions (Figure 10.9*A*). These latter molecules connect actin to proteins such as tropomodulin and tropomyosin (see below) that regulate microfilament function in cells such as erythrocytes (Figure 10.9*B*) and myocytes (Figure 10.9*C*). The family of elastomeric homologs mediating actin cross-linking includes:

1. **Spectrin**.
2. **α-Actinin**.
3. **Dystrophin**.
4. **Fimbrin**.

These spectrin-family proteins consist of two zipper-like antiparallel chains containing repetitive 106-residue units that form a three-helix bundle stabilized by hydrophobic and electrostatic interactions. While spectrin itself exists as a heterodimer (α- and β-chains) or tetramer, other members of the family are homodimeric. The β-subunit of spectrin binds a conserved membrane protein called **ankyrin**, which acts as an adaptor between the spectrin skeleton and membrane ion channels (Figure 10.10).

Different ankyrins occur in different cell lineages, an example being the 206-kDa ankyrin$_B$ which predominates in brain tissue. Note, however, that the 202-kDa red-cell ankyrin, or ankyrin$_R$, is also expressed at high level in the cerebellum. **Ankyrin-like domains** occur in a large number of multisubunit proteins where they act as molecular clothes-pegs for protein binding. Transmembrane molecules linked to spectrin by ankyrin include:

1. The **anion exchanger** (band 3; Figure 10.9*B*)
   • In red blood cells and renal collecting ducts.
2. The **voltage-sensitive sodium channel**
   • In brain, nodes of Ranvier, and neuromuscular junctions.
3. The **amiloride-sensitive sodium channel** and the **Na⁺/K⁺-ATPase**
   • In renal distal tubular cells.

Ankyrins may thus help position ion channels and other integral membrane proteins. Since the cellular distribution of spectrin can be sharply polarized – in lymphocyte caps, for example, or in association with acetylcholine receptors in neuromuscular junctions – spectrin and ankyrin may define membrane domains for co-localization of signaling molecules such as protein kinase C. Another important actin-crosslinking protein is **dystrophin**, a molecule linking glycoproteins and calcium channels that is mutated in certain X-linked **muscular dystrophies** (see below).

A. Focal adhesion

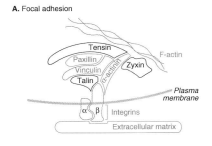

B. Red blood cell

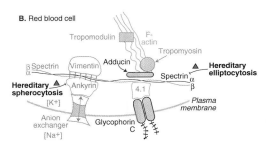

C. Muscle fiber

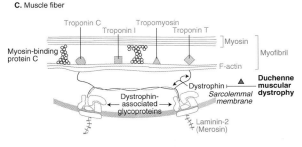

Figure 10.9 F-actin-based cytoskeletal arrangements in three different cellular contexts: *A*, Focal adhesions; *B*, Red blood cells, and *C*, Muscle cells.

Spectrin and ankyrin in hemolytic anemias

Red blood cells lack tubulin and intermediate filaments, thereby providing a simplified model of cytoskeletal organization. Hence, it may not be a coincidence that the phenotypes so far associated with spectrin and ankyrin abnormalities are hematological. Spectrin mutations are responsible for some cases of hemolytic anemia due to **hereditary elliptocytosis**, reflecting the disruption of side-chain interactions with the repetitive three-helix bundle in red cell membranes.

Erythrocyte spectrin deficiency is also associated with **hereditary spherocytosis**, but it is the *ANK1* (ankyrin$_R$) locus on chromosome 8p11 that has been most convincingly linked to this common hemolytic disorder. This suggests that spectrin deficiency may sometimes occur secondary to ankyrin dysfunction. However, gene mutations affecting both α-spectrin (on chromosome 1q22) and β-spectrin (on chromosome 14q23) have also been reported to occur in human and murine spherocytosis. Both the spectrin-binding domain and the band-3-binding domain of ankyrin are likely sites for pathogenetic mutations.

Dystrophin contacts the extracellular matrix via DAGs

Measuring in at 2400 kb – over two million base pairs – dystrophin is encoded by one of the largest known genes in the human genome. The dystrophin gene is a member of the actin-crosslinking protein superfamily that includes spectrin and α-actinin. To gain some idea of the size of this gene, consider that the cytoskeletal protein actin is encoded by a gene 3.5 kb in genomic length whereas that encoding the muscle-specific myosin heavy chain (another filamentous protein) is about 30 kb. Hence, the gene encoding dystrophin is almost a thousand-fold larger than the actin gene, and can take an entire day to transcribe. Over 98% of this gene length comprises 84 introns, some of which exceed 300 kb in length. The dystrophin mRNA transcript measures a mere 14 kb – an extremely large message (corresponding to a coding region of 11 kb) but tiny in comparison with its genomic DNA. Taking into account the size of the gene, the multiplicity of exon-intron splice junctions, and the correspondingly high likelihood of processing and replicative errors, neither the prevalence of dystrophin mutations (manifesting most notoriously as **Duchenne muscular dystrophy**, DMD) nor the 30% frequency of new mutations underlying the latter is surprising.

Dystrophin mRNA encodes an amino-terminal actin-binding polypeptide domain, a long stretch of spectrin-like repeats forming a central triple-helical rod-shaped domain, an α-actinin-like cysteine-rich domain, and a carboxy-terminal domain. Immunocytochemical studies localize this 427-kDa α-helical protein to the inner face of the myofibril cell membrane near the triad junctions uniting T-tubules and the sarcoplasmic reticulum, consistent with a role in sarcolemmal reinforcement (Figure 10.9*C*). In contrast to the length of the genomic DNA, 10 000 dystrophin proteins can be laid end-to-end across the span of a pinhead.

The membrane-anchored dystrophin carboxy-terminal domain binds an oligomeric complex of five membrane-spanning **dystrophin-associated glycoproteins** (DAGs). These DAGs connect dystrophin molecules with the extracellular matrix protein laminin, indicating that the dystrophin–DAG complex acts as a link between the sarcolemma and the extracellular matrix. One such DAG, **α-dystroglycan**, is a cell-surface receptor for the causative organism of

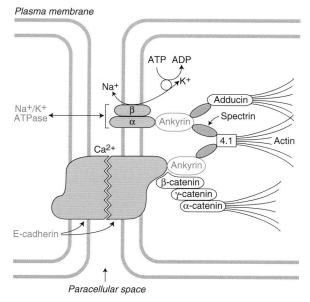

Plasma membrane

Figure 10.10 Role of ankyrin as a connecting molecule between cytoskeletal proteins such as spectrin, and surface proteins such as the anion exchanger.

leprosy, **Mycobacterium leprae**, as well as for the **Lassa** fever and **lymphocytic choriomeningitis viruses**.

Why is the dystrophin gene so large? Even massive deletions obliterating almost 50% of the amino acid sequence may cause clinically mild disease, suggesting that much of the gene is not essential for its function. Moreover, despite its size, the dystrophin polypeptide accounts for less than 0.001% of total muscle protein. What is thought of as muscle dystrophin is in fact expressed in other human tissues – notably in glial cells.

CLINICAL KEYNOTE

Duchenne and Becker muscular dystrophies

Patients with Duchenne muscular dystrophy (DMD) exhibit marked reductions of **dystrophin-associated glycoproteins** (DAGs) that parallel the primary deficiency of dystrophin, consistent with a role for dystrophin in mediating the assembly and/or integration of sarcolemmal DAGs. Conversely, the severe congenital muscular dystrophy **Fukuyama disease** arises because of a primary DAG defect that may be associated with secondary dystrophin deficiency.

A less common (1/20 000) and clinically milder syndrome than DMD is the allelic disorder **Becker muscular dystrophy** which is characterized by later onset and slower progression. Many cases present with only intermittent cramps, myalgias and elevated **creatine phosphokinase** (CPK), and affected subjects may remain ambulatory until well past middle age. In both Becker and DMD, 60–70% of cases arise because of deletions. In contrast to DMD, however, deletions in the Becker variant are almost always in-frame, whereas DMD is often characterized by truncating out-of-frame (frameshift; pp. 79–80) deletions.

DMD is characterized by the absence of dystrophin protein production: immunohistochemic confirmation of this absence generally suffices for diagnosis. Becker dystrophy, on the other hand, may be associated with normal quantities of functionally abnormal dystrophin (often suggested by an abnormal size of the message or protein on gel electrophoresis) and/or reduced quantities of normal dystrophin. In the Becker variant, amino-terminal (5′) deletions tend to be associated with more severe phenotypic deficits than are carboxy-terminal (3′) deletions; Becker patients with less than 20% normal dystrophin levels may be clinically confused with the DMD phenotype. Autosomal recessive congenital muscular dystrophy arises because of deficiencies of **merosin** (laminin α2 chain) or its receptor **integrin α7**.

Male patients with a clinical diagnosis of **limb-girdle muscular dystrophy** – a genetically heterogeneous disorder in which CPK levels tend to be elevated – should be routinely screened with dystrophin cDNA probes to exclude Becker dystrophy. **Facioscapulohumeral dystrophy** is linked to a gene on chromosome 4, whereas **oculopharyngeal muscular dystrophy** is linked to a gene on chromosome 14.

Molecular motors

NTPases regulate the movement of motor proteins

The transduction of extracellular signals to intracellular microfilaments modifies cytoskeletal organization and cell motility. Such conformational changes are driven by multisubunit proteins fueled by nucleoside triphosphate (**NTP**) hydrolysis – i.e., by dephosphorylation of ATP or GTP. By releasing this chemical energy in a controlled fashion, ATPases or GTPases

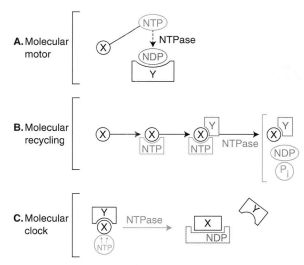

A. Molecular motor

B. Molecular recycling

C. Molecular clock

Figure 10.11 Three different usages of an NTPase. *A*, As a molecular motor; *B*, as a recycling mechanism; and *C*, as a molecular clock (see text).

(**NTPases**) act as **molecular timers** within cells. For example, ribosomal binding of aminoacylated tRNA is followed by the dissociation of a GDP-bound complex from the ribosome-bound tRNA; the correct amino acid is only incorporated into the nascent polypeptide after a proofreading delay caused by the hydrolysis of tRNA-bound GTP. Similarly, NTPase-dependent allosteric alterations may trigger changes in heterologous protein binding, leading in some instances to protein recycling.

ATP/GTP-dependent molecules can directly affect cytoskeletal contractility by acting as **protein motors** (Figure 10.11). The archetype of these motor protein complexes is **ATP synthase**, a bifunctional mitochondrial multidomain enzyme that can either synthesize or hydrolyze ATP. The water-soluble F_1 region of ATP synthase contains a rotary γ-subunit that produces three ATP molecules (from ADP) each full turn; this is functionally linked to the platform-like membrane-embedded F_0 channel which transmits protons. Energy for the F_1 synthesis reaction is provided by the F_0 transmembrane proton-motive force generated during mitochondrial oxidative phosphorylation. Under conditions of ambient ATP abundance, however, protons may be pumped through F_0 in the reverse direction to drive enzymatic ATP hydrolysis via counter-rotation of the γ-subunit. In functional terms, then, the enzyme consists of two counter-rotatory complexes (the "stator" and the "rotor") in which open, loose, and tight states correspond to absent binding, ADP binding, and ATP binding respectively.

NTPase-containing protein motors are thus **mechanoenzymes** which convert afferent chemical energy (ATP) to efferent movement, e.g., of cytoskeletal proteins. This is the converse of mechanotransduction, in which cells convert afferent kinetic energy into efferent chemical signals (p. 504). Such motor proteins include:

1. Microtubule-based motors: **kinesin, dynein, dynamin**.
2. Actin-based motors: **myosin**.

Myosin is a ubiquitous motor protein with contractile functions in muscle and nonmuscle cells alike. One myosin isoform, **myosin I**, controls membrane movement of intestinal microvilli, each of which contains a core of myosin-crosslinked actin microfilaments rooted in the terminal web of the cytoskeleton; a nuclear isoform of myosin I complexes with RNA polymerase II and may thus help to power transcription. A distinct myosin isoform, **myosin V**, regulates the movement of vesicles attached to actin microfilaments. In addition to its role in cytoskeletal contraction and cell motility, myosin-dependent ATP hydrolysis (accompanied by myosin phosphorylation) is essential for chromosomal segregation during anaphase.

MOLECULAR MINIREVIEW

Myosin, myocilin, and ciliary function

At least a dozen distinct myosin proteins are recognized, including some that mediate functions such as organelle transport, endocytosis, hearing, balance, and vision. Mutations of certain myosin subtypes (e.g., **myosins VI, VIIa, Iβ**) have been linked to heritable deafness and/or vertigo syndromes in experimental animals (e.g., Snell *waltzer* mouse). The finding of myosin mutations in **Usher 1B syndrome** supports the probable importance of these molecules in hair-cell stereocilia func-

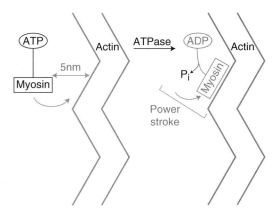

Figure 10.12 ATP-dependent mechanotransduction by actomyosin. The direction of the power stroke is indicated.

tion; in this context myosin supplies the "rope" supporting an ion channel "trap-door" required for normal auditory function (p. 505).

Primary open-angle glaucoma may be associated with *GLC1A* mutations on chromosome 1 affecting the trabecular meshwork protein **myocilin**, which is also expressed in the ciliary body, retina and muscle; the trabecular meshwork regulates aqueous humor outflow from the eye, hence determining intraocular pressure. Myocilin expression increases in parallel with intraocular pressure in response to ocular or systemic treatment with glucocorticoids.

Myosin powers muscle contraction

The contractile properties of actin are not conferred by polymerization alone, but rather depend on myosin-dependent power strokes delivered via a lever arm mechanism. During muscle contraction actin-dependent ATP hydrolysis is triggered by filamentous myosin: thin-filament F-actin molecules interact cyclically with two-headed myosin (myosin A) molecules protruding from thick filaments, forming a viscous chemomechanical transducing complex termed **actomyosin** (myosin B). Actomyosin-induced ATP hydrolysis powers the movement of myosin heads along the actin microfilament in 5-nm steps; these working strokes may be accompanied by changes in the myosin crossbridge structure that reduce intermolecular viscosity and thus enable thick and thin muscle filaments to slide past each other (Figure 10.12).

In relaxed muscle the elongated protein dimer **tropomyosin** sterically inhibits actomyosin formation. Nerve action potentials increase calcium levels within the muscle cell, releasing tropomyosin inhibition via activation of **troponin** – a regulatory complex consisting of **troponin C** (calcium-binding subunit), **troponin I** (inhibiting actomyosin ATPase subunit and, hence, crosslinking) and **troponin T** (tropomyosin-binding subunit). Each troponin molecule inactivates one tropomyosin dimer. Plasma levels of cardiac-specific troponin isoforms such as cardiac troponin-T correlate with the timing (detectable rise at 3–12 hours, peaks at 24 hours, normal after 1–2 weeks) and severity of myocardial infarction. Serum troponin levels may also be used to monitor the cardiotoxicity of anticancer drugs such as doxorubicin and the ErbB2 antibody trastuzumab. Other molecular markers of cardiac muscle necrosis following infarction include (in order of appearance) **myoglobin** (detectable after 1–3 hours), **creatine kinase** (3–12 hours), **enolase** (5–10 hours) **myosin light chain** (6–12 hours), **lactate dehydrogenase** (LDH; 10–12 hours) and **myosin heavy chain** (36–48 hours).

The largest known (molecular weight 3000 kDa, 3 megadaltons; 27000 amino acids) human protein, **titin** or connectin, prevents the overstretching of cardiac and skeletal muscle sarcomeres during adult life. Each titin molecule within the sarcomere stretches over a micrometer in length. Titin contains a catalytic (kinase) domain that phosphorylates the muscle protein **telethonin** in differentiating myocytes, thereby regulating the assembly of myosin-containing thick filaments (myofibrillogenesis). Titin may also be involved in chromosome condensation in nonmuscle cells. An analogous molecule is the 700-kDa sarcomeric protein **nebulin**, which is expressed exclusively in skeletal muscle where it is involved in thin filament assembly and maintenance.

Familial hypertrophic cardiomyopathy

Human diseases affecting voluntary (skeletal) or involuntary (smooth) muscle may reflect primary or secondary abnormalities of cytoskeletal-associated molecules involved in muscle contraction. One such condition, **familial hypertrophic cardiomyopathy** (HCM), results from missense mutations affecting a variety of sarcomeric proteins:

1. **β-myosin heavy chain** (βMHC) in 30% cases.
2. **Cardiac myosin binding protein C** (MyBPC) in 15% cases.
3. **Troponin T** in 10% cases.
4. **α-Tropomyosin** in 5% cases.
5. Rare.
   - **Myosin light chains** (regulatory or essential).
   - **α-Cardiac actin**.
   - **Troponin I**.

The prognosis of *βMHC* mutations varies with the genotype; for example, the Arg403Gln mutation is associated with 50% mortality by the age of 40. MyBPC mutations tend to be variably penetrant, present later in life (after age 50), and are associated with a relatively low risk of sudden death. Troponin T mutants can also present late, but are associated with a high risk of sudden death despite minimal hypertrophy. Chronically increased cardiac muscle cell calcium levels may contribute to sarcomere hypertrophy by activating the calcium-dependent phosphatase **calcineurin**; hence, use of the calcineurin-inhibiting immunosuppressants ciclosporin and tacrolimus (p. 487) could limit hypertrophy.

Familial myofibrillar cardiomyopathies may result from mutations affecting the intermediate filament protein **desmin**. **Congestive (dilated) cardiomyopathies** may be associated with mutations of **α-cardiac actin** (which can cause either hypertrophic or congestive cardiomyopathy), missense mutations of **cardiac β-myosin heavy chain** (Ser532Pro or Phe764Leu; no hypertrophy), deletions of **cardiac troponin T** (ΔLys210), **lamins A** and **C, dystrophin** (e.g., exon 29 deletions in X-linked cases) or **adhalin** (α-sarcoglycan), or mutations affecting the X-linked nuclear envelope protein **emerin**.

Creatine and creatinine

Muscle cells require a high-energy ATP/ADP buffering system that is provided by **creatine**, a metabolite of the amino acid arginine. **Creatine phosphate** is hydrolyzed to yield the free energy for ATP production from ADP. Creatine phosphate thus acts as a short-term muscle energy store – following its consumption, ATP is generated from aerobic metabolism (oxidative phosphorylation) or from anaerobic processes such as glycolysis and glycogenolysis.

The replenishment of creatine phosphate stores following conversion to creatine/ATP is catalyzed by **creatine kinase** (CK). Creatine kinase is an abundant enzyme in muscle, and detection of muscle-specific isozymes in serum is useful for the diagnosis of disorders such as myocardial infarction, polymyositis, and Duchenne muscular dystrophy.

Nuclear magnetic resonance (NMR) spectroscopy can detect creatine levels and phosphorylation in tissues (p. 559). NMR can thus be of diagnostic use in disorders such as the rare inborn error of metabolism **guanidinoacetate methyltransferase deficiency** – a severe infantile creatine-deficiency disorder in which creatine levels can be restored using arginine supplements.

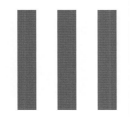

From molecular biochemistry to human cell biology

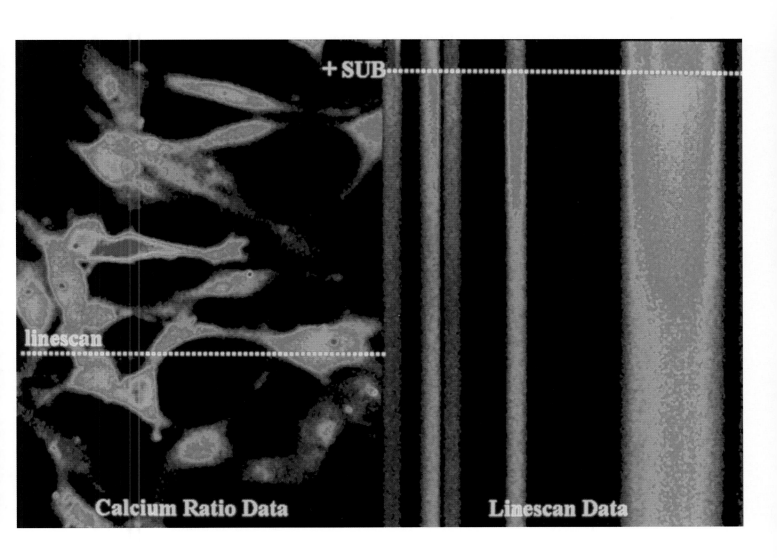

Figure 11.1 (previous page) Calcium signaling imaged by Fura-2 fluorescence (Wellcome Medical Photographic Library, no. B000462C01).

Cells communicate with each other using a simple biochemical language. If the letters of this molecular alphabet are represented by elementary constituents such as pH and reactive ions, and the words by molecules such as glucose (food) and ATP (energy), then primitive sentences – e.g., stop dividing, start moving, change metabolic state – can be thought of as the sequential interaction of signaling molecules with their receptors. Much has been learnt about the spelling (structure) of these signaling molecules, but far less is known about the grammar of the intermolecular interactions that determine the outcome of cellular conversations. This section describes the basic vocabulary of cell signaling conversations.

Signal initiation

Proteins signal via inducible phosphorylation events

Molecules transmit information to other molecules. This process, termed **signal transduction**, comprises a cascade of on–off molecular switches involving the reversible phosphorylation of tyrosine, serine or threonine residues. Such phosphorylation events (which always occur intracellularly) may affect a single critical amino acid or multiple sites within target molecules. Transferred phosphates usually originate from ATP or GTP, depending upon the specificity of the signaling superfamily involved. Molecules regulating signal transduction cascades most often belong to one of the following groups (Figure 11.2):

1. Extracellular **ligands**.
2. Cell surface **receptors**.
3. Signaling enzyme **effectors** immediately downstream of receptors.
4. Nonenzymatic cytosolic **second messengers**.
5. Nuclear **transactivators**.

The interaction of these molecules determines the tissue specificity of their effects in vivo. For example, an increase in visceral size induced by overexpression of an extracellular ligand would imply that complementary cell surface receptors are co-expressed in the target tissue.

The net outcome of phosphorylation reactions is determined by two sets of functionally opposed catalytic molecules: enzymes that catalyze phosphorylation, or **kinases**, and enzymes that catalyze dephosphorylation termed **phosphatases** (Figure 11.3). A striking genotypic difference between bacteria and humans is that the former encode very few kinases, whereas over 1% of all human genes do so.

A common feature of cell signaling cascades is that the initial stimulus is amplified by a succession of downstream events. This is particularly true of **tyrosine phosphorylation** events, which – compared with **serine-threonine phosphorylation** events – occur with relative rarity within the cell, accounting for as few as 2% of all phosphorylations. Tyrosine phosphorylation thus tends to be a decisive signaling event for cell growth. The molecules that mediate this post-translational modification are termed **tyrosine kinases**.

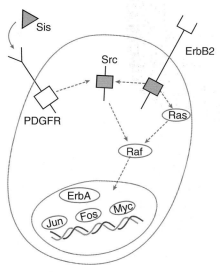

Figure 11.2 Signal transduction. A hypothetical signaling cascade involving a ligand (Sis), receptors (PDGFR and ErbB2), intermediary molecules (Ras, Src, Raf), transcription factors (ErbA), and target gene proteins (Jun, Fos, and Myc) is shown.

Figure 11.3 Cartoon depicting the reciprocal functional relationship between kinases and phosphatases. Substrate X is phosphorylated by the former and dephosphorylated by the latter.

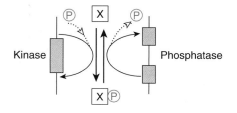

MOLECULAR MINIREVIEW

Tyrosine kinases

Two kinds of protein contain the catalytic tyrosine kinase domain: cytosolic (nonreceptor) tyrosine kinases, and receptor (transmembrane) tyrosine kinases.

Nonreceptor tyrosine kinases are intracellular proteins that lack extracellular domains but contain conserved catalytic domains. Soluble ligands modulating the activity of these nonreceptor kinases have not been isolated. There are at least ten families of cytosolic tyrosine kinases that account for about 50 proteins. These kinase families act as downstream effectors of receptor tyrosine kinases, and differ in terms of their cell localization motifs. Examples of cytosolic tyrosine kinases include the potent transforming protein **Src**, the lymphocyte signaling proteins **Lck**, **Fyn**, and **Lyn**, and the nuclear tyrosine kinase **Abl**. As noted earlier, the 125-kDa membrane-associated tyrosine kinase **Fak** (focal adhesion kinase) clusters in adhesion plaques where it is activated by cell contact in the presence of extracellular matrix proteins such as fibronectin.

Tyrosine kinases rank amongst the most potent mitogenic and transforming molecules known. Tyrosine phosphorylation of cytoskeletal-associated proteins such as **paxillin**, **tensin** and **ezrin** can cause the cell to change shape, leading to a loss of adhesion that may play a role in tumor invasion. Conversely, genes encoding other tyrosine-phosphorylated substrates – such as **β-catenin** or **α-catenin**, which positively regulate adhesion – may be mutated or deleted in **colon cancer** or **prostate cancer** respectively.

Phosphorylated amino acids bind specific target motifs

Signals are transmitted to downstream signaling molecules by two key mechanisms: allosteric switching of substrate function, or recruitment of the modified substrate to a discrete cell compartment where it will interact with other key molecules. One example of a phosphorylation-induced allosteric event is that involving the membrane enzyme **phospholipase C-γ** which becomes catalytically active following the phosphorylation of a specific tyrosine.

Phosphoprotein recruitment is a more common signal transduction mechanism than allosteric activation. Tyrosine kinases autophosphorylate (i.e., transphosphorylate within dimers) tyrosine residues on the same protein, and mutagenesis of these **autophosphorylation sites** can cause a loss of function similar to that induced by abolition of kinase activity. Receptor autophosphorylation sites recruit signaling proteins of two main kinds:

1. Enzyme substrates with signaling activity
   - e.g., Phospholipase C-γ (PLC-γ), GTPase-activating proteins (GAPs), Src.
2. Noncatalytic receptor-binding molecular **adaptors**.
   - e.g., Growth factor receptor-binding (GRB) proteins such as **Grb2**, **Grb7**, **Crk**, **Nck**, and the **p85** subunit of **phosphatidylinositol-3′-kinase** (PI3K).

Peptide recognition events focus on amino acid targeting cassettes as short as four to seven residues in length. For example, phosphorylated tyrosine residues within signaling proteins may bind substrates that are recruited to the membrane, Golgi apparatus or lysosome. A graphic example of this recruitment mechanism is provided by the microanatomy of the platelet-derived growth factor receptor (Figure 11.4). For example, tyrosine autophosphorylation of Y*XX*M motifs within such receptors leads to specific recruitment of PI3K and, hence, to all of the downstream effects associated with that signaling enzyme (p. 290).

Peptide-binding domains of this kind (Figure 11.5 and Table 11.1) are clinically relevant. Mutations of the PH domain in the **Btk tyrosine kinase** prevent correct membrane localization of this protein, for example, thus causing **Bruton agammaglobulinemia**. Similarly, mutations affecting the 40-residue WW domain in the **amiloride-sensitive epithelial sodium channel** impair its degradation, causing the hypertensive disorder **Liddle syndrome**.

Figure 11.4 Intracellular microanatomy of the platelet-derived growth factor (PDGF) β-receptor, showing the positions of critical tyrosine residues which, when phosphorylated, become binding sites for SH2-containing downstream signaling molecules. GAP, GTPase-activating protein; PI3K, phosphatidylinositol-3′-kinase; PLC-γ, phospholipase C-γ; SH-PTP2, SH₂-containing protein tyrosine phosphatase-2.

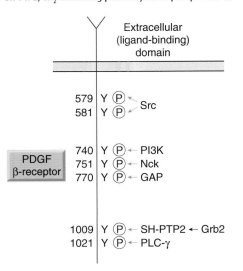

Table 11.1. Protein-sorting domains

Domain type	Target binding sequence	Function
SH2 (Src homology 2)	Phosphotyrosine + carboxy-terminal 3–5 amino acids	Recruitment of tyrosine phosphoproteins (especially to tyrosine kinases)
SH3 (Src homology 3)	Proline-rich sequences	Binding and orientation of docked proteins (especially cytoskeletal proteins)
PTB (phosphotyrosine binding)	(Phospho)tyrosine + amino-terminal β-turn, e.g., NPXY	Formation of multiprotein complexes involved in metabolism or protein degradation
PDZ (postsynaptic density protein, disks large, zona occludens)	Short serine/threonine-phosphorylated peptides with carboxy-terminal hydrophobic group (e.g., E-S/T-D-V-COOH)	Clustering of transmembrane multiprotein complexes (e.g., ion channels in synapses)
PH (pleckstrin homology)	Phosphoinositide-2/3-phosphates	Membrane association
FYVE	Phosphoinositide-monophosphates	Membrane association
WW (double tryptophan)	Phosphoserine-polyproline (PPXY, PPLP) motifs in E3 ubiquitin ligases	Ubiquitin-dependent protein degradation
WD40 (leucine-rich repeats in F-box proteins)	Phosphoserine	Ubiquitin-dependent protein degradation
FHA (forkhead-associated)	Phosphothreonine	Kinase binding and apoptosis induction as part of DNA damage response
14–3–3 (protein dimers)	Phosphoserine (or phosphothreonine), e.g., R-S-X-S-X-P	Prevention of nuclear translocation

There are many other peptide-binding domains, including **DED domains** (which mediate cell death) and **bromo domains** (which bind lysine-acetylated histones). However, the best characterized peptide-binding domains are the **SH2** and **SH3** domains.

SH2 and SH3 domains form plug-in binding sites

Src (pp60^{Src}) is an ancestral member of the tyrosine kinase superfamily. The bilobed tyrosine kinase domain is tightly conserved throughout the tyrosine kinase superfamily, and was formerly known as the SH1 (**Src homology 1**) domain. Two other conserved Src domains, which often occur within in the same molecule, are:

1. **SH2 domains**
   - Phosphotyrosine-binding sequences ≈100 amino acids long.
2. **SH3 domains**
   - Proline-binding sequences ≈60 amino acids long, which link tyrosine phosphoproteins with the downstream signaling system.

The binding of phosphotyrosine by SH2 domains involves (1) an induced fit of lysine/arginine amino groups with the aromatic tyrosine ring, and (2) hydro-

A.

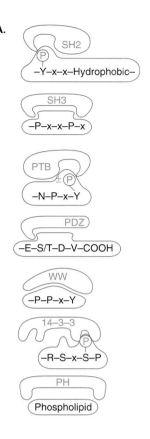

B.

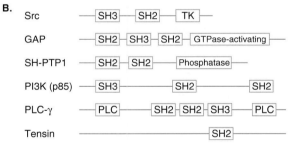

Figure 11.5 Signal domain motifs. *A*, Structure of (from top) SH2, SH3, PTB, PDZ, WW, 14–3–3, and PH domains. *B*, Domain structures of selected SH2- and SH3-containing signaling proteins, showing the multiplicity of sites.

gen bond formation between the phosphate and the SH2 sequence. The specificity of the SH2-domain binding is determined by the three to five amino acids on the carboxy-terminal side of the phosphotyrosine: for example, PI3K likes to bind Y*XX*M (phosphotyrosine-variable-variable-methionine) sequences, whereas Grb2 prefers EYINQ. This SH2-phosphotyrosine interaction resembles that between a two-pronged plug and a two-hole socket. In contrast, the binding of SH3 domains to polyproline helices resembles that of a three-pin plug. Over 125 SH2 domains have been identified by the human genome project.

Non-SH2 phosphotyrosine-binding (**PTB**) domains – often implicated in metabolic processes – bind NP*X*Y consensus sequences which mediate protein degradation. However, the phosphorylation-dependence of PTB domain binding to these tyrosine-containing target sequences is less clearcut than for SH2 domains.

SH3 domains may occur alone in some molecules, particularly in cytoskeletal proteins such as α-spectrin and myosin-1b. SH3 domains are more often sited close to an SH2 sequence, however, consistent with an adaptor function. In contrast to the behavior of SH2 domains, serine phosphorylation of SH3 domain recognition sites may cause bound proteins to uncouple. More than 250 SH3 domains have so far been identified in the human genome.

The superfamily of SH2- and SH3-containing gene products is shown in Figure 11.5*B*. Note that not all tyrosine kinase substrates contain SH2 domains, and not all SH2-containing molecules are signaling enzymes.

MOLECULAR MINIREVIEW

Src and Csk: yin and yang

Being a myristoylated protein, Src localizes to the inner leaflet of the cell membrane. Tyrosine 527 is phosphorylated when Src is present on endosomal membranes; this phosphorylation event is associated with the closed conformation of the activation loop (p. 259). In contrast, tyrosine 416 phosphorylation is associated with the open conformation of the loop, usually when Src is sited within focal adhesions. **Csk** (c-src kinase) is an SH2-containing kinase that is recruited to the membrane by a transmembrane phosphoprotein (**Cbp**, Csk-binding protein).

Phosphorylation of the Src carboxy-terminal tyrosine-527 site by Csk in turn causes snapback binding of the Src SH2 domain, thereby creating an inactivation helix that stiffens the Src kinase domain and obstructs the tyrosine-416 phosphoacceptor site, reducing kinase domain accessibility and preventing the phosphorylation of further substrates (Figure 11.6). High-affinity binding molecules such as the activated PDGF receptor may also displace Csk.

The brains of transgenic Csk knockout mice become necrotic; these mice die in utero because of the constitutive activation of Src and Fyn within the nervous system. Like Src, Fyn is strongly expressed in the central nervous system where it modulates pheromonal feeding behavior in rodents: transgenic mice with defective Fyn expression have major learning disabilities, confirming a key role for such molecules in normal brain development. Embryonic knockout of Src activity results in the phenotype of **osteopetrosis** (marble bone disease), implying a developmental role for Src in normal osteoclast function.

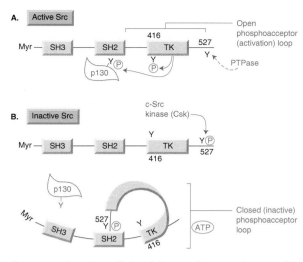

Figure 11.6 Allosteric regulation of the cytosolic tyrosine kinase Src by c-Src kinase (Csk). *A*, Active (open) configuration. *B*, Snapback (inactive) configuration due to SH2 domain binding to phosphorylated Tyr-527, preventing accessibility of substrates (e.g., p130^{Cas}) to the kinase domain. Myr, myristoylated Src terminus.

Antigens activate immune cells via cytosolic tyrosine kinases

The recognition of antigens by lymphocytes unleashes a signal transduction cascade capable of triggering both clonal expansion (proliferation) and differentiation. Key molecules in this process include:

1. Cell-surface antigen receptors
   - Surface immunoglobulins.
   - T cell receptors.
   - Fc receptors.
2. Nonreceptor tyrosine kinases downstream of antigen receptors
   - Fyn, Lck, Lyn, Btk,
   - Csk (inactivates Src, Fyn, Lck).

Unlike the secreted antibodies produced by plasma cells, B cells express membrane-bound surface immunoglobulins with vestigial cytoplasmic tails. Antigen binding to surface immunoglobulins initiates the assembly of a multisubunit complex which includes accessory molecules termed Igα and Igβ. These latter molecules contain immunoreceptor tyrosine-based activation motifs (**ITAMs**) which become phosphorylated by the Src-family tyrosine kinases **Lyn**, **Lck** and **Fyn**. Recruitment of additional tyrosine kinases (e.g., **Syk**) to these ITAMs then occurs, unleashing a self-amplifying activation cascade (Figure 11.7). A similar tyrosine kinase signaling cascade occurs in response to the ligation of Fc receptors by antigen–antibody complexes (p. 201), leading to phagocytosis, superoxide production, and the release of inflammatory mediators.

Like surface immunoglobulins, catalytically inactive T cell receptors (**TCRs**) participate in a tyrosine kinase signal transduction cascade. The crosslinking of TCRs to antigens activates independent ε- and ζ-mediated T cell activation pathways that involve the CD3-associated tyrosine kinase Fyn, the CD4/8-associated tyrosine kinase Lck, and the membrane-bound tyrosine phosphatase **CD45**. The dimeric transmembrane ζ subunit of the TCR–CD3 complex is a target of p56^{Lck} and p59^{Fyn}, with phosphorylation of ζ in turn recruiting the amplifying tyrosine kinase **ZAP-70** (zeta-associated protein) – mutations of which are responsible for CD8 lymphopenia.

Antigen-dependent T cell activation is enhanced by **B7** ligand co-stimulation (expressed by activated antigen-presenting cells) as well as by CD28 (expressed by resting T cells). In contrast, T cells may be silenced by B7-induced activation of the transmembrane T cell inhibitor **CTLA-4** which triggers intracellular phosphatase activity. Following activation by antigen or by the interleukin-2 receptor (**IL-2R**), p56^{Lck} associates noncovalently with the cytoplasmic tails of CD4, CD8 or class II major histocompatibility complex (MHC) proteins prior to downstream signaling.

Natural killer (NK) cells sense class I MHC molecules through cell-surface lectins termed **killer-cell inhibitory receptors** (KIR). These latter receptors of the immunoglobulin superfamily inhibit NK-cell-dependent cytolysis when activated: such inhibition is mediated by immunoreceptor tyrosine-based inhibitory motifs (**ITIMs**), which recruit tyrosine phosphatases. Tumors and viral infections may downregulate class I MHC proteins, leading to ITIM dephosphorylation, NK cell disinhibition, and cytotoxic killing.

Figure 11.7 Antigen-dependent signaling involving the T cell receptor (TCR). Recruitment of the cytosolic kinases Fyn and Lck to the TCR intracellular domain leads to tyrosine phosphorylation of the latter, followed by recruitment of further molecules such as ZAP-70.

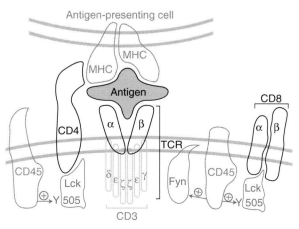

Figure 11.8 Dimeric interactions amongst different growth factor receptors. *A,* Ligand-dependent dimerization of the epidermal growth factor receptor (EGFR). *B,* Insulin receptor predimerized by extracellular domain disulfide bond formation; however, full kinase activation still requires ligand binding. *C,* Constitutive dimerization of rodent *neu* (wild-type homolog is human ErbB2) due to a carcinogen-induced mutation affecting transmembrane amino acids, thus relieving the negative constraint of the normal extracellular domain on dimerization. *D,* Constitutive dimerization of the Met (hepatocyte growth factor) receptor due to chromosomal translocation involving the Tpr gene product, leading to intracellular retention of the dimer and ligand-independent signaling.

A.

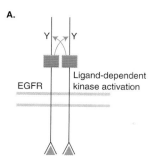

B.

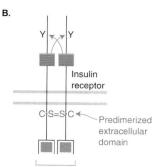

C.

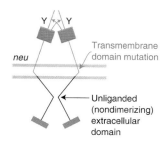

D.

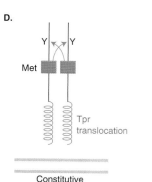

CLINICAL KEYNOTE

Bruton agammaglobulinemia

The nonreceptor **Btk** tyrosine kinase is mutated in the immunodeficiency syndrome of **X-linked** (Bruton) **agammaglobulinemia**. The Bruton tyrosine kinase (*Btk*) mutation does not directly affect kinase activity, but rather disrupts a pleckstrin homology (PH) domain linked to membrane localization; such domains are binding sites for phosphatidylinositol phosphate (PIP) membrane phospholipids. Impaired function of Btk may thus reflect a trafficking defect rather than a null mutation, in turn suggesting that the correct membrane localization of Btk plays a central role in B cell development. This phenotype illustrates that tyrosine kinases may serve functional roles distinct from cell growth.

Growth factors cause receptor tyrosine kinases to dimerize

Receptor tyrosine kinases consist of an extracellular (ligand-binding) domain, a short (20–25 residue) hydrophobic transmembrane domain, and an intracellular domain containing an ATP-binding catalytic subdomain. Such receptors are activated by polypeptide ligands, triggering a conformational change in the extracellular domain that permits adjacent receptors on the plasma membrane to cluster and oligomerize (Figure 11.8).

Ligand-dependent receptor dimerization activates intracellular kinase domains by causing the autophosphorylation of three tyrosine residues within the 30-amino-acid **activation loop**, thereby opening the conserved G–X–G–X–X–G ATP-binding site to heterologous substrates. As few as 5% of ligand-bound receptors can transmit the maximal signal, with the half-life of this response being as short as 2 min. Ligands may induce the formation of either receptor **homodimers** or **heterodimers**, with the latter being an important mechanism of signal diversification.

Autophosphorylated tyrosine residues within the receptor's cytoplasmic domain become sequence-specific binding sites for signaling substrates which may then be presented to the kinase domain for tyrosine phosphorylation. For example, phosphorylation of Tyr-992 in the EGF receptor creates a binding site for PLC-γ (in turn activated by tyrosine phosphorylation); phosphorylation of Tyr-1173 permits receptor binding of the docking protein **Shc**; and phosphorylation of Tyr-1068 allows binding of the adaptor molecule **Grb2** which in turn links to the **Ras** signaling pathway (p. 283).

Tyrosine phosphorylation cascades of this kind may culminate not only in the activation of nuclear growth genes, but also in the phosphorylation of membrane-associated proteins (e.g., β-catenin), reducing cell adhesion and increasing motility (Figure 11.9). Constitutive growth factor receptor signaling may thus promote tumor cell invasion and metastasis in addition to growth.

Over 60 receptor tyrosine kinases from 20 structural subfamilies are characterized. Receptor tyrosine kinases are usually referred to as **growth factor receptors**, but not all growth factor receptors are receptor tyrosine kinases: certain hematopoietic growth factor receptors belong instead to the cytokine receptor superfamily (pp. 303–4). By the same token, not all growth factor receptors trigger growth: the ligand for the receptor tyrosine kinase **Axl**, for example, is a vitamin-K-dependent growth-arrest-specific (*gas*) gene product. The largest single subfamily of receptor tyrosine kinases is the **Eph** kinase group, which mediates axonal guidance and fasciculation in response to membrane-anchored **ephrin** ligands.

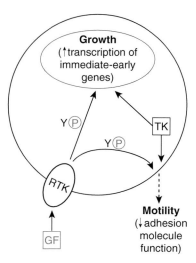

Figure 11.9 Dual targets of receptor tyrosine kinase (RTK) activity: activation of nuclear growth-regulatory genes involved in the initiation of DNA synthesis, and functional modification of membrane-associated proteins involved in intercellular adhesion and growth control. GF, growth factor; TK, tyrosine kinase.

Figure 11.10 Interaction of platelet-derived growth factor (PDGF-A or PDGF-B) ligands with PDGF receptors α or β. *A*, Binding of both ligands by PDGF receptor α, and of both receptors by PDGF-B. *B*, Receptor binding of ligand dimers by receptor dimers. Both PDGF-BB, PDGF-AA and PDGF-AB bind the α-receptor homodimer; binding of the $\alpha\beta$-receptor heterodimer requires at least one B ligand; whereas binding of β-receptor homodimers is exclusive to the BB ligand homodimer.

A.

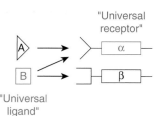

B. Dimerizing ligand combinations

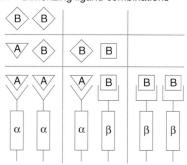

Polypeptide growth factors

Polypeptide ligands or **growth factors** (more accurately termed **peptide signaling molecules** comprise a number of structural families:

1. The **cystine knot** group
   - Nerve growth factor (NGF) group,
   - Transforming growth factor β (activin, inhibin) group,
   - PDGF, vascular endothelial growth factor (VEGF) group,
   - Human chorionic gonadotrophin (HCG) [peptide hormone: follicle-stimulating hormone (FSH), luteinizing hormone (LH), thyroid-stimulating hormone (TSH)] group.
2. The **EGF-like** growth factors
   - Epidermal growth factor (EGF), transforming growth factor α (TGFα), amphiregulin, etc. (p. 329).
3. The **β-trefoil** group (p. 333)
   - pS2; intestinal trefoil factor (ITF); spasmolytic polypeptide (SP).
4. The **four-helix bundle** group
   - Granulocyte colony-stimulating factor (G-CSF), ciliary neurotrophic factor (CNTF), interleukin-2 (IL-2), growth hormone (GH).

Receptors may have more than one ligand, and ligands more than one receptor. For example, the EGF receptor binds nine distinct ligands including not only EGF but also transforming growth factor α (TGFα) and amphiregulin. Similarly, the ligand produced by v-*sis*-transformed fibroblasts (the BB isoform of platelet-derived growth factor, PDGF) activates both the PDGFα and the PDGFβ receptors, whereas PDGF-AA activates only the α receptor (Figure 11.10). Still other "receptors" appear to have no ligand: this applies to the internalization-defective EGF receptor homolog **ErbB2**, which promotes tumor growth by impairing the degradation of heterodimerized ligand-activated receptors.

Receptor downregulation short-circuits ligand signaling

Growth factor signaling is normally terminated by the ligand-dependent degradation of catalytically activated receptors. In the unligated state, receptor activation is prevented by the extracellular domain. This constraint is relieved by ligand-induced conformational changes affecting the extracellular domain, as illustrated by mutations that constitutively activate receptors (Figure 11.11). The process of downregulation involves a series of steps:

1. Receptor tyrosine autophosphorylation (induced by dimerization) of certain sites that bind targeting proteins.
2. Receptor internalization into the cytoplasm by vesiculation.
3. Receptor trafficking through the endosomal system.
4. Receptor targeting to acidic lysosomes or proteasomes for degradation.

Receptor trafficking to lysosomes is mediated by coated-pit-related structures called **adaptins**; the hijacking of adaptins by viral proteins is implicated in tumorigenesis. But not all internalized receptors are degraded; instead, some are recycled through the Golgi and back to the cell surface.

A critical molecule determining whether a receptor is degraded is the docking of the SH2-containing RING finger protein **Cbl**, which is a ubiquitin ligase that tags proteins for proteasomal destruction. In contrast, the viral transforming protein v-Cbl fails to trigger receptor downregulation (i.e., it permits receptor recycling) and is thus implicated in the pathogenesis of certain **myeloma** and **lymphoma** cases.

The physiologic and pathologic significance of receptor downregulation

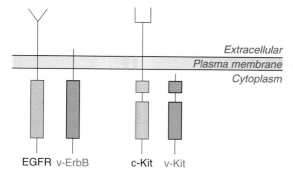

Figure 11.11 Viral transforming homologs of wild-type human gene products. On the left, the epidermal growth factor receptor (EGFR) and its (avian) virus-encoded mutant v-ErbB; and on the right, the wild-type human stem cell factor receptor c-Kit, and its viral transforming homolog v-Kit. Both viral gene products acquire transforming activity through constitutive activation of their intracellular catalytic domains, in turn reflecting deletions that eliminate the respective extracellular domains.

is further illustrated by the biology of the EGF receptor ligand transforming growth factor α (**TGFα**) (Figure 11.12). The EGF receptor (**EGFR**) is curious for having multiple ligands, amongst which TGFα is notable for its association with rapid cell growth during embryogenesis and carcinogenesis. TGFα is exquisitely sensitive to degradation by a low pH; since endosomal pH is lower than extracellular pH, TGFα dissociates from internalized EGFRs more readily than does EGF, thereby allowing EGFRs to de-dimerize and tyrosine-dephosphorylate. Since an EGFR tyrosine phosphorylation motif binds Cbl, TGFα-activated EGF receptors may preferentially recycle to the cell membrane, permitting prolonged signaling. This potentiation of ligand-dependent EGFR downregulation by TGFα may explain why tumors preferentially overexpress TGFα rather than EGF.

CLINICAL KEYNOTE

Ret, endocrine tumors, and Hirschprung disease
The *Ret* gene encodes a receptor tyrosine kinase essential for the development of neural crest cell lineages, including those that give rise to neuroendocrine lineages. *Ret* is prominently expressed in calcitonin-producing (C) cells of the thyroid gland, as well as in the parathyroid glands and adrenal medulla. The receptor is activated by the ligand **GDNF** (glial-derived neurotrophic factor) which, in structural terms, is a member of the TGFβ superfamily (though other members of this family activate serine-threonine kinases; pp. 333–4). *Ret* mutations are responsible for two unrelated groups of heritable disorders:
1. Gain-of-function mutations
   - Familial endocrine tumor syndromes, especially multiple endocrine neoplasia (**MEN**) syndromes.
2. Loss-of-function mutations
   - **Hirschprung disease**.
The following dominantly inherited syndromes of endocrine cancer are associated with germline point mutations in the *Ret* gene:
1. MEN type 2A (**MEN 2A**)
   - Medullary carcinoma of the thyroid (MTC) in 95%,
   - Pheochromocytoma (catecholamine-secreting tumor; Figure 11.13) in 50%,
   - Gliomas (brain tumors), hyperparathyroidism in 10%.
2. MEN type 2B (**MEN 2B**)
   - Pheochromocytoma, MTC, mucosal and gut neuromas.

Figure 11.12 Differential effects on EGF receptor downregulation by EGF and TGFα. Unlike the former (at left), the acid-labile TGFα ligand dissociates early from the endosomal receptor (at right) – thereby dissolving the receptor dimer and permitting receptor recycling back to the cell surface.

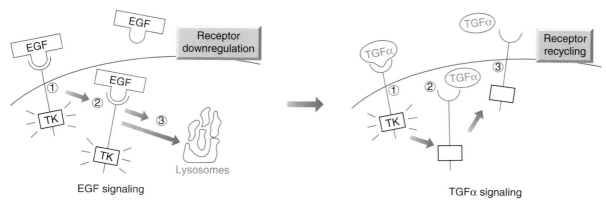
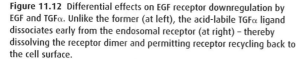

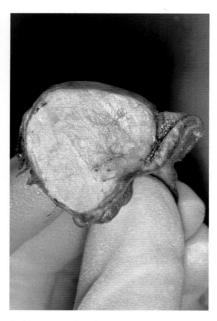

Figure 11.13 Adrenal tumor (pheochromocytoma) resected from a patient with a *Ret* mutation causing multiple endocrine neoplasia (Wellcome Medical Photographic Library, no. N0004727C).

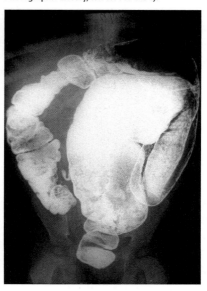

Figure 11.14 Barium enema of patient with congenital aganglionic megacolon (Hirschprung disease) due to null mutations of *Ret*, showing enormous dilatation of the left colon (Wellcome Medical Photographic Library, no. N0007447C).

3. Familial medullary carcinoma of the thyroid (**FMTC**).

The importance of normal Ret function in neuroendocrine tissues reflects its tissue-specific expression in these sites. Of note, *Ret* is the only dominantly transforming gene thus far to have been implicated in a familial cancer syndrome (most other syndromes of this kind arise because of loss-of-function mutations; p. 367).

For children of known MEN2 families, prophylactic thyroidectomy may be undertaken after the age of six following two independent confirmations of a Ret mutation, and annual biochemical screening for **pheochromocytoma** (which secretes catecholamines) and/or **parathyroid adenomas** (which secrete parathyroid hormone, thus causing hypercalcemia) is continued lifelong.

Ret mutations also account for 75% cases of Hirschprung disease (**congenital aganglionic megacolon**), a pediatric disorder of colonic motility. In this case the phenotype is recessive, resulting in loss of *Ret* function – and implying a role for *Ret* in embryonic maturation of the gut nervous system (Figure 11.14). Note, however, that extracellular domain *Ret* mutations may cause Hirschprung disease via a dominant negative mechanism. Other gene mutations which may cause Hirschprung disease include those affecting the Ret ligand GDNF, the endothelin 3 signaling system (p. 350), and the Sox10 embryonic morphogen (p. 413).

MOLECULAR MINIREVIEW

Genotype-phenotype correlations in MEN

An instructive feature of *Ret* diseases is the relationship between phenotypic and genotypic changes. Both FMTC and MEN 2A are associated with mutations that affect cysteine residues immediately extracellular to the membrane; these mutations probably relieve the negative constraint on receptor dimerization normally imposed by the unliganded extracellular domain, thereby constitutively enhancing receptor activity. Mutations in sporadic papillary thyroid carcinoma (PTC) tend to affect the juxtamembrane domain, and are again associated with constitutive tyrosine kinase activity (Figure 11.15). Tyr-1062 is the Ret-binding site for Shc and Enigma, and phosphorylation at this site is required for the Ret-transforming activity of MEN 2A/B tumors.

The mutation underlying most MEN2B cases is an exon 16 point mutation disrupting methionine-918 in the kinase domain of the receptor. Conversion of this residue to a threonine alters the specificity of substrate phosphorylation to resemble that of nonreceptor tyrosine kinases such as Src; this change in phosphorylation substrate specificity has potent neoplastic consequences.

Certain sporadic (nonfamilial) thyroid cancers, notably **PTC**, arise in 10–50% cases from *Ret* mutations involving the formation of constitutively activated fusion proteins (**Ret/PTC** types 1–5 consisting of the 3′ tyrosine kinase Ret domain) rather than point mutations. These Ret/PTC tumors may be associated with radiation exposure (Ret/PTC1 and 3) and an early age of onset.[1]

Ret is located on chromosome 10, whereas the *Menin* gene responsible for **MEN1** lies on chromosome 11q13. The **Menin** protein normally resides within the cell nucleus where it regulates transcription; in MEN1 patients, mutations (of which more than 300 are known) tend to delete both nuclear localization signals, thereby impairing nuclear translocation of Menin. Hyperparathyroidism is the initial presentation in 90% of MEN1 patients, though pituitary and enteropancreatic tumors also occur often.

---

[1] Note that although *Ret* mutations can cause either medullary or papillary thyroid cancers, other histological subtypes have a distinct molecular pathogenesis. Hence, **follicular thyroid carcinomas** may be induced by either constitutively activating K-*Ras* gene mutations or translocations that inhibit peroxisome proliferator-activated receptor-γ (p. 441); **benign toxic thyroid adenomas** arise because of mutations affecting thyrotropin receptors or G-proteins; and **undifferentiated (anaplastic) thyroid cancers** are usually characterized by loss-of-function mutations affecting the *p53* growth control gene.

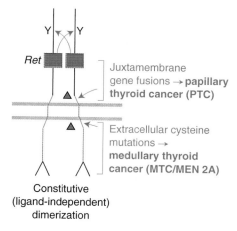

Figure 11.15 Schematic illustration of *Ret* mutations. Extracellular domain mutations mainly cause medullary thyroid cancers (MTC) due to constitutive receptor activation; juxtamembrane domain fusions, in contrast, mainly cause papillary thyroid cancer (PTC (see above)). The more severe MEN 2B phenotype arises through catalytic domain mutations that may alter the substrate specificity of the kinase.

Figure 11.16 Density-dependent cell growth inhibition mediated by the activation of receptor tyrosine phosphatases (RPTPs). In the absence of cell contact (top) RPTPs remain inactive and growth proceeds; cell contact activates RPTPs, however, leading to intracellular tyrosine dephosphorylation of specific substrates and consequent growth inhibition (bottom).

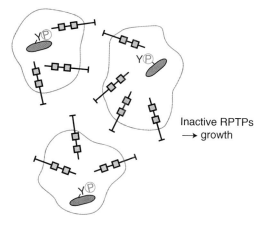

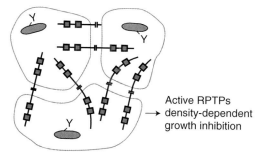

Signaling cascades

ATP-dependent kinase signaling is reversed by phosphatases

In physics, every action has an equal and opposite reaction; in human biology, every on switch has an off. Most of these on and off switches consist of reversible phosphorylation events in which the off switches are usually phosphatases. Such phosphatases fall into two main groups: **serine-threonine phosphatases** and **tyrosine phosphatases**.

Unlike serine-threonine and tyrosine kinases, which exhibit homology in their catalytic domains, serine-threonine and tyrosine phosphatases are structurally unrelated. Serine-threonine phosphatases such as **PP1**, **PP2A**, and **PP2B** are metallophosphoesterases which require divalent cations (Zn^{2+}, Mn^{2+}, Fe^{2+}) for activity. The anabolic effects of **insulin** – the antidiabetic hormone – are mediated by PP1-dependent dephosphorylation (and hence activation) of **glycogen synthase**. Like PP1, PP2A is inhibited by the tumor-promoting chemical okadaic acid; since mutations impairing the function of PP2A have been implicated in the progression of human lung and colon cancer, PP2A may have a role in growth control. Certain immunosuppressant drugs act by inhibiting PP2B, better known as calcineurin (p. 487).

An off switch for certain tyrosine kinases and their substrates is provided by **protein tyrosine phosphatases** or **PTPases**. These molecules share a phosphate-binding site containing a nucleophilic cysteine residue that recognizes the negatively charged phosphotyrosine target. Like tyrosine kinases, PTPases form a superfamily of about 100 members from two broad groupings:

1. **Transmembrane tyrosine phosphatases**
   - Contain two catalytic subdomains (of which the carboxy-terminal one exhibits no phosphatase activity).
   - Mediate contact inhibition of cell growth (Figure 11.16).
   - Include the leukocyte common antigen **CD45** and the placental leukocyte common antigen-related (**LAR**) molecule.
2. **Cytosolic tyrosine phosphatases**
   - May contain SH2 domains (SH-PTPs, e.g., placental **PTPase 1B**).
   - Can be catalytically activated by tyrosine phosphorylation, consistent with a negative feedback role.
   - Include the cytoskeletal protein homolog **PTPH1** which binds adaptor proteins in response to serine phosphorylation events.

PTPases tend to be more potent than their counterpart kinases (by 10- to 1000-fold on a molar basis) and also more diverse in function. Inhibition of tyrosine kinase activity by PTPases may induce differentiation in either adult or embryonic tissues; for example, a germline loss-of-function PTPase mutation leads to severe developmental hematopoietic defects in the *motheaten* mouse. Additional PTPase effects include homotypic cell adhesion (for certain receptor-like phosphatases) and downstream adaptor signaling (for SH2-containing cytosolic PTPases). Knockout of PTP-1B produces mice that hyperphosphorylate the insulin receptor and its major substrate IRS-1, leading to increased sensitivity to insulin.

Just as not all phosphotyrosines have the same mitogenic properties, not all PTPases are growth-inhibitory; this may account for the phenomenon of PTPase overexpression (e.g., **prostatic acid phosphatase**) in certain human cancers. **PTEN** (phosphatase and tensin homolog deleted on chromosome ten) is a dual-specificity lipid phosphatase and PTPase that antagonizes the growth-promoting effects of PI3K and receptor tyrosine kinases respectively;

severely affected individuals (e.g., those with congenital myotonia) may have anywhere from 200 to 3000 repeats. This variation in fragment length may also explain the variability in age of disease onset. Incomplete penetrance of the disease may reflect the transmission of a triplet expansion segment reduced in size; **reverse mutations** may abolish the phenotype, reflecting recombination of the expanded repeat with the homologous region of the wild-type chromosome.

Expression of an expanded CTG repeat in the 3′-untranslated region of an unrelated (actin) gene in transgenic mice also leads to myotonia and myopathy, implying a direct (gain-of-function) role for myotonin mRNA CUG repeats in the development of these latter pathologies; this is consistent with the autosomal dominant mode of transmission. In contrast, reduced expression of the 5′ *DMPK* gene appears responsible for cardiac arrhythmias, whereas reduced expression of the 3′ *SIX5* gene may cause cataracts. A second genetic locus for myotonic dystrophy, named *DM2*, has been identified on chromosome 3.

Cell growth is driven by the Ras-Raf-MAP kinase pathway

Mitogen stimulation unleashes a phosphorylation cascade involving numerous downstream growth-stimulatory proteins, including:

1. Effector kinases
   - Raf.
   - Mos (in germ cells).
2. Transcription factors
   - Myc.
   - Fos, Jun (AP1).
   - Myb (in hemopoietic tissues).

A key molecule in this cascade is the 74-kDa serine-threonine kinase **Raf** which is the immediate downstream target of the potent mitogen p21^{Ras}. Like PLC-γ, PI3K and GAP, Raf binds to tyrosine kinases via its SH2 domain, leading to phosphorylation of Raf and activation of its serine-threonine kinase activity. Several different Raf families exist – A-Raf, B-Raf, and Raf-1 – which vary in their tissue-specificity and upstream regulation.

Mos is a serine-threonine kinase like Raf. Unlike Raf, pp39^{Mos} (cytostatic factor) is expressed only in germline tissue where it controls cell-cycle progression via tubulin phosphorylation during meiotic oocyte maturation.

Raf activity is supported by the phosphoserine-dependent binding of grooved **14-3-3** protein dimers (Table 11.1). These are acidic 30-kDa adaptor proteins which also interact with PI3K, protein kinase C (PKC), Bcr (see below), the growth control protein Cdc25 (p. 361), and the cell death regulator Bad (p. 380).

Activation of Raf leads to phosphorylation and nuclear translocation of ERKs. Activation of both Raf and ERKs is induced by PKC but not by PKA. There are a dozen different PKC isoforms: for example, **PKCα** localizes to the ER and cell periphery, **PKCγ** to the Golgi, and **PKCε** to the nuclear membrane. PKC is activated by the hydrolysis of membrane lipid (p. 289), and is recruited to the membrane where anchoring proteins termed **RACK**s (receptor for activated C-kinase) bind the enzyme following its translocation from the cytosol.

ERKs are activated by dual-site phosphorylation induced by MAPK kinases termed **MEK**s (MAP/ERK kinases). These latter molecules are themselves phosphorylated and activated by MAP kinase kinase kinases, of which at least a dozen (including Raf) are known. The notorious germ warfare toxin **anthrax** contains a metalloprotease domain which acts in part by cleaving MEK.

Via the intermediary activation of 90-kDa **Rsk** (ribosomal S6, MAPKAP) kinases (i.e., Ras-Raf1-MEK1-ERK2-Rsk), ERK activation can induce the nuclear transactivation of Fos, CREB, NFκB, or estrogen receptors. Expression of these mitogenic transactivators causes quiescent cells to emerge from metabolic inactivity into DNA synthesis. Rsk may also modulate protein synthesis by phosphorylating glycogen synthase kinase-3β (**GSK-3β**), and can inhibit Ras-Raf-ERK signaling via phosphorylation of the GTP exchanger Sos (p. ***). Cell division is thus controlled by the kinetics of ERK signaling (Figure 11.17). However, other stress response pathways involve different molecules, including MEKK, Sek, Hog, and hsp27.

Figure 11.17 Overview of signaling pathways culminating in activation of mitogen-activated protein kinases (MAPK) and transcription factors. Signal cascades downstream of three receptor classes – receptor tyrosine kinases (RTKs), G-protein-coupled receptors (GPCRs: p. 278), and integrins (extracellular matrix protein receptors) – are shown. RTKs activate the Ras-Raf-MAP kinase pathway as well as pathways downstream of Src, PI-3′-kinase/protein kinase B (PI3 K/PKB), protein kinase C (PKC), and calcium; GPCRs activate pathways involving PKA, CREB, PKC and calcium; whereas integrins activate Fak-dependent signal pathways including that involving Jnk signaling. These signals result in the nuclear activation of a panel of oncogenes including not only Jun, Fos and Myc, but also NFAT, NFκB, SRF, TCF4 and GHF1. CaM, calmodulin; cAMP, cyclic adenosine monophosphate; CREB, cAMP response element binding protein; DAG, diacylglycerol; GSK, glycogen synthase kinase; IP_3, inositol 1,4,5-trisphosphate; MEK, MAP/ERK kinase; NFAT, nuclear factor of activated T cells; NFκB, a gene regulatory protein; PIP_2, phosphatidylinositol (4,5)-bisphosphate; PIP_3, phosphatidylinositol (1,4,5)-trisphosphate; PKA, protein kinase A; PLC, phospholipase C; SRF, serum response factor.

CLINICAL KEYNOTE

Chronic myeloid leukemia and the Philadelphia chromosome

Chromosomal translocation events may lead to juxtaposition of heterologous gene sequences, generating a fusion protein with constitutive proliferative (tumorigenic) activity. A classic example of this occurs in chronic myeloid leukemia (**CML**), a malignancy inducible by ionizing radiation. Bone marrow from patients with this disease yields a subset of metaphase cells containing a short chromosome 22, which represents a reciprocal translocation between chromosomes 22 and 9. This cytogenetic anomaly is known as the **Philadelphia chromosome (Ph[1])**. Of note, it is usually the paternally derived chromosome 9 that is translocated to the maternal chromosome 22 to form Ph[1], suggesting an imprinting effect (p. 406).

The clonal growth advantage implied by Ph[1]-positivity has been confirmed using **glucose-6-phosphate dehydrogenase** (**G6PD**) isoenzyme analysis based on X-chromosome inactivation (p. 410). In female (XX) patients heterozygous for the *G6PD* gene, the product of the variant X-linked allele (Gd[A]) is distinguishable from

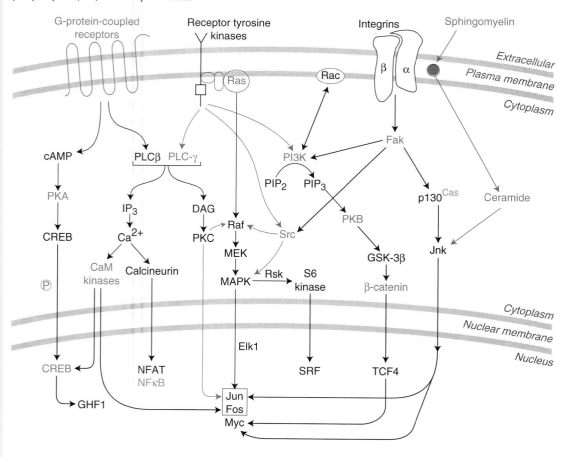

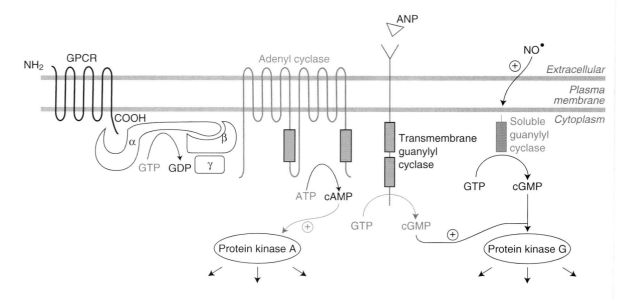

Figure 11.24 Activation of protein kinase A and protein kinase G by GTP-dependent signaling, including transmembrane and soluble guanylyl cyclases. ANP, atrial natriuretic peptide; cGMP, cyclic guanosine monophosphate; GPCR, G-protein-coupled receptors; GTP, guanosine triphosphate; NO•, nitric oxide.

G-proteins

Fluid balance is regulated by guanylyl cyclases

The formation of cyclic guanosine monophosphate (cGMP) is catalyzed by **guanylyl cyclases**, leading in turn to the activation of cGMP-dependent protein kinases, phosphatases, ion channels, and phosphodiesterases. In addition to other functions, guanylyl cyclases regulate fluid balance within body compartments; e.g., synovial fluid, seminal plasma, and cerebrospinal fluid. The main types of guanylyl cyclase (Figure 11.24) are:

1. Soluble (heterodimeric) guanylyl cyclases
   - Contain catalytic (but not kinase or transmembrane) domains.
   - Are activated by vasoactive gases: **nitric oxide** (hence, soluble guanylyl cyclases are nitric oxide receptors) and **carbon monoxide**.
2. Membrane/receptor guanylyl cyclases
   - Guanylyl cyclase A (**GC-A**).
       Activated by A-type (atrial) natriuretic peptide (**ANP**).
   - Guanylyl cyclase B (**GC-B**).
       Activated by C-type natriuretic peptide (**CNP**).
       Not activated by B-type natriuretic peptide (**BNP**; see below).
   - Guanylyl cyclase C (**GC-C**)
       Intestinal guanylyl cyclase; may activate the cystic fibrosis transmembrane conductance regulator (p. 190).
       Binds all natriuretic peptide ligands: ANP, BNP, CNP.
       Activated in disease by heat-stable enterotoxin of *Escherichia coli*.
       Enterotoxigenic secretory diarrhea reflects increased cGMP.
3. Retinal guanylyl cyclase
   - Activated by recoverin (p. 516).

ANPs circulate as either 98-amino-acid amino-terminal peptides and/or 28-amino-acid (mature) carboxy-terminal peptides originally secreted as precursor molecules by the cardiac atria in response to atrial distension. The kidney processes ANP precursors differently, releasing a 32-amino-acid fragment termed **urodilatin**, which maintains renal blood flow. BNP was first isolated from brain and hence initially called brain natriuretic peptide. In fact, BNP is most abundantly secreted from the cardiac ventricles and the mature 32-amino-acid fragment only activates GC-C. Discovery of CNP (the ligand for

GC-B) led to its characterization as the most abundant natriuretic peptide in the brain. The 22-amino-acid mature CNP peptide is the most potent venodilator of all the ligands, but has little natriuretic activity because there are so few type B receptors in the kidney. An addition to the family, **DNP**, occurs in certain snake venoms.

Cross-activation of cGMP-dependent protein kinases can sometimes be induced by cAMP. However, most cGMP-dependent signaling is triggered by the activation of guanylate cyclases downstream of either nitric oxide or ANP. The anti-impotence drug **sildenafil** (Viagra™) potentiates guanylyl cyclase by antagonizing its functional inhibitor, phosphodiesterase 5 (p. 354).

Atrial natriuretic peptide

Atrial natriuretic peptide (ANP) is the most natriuretic of the guanylyl cyclase ligands. ANP directly activates a guanylyl cyclase catalytic domain within its receptor – a single-transmembrane-domain (like a receptor tyrosine kinase) rather than a seven-transmembrane-domain (G-protein-coupled) receptor. The binding of ANP leads to marked increases in cGMP production by the intracellular domain of this receptor.

ANP release is induced by blood volume expansion as detected by peripheral vascular baroreceptors in either the atrium itself (atrial stretch causing the release of atrial cell granules) or the central nervous system. The effects of ANP include inhibition of renin secretion, stimulation of natriuresis (partly via direct renal action), and thirst quenching (by indirectly antagonizing the hypothalamic effect of angiotensin II; p. 349). Plasma levels of ANP and BNP are elevated in **congestive heart failure**. Synthetic analogs of these molecules may thus prove of therapeutic value in this context.

GTP-binding heterotrimers are molecular switches

Guanine nucleotides include cyclic guanosine monophosphate (cGMP), guanosine triphosphate (GTP) and guanosine diphosphate (GDP). Guanine-nucleotide-binding proteins are collectively called **G-proteins**. Proteins that bind GTP do so via a helical 21-kDa core motif termed a **G domain**: the guanine moiety of GTP protrudes from the G domain cleft, whereas the γ-phosphates are buried deep within the G domain. GTP-binding proteins serve many different functions:

1. **Heterotrimeric G-proteins**
   - Membrane-associated regulators of intercellular signal transduction.
2. **Small GTP-binding GTPases**
   - Regulate cell proliferation, morphology, and motility.
3. **Transport GTPases** (e.g., kinesin, dynamin)
   - Function as mechanochemical enzymes.
4. **Tubulins**
   - Responsible for microtubule polymerization.
5. **Initiation/elongation factors** in protein synthesis
   - Mediate aminoacyl-tRNA transport to ribosomes.

Heterotrimeric G-proteins consist of α, β and γ subunits. These heterotrimers associate with the plasma membrane via binding of α-subunits to hydrophobic myristate lipid anchors within the phospholipid bilayer. GTP binding to the large (40 kDa) G-protein **α subunit** (G_α) causes dissociation of the

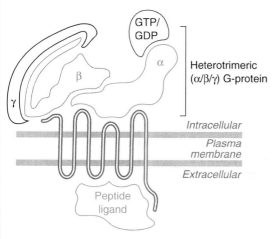

Figure 11.25 Heterotrimeric structure of G-proteins associated with heptahelical receptors. GTP binds to the α-subunit of the G-protein heterotrimer in response to ligand binding, leading to release of the βγ heterodimer followed by downstream signaling.

Table 11.2. G-protein-coupled receptors

1. Sensory receptors
   - Opsins (e.g., the photoreceptor rhodopsin; p. 513)
   - Olfactory and taste receptors

2. Adrenergic receptors and other biogenic amine receptors
   - e.g., Receptors for dopamine and histamine

3. Glycoprotein hormone receptors
   - e.g., Receptors for ACTH, TSH, FSH/LH/HCG
   Peptide hormone receptors
   - e.g., Receptors for PTH – PTHrP, calcitonin and glucagon
   Brain/gut peptide hormone receptors
   - e.g., Receptors for vasopressin, secretin, VIP, and TRH

4. Arachidonic acid derivative receptors
   - e.g., Receptors for prostaglandins, leukotrienes, thromboxane A_2

5. Voltage-gated ion channel receptors
   - e.g., Receptors for K^+, Ca^{2+} and Na^+ channels

6. Amino acid receptors
   - e.g., Receptors for GABA and glutamate

7. Purine receptors
   - e.g., Receptor for adenosine and ATP

8. Tachykinin receptors
   - e.g., Receptor for substance P

9. Complement receptors
   - Receptor for C5a

10. Antigen receptors
   - Receptor for IgE–antigen complexes

Notes:
ACTH, adrenocorticotrophin; PTH, parathyroid hormone; TRH, thyrotropin-releasing hormone; VIP, vasoactive intestinal polypeptide.

Figure 11.26 Profile and cross-section structures of G-protein-coupled receptors. TM, transmembrane (domain).

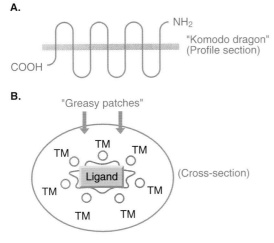

A.

NH$_2$

"Komodo dragon"
(Profile section)

COOH

B.

"Greasy patches"

TM TM TM

TM Ligand TM

TM TM

(Cross-section)

Peptide hormones activate G-protein-coupled receptors

Cell signals occur either as a discrete regulatory pulse (e.g., all-or-nothing activation of a nerve synapse, or transactivation of a single-copy gene) or else as wavelike variations in steady-state levels of a regulatory molecule (e.g., expression flux of a housekeeping protein). Accordingly, a given receptor class tends to respond more sensitively to ligand concentrations that are either (1) low but increasing or (2) always detectable but changing in intensity. For example, growth factor receptors (usually receptor tyrosine kinases or cytokine receptors) tend to exhibit high affinity for low-concentration ligands.

In contrast, neurotransmitter receptors may be more finely tuned to directional changes in ligand concentrations; these latter receptors are most often **G-protein-coupled receptors** (GPCRs), and may be functionally linked to ion channels (Table 11.2). GPCRs are a massive receptor superfamily which is structurally defined by seven transmembrane α-helices. Though this heptahelical feature is often profiled in diagrams as if serpentine in conformation, the transmembrane domains are in fact arranged as a circular array forming a central nest to which extracellular peptide ligands (including neurotransmitters; Figure 11.26) can bind. Lipophilic cytoplasmic molecules, on the other hand, may interact directly with receptor transmembrane domains via membrane pockets. Newly synthesized receptors are escorted to the plasma membrane by proteins termed **RAMPs** (receptor activity-modifying proteins).

A consequence of the large number of GPCRs is that the numerous ligands for these receptors form structural subfamilies. For example, the **tachykinin** family is characterized by a carboxy-terminal sequence Phe-*X*-Gly-Leu/Met-Met where the identity of *X* modifies the specificity of receptor binding. Other such peptide hormone families include the **VIP-glucagon-secretin** (where VIP is vasoactive intestinal polypeptide) and the **calcitonin-CGRP-amylin-adrenomedullin** ligand families (where CGRP is calcitonin gene-related peptide). The same receptor for the latter family can alter its specificity depending on whether it is presented to the cell surface by **RAMP1** (a CGRP receptor) or **RAMP2** (an adrenomedullin receptor).

These ligands tend to be small (e.g., 8–12 amino acids) and hence capable of circulating in plasma without being proteolysed. This feature distinguishes peptide hormones from larger (50–400 amino acids) polypeptide growth factors, which generally restrict their action to the extracellular matrix (insulin and the insulin-like growth factors are the exceptions). However, peptide ligands are not always required for receptor activation: the retinal GPCR rhodopsin is activated by photons of light, whereas the procoagulant thrombin receptor is activated by proteolytic cleavage of its extracellular domain to reveal a tethered ligand (p. 468).

Like G-proteins, GPCRs lack intrinsic catalytic activity. Ligand binding to GPCRs leads to noncovalent association of the receptor's cytoplasmic domain with membrane-associated GDP-bound G-proteins. The receptor-bound heterotrimer releases GDP and binds GTP, in turn causing dissociation of the α-subunit from the heterotrimer and thus revealing a binding site on Gα for the effector (e.g., adenyl cyclase). GTP hydrolysis then catalyzes activation of the effector, with Gα reverting to the GDP-bound state (Figure 11.27).

Although lacking the structural complexity of growth factor receptors, the flexibility of GPCR signaling derives from their sheer number. This combination of structural simplicity and functional diversity is reflected in the large number of drugs that act as GPCR agonists or antagonists, with as many as 50% of all new drugs now targeting the GPCR superfamily.

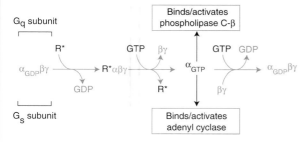

Figure 11.27 Differential regulation of effector signaling by different G-protein subunits. G_q binds and activates phospholipase C-β, whereas G_s stimulates adenyl cyclase; both result in conversion of GTP to GDP. R, receptor subunit.

Signal control and termination

Downstream signaling may be inhibited by G-proteins

G-protein-mediated signaling most commonly involves the stimulatory G-protein G_s which activates adenyl cyclase, thereby initiating a cAMP-dependent signal transduction pathway. However, some receptors may activate either G_s or G_i – the **calcitonin** receptor is an example. GPCRs that consistently inhibit adenyl cyclase by activating α_i-containing (G_i) G-proteins include:

1. $\boldsymbol{\alpha_2}$**-adrenergic** receptors.
2. **β-endorphin** (opiate) and **tetrahydrocannabinol** (THC, cannabinoid) receptors.
3. **Acetylcholine** (muscarinic) receptors.
4. **Angiotensin II** receptors.
5. **Somatostatin** receptors.

The physiologic effects of activating these receptors are mediated by inhibition of downstream signaling (Figure 11.28). This means that signals can be actively terminated by ligand secretion – not merely allowed to decay – which can be important for rapid cellular responses such as those involving adaptation to environmental stimuli (e.g., changes in blood pressure or neurotransmission). G-protein-mediated cell signaling is terminated in other contexts by activation of GTP-catabolizing **GTPases**, which return the G-protein α-subunit to the inactive GDP-bound form. Ligand-dependent receptor signaling may also be terminated by negative feedback loops involving kinases, a process termed desensitization (see below).

This remarkable ability of GPCRs to switch themselves off via a number of synergistic mechanisms explains their utility as membrane-associated sensory and timing devices. In contrast, autocatalytic receptor protein kinases send powerful signals to the cell nucleus, which are primarily involved in the regulation of cell growth decisions. Mutations affecting the latter receptors are therefore more heavily implicated in cancer development, although benign tumors may result from mutations affecting GPCRs.

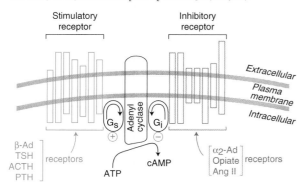

Figure 11.28 Agonist and antagonist G-proteins. Receptors activating inhibitory G-proteins (G_i), shown at right, prevent conversion of ATP to cAMP. Ang II, angiotensin II; α_2-Ad, α_2-adrenergic (receptor).

G-protein-coupled receptor mutations in human disease

As with G-proteins, mutations (usually germline) affect GPCRs. For example, a single mutation affecting the **melanocyte-stimulating hormone receptor** can cause pale skin, whereas a double mutation can cause red hair and freckles. Numerous clinical disorders may also result from such mutations, including:

1. Mutations affecting cone opsin (**iodopsin**) genes
   - Usually associated with **color-blindness** (p. 515).
2. Mutations affecting the **rhodopsin** gene
   - Responsible for some cases of night-blindness (**nyctalopia**) and others of **retinitis pigmentosa**.
3. Mutations affecting the V2 (**vasopressin**) receptor gene
   - Responsible for **nephrogenic diabetes insipidus**.
4. Mutations affecting the TSH (thyrotropin) receptor
   - Responsible for most **hyperfunctioning** (toxic) **thyroid adenomas**.
5. Mutations affecting the **luteinizing hormone** receptor
   - Responsible for **male precocious puberty**.
6. Mutations affecting the **follicle-stimulating hormone** receptor

tivity to agonist ligand exposures. Recognized syndromes of receptor supersensitivity include:

1. **Tardive dyskinesias**.
2. **Caffeine withdrawal**.

Long-term administration of dopamine receptor antagonists such as **chlorpromazine** (e.g., for institutionalized schizophrenics) may cause dopamine receptor upregulation and dopaminergic hypersensitivity. This manifests clinically with involuntary movements (tardive dyskinesias) distinct from the dystonias associated with short-term treatments.

Caffeine, like its fellow methylxanthine **theophylline**, is an adenosine receptor (A_1, A_2) antagonist and hence a phosphodiesterase inhibitor. Acute exposures to these drugs thus increase cellular cAMP levels, leading to the familiar caffeine/theophylline side-effects of tremor, palpitations, diarrhea, and insomnia. In contrast, chronic caffeine ingestion leads to adenosine receptor upregulation associated with increased $G_{i\alpha}$ and enhanced adenyl cyclase inhibition. Of note, chronic caffeine administration also inhibits the expression of β-adrenergic receptors. Abrupt caffeine cessation under these circumstances leads to a sharp fall in brain cAMP (reflecting sensitization to the physiologic ligand, adenosine, leading to excess phosphodiesterase release) and the familiar withdrawal syndrome.

Crosstalk between unrelated signaling molecules may be either inhibitory or potentiating. For example, the adrenergic-receptor-mediated signal transduction system may be sensitized by thyroid hormone excess in **thyrotoxicosis**, a clinical condition characterized by sympathetic nervous system overactivity (e.g., anxiety, eyelid retraction, hyperreflexia). A related interaction occurs in patients with hypercortisolism (**Cushing syndrome**) in whom elevated blood pressure reflects not only sodium retention but also a synergistic pressor effect between the glucocorticoid and adrenergic receptor systems. Inhibitory interactions also take place between heterologous receptor pathways, with one example involving the antagonistic interactions of insulin and catecholamines on carbohydrate metabolism. Relevant to this, the G-protein-coupled receptor ligand **somatostatin** may inhibit cell growth by indirectly activating a tyrosine phosphatase.

CLINICAL KEYNOTE

Adrenergic receptor function in human disease

Many clinical conditions are associated with changes in adrenergic receptor expression and/or function. These include:

1. **Hypertension**
   - β receptor downregulation.
   - α receptor upregulation.
2. **Congestive cardiac failure**
   - β_1 receptor downregulation.
   - β_2 receptor uncoupling due to increased βARK activity.
3. **Pheochromocytoma**
   - Both α- and β-receptor downregulation.

Congestive cardiac failure is characterized by a compensatory increase in the sympathetic nervous drive to the heart, with increased βARK (leading to receptor uncoupling) and reduced **β_1 receptor** transcription being the deleterious consequences.

Polymorphisms of adrenergic receptors have been associated with susceptibility

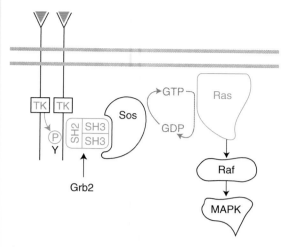

Figure 11.30 Activation of cell growth by Ras. Ligand-dependent growth factor receptor activation is followed by receptor tyrosine autophosphorylation, binding of the Grb2 adaptor protein, recruitment of Grb2 by the membrane-associated GTP exchange protein Sos which in turn binds Ras. GTP hydrolysis triggers Ras-dependent activation of Raf, leading (via MEK) to MAP kinase activation with nuclear translocation of the latter.

to certain diseases: some cases of **morbid obesity** have been linked with codon 64 polymorphisms of the β_3 **receptor** gene (e.g., in Pima Indians), while **nocturnal asthma** has been associated with codon 16 β_2 **receptor** polymorphisms. However, the pathogenetic significance of these reports remains controversial.

Small GTP-binding proteins diversify membrane signaling

Small monomeric GTP-binding proteins form a key group of signaling proteins. These G-proteins, which are usually prenylated and hence associated with the plasma membrane, contain intrinsic GTPase activity that inactivates the protein as a negative feedback mechanism. These molecules are critical downstream targets of receptor tyrosine kinases, though not of G-protein-coupled receptors. Such molecules include:

1. Mitogenic proteins linking membrane signals and the nucleus
   • **H-Ras** (Ha-Ras, Harvey Ras).
   • **K-Ras** (Ki-Ras, Kirsten Ras) A and B.
   • **N-Ras** (neuroblastoma-associated Ras).
2. Cytoskeletal-associated GTP-binding proteins
   • **Rho, Rac.**
3. Intracellular transport GTP-binding proteins
   • **Rab** family (recruitment of vesicle docking proteins).
   • **Ran** family (nucleocytoplasmic transport).

The prototype of this class of proteins is the 21-kDa **Ras (p21^{Ras})**, a small GTP-binding protein with potent mitogenic activity associated with weak intrinsic GTPase activity. The 189-amino-acid p21^{Ras} protein contains a farnesylated lipid tag with a CAA*X* sequence that is cleaved by membrane-bound proteases to reveal a hydrophobic binding site (pp. 133–4).

The Ras isoforms differ in their carboxy-terminal sequences and lipidation. Unlike K-Ras which contains a polybasic region, H-Ras is palmitoylated and hence targeted to caveolae (in which growth factor receptors reside during quiescent growth periods). Such differences may help account for the divergent signaling properties of these isoforms: PI3K is more potently activated by H-Ras than by K-Ras, for example, whereas the reverse appears true for Raf. Similarly, *N-Ras* knockout mice have no phenotype, whereas *K-Ras* knockouts are embryonic lethal.

Growth factor receptor activation leads to Ras co-activation via initial tyrosine phosphorylation of the SH2/SH3-containing adaptor protein **Grb2** (growth factor receptor-binding protein 2). The SH3 domain of Grb2 forms a high-affinity bond with proline-rich regions of **guanine nucleotide exchange proteins** (Ras exchangers, GDP-dissociation stimulators), which promote exchange of GDP for GTP, increasing Ras-GTP and promoting mitogenesis. The GDP-dissociation stimulator **Sos** (named after the *Drosophila* protein Son of sevenless) complexes with Grb2 (which is in turn SH2-bound to the ligand-activated growth factor receptor), recruiting Sos to the membrane. Sos inserts an α-helix into Ras, thereby forcing open the nucleotide- (GTP/GDP-) binding site; the latter remains open for GTP-GDP exchange for as long as Sos is around. **Raynaud disease** is a vasospastic disorder affecting the fingers in which the propeller-shaped guanine nucleotide exchange protein **RCC** (regulator of chromosome condensation) is the target of autoantibodies.

Ras proteins become mitogenic following GTP binding and phosphatidylcholine hydrolysis. The consequences of Ras activation depend upon the cell context: epithelial cells are most often induced to proliferate, but neurons may differentiate, and T lymphocytes may undergo negative selection (clonal

12

Bioactive lipids and inflammatory cytokines

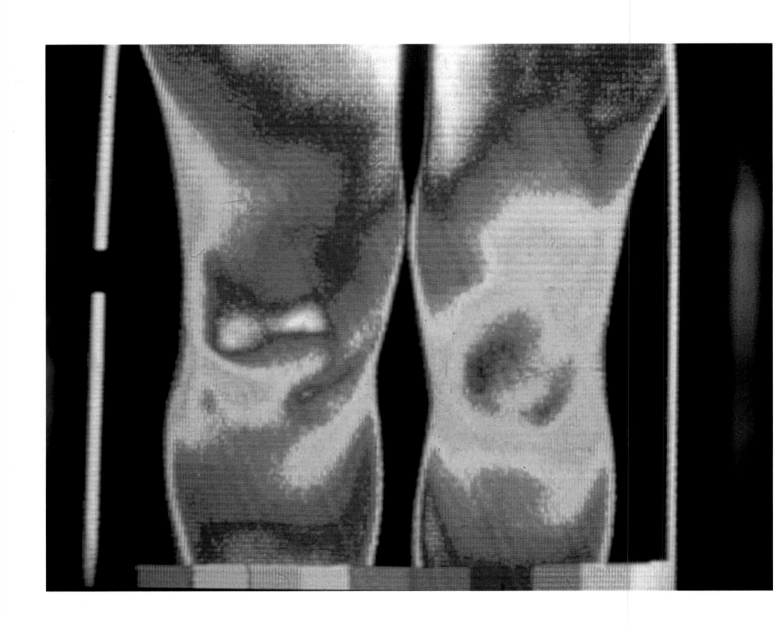

Dietary fats and oils – the lipids best known to most of us – get a bad press. As it happens, endogenous lipids are essential for normal cell behavior: partly on account of their hydrophobic properties, which make them essential membrane constituents, and partly by virtue of their signaling abilities. In this section we discuss how the hydrolysis of lipid-containing membrane constituents regulates the production of molecules that mediate inflammatory responses.

Lipid signaling

Lipids transduce signals from membranes

Although widely regarded as inert, lipids are in fact potent mediators of signal transduction. A striking example is the **lipid A** domain of bacterial **lipopolysaccharide** (LPS; also known as **endotoxin**) – a modified membrane phospholipid in Gram-negative organisms that contributes to septic shock (p. 299). A serum LPS-binding protein presents the endotoxin molecule to CD14-expressing monocyte-macrophages and neutrophils, leading to nonspecific immune recognition followed by activation of blood clotting and host defenses. Non-LPS immunogenic microbial lipids include **lipoteichoic acid** and **lipoarabinomannan**.

Lipid signaling molecules often have composite structures that include sugar and/or protein regions. The latter may include SH2 domains, which provide a mechanism for integrating lipid signaling with other biochemical response pathways. Signaling molecules may thus be formed from a variety of membrane-associated lipids including **phosphatidylinositol**, **PIP$_2$**, **phosphatidylcholine** (lecithin), and **phosphatidic** and **lysophosphatidic acid**. The most abundant of these lipid phosphates is the monophosphorylated **phosphatidylinositol-3-phosphate** (PIP), which recruits endosomal and signaling proteins to the membrane via its interaction with a specific PIP-docking motif termed a FYVE domain. Metabolically active phosphoinositols are derived in part by hydrolysis of membrane-bound GPI anchors (p. 134).

Intracellular phosphoinositides form Golgi secretory vesicles which are exported to the cell surface where they fuse with the membrane, discharging their contents into the extracellular space. Phosphatidylinositol is also a catabolic substrate in many mitogenic signaling pathways, however, and regulates the activity of membrane-bound enzymes. Such membrane phosphoinositols are modified by SH2-containing enzymes ("fat controllers"), prominent amongst which are:

1. **Phospholipase** (especially A, C-β, C-γ, and D) lipid-cleaving enzymes.
2. **Phosphatidylinositol-3′-kinase** (PI3K – pronounced "pee eye three kinase") lipid kinases.

Phospholipases produce the second messengers **arachidonate**, **diacylglycerol** (DAG) and **IP$_3$** (Figure 12.2). Growth-factor-inducible tyrosine phosphorylation of **phospholipase C-γ** (PLC-γ) directly confers catalytic activity on the enzyme via an allosteric mechanism: PIP$_2$ is hydrolyzed by tyrosine-phosphorylated PLC-γ, yielding DAG and IP$_3$ which in turn mediate protein kinase C (PKC) activation and calcium mobilization respectively. Activated PKC localizes to the plasma membrane, whereas IP$_3$ binds receptors in the endoplasmic reticulum (Figure 12.3). Hydrolysis of PIP$_2$ is also inducible by **phospholipase C-β** (PLC-β) activation triggered by G-protein-coupled receptor ligands such as substance P, histamine, and thromboxane A$_2$. Moreover, PKC can be activated by DAG agonists called **phorbol esters** which are potent

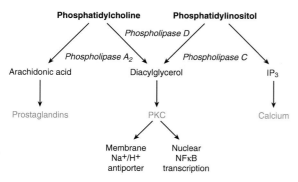

Figure 12.2 The hydrolysis of membrane phospholipids by phospholipases. PKC, protein kinase C; IP_3, inositol 1, 4, 5-trisphosphate.

tumor promoters. DAG may also be formed by de novo synthesis from fatty acyl CoA within the endoplasmic reticulum rather than through PIP_2 hydrolysis. PLC-γ-mediated hydrolysis of phosphatidylcholine, the principal cell membrane phospholipid (which is also metabolized by phospholipase D), is yet another pathway of DAG biosynthesis.

PIP_2 may be shielded from PLC-dependent hydrolysis by binding of the actin-binding ADP/ATP exchange protein **profilin** (p. 240) which can thus inhibit signal transduction. Growth-factor-induced phosphorylation events cause disassembly of this complex, resulting in cytoskeletal reorganization.

Inhibition of PIP_2 precursor synthesis by inositol monophosphatase antagonism is one of several mechanisms implicated in the therapeutic action of the antipsychotic drug **lithium** (Figure 12.4). Since inositol is unable to cross the blood-brain barrier and reactivate PIP_2 synthesis, the signaling pathway is selectively muted within the brain.

MOLECULAR MINIREVIEW

PI-3′-kinase (PI3K)

Phosphatidylinositol-3′-kinase (**PI3K**) is a bipartite molecule consisting of an 85-kDa SH2-containing domain (p85) and a 110-kDa catalytic domain (p110). PI3K activity can be triggered by tyrosine phosphorylation events due to growth factors or $\alpha_6\beta_4$ integrins (which activate Fak; p. 226). Catalytic activation and the membrane recruitment of PI3K have several outcomes relating to the dual lipid kinase and protein kinase activities of PI3K (Figure 12.4):

1. Phosphoinositide production of PIP_3 from PIP_2. Conversion to PIP_3 activates the pro-survival enzyme, protein kinase B or **PKB** (Akt; see below).
2. The actin-controlling **Rac** protein controls PIP_2 synthesis. By depleting PIP_2 stores, PI3K triggers the activation of Rac, leading to disruption of actin structures, increased motility, chemotaxis, and tissue invasion (p. 284).

In addition, PI3K-dependent protein phosphorylation may activate cell growth by co-activating the Src, PKC and mitogen-activated protein (MAP) kinase signaling pathways. However, knockout studies have shown that this latter pathway is not required for the PI3K-dependent action of insulin on glucose homeostasis (p. 429), indicating that lipid kinase pathways are more central to PI3K action in certain contexts. The survival-enhancing properties of PI3K or its homologs may also derive in part from actions within the nucleus: in yeast, PI3K-dependent phosphorylation of histone H2A enhances DNA repair of double-strand breaks by altering chromatin structure.

PI3K is thus a signaling enzyme that favors cell growth and is also implicated in tissue invasion. Consistent with this, the PIP_3-producing activity of PI3K is antagonized by the growth-regulatory lipid phosphatase **PTEN** which is mutated in premalignant syndromes such as **juvenile polyposis** or **Cowden syndrome** (pp. 364–5), as well as in **endometrial hyperplasia** (50%) and **endometrial cancer** (75%). Dietary fatty acids differentially affect PI3K activity – oleic acid activates it, whereas palmitic acid inhibits it – consistent with dietary carcinogenesis. PI3K inhibitors of the **wortmannin** variety could thus prove useful for either prevention or treatment of cancers of the colon, endometrium, and ovary.

Cells relieve stress by activating a lipid-protein kinase cascade

Most of us think stress is all in the mind, but cells experience stress as a direct physical phenomenon. A variety of noxious stimuli induce cell stress, including inflammation, heat, radiation, hypoxia, and hyperosmolality. This deranges cellular constituents such as membranes and DNA. Cells have thus evolved

Figure 12.3 Membrane recruitment of protein kinase C (PKC) following activation by its endogenous ligand diacylglycerol (DAG). Following allosteric activation of phospholipase C-γ (PLC-γ) by tyrosine phosphorylation, phosphatidylinositol bisphosphate (PIP_2) undergoes hydrolysis to the bioactive lipids DAG and IP_3; the latter induces mobilization of calcium stores in the endoplasmic reticulum (p. 272).

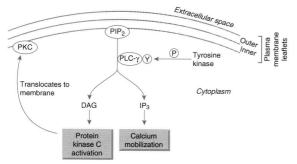

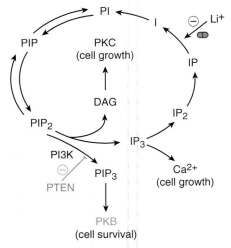

Figure 12.4 The phosphatidylinositol cycle. Phosphatidylinositol (PI) is phosphorylated first to PI monophosphate (PIP), then to the bisphosphate (PIP₂) and ultimately to the trisphosphate (PIP₃). Hydrolysis of PIP_2 yields inositol 1, 4, 5-trisphosphate (IP_3), which is sequentially dephosphorylated to the bisphosphate (IP_2), monophosphate (IP) and eventually to inositol alone (I); the latter reaction is inhibited by lithium (Li^+). DAG, diacylglycerol; PKC, protein kinase C; PI3K, phosphatidylinositol-3′-kinase; PKB, a serine-threonine kinase; PTEN, growth-regulatory lipid phosphatase.

Figure 12.5 Sphingomyelin metabolism and signaling. Hydrolysis of sphingomyelin by sphingomyelinase produces choline (p. 174) and ceramide; the latter activates the Jnk signaling pathway. Hydrolysis of lecithin (phosphatidylcholine) to diacylglycerol (DAG) by phospholipases A or D may be linked to the reconversion of ceramide to sphingomyelin.

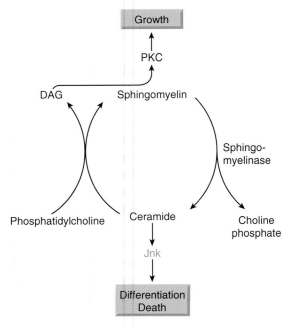

adaptive response pathways which are triggered by damaging stressors.

Inflammatory and other membrane-damaging stimuli trigger a cell stress pathway that is propagated by the hydrolysis of membrane phospholipids. Stress kinases belong to the MAP kinase superfamily:

1. **ERKs** (extracellularly regulated kinases)
   - Are activated by the Ras-Raf pathway (p. 266).
   - Usually induce growth, but the outcome varies with signaling kinetics.
2. **p38 MAP kinase**
   - Activated either by cell stress or by growth factors.
3. **Jnk** (pronounced "junk"; Jun kinase)
   - Is activated by membrane-derived sphingolipids or DNA damage.
   - May induce diverse cell outcomes including cell death.

Jnk activation is triggered by the glycosphingolipid **ceramide**, a sphingomyelin hydrolysis product. Choline deficiency can also deplete membrane phosphatidylcholine and thus trigger an increase in ceramide, but de novo synthesis of ceramide occurs most notably as a prelude to ganglioside biosynthesis in neural tissues. Sphingomyelinase-dependent release of ceramide by membrane damage may thus lead to Jnk-induced cell cycle arrest, differentiation or death (Figure 12.5). Note, however, that cell growth can also be induced by Jnk in some circumstances.

Medical treatments may increase ceramide concentrations via different mechanisms. For example, increased de novo ceramide synthesis is induced by anticancer drugs such as paclitaxel, etoposide, doxorubicin and vincristine; increased sphingomyelinase activity is induced by ionizing radiation; whereas reduced glycosylation of ceramide may be induced by tamoxifen, ciclosporin, ketoconazole, verapamil or mifepristone.

Other MAP kinase family members (such as ERK2 or p38 MAP kinase) activate a distinct serine-threonine kinase: ribosomal S6 kinase, or **Rsk** (pronounced "risk"). The rare X-linked **Coffin–Lowry syndrome** of mental retardation and skeletal deformities arises because of *Rsk* mutations, and the mutant protein in the hamartomatous **Peutz–Jeghers syndrome**, **LKB1** (p. 367), contains a Rsk-like catalytic domain that is implicated in the normal cell death of gut mucosal cells.

The effects of Jnk signaling are opposed by the survival kinase **PKB** (Akt). The pleckstrin homology (PH) domain of PKB binds PIP_3 produced by PI3K, leading to membrane translocation of PKB where it is catalytically activated by transphosphorylation of threonine-308/9 and serine-473/4. PKB promotes cell survival by phosphorylating (and inactivating) cell death proteins such as Bad and caspase-9 (pp. 380–2). In addition, PKB phosphorylates and inactivates glycogen synthase kinase-3-beta (GSK3β), permitting dephosphorylation of β-catenin and thus decoupling it from the adenomatous polyposis coli gene product **APC** to allow its nuclear translocation; the transcription factor TCF4 is then induced by β-catenin, together with its main downstream target, the immediate-early *Myc* gene (pp. 213–14).

Jaks and STATs in disease states

Jak3 mutation can cause autosomal recessive **severe combined immunodeficiency** (SCID) – as noted above, γ-chain mutation is the usual cause of X-linked SCID – raising the possibility of developing *Jak3* gene therapy for this disorder. *STAT4* knockout mice are defective in one kind of T cell helper activity (T_H1; p. 479), whereas *STAT6* knockouts are defective in T_H2 activity such as may predispose to **bronchiolitis** and **lepromatous leprosy.**

Constitutive activation of STAT1 leads to premature cartilage maturation in **thanatophoric dwarfism** due to *FGFR3* mutation (p. 345).

Constitutive STAT activation is implicated in many leukemias. **Acute promyelocytic leukemia**, which arises via chromosomal 17q translocation events affecting retinoic acid receptor-alpha (RARA; pp. 55–6), may on occasion be caused by a duplication event yielding the fusion gene *STAT5b-RARA*. Therapeutic inhibition of Jak2 activity may cause clinical remission of refractory **acute lymphoblastic leukemia** – a malignancy associated with constitutive Jak2 activity. Inhibition of this tyrosine kinase selectively kills leukemic cells but does not affect normal hemopoiesis. Similar drugs may thus emerge with the potential to treat other cancers associated with constitutive signaling abnormalities.

Nonimmune host defences

Complement proteins tag antigens for phagocytosis

The human body produces circulating molecules that stick to microbial surfaces, thereby tagging such organisms for destruction by cell-mediated processes. These tags comprise two main families of host defense proteins, which mediate antigen-specific and nonspecific immunity respectively: antibodies and **complement**. The latter term designates a family of over 30 proteins that trigger a cascade of amplifying reactions (Figure 12.13) required for host defence, antigen processing, or waste disposal.

As in the coagulation cascade (p. 465), complement proteins are sequentially activated by proteolysis. This leads to serial generation of proteases that have other complement components as their substrates. For all complement components except C2, the smaller proteolytic fragment from such reactions is labelled "a" (e.g., C3a) whereas the larger remnant is termed "b" (e.g., C3b). Activation of this proteolytic cascade leads to **opsonization** of complement-bound particles followed by lysis of target cell membranes. Opsonization is a process in which extracellular particles are softened and made sticky for phagocytosis either by the classical pathway (initiated by the binding of circulating immune complexes) or else by the alternate pathway (initiated by IgA or endotoxin-activated C_3) of complement action.

The classical pathway of complement activation is initiated by C_1, a tripartite protein complex consisting of C_{1q}, C_{1r}, and C_{1s}. The hexavalent **C_{1q}** molecule contains Fcγ and Fcμ receptors which bind IgG/IgM-containing immune complexes. Activation of C_{1q} leads to production of activated C_{1s} which in turn activates C_4 and C_2. The **C_4/C_2 complex** cleaves C_3 – which, at plasma concentrations of 1 mg/ml, is the most abundant complement protein – to form the key opsonin **C_{3b}**. Complement-coated organisms are then recognized by **complement receptors** (CRs; Table 12.4) on the surface of phagocytic leukocytes, most of which bind C3b. The CR2 complement receptor, which is selectively expressed in both B cells and nasopharyngeal epithelial cells, represents the portal of entry for Epstein-

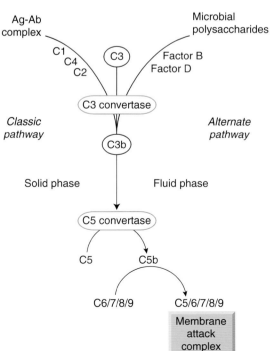

Figure 12.13 The complement cascade: classical and alternate pathways.

Table 12.4. Complement receptors, ligands and function

Complement receptor (CR)	Main ligands	Function and significance
CR1	C3b, C4b	Present on red blood cells, leukocytes, kidney cells Triggers Fc receptor-mediated phagocytosis Clears circulating immune complexes
CR2	C3b, C3d	Present on B cells and nasopharyngeal epithelium
	EBV	Portal of entry for EBV
CR3	C3b	Present on macrophages, neutrophils, NK cells Involved in cell adhesion, chemotaxis, phagocytosis
CR4	C3b	Present on monocytes, neutrophils, platelets Promotes Fc receptor-mediated phagocytosis
CR5a	C5a	Present on basophils, neutrophils, mast cells, monocytes, endothelium Enhances histamine release, vascular permeability, and chemotaxis

Notes:
EBV, Epstein–Barr virus; NK, natural killer.

Barr virus in **infectious mononucleosis** and **nasopharyngeal carcinoma** respectively.

Activation of phagocyte C_{3b} receptors leads to endocytosis of complement-coated complexes into phagocytic vacuoles, whereupon the offending organism is lyzed. Nonphagocytic microbial lysis may occur when multiprotein complement **membrane attack complexes** (MACs: $C_{5b,6,7,8,9}$) insert the hydrophobic tails of C_8 and C_9 through target cell membranes. As noted below, *Neisseria* spp. (meningococci and gonococci) evade MAC attack by sialylating their polysaccharide capsule (p. 135 and Figure 5.17) and sequestering factor H, thereby aborting the complement cascade.

The lesions induced by MACs are similar to those induced by the 70-kDa pore-forming protein **perforin** (cytolysin) which structurally resembles C_9. Perforin is released from cytoplasmic granules by activated killer cells; these granules also contain neutral serpins termed **granzymes** (A and B). Perforin attaches and inserts into the plasma membrane of target cells where it aggregates in the presence of calcium, causing the formation of multimeric 10- to 20-nm diameter pore complexes which permit lethal osmotic equilibration between the cytoplasm and extracellular space (Figure 12.14). Granzymes also initiate a pathway activating DNA endonucleases, thus potentiating the cell-killing effect of perforin (p. 383). The granules of cytotoxic T cells contain a saposin-like enzyme termed **granulysin** which kills intracellular organisms such as *Mycobacteria*, *Listeria* and *Trypanosoma* spp.

In addition to its direct antimicrobial effects, complement may modulate neutrophil chemotaxis ($C_{5,6,7}$) and anaphylaxis (C_{3a}, C_{5a}). Since complement proteins are also acute phase reactants, plasma complement levels (C_3 and C_4) may be nonspecifically elevated in conditions such as **trauma** and **myocardial infarction**. In contrast, C_3 and C_4 levels are reduced by activation of the classical pathway such as occurs in collagen-vascular diseases like **systemic lupus erythematosus** (SLE). Low C_3 with normal C_4 levels usually indicates alternate pathway activation associated with disorders such as **postinfective glomerulonephritis**. Hence, measurement of serum complement levels can be of diagnostic value.

Figure 12.14 Cell permeabilization by perforin-dependent membrane perforations.

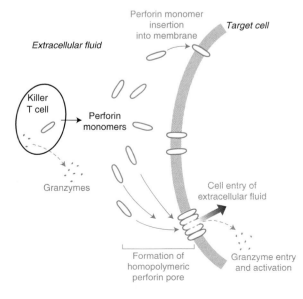

Killer T cell — Perforin monomers — Granzymes — Extracellular fluid — Perforin monomer insertion into membrane — *Target cell* — Cell entry of extracellular fluid — Formation of homopolymeric perforin pore — Granzyme entry and activation

CLINICAL KEYNOTE

Complement deficiency and human disease

Activation of C_1 (and hence of the classical pathway) is controlled by host-protective complement antagonists such as C_1-**esterase inhibitor** and **decay accelerating factor**. Relevant to this, only three human complement pathway dysfunctions are at all common:

1. C_1-**esterase inhibitor** (C_1-INH) **deficiency**
   - Results in **hereditary angioedema**.
2. C_2 **deficiency**
   - Causes collagen-vascular disorders such as **lupus**.
3. **Decay accelerating factor** (DAF) **deficiency**
   - Associated with **paroxysmal nocturnal hemoglobinuria**.

C_1-INH deficiency leads to uncontrolled complement activation with measurable plasma levels of the activated C_1 protease subunit, C_{1s}. Excessive complement activation in this disorder is responsible for the clinical syndrome of hereditary angioedema, which manifests as episodic skin swellings associated with recurrent gastrointestinal and/or respiratory tract obstruction (Figure 12.15). Although the clinical presentation suggests hypersensitivity, signs of histamine-mediated effects (e.g., pruritus, urticaria) are conspicuously absent. Such patients may

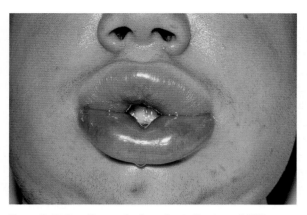

Figure 12.15 Hereditary angioedema due to C1-esterase inhibitor deficiency (Wellcome Photo Library, N0007575C).

present with recurrent abdominal pain, or may require urgent tracheostomy for asphyxiation secondary to glottal edema.

Reduced cell-surface expression of the complement inhibitor DAF is implicated in the pathogenesis of paroxysmal nocturnal hemoglobinuria (PNH) – a clinical syndrome of hemolysis caused by red blood cell hypersensitivity to complement. The underlying defect in PNH does not appear to be specifically related to DAF, however, but more generally related to the defective synthesis of GPI-containing membrane proteins (p. 134).

C_2 deficiency is the commonest hereditary cause of hypocomplementemia, affecting 1 in 10000 people. About half of these individuals are asymptomatic; the remainder may present with collagen-vascular diseases such as **systemic lupus erythematosus**, **Henoch–Schönlein purpura**, and **polymyositis**. Even heterozygotes are prone to develop lupus, as are those primarily deficient in other complement proteins (e.g., C_{1q} deficiency, C_4 deficiency).

The most serious deficiency is **C_3 deficiency**, which is accompanied by recurrent life-threatening infections with encapsulated bacteria (e.g., pneumococcus, meningococcus, gonococcus, *Hemophilus influenzae*) similar to those seen in patients with splenic dysfunction. Since C_3 represents the convergence of both the classical and alternate complement pathways, the severity of this phenotype is unsurprising.

A deficiency of terminal complement components is characterized by particular susceptibility to **Neisserial infections**. Paradoxically, such patients may incur milder morbidity from such infections than do immunocompetent individuals because the release of bacterial endotoxin – and the accompanying severity of tissue damage – is impaired by low complement levels (hypocomplementemia). Other presentations of complement deficiency such as **Raynaud phenomenon** (in C_7 deficiency) and **hemolytic uremic syndrome** (in factor H deficiency) are rare.

Defensins kill microbes by permeabilization

Neutrophils are phagocytic cells – cellular garbage disposals, if you will – which exert their antimicrobial actions via one of two main strategies:

1. Oxidative generation of **free radicals** and **peroxides**
   - e.g., H_2O_2; OH^-.
2. Nonoxidative generation of peptide microbicides
   - e.g., Lysozyme, cathepsin G, azurocidin or defensins.

Like interferons, **defensins** provide a constitutive level of host resistance to microbiological attack. Defensins are small (~30 amino acids) membrane-active peptides expressed in phagocytic cells which participate in oxygen-independent host defense against bacteria, fungi, and viruses. These cationic cysteine-rich proteins (which include HNP-1, 2 and 3) make up about 5% of total neutrophil protein, reaching concentrations up to 100 mg/ml in phagocytic vacuoles, and stimulate monocyte chemotaxis. Human β-defensins are expressed in vaginal and skin epithelium in response to pathogens such as *Candida* spp., whereas other defensins antagonize the action of corticosteroids by binding the adrenocorticotrophic hormone receptor.

Major antimicrobial targets of defensins include Gram-positive bacteria, fungi, enveloped viruses (especially herpes simplex and influenza A) and Gram-negative bacteria. In contrast, cytokines such as interferons are mainly responsible for viral defense.

All defensins contain an invariant octapeptide sequence responsible for their antimicrobial activity. Defensins enter microbes via **defensin pores** which they create by disrupting membranes. These pores appear to be non-selective voltage-gated membrane channels that permeabilize (and thus kill) target cells. Similar induction of lethal pores is the mechanism of action for several infectious toxins.

MOLECULAR MINIREVIEW

Acute phase proteins
Cytokines such as IL-6 may trigger increased plasma levels of inflammatory marker proteins termed **acute phase reactants**. Two such proteins are members of the pentraxin superfamily, **C-reactive protein** (CRP) and **amyloid P component** (see below). Plasma CRP varies with the activity of inflammatory diseases such as **rheumatoid arthritis**. Other acute phase reactants include serum amyloid A (see below), haptoglobin, hemopexin, ceruloplasmin, fibrinogen, fibronectin, ferritin, α_1-antitrypsin, plasminogen (activator), and the C3 and C4 complement proteins. Plasma proteins that decrease during inflammation include albumin, α-fetoprotein, factor XII, insulin-like growth factor I, transferrin, transthyretin and thyroid-binding globulin (TBG).

Chronic inflammation causes amyloid deposition

Amyloid is a structurally heterogeneous material that is deposited in body organs as fibrils consisting of antiparallel β-pleated sheets. These fibrillar proteins occur in heterogeneous forms variously designated as AP, AL, AA, SAA and others. The clinical syndromes that result from amyloid fibril deposition are collectively termed **amyloidosis** (see also pp. 139, 474). Once deposited, amyloid fibrils interfere with organ function, leading to complications such as renal failure, cardiomyopathy, neuropathy, and arthropathy. The fibrils are nonimmunogenic and resist digestion with proteases, though synthetic peptides (so-called β-sheet breakers) may prove clinically useful. However, amyloid P (**AP**) fibrils, which consist of ten glycosylated chains assembled as two noncovalently joined pentameric discs, are notably resistant to degradation by scavenger cells. AP amyloid occurs in all amyloid deposits with the exception of the **cerebral amyloidoses**.

Fibril composition tends to vary with different etiologies of amyloidosis. For example, **primary amyloidosis** is a dysproteinemic state (i.e., akin to myeloma) characterized by excess immunoglobulin light chain production. Such amyloid light chain disorders exhibit "amyloid light" (**AL**) fibril deposition. In contrast, chronic inflammatory states (including not only chronic infections, but also **familial Mediterranean fever**) may cause **secondary amyloidosis** consisting of amyloid A (**AA**) fibrils. Serum amyloid A (**SAA**) is an HDL-binding apolipoprotein family that promotes phagocytic cell adhesion to vascular endothelium. A 37-amino-acid peptide termed **islet amyloid polypeptide** may be responsible for the destruction of pancreatic β-cells in **type 2 diabetes mellitus**.

CLINICAL KEYNOTE

Familial Mediterranean fever
Periodic fevers separated by symptom-free intervals occur as four syndromes:
1. Autosomal recessive

- Familial Mediterranean fever (FMF).
- Hyper-IgD syndrome.
2. Autosomal dominant
   - Familial Hibernian fever, or TRAPS (see below).
   - Muckle–Wells syndrome.

An autosomal recessive syndrome of recurrent fevers lasting one to four days associated with severe abdominal pain (peritonitis), arthritis, pleuritis, and/or secondary (AA) amyloidosis, FMF affects Middle Eastern ethnicities (Sephardic Jews, Turks, Armenians, and Arabs) in whom the carrier frequency may be as high as 1:10. **C5a inhibitor** activity is reportedly low in joint and peritoneal fluid, suggesting that this deficiency could predispose to acute attacks.

The 10 exon gene responsible for FMF, which produces a protein dubbed **pyrin**, is located on chromosome 16p near the α-globin gene locus. The 3.7-kb mRNA encodes a highly basic 781-amino-acid protein with a nuclear localization sequence and bZIP domain, which is thus believed to be a transcription factor. Three mutations clustering around exon 10 account for 85% of cases: M694V, M680I, and V726A; exon 2 is responsible for most of the remainder. Hence, polymerase chain reaction (PCR) assays can now be used for diagnostic purposes in 80% cases. Homozygosity for M694V is seen in 95% of African patients and is associated with a more aggressive clinical course (higher incidence of **amyloidosis**, and higher therapeutic requirement for **colchicine**).

The hyper-IgD syndrome gene product, **mevalonate kinase**, is encoded on chromosome 12q24; this is the enzyme that catalyzes the step after HMGCoA reductase in cholesterol biosynthesis. Familial Hibernian fever is caused by gain-of-function mutations affecting 55-kDa type I tumor necrosis factor receptor, and is therefore sometimes called TRAPS, or **TNF receptor-associated periodic syndrome**. The gene underlying Muckle–Wells syndrome is located on chromosome 1q44.

Summary

Lipids transduce signals from membranes. Cells relieve stress by activating a lipid/protein kinase cascade.

Arachidonic acid is oxidized to eicosanoids. Prostaglandins and leukotrienes regulate local inflammation. Eicosanoid biosynthesis is a key therapeutic drug target. Cyclooxygenase isoforms exert different effects.

Interleukins control leukocyte function during inflammation. Tumor necrosis factor contributes to septic shock. Interferons are antiproliferative cytokines.

Host antiviral gene products are induced by viral RNAs. Hemopoietins and cytokines bind noncatalytic receptors. Cytokine receptors activate the Jak-STAT signaling pathway.

Complement proteins tag antigens for phagocytosis. Defensins kill microbes by permeabilization. Chronic inflammation causes amyloid deposition.

Enrichment reading

Bedtime reading

Cantell K. *The story of interferon: the ups and downs in the life of a scientist.* World Scientific Publishing, 1998

Cheap'n'cheerful

RE, Gearing A. *The cytokine factbook.* Academic Press, New York, 2000

Library reference

Laychock SG, Rubin RP (eds). *Lipid second messengers.* CRC Press, Boca Raton, FL, 1999

Meager T. *The molecular biology of cytokines.* John Wiley & Sons, New York, 1998

Morgan BP, Harris CL (eds). *Complement regulatory proteins.* Academic Press, New York, 1999

Serhan CN, Ward PA (eds). *Molecular and cellular basis of inflammation.* Humana Press, Champaign, IL, 1998

QUIZ QUESTIONS

1. Explain how membrane phospholipids can become involved in intracellular signaling.
2. Describe how arachidonic acid modulates tissue inflammation.
3. What are the beneficial and toxic effects of nonsteroidal anti-inflammatory drugs, and by which biochemical pathways are they mediated?
4. How do eicosanoids induce changes in blood vessel caliber?
5. Describe how leukotrienes may be involved in the pathogenesis of asthma, and explain the potential therapeutic relevance of this.
6. Speaking biochemically, why do people take aspirin?
7. What are interleukins, and what is the structural nature of the molecules they bind?
8. Explain the pathogenesis of septic shock.
9. Which cell types produce which interferons, and with what effects?
10. Describe how interferons inhibit viral proliferation.
11. Using an example, explain how cytokines activate cytokine receptors, and name a disease resulting from dysfunction of this pathway.
12. Define what is meant by the term "acute phase reactant".
13. What is opsonization?
14. Which complement components are differentially involved in the classical and alternate pathways?
15. Name and describe some diseases associated with abnormalities of the complement pathway.

13 Hormones and growth factors

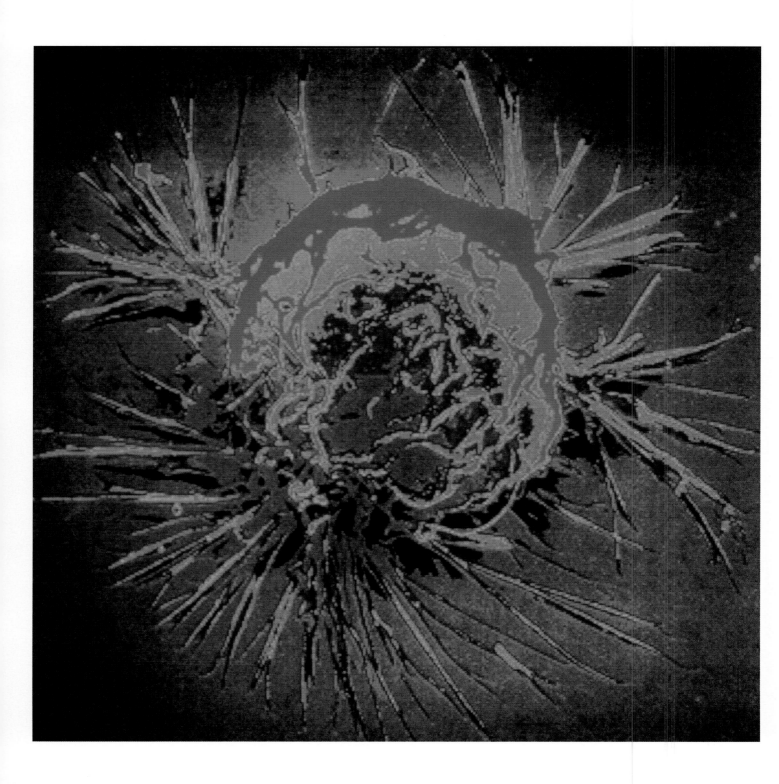

Figure 13.1 (*previous page*) Immunohistochemical demonstration of massive cell surface receptor overexpression in a human breast cancer cell line. Color-enhanced modified image, showing growth factor receptor in red, and digitized (Wellcome Trust Medical Photographic Library, no. N0013284C).

Hormones, growth factors, cytokines and neurotransmitters are extracellular molecules that bind receptors which initiate pathways leading to gene expression. In recent years the fields of biochemistry and endocrinology have merged with the mainstream of signal transduction. As detailed in this section, both intracellular signaling and intercellular communication are essential for coordinating the behavior of human cells and tissues.

Hormone biosynthesis

Hormones are derived from cholesterol or amino acids

Glands secrete molecules called **hormones**, which trigger changes of gene expression in distant parts of the body; hormones are thus defined functionally rather than structurally. Nonetheless, there are two main structural classes of hormone:

1. **Steroid hormones** (plus sterols and thyroid hormones)
   - Long plasma half-life; mainly bound to carrier proteins.
   - Fat-soluble (lipophilic; free hormone enters cells directly).
   - Transform intracellular receptors that act in the nucleus.
2. **Peptide hormones** (plus catecholamines)
   - Short plasma half-life; no carrier proteins.
   - Water-soluble (hydrophilic; unable to cross membranes).
   - Activate cell-surface receptors.

Steroid hormones are synthesized from cholesterol, a primitive lipid which is cleaved to yield pregnenolone (Figure 13.2). This is in turn metabolized to aromatic four-ring hormones such as estradiol, progesterone, testosterone, cortisol, and aldosterone (Figure 13.3). These hormones are too small to convey much information and thus need to transduce their message via a larger receptor protein. Not all members of the steroid hormone receptor superfamily bind steroid hormones, however. For example, the ligand for the vitamin D_3 receptor – 1,25-dihydroxy-cholecalciferol, or calcitriol – is a photolytic derivative of cholesterol that is not a steroid but rather a **sterol**. Similarly, vitamin A (retinoic acid; Figure 13.3) is a cholesterol-derived nonsteroid ligand for a family of steroid-related receptors called the retinoic acid receptors (pp. 148–9).

Other steroid receptor superfamily members include **xenobiotic receptors** such as the dioxin receptor (aryl hydrocarbon receptor) and the peroxisome proliferator activator receptors. The latter receptor family may be mutated in diabetic kindreds, and is targeted by hypolipidemic, antidiabetic and anti-inflammatory drugs. Additional orphan receptors of this class include the farnesoid X receptor, pregnane X receptor, and the liver X receptor. An unusual member of this grouping is the constitutive androstane receptor, which is activated in the absence of ligand but inactivated by the binding of weak androgenic ligands (p. 439).

Many cell signaling molecules are derived from single amino acids, with some (e.g., the neurotransmitters glutamate, aspartate and glycine; p. 495) being bioactive in the unmodified state. An example of a signaling molecule based on a modified amino acid is that for thyroid hormone (**triiodothyronine**, T_3, the active metabolite of **thyroxine**, T_4) which is derived in turn from tyrosine (p. 159). Like vitamins A and D, T_3 is not a steroid hormone (Figure 13.3) yet it binds a steroid receptor superfamily member.

Peptide hormones range in size from three amino acids (thyrotropin-releasing hormone or TRH) to 8- to 14-residue oligopeptides (oxytocin, vasopressin/antidiuretic hormone, and somatostatin) through to 50- to

Figure 13.2 Overview of steroid hormone biosynthesis: derivation of steroids from acetyl CoA.

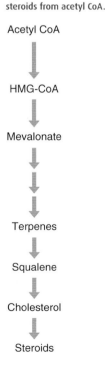

Acetyl CoA

↓

HMG-CoA

↓

Mevalonate

↓
↓
↓

Terpenes

↓

Squalene

↓

Cholesterol

↓

Steroids

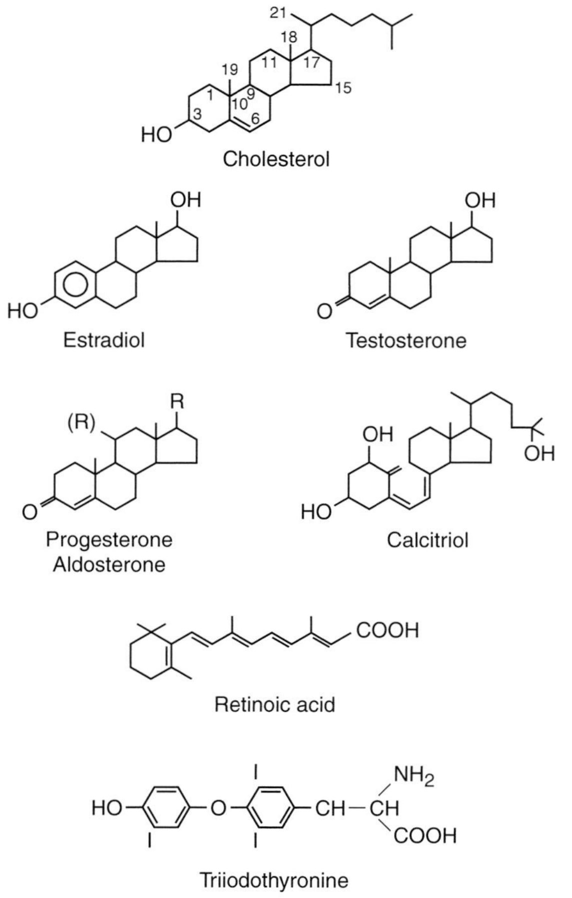

Figure 13.3 Steroid hormone family members: the parent molecule cholesterol (top); estradiol, testosterone, progesterone, aldosterone (with 11-hydroxyl side-chain bracketed), calcitriol; retinoic acid and T₃ (a sterol; at bottom).

200-residue proteins (insulin, parathyroid hormone, thyrotropin, and growth hormone). Most peptide hormones activate G-protein-coupled receptors, but cytokine receptors (e.g., prolactin receptors) and receptor tyrosine kinases (e.g., insulin receptors) are occasionally the target.

MOLECULAR MINIREVIEW

Hormone carrier proteins

Hydrophobic steroid hormones circulate in plasma complexed to transport proteins. With the prominent exceptions of growth hormone and the insulin-like growth factors, most peptide hormones do not circulate bound to such complexes. The primary function of carrier proteins may be to act as a hormone reservoir: since only a small percentage of free (non-protein-bound) plasma hormone is available for cell entry, these plasma transporters minimize fluctuations in hormone availability. Such carrier proteins include:

1. **Sex-hormone binding globulin** (SHBG)
   - Transports estrogens and androgens.
2. **Corticosteroid-binding globulin** (CBG)
   - Transports cortisol and progesterone.
3. **Thyroid-binding globulin** (TBG)
   - Transports thyroid hormones, especially T_4.

Thyroid-binding globulin, or TBG, is a 54-kDa glycoprotein secreted by the liver. Point mutations or deletions of the X-chromosomal *TBG* gene are associated with sex-linked human syndromes of TBG deficiency or excess. These syndromes may be responsible for diagnostic errors based on total plasma hormone levels. For example, abnormally high levels of TBG – which arise not only from mutations but also from self-limiting conditions or drugs – lead to high plasma T_4 levels despite clinical euthyroidism (**euthyroid hyperthyroxinemia**). Hence, if no estimate of free T_4 is undertaken, such patients are at risk of inappropriate antithyroid therapy. Conversely, patients with TBG deficiencies exhibit low plasma total T_4 levels despite having normal free thyroid hormone concentrations.

[Note that **thyroglobulin** is a 660-kDa tyrosine-binding glycoprotein that makes up most of the thyroid follicular colloid protein and binds T_3/T_4 during the organification step of thyroid hormone biosynthesis. Plasma thyroglobulin is monitored as a tumor marker in patients with differentiated thyroid cancer.]

Mutations affecting other T_4 carrier proteins such as **transthyretin** also result in euthyroid hyperthyroxinemia. Interestingly, transthyretin mutations underlie a distinct autosomal dominant disorder, **familial amyloidotic polyneuropathy**.

Inactive precursors may be converted to active hormones

Hormones are synthesized in a number of steps. Variables affecting the functional activity of a hormone include:

1. The net rate of hormone biosynthesis.
2. The expression of endogenous synergistic or antagonistic molecules.
3. The metabolic activation of inactive hormone precursors.

The end-organ metabolic activation of precursor hormones is carried out by enzymes termed **convertases** or **maturases**. Many of these inactive precursors or **prohormones** (including prorenin and proinsulin) are cleaved by serine proteases homologous to the yeast subtilisin enzyme family, and examples of such prohormone activation are summarized in Table 13.1. Many other hormones are initially produced as inactive precursors, including **pro-opiomelanocortin** (**POMC**) which is of particular interest since its mature proteolytic cleavage

Table 13.1. Prohormones and convertases

1. Thyroid hormone metabolism
   - Thyroxine (T_4) is peripherally monodeiodinated to the more active triiodothyronine (T_3) by the enzyme T_4 5′-deiodinase. A biologically inactive form of T_3, reverse T_3, is also produced by extrathyroidal T_4 deiodination
   - Drugs used in hyperthyroidism (such as propylthiouracil, propranolol, and dexamethasone) may act partly by inhibiting T_4 5′-deiodinase

2. Androgen metabolism
   - Circulating testosterone is reduced in androgen target tissues to active dihydrotestosterone (DHT) by the enzyme 5α-reductase, hereditary deficiencies of which result in one variety of male pseudohermaphroditism. DHT is 50-fold more potent than testosterone in promoting prostate growth, but testosterone may directly promote muscle growth and spermatogenesis
   - Androgens are also prohormones for the bioactive estrogens estradiol, estrone, and estriol, which are derived by aromatization of the androgens testosterone, androstenedione and dihydroepiandrosterone (DHEA) respectively; the latter is reputed to be an "anti-ageing hormone" which restores self-esteem and mood while also increasing bone density and sexual function. The responsible aromatases for estrogen biosynthesis occur not only in the ovary and placenta, but also in peripheral tissues such as fat, liver and muscle

3. Vitamin D metabolism
   - Dietary vitamin D undergoes hepatic conversion to 25-OH cholecalciferol
   - In the kidney, this 25-hydroxy vitamin D metabolite undergoes 1-hydroxylation to yield the bioactive form, 1,25-dihydroxy-vitamin D (calcitriol)
   - Deficiency of renal 1-α hydroxylase causes type I vitamin-D-dependent rickets

4. Angiotensin metabolism
   - The vasoactive intermediary in the renin-angiotensin-aldosterone system originates in the liver as angiotensinogen, overexpression of which is genetically linked to hypertension. This molecule is first cleaved by the acid protease renin to form an inactive decapeptide, angiotensin I
   - Angiotensin I is metabolized by angiotensin-converting enzyme (ACE) in pulmonary endothelia to the active octapeptide, angiotensin II. ACE inhibitors are used to treat hypertension and heart failure

5. Insulin metabolism
   - Insulin is synthesized as an inactive 110-kDa precursor termed preproinsulin which is converted by a signal peptidase to proinsulin
   - Proteolytic cleavage of a connecting peptide (C-peptide) by a subtilisin-like endopeptidase leaves the bioactive insulin molecule composed of a 21-residue A chain and 30-residue B chain linked by disulfide bonds
   - Plasma proinsulin/C-peptide levels are used in the differential diagnosis of recurrent hypoglycemic attacks: high levels during an attack are consistent with underlying insulinoma, whereas low levels suggest factitious self-administration of synthetic insulin

products include adrenocorticotrophic hormone (ACTH), melanocyte-stimulating hormone (MSH), β-endorphin, and met-enkephalin (Figure 13.4). For this reason POMC is sometimes termed **big ACTH**. The excessive pigmentation (MSH- and ACTH-induced) and hypokalemia (cortisol-induced) sometimes seen in small-cell lung cancer reflects paraneoplastic overproduction of this ACTH precursor.

Steroid hormones

Steroid hormones are synthesized by metabolic interconversion

Steroidogenesis takes place predominantly in the adrenal cortex, testis, ovary, and placenta. Whereas the adrenal medulla produces all catecholamines (p. 433), distinct regions of the adrenal cortex produce steroid hormones:

1. The outer cortex is where **aldosterone** (mineralocorticoid) synthesis takes place, mainly regulated by the pressor peptide angiotensin II (p. 348).
2. The inner cortex is where **cortisol** (glucocorticoid) synthesis takes place. Cortisol synthesis is mainly regulated by pituitary ACTH.

Both cortisol and aldosterone have pressor effects. In contrast, interconversion reactions between gonadal steroids produce striking differences in sexual phenotype:

1. Testicular Leydig cells synthesize **testosterone**.
2. Ovarian outer (theca) cells synthesize **androgens**. Thecal steroidogenesis is controlled by the pituitary hormone **luteinizing hormone** (LH).
3. Ovarian inner (granulosa) cells convert androgens to **estradiol**. Granulosa cell steroidogenesis is controlled by the pituitary hormone **follicle-stimulating hormone** (FSH).
4. **Progesterone** is synthesized in the ovarian corpus luteum.

In pregnant women the placenta produces **human placental lactogen** (HPL) and **human chorionic gonadatrophin** (HCG) in addition to progesterone, and also converts androgens to estrogens (especially estriol; see below). Estrogens are present in high concentration in male semen where they regulate epididymal fluid resorption, and estrogen receptors (p. 317) are co-expressed with androgen receptors throughout the male genital tract.

MOLECULAR MINIREVIEW

Steroid hormone biosynthesis

Most enzymes involved in steroid synthesis are P_{450} cytochrome oxidases. The rate-limiting step in steroid hormone synthesis is the conversion of the 27-carbon cholesterol molecule to the 21-carbon **pregnenolone** by a cholesterol side-chain cleavage enzyme called **desmolase**. Subsequent enzymatic steps lead to the synthesis of various steroids based on the following structure–function relationships:

1. **C21** (21-carbon) **steroids**
   - Progesterone
     is the precursor of all other steroid hormones,
     3β-dehydrogenase is required for pregnenolone oxidation,
   - Glucocorticoids and mineralocorticoids
     both require **21-hydroxylase** and **11-β-hydroxylase**.
     glucocorticoids also require **17-hydroxylase**.
     mineralocorticoids also require **18-hydroxylase**.

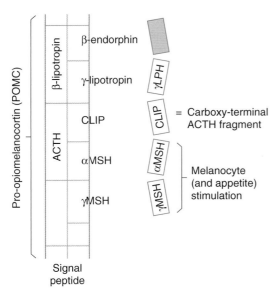

Figure 13.4 Biosynthesis of adrenocorticotrophic hormone (ACTH), melanocyte-stimulating hormone (MSH) and β-endorphin from pro-opiomelanocortin (POMC) proteolysis (see pp. 321, 426).

2. **C19 steroids**
   - Androgens
       require 17-hydroxylase and 2-carbon cleavage (lyase),
       pregnenolone is converted to the androgen **dihydroepiandrosterone (DHEA)**,
       progesterone is converted to **androstenedione**.
3. **C18 steroids**
   - Estrogens
       derived from androgens by A ring aromatization and C19 demethylation
       i. **estrone** (E_1), the major postmenopausal estrogen, is derived by the peripheral aromatization of androstenedione.
       ii. **estradiol** (E_2), the major premenopausal postpubertal estrogen, is derived by ovarian aromatization of testosterone.
       iii. **estriol** (E_3), the major pregnancy-associated estrogen, is derived by placental aromatization of DHEA.

Heritable deficiencies of any of these enzymes (e.g., caused by a mutation of the *CYP21* gene on 6p21.3 that encodes 21-hydroxylase) can cause the clinical syndrome of **congenital adrenal hyperplasia**.

Transformed steroid receptors translocate to the nucleus

Steroid hormone receptors are ligand-dependent transcription factors that consist of three main domains (Figure 13.5):
1. A carboxy-terminal **hormone-binding domain**
   - Well conserved (≅90% cross-species).
2. A central 66- to 68-amino-acid **DNA-binding** (zinc finger) **domain**
   - Most strongly conserved (approaches 100% cross-species).
3. An amino-terminal **modulating domain**
   - Highly variable structure (formerly termed immunodomain).

In addition, there may exist overlapping subdomains with additional functions such as a dimerization domain, one or more transactivation domains, a nuclear localization domain, and an Hsp90-binding domain. Note that some of the latter domains are sited within the former (especially ligand-binding) domains. Ligand binding to receptors may sometimes take place in the cytoplasm (as reported for the glucocorticoid receptor) but activated receptors invariably localize to the nucleus (e.g., estrogen/progesterone/T_3 receptors). Since cytoplasmic receptors are actively transported across the nuclear envelope and then shuttle back to the cytoplasm, the molecular superfamily comprising steroid hormone receptors and T_3/sterol receptors is designated the **nuclear receptor superfamily**. As noted above, this superfamily includes not only steroid and sterol hormone receptors, but also orphan receptors for which high-affinity endogenous ligands remain poorly defined.

Hormone binding induces a structural change termed receptor **transformation**, which triggers a sequence of molecular events comprising Hsp90 dissociation, dimerization, nuclear translocation, DNA binding, and transactivation of hormone-specific gene expression. Untransformed (8S) receptors remain complexed with Hsp90 heat-shock proteins in the cytoplasm. Hormone-dependent receptor transformation gives rise to serine phosphorylation events that permit the swinging of a **hinge region** between the hormone- and DNA-binding domains, thus permitting receptor dimerization. These conformational changes may in turn expose the zinc fingers of the DNA-binding domain to intranuclear upstream (5′) enhancer sequences termed **hormone response elements (HREs)**. Steroid receptor HREs are usually palindromic, consistent with dimeric receptor binding, and receptor specificity for these HREs depends not

Figure 13.5 Microanatomy of a steroid hormone receptor, showing the amino-terminal transactivating domain, the carboxy-terminal ligand-binding domain, and the zinc finger-containing DNA-binding domain. NLS, nuclear localization sequence; HRE, hormone response element.

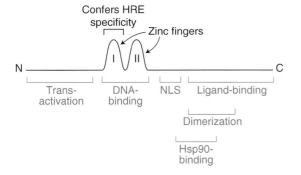

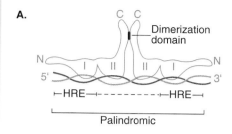

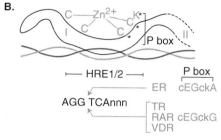

Figure 13.6 Interaction of steroid hormone receptors with hormone response elements (HREs). *A*, Ligand-dependent receptor dimerization permits DNA binding of the dimer to a palindromic HRE. *B*, Demonstration of how the HRE half-site spacing and the structure of the P-box domain interact to regulate the specificity of receptor binding. RAR, retinoic acid receptor; TR, thyroid hormone receptor; VDR, vitamin D receptor.

only on the nucleotide half-sequence but also on the length between the half-sequences (Figure 13.6*A*). Of the two zinc fingers present in steroid hormone receptors, the first contains a three-amino-acid subdomain which distinguishes the HRE half-site nucleotide sequence. A five-amino-acid subdomain in the second zinc finger distinguishes the spacing between the half-sites by acting as a DNA length sensor between dimerized receptors (Figure 13.6*B*).

Unlike classic steroid receptors, vitamin D (VDR), thyroid hormone (TR), and retinoic acid receptors (RAR) bind DNA half-sites arranged as nonpalindromic direct repeats with base-pair spacings of 3, 4, and 5 respectively. These receptor–DNA interactions may be further regulated by heterodimer formation with ligand-activated adaptor receptors. Mutant receptors lacking the hormone-binding domain may be constitutively activated. Certain variant forms of the T_3 receptor bind DNA in the absence of hormone, acting in these circumstances as negative transcription factors that inhibit T_3-dependent gene expression.

MOLECULAR MINIREVIEW

Female sex hormone receptors

The **estrogen receptor** (ER) exists as alpha (**ERα**) and beta (**ERβ**) isoforms, providing a further dimension of tissue specificity. The ERα isoform may signal not only by transactivation of specific genes, but also via ligand-dependent binding to the p85 subunit of the SH2-containing effector phosphatidylinositol-3′-kinase (PI3K); this latter interaction triggers the activation of protein kinase B (PKB) and endothelial nitric oxide synthase (eNOS; p. 352), thus contributing to the vascular protective effects of estrogens. ERβ expression is normally high in colorectal epithelium but is reduced in **colorectal cancer**, suggesting that the protective effects of estrogens on colorectal cancer incidence in females may reflect ERβ actions. ERβ is also abundantly expressed in normal breast and prostatic tissue, but declines during malignant transformation; a reciprocal relationship with ERα expression levels may characterize estrogen-dependent tumor evolution.

Progesterone likewise activates two intracellular receptors, **PR-A** and **PR-B.** The former mediates uterine epithelial involution, whereas the latter mimics the uterotrophic (and carcinogenic) effects of estrogen. However, progesterone may activate transcription not only by sequence-specific receptor-DNA binding, but also via "nongenomic" actions of the receptor including activation of the breast-regulatory cytokine **Stat5**, MAP kinase stimulation, or Jnk kinase inhibition. A further nongenomic action of progesterone involves low-affinity interference with cell-surface **oxytocin receptor** activation, which may help to suppress premature labor during late pregnancy. Since steroid hormones may have neuroactive effects – with one example being modulation of brain $GABA_A$ receptors by progesterone (p. 499) – mood changes during the menstrual cycle may arise in part via this mechanism.

Hormone blockade may cause or revert disease

There are many recognized clinical syndromes of hormone resistance caused by defective hormone receptor synthesis. Affected individuals have normal or elevated levels of circulating hormone, supplements of which are relatively ineffective in correcting the deficiency phenotype. Mutations affecting members of the steroid hormone receptor superfamily include:

1. **Testicular feminization syndrome** – mutant androgen receptors.
2. **Pseudohypoaldosteronism** – mutant mineralocorticoid receptors.
3. **Vitamin-D-resistant rickets** – mutant vitamin D receptors.

4. **Thyroid hormone resistance** – mutant T_3 receptors.

Complete androgen insensitivity may occur because of over 300 loss-of-function mutations affecting the 8-exon Xq11-12 chromosomal locus. A variety of activating mutations affecting the androgen receptor gene have also been reported in prostate cancer, though late-stage disease is more often associated with gene inactivation caused by promoter hypermethylation. Still other mutations may cause resistance to androgens (and hence to anti-androgens).

The X-linked coagulopathy **hemophilia B Leyden** (not to be confused with factor V Leiden; p. 471) arises because of a factor IX promoter mutation. The inhibitory effects of this mutation are reduced following the androgen surge of puberty due to a coexisting androgen-responsive element six nucleotides downstream in the same promoter. Nonsteroid hormone receptors also participate in the pathogenesis of resistance syndromes. For example, inactivating mutations of the luteinizing hormone receptor have been associated with one form of **male pseudohermaphroditism.**

All hormonal agonists activate receptors in the same way, whereas hormonal antagonists inactivate receptors in all sorts of different ways. The potency of hormonal agonists (including synthetic derivatives such as the glucocorticoid dexamethasone) is primarily a function of receptor affinity – in other words, potency is inversely proportional to the rate of agonist/receptor dissociation. In contrast, anti-hormonal drugs may act by a multiplicity of mechanisms: by providing dysfunctional ligands (which may also exhibit high receptor affinity), by inhibiting prohormone activation, or by disrupting the circadian rhythm (pulsatility) of hormone release. Uncontrolled cell growth is responsible for many human diseases, making therapeutic reversal of hormone-dependent growth an attractive pharmacologic strategy.

The abortifacient **mifepristone (RU486)** is a partial progesterone agonist that inhibits Hsp90 dissociation from inactive progesterone receptor heterooligomers. Changes in receptor conformation induced by RU486 are distinct from those induced by progesterone. Similarly, **5-α-reductase inhibitors** (e.g., **finasteride**) inhibit the conversion of testosterone to dihydrotestosterone, thus inhibiting growth in benign prostatic hyperplasia. The thyroid hormone antagonist **propylthiouracil** has several different mechanisms of action, including inhibiting the organification and coupling steps of thyroid hormone biosynthesis, and impairing extrathyroidal conversion of T_4 to T_3.

PHARMACOLOGIC FOOTNOTE

Breast cancer hormonal therapies

Tamoxifen is a weak estrogen agonist that binds ER and thus antagonizes the effects of estradiol-induced receptor activation. Tamoxifen does not alter the DNA binding of ER, but may antagonize the transactivating properties of the receptor by changing its tertiary structure. Curiously, tamoxifen opposes the action of estrogen in breast tissue and yet mimics the carcinogenic effect of estrogen on the uterus. ER splice-variants may cause tamoxifen resistance in ER-positive breast cancer cases, as may overexpression of the **p130**[Cas] (Crk-associated substrate) adaptor protein. **Raloxifene** is an anti-estrogen that blocks estrogen in the breast while mimicking its beneficial effects on bone mineralization. The anti-estrogen ICI 164,384 inhibits ER binding to DNA and may also prevent ER dimerization, whereas ICI 182,780 activates and thus downregulates the receptor. Such ER-binding drugs are termed **selective estrogen receptor modulators** or **SERMs** (p. 422).

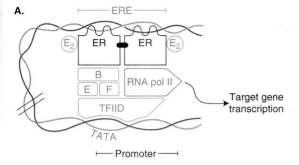

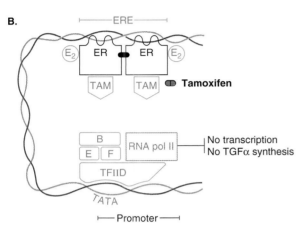

Figure 13.7 Estrogen receptor (ER) interaction with DNA in the presence of estrogen and its pharmacologic antagonist tamoxifen. *A,* Binding of the estrogen-activated ER dimer to its upstream hormone response element (HRE), followed by DNA looping and assembly of the multiprotein transcription apparatus. *B,* Binding of tamoxifen to ER prevents assembly of the transcription complex, thereby preventing estrogen-inducible gene activation. ERE, estrogen-response elements; E_2, estradiol; TAM, tamoxifen; TGFα, transforming growth factor alpha.

Aromatase inhibitors (e.g., anastrozole, letrozole), which inhibit the peripheral conversion of androgens to estrogens, form another class of drugs used to treat breast cancer. Declining estradiol levels remove negative feedback from pituitary LH/FSH (an effect that may be mediated via an estrogen-response element upstream of the **gonadotropin-releasing hormone** – GnRH – gene) and thus preclude effective suppression of ovarian estrogens in premenopausal women. For this reason aromatase inhibitors are usually prescribed only for **postmenopausal breast cancer** patients.

Disrupting pulsatile trophic hormone secretion by continuous agonist application suppresses hormone action. The best example of this is glucocorticoid-inducible ACTH suppression, which leads to adrenal gland atrophy in patients on long-term synthetic steroids. Similarly, GnRH agonists (e.g., goserelin, leuprolide) stimulate the continuous secretion of LH or FSH, inhibiting gonadal testosterone or estrogen release. Hence, these drugs are used in **prostate cancer** and in **premenopausal breast cancer**.

Receptor–DNA interactions determine gene expression

Many differentiated cell and tissue phenotypes are critically determined by steroid hormone receptor binding to DNA. However, many hormone response elements (HREs) – such as those of the glucocorticoid, mineralocorticoid, androgen, and progesterone receptors – are identical, indicating that the specificity of gene expression is not attributable to DNA-receptor binding alone. Tissue-specific receptor expression is thus a critical factor in conferring specificity of hormone action: even if downstream gene expression patterns are identical, tissues expressing different receptors will only express those genes if and when the appropriate hormone is released into the bloodstream. The regulation of steroid hormone action is more complex than this, however, involving as it does many other regulatory variables:

1. Agonist or antagonist ligand binding
   - e.g., Tamoxifen (Figure 13.7).
2. Receptor homo- or heterodimerization
   - e.g., Heterodimeric interactions within the nonsteroidal side of the nuclear receptor superfamily. Steroid hormone receptors may also interact with other dimeric transcription factors such as NFκB and the Fos-Jun complex, co-occupying composite HREs with these factors (see Figure 3.14). Steric hindrance from adjacent DNA binding to such sites may produce antagonistic interactions.
3. Receptor isoform expression
   - e.g., The retinoic acid receptor (RAR) exists as α, β and γ isoforms encoded on separate chromosomes, with the RARα isoform having tenfold lower affinity for retinoic acid. Chromosomal translocations cause the *RARα* gene to fuse with one of two zinc finger genes in **acute promyelocytic leukemia** (*PML* or *PLZF*), thereby inhibiting retinoic-acid-(RA-) dependent neutrophil maturation while abolishing TNF-inducible blast cell death. Similarly, the T_3 receptor has α and β isoforms encoded by the *ErbA* gene: an alternatively spliced α-receptor, ErbAα2, does not bind T_3 and thus exerts negative effects similar to the viral transforming protein v-ErbA.
4. Positive or negative HREs
   - e.g., Negative glucocorticoid response elements (nGREs) differ in sequence not only from positive GREs but also from each other. Negative GREs bind receptors with lower affinity than do positive GREs, and may

function as negative regulators in some tissues while positive in others. Negative thyroid hormone HREs also occur. Conversely, T_3 receptors may bind and negatively regulate estrogen-response elements (EREs).

The regulatory flexibility conferred by these multiple variables is enormous. The necessity for this flexibility is clear – whereas cell-surface receptors transduce their signals to the nucleus via a morass of intermediary molecules, the ancient nuclear receptor family communicates directly with DNA in response to signals transmitted from distant organs.

MOLECULAR MINIREVIEW

RXRs: hormone receptor co-regulators

Receptors from the nonsteroidal side of the nuclear receptor superfamily – the receptors for vitamin A (retinoic acid, RA), vitamin D, and thyroid hormones – can heterodimerize either with each other or with intranuclear accessory molecules including the **retinoid X receptors** RXRα and RXRβ. RXRs are homologous to the retinoic acid receptors (RARs, see above), especially in their DNA-binding domains. The pharmacologically active drug **all-trans-retinoic acid (ATRA)** binds RARs with high affinity, whereas the RA metabolite **9-cis-retinoic acid** is a high-affinity natural ligand for both RARs and RXRs. Such RXR agonists or **rexinoids** regulate RXR heterodimerization with a variety of nuclear hormone receptors, including those controlling lipid, sugar and xenobiotic metabolism (p. 439).

RXRα is abundantly expressed in the liver (where it may transactivate hepatitis B virus genes). **RXRβ** heterodimerizes not only with RARs, but also with vitamin D receptors and thyroid hormone receptors. With respect to the latter interaction, treatment of T cell lymphoma patients with RXR ligands (**bexarotene**) can cause pituitary hypothyroidism due to thyrotropin suppression. Selective knockout of RXRα in adult transgenic mice disrupts heterodimers of RXRα and the vitamin D receptor, causing hair follicle degeneration and hyperplastic skin lesions.

Rexinoids can **squelch** the activity of heterologous sterol receptors by driving the formation of RXR homodimers. This reduces the formation of RXR-containing heterodimers – the main DNA-binding form of RARs and related receptors. RXRs are thus **co-regulatory transactivators**, which form heterodimers with other nuclear receptors. 9-cis-retinoic acid may also modulate lipid homeostasis by activating RXR heterodimers incorporating peroxisome proliferator-activated receptors (pp. 439–40). RXRα is a critical regulator of adipocyte differentiation, and is a candidate gene for a rare recessive variety of diabetes, congenital generalized lipodystrophy (**Seip–Berardinelli syndrome**).

Peptide hormones

Most brain hormones activate G-protein-coupled receptors

Unlike the gonads, adrenals and thyroid, the human brain and pituitary gland synthesize predominantly nonsteroidal (peptide) hormones. Many such hormones function in both the central nervous system and periphery. Most brain hormones fall into the following groups:

1. **Neurotransmitters**
   - Cholecystokinin (CCK), vasoactive intestinal polypeptide (VIP), bombesin, substance P, β-endorphin.
   - Somatostatin (primarily present in the hypothalamus).
2. **Hypothalamic releasing hormones**

- TRH (thryotropin-releasing hormone; releases TSH, prolactin).
- GnRH (gonadotropin-releasing (LH, FSH) hormone).
- CRH (corticotropin-releasing (ACTH) hormone).
- GHRH (growth-hormone-releasing hormone).
3. **Posterior pituitary peptide hormones**
   - Vasopressin (antidiuretic hormone (ADH)).
   - Oxytocin.
4. **Anterior pituitary hormones**
   - Dimeric glycoproteins: TSH, LH, and FSH.
   - Pro-opiomelanocortin (POMC) derivatives: ACTH, melanocyte-stimulating hormone (MSH) and met-enkephalin.
   - Somatomammotropins: prolactin and growth hormone (GH).
5. **Pineal gland** (indoleamine) **hormones**
   - Serotonin (5-hydroxytryptamine).
   - Melatonin (N-acetyl-5-methoxytryptamine).

The above anatomic groupings of these hormones are accompanied by functional heterogeneity. TRH and met-enkephalin are neurotransmitters, for example, whereas β-endorphin is a proteolytic derivative of POMC. One feature uniting these hormones is that most interact with G-protein-coupled receptors – exceptions to this are the somatomammotropins GH and prolactin, which activate cytokine receptors.

G-protein-coupled receptors activated by brain hormones usually stimulate adenyl cyclase and thus cyclic AMP. This is the signaling mode of the heterodimeric pituitary glycoproteins **FSH**, **LH**, and **TSH**, which contain identical α-subunits. The placental hormone β human chorionic gonadotrophin (**β-HCG**) is a structurally related molecule that shares not only the same α-subunit as LH but also an LH-like β-subunit, thereby enabling β-HCG to bind the LH receptor. Androgen-secreting Leydig cell tumors may arise because of activating mutations of the LH receptor (D578G), leading to precocious puberty due to **testotoxicosis**.

Oxytocin and **vasopressin** (antidiuretic hormone, ADH) are structurally related hypothalamic nonapeptides that act via G-protein-coupled receptors, as do other small peptides including bradykinin and the endothelins. Whereas hypothalamic oxytocin is responsible for **milk ejection** during lactation, de novo synthesis of uterine oxytocin is implicated in **labor induction**. The distinct pressor effects of vasopressin are mainly due to the presence of a hydrophilic **arginine** residue (in place of the hydrophobic leucine in oxytocin) at position 8 in the molecule. The long-acting vasopressin analog used to treat hypothalamic deficiency states (diabetes insipidus) is **1-deamino-D-arginine vasopressin (DDAVP)**. **Nephrogenic diabetes insipidus** is an inherited end-organ resistance to vasopressin caused by mutations affecting the **vasopressin type 2 receptor**.

Gestational tumors termed **choriocarcinomas** often express huge quantities of β-HCG. Such patients may develop mild hyperthyroidism due to weak TSH agonism by look-alike HCG molecules; TSH receptor mutants hypersensitive to β-HCG may also cause familial gestational hyperthyroidism. So-called nonfunctioning pituitary adenomas (adenomas unassociated with symptoms of hormone overproduction) can secrete glycoprotein α-subunits alone. Overproduction of β-HCG by **testicular germcell tumors** may be heralded by the development of gynecomastia in young men, whereas constitutive secretion of prolactin by **pituitary (micro)adenomata** can present with galactorrhea in nonpuerperal individuals (Figure 13.8).

Figure 13.8 Clinical consequences of hormone overproduction. A, Hypersecretion of β human chorionic gonadotrophin (β-HCG) by a testicular tumor, manifesting as gynecomastia in a young male. B, Constitutive prolactin secretion from a pituitary tumor, manifesting as galactorrhea (Wellcome Medical Photographic Library, N0008983C and N0008970C).

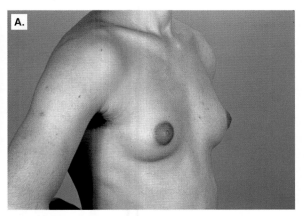
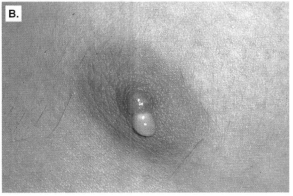

MOLECULAR MINIREVIEW

Growth hormone and prolactin

The pituitary somatomammotropins **prolactin** and **growth hormone** (GH) act via cytokine receptors, which signal by activating nonreceptor Jak tyrosine kinases (p. 305). G-protein-mediated pathways are important in regulating the growth of pituitary somatotrophic cells, with the result that mutations activating G-protein-dependent cAMP production may cause GH-secreting pituitary tumors (p. 277). The placental hormone human placental lactogen (HPL, formerly human chorionic somatomammotropin) is homologous to GH and, to a lesser extent, prolactin.

The 5-exon gene encoding prolactin diverged from the GH/HPL locus about 400 million years ago, whereas the duplication event leading to divergence of GH and HPL occurred as recently as 50 million years ago. This is reflected in the 85% amino acid homology between the two hormones (compared with only 20% for GH and prolactin) and in the juxtaposition of their encoding genes within the same 50-kb stretch of chromosome 17. In functional terms HPL combines the lactogenic and growth-promoting features of prolactin and GH respectively.

Prolactin is synthesized in an alternative nonpituitary form by decidual (luteal-phase or pregnant) endometrium, and a prolactin-releasing pituitary hormone analogous to GHRH has been identified. A structurally unrelated decidual hormone is **relaxin**, a G-protein-coupled receptor ligand which prepares the blastocyst for invasion, and causes cervix softening, pelvic joint destabilization, myometrial quiescence and (perhaps) diabetes-associated sequelae during pregnancy.

CLINICAL KEYNOTE

Creativity, depression, and hormone feedback loops

Feedback regulation is central to the biology of hypothalamic releasing hormones. Processes related to reproduction, such as pregnancy, menstruation, puberty and menopause, as well as normal thyroid and adrenal hormone homeostasis, rely upon the inhibition of hypothalamic hormone release in response to serum levels of the target hormone (Figure 13.9). Active **pulmonary tuberculosis** is associated with activation of the hypothalamo-pituitary-adrenal (HPA) axis, leading to hypercortisolemia. This may contribute to the immune paresis observed in progressive tuberculosis, and could also account in part for the creativity of consumptive writers such as Keats, Lawrence, Proust, Mansfield, and Orwell.

Pituitary release of growth hormone (GH) is controlled not only by hypothalamic GH-releasing hormone but also by the secretagogue **ghrelin**, which is released in the stomach and activates a pituitary G-protein-coupled receptor. Increased feeding and body mass are observed following ghrelin administration, suggesting that this molecule could be used to treat wasting and cachexia syndromes. Blunted release of GH in response to GHRH in childhood has been associated with an increased risk of **depression** in later life.

Brain and gut hormones may be identical

Many peptide hormones are co-expressed in the gastrointestinal tract and central nervous system, suggesting a common role for neurotransmitters in brain and gut. Such co-expressed peptides include:

1. **Cholecystokinin** (CCK), **neurotensin**.
2. **Somatostatin**.
3. Vasoactive intestinal polypeptide (VIP), **substance P**, **bombesin**, and **endorphins**.

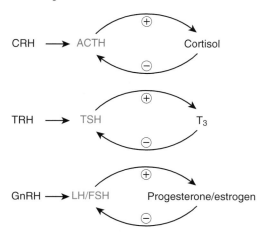

Figure 13.9 Feedback loops operating between hypothalamic releasing hormones, their pituitary effectors, and peripheral target hormones. ACTH, adrenocorticotrophic hormone; CRH, corticotropin-releasing hormone; FSH, follicle-stimulating hormone; GnRH, gonadotropin-releasing hormone; LH, luteinizing hormone; T_3, triiodothyronine; TRH, thyrotropin-releasing hormone; TSH, thyroid-stimulating hormone.

Like the anterior pituitary hormones, **cholecystokinin** (CCK) – the so-called **hormone of satiety** which acts on both the gut and central nervous system – activates G-protein-coupled receptors which in this case activate the second messenger phospholipase C (as do the hypophysiotropic hormones TRH and GnRH, the posterior pituitary hormone ADH, and the neurotransmitter bombesin). CCK is structurally very similar to **gastrin** (a gastrointestinal hormone that increases gastric acidity) and insulin. Plasma CCK levels may be low in **celiac disease**, a disorder causing villous atrophy of the CCK-containing small intestinal mucosa.

A structurally distinct brain-and-gut peptide hormone family is that including **VIP**, **GHRH**, **secretin**, and **glucagon**. As with CCK and VIP, the central nervous system contains detectable amounts of insulin, glucagon and secretin, but a neurotransmitter role for these gut hormones remains poorly defined. In addition to its other actions, VIP exerts an anti-inflammatory effect via inhibition of type I helper T cells, and could thus prove useful in disorders such as **rheumatoid arthritis**.

MOLECULAR MINIREVIEW

Melatonin

Melatonin is a light-inhibited pineal gland hormone involved in maintaining circadian rhythm (p. 517) and is thus implicated in the pathogenesis of jet-lag and seasonal affective disorder (SAD). Synthesized by the enzyme *N*-**acetyltransferase** (**NAT**, which resembles a bacterial photosynthetic enzyme), melatonin is a hypnotic hormone produced exclusively during darkness when NAT levels rise 10- to 100-fold. In neuroanatomic terms the light–dark circadian cycle is generated by the suprachiasmatic nucleus (SCN) of the hypothalamus, which is synchronized via a monosynaptic pathway between the retina and the hypothalamus. The SCN contains melatonin receptors, whose activity depends upon the synthesis of pineal melatonin as regulated by the superior cervical ganglion. Neural induction of melatonin is inhibited not only by bright lights but also by β-adrenergic blockade. The pineal gland synthesizes other indoleamine hormones that act via G-proteins, including the structurally related neurotransmitter **serotonin**. However, whereas melatonin arises via tryptophan decarboxylation, serotonin results from tryptophan hydroxylation.

Unrelated to melatonin (in case you were wondering) is the **melanocortin** hormone family – including melanocyte-stimulating hormone, MSH, and adrenocorticotrophic hormone, ACTH – which regulates skin pigmentation by enhancing melanocyte growth and **melanin** production. MSH receptor mutations may contribute to some skin cancers. The **cannabinoid receptor** (pp. 509–10) is a distant relative of the melanocortin receptor.

Inhibitory hormones regulate hypothalamo-pituitary function

The intracranial hormone command center is replete with negative feedback control loops. **Somatostatin** (also known as growth hormone release-inhibiting peptide) is a 14-amino-acid polypeptide (except in the intestine, where it contains 28 amino acids) that inhibits, GH, TSH, ACTH and gonadotropin-releasing factor (GnRF) as well as insulin, renin and many gut hormones. Its antiproliferative effects relate to the activation of tyrosine phosphatases by a G-protein-mediated mechanism; additional inhibitory signals include the inactivation of adenylate cyclase and calcium influx. A nonhydrolyzable synthetic analog, **octreotide**, is used to control diarrhea in

VIP-secreting tumors (**VIPomas**) as well as for the medical management of GH-secreting pituitary tumors (**acromegaly**) and intestinal obstruction.

Pituitary gonadotropin (LH/FSH) release may be modulated by the biologically opposed TGFβ-like gonadal hormones **inhibin** and **activin**. Inhibin antagonizes FSH release with little effect on LH. Activin is a dimer of inhibin β-subunits (β_A and β_B) which, unlike inhibin, stimulates FSH release and is also an important embryonic morphogen. Another example of negative feedback is the inhibition of GnRH secretion by prolactin, which accounts for the amenorrhea seen in breast-feeding mothers and women with prolactin-secreting pituitary tumors. Since the major endogenous inhibitor of prolactin (and GH) release is **dopamine**, hormonal hypersecretion from GH- or prolactin-secreting pituitary adenomas may be suppressed by the dopamine receptor agonist **bromocriptine**.

Endogenous opioids such as **β-endorphin** and **met-enkephalin** are hypothalamic neurotransmitters that bind G-protein-coupled receptors, inhibiting net cAMP synthesis by antagonizing adenyl cyclase and activating phosphodiesterase. This leads in turn to inhibition of hypothalamic GnRH secretion. The stress-inducible hypothalamic corticotropin-releasing hormone (CRH) may also inhibit GnRH secretion.

CLINICAL KEYNOTE

Autoantibodies in human endocrinopathies

Human autoimmune disease includes not only collagen-vascular diseases (the so-called lupus cluster) but also a number of endocrinopathies in which circulating autoantibodies play diagnostic and/or pathogenetic roles:

1. **Diabetes mellitus** may arise because of a rare syndrome of insulin resistance (type B) caused by antibodies to the insulin receptor; coexisting acanthosis nigricans skin lesions are typical of this syndrome. Autoantibodies to antigens such as the 64-kDa GABA-synthesizing enzyme glutamic acid decarboxylase remain of unclear pathogenetic significance (p. 430).
2. Sporadic **Addison disease** (primary hypoadrenalism) may sometimes be caused by autoantibodies to the cortisol biosynthetic hormones 21-hydroxylase or 17-hydroxylase.
3. In a subset of patients with **Hashimoto thyroiditis** – the major cause of goitrous hypothyroidism – levels of blocking antibodies to the glycoprotein hormone thryotropin (also known as thyroid-stimulating hormone or TSH) correlate with the clinical course. However, a more common class of autoantibodies reactive with thyroid microsomal antigens specifically targets the biosynthetic enzyme **thyroid peroxidase** which catalyzes iodine oxidation. The pathogenicity of these latter antibodies is in doubt.
4. **Graves disease** of autoimmune thyrotoxicosis arises because of an agonistic autoantibody that constitutively activates TSH. This antibody is sometimes called **thyroid-stimulating immunoglobulin** or **TSI**.

To understand the language of cells it is necessary to translate all parts of the text together rather than focusing only on one section. Hence, labeling a group of molecules with a sweeping designation such as growth factors can be a risky exercise: the creation of a separate category for these molecules does not mean that they can be considered in isolation from hormones, cytokines and other components of the cell signaling machinery. As discussed below, these different molecular groupings actually share many structural and functional features.

Polypeptide growth factors

Body size is controlled by circulating factors

Hormones may act like growth factors and growth factors like hormones. This is illustrated by the functional overlap between three molecules: **growth hormone (GH)**, **insulin**, and **insulin-like growth factor-1 (IGF1)**.

Human GH is a 22-kDa monomer of 191 amino acids that is stored in anterior pituitary granules from where it is secreted into the circulation every three hours and during stage-4 sleep. Three GH gene copies map in tandem with three copies of the gene for human placental lactogen (HPL) to the same region of chromosome 17q, while a second GH-variant gene expressed in the placenta may contribute to fetal growth. The pituitary-specific POU-domain transactivator **Pit-1** (GHF1) regulates the expression both of GH genes and also of a G-protein-coupled receptor for the gastric GH-releasing factor ghrelin which acts by increasing pituitary cAMP levels. Of note, Pit-1 activates GH expression in some pituitary cells (somatotropes) but represses it in others (lactotropes), reflecting a two-base-pair difference in spacing of the bipartite POU domain response element within the respective promoters. This illustrates how tissue differentiation may involve variable effects of the same effector in different cell lineages.

GH exerts two qualitatively distinct types of metabolic effect:

1. Insulin-like (anabolic, pro-growth) effects – on protein metabolism and bone growth.
2. Anti-insulin (catabolic, diabetogenic) effects – on fat and carbohydrate metabolism.

With respect to glucose metabolism, GH is the **hormone of fast** (starvation) since it promotes lipolysis, hyperglycemia, and insulin resistance (i.e., an anti-insulin effect). In contrast, the glucose-inducible pancreatic hormone insulin – which like GH promotes growth, but unlike GH inhibits lipolysis – is the **hormone of feast**. This designation reflects the fact that insulin receptor activation induces expression of postprandial gene products (such as immediate-early proteins, glucose transporters, and glycolytic enzymes) while repressing catabolic enzymes, such as **phosphoenolpyruvate carboxykinase**, which mediate glucose production from long-term energy stores (Table 6.4).

Insulin-dependent phosphorylation activates glycogen synthesis by triggering downregulation of the serine-threonine kinase **glycogen synthase kinase-3β** (GSK-3β). Of note, the latter enzyme participates in many processes other than glycogen synthesis, including hyperphosphorylation of the **Alzheimer disease** microtubule-associated **tau** protein (therapeutically inhibited by **lithium**, a GSK-3β blocker) and nuclear translocation of the membrane-associated transcription factor **β-catenin**. The ribosomal protein **PHAS-1**, which binds translational elongation initiation factors (eIFs; p. 110), represses protein synthesis unless phosphorylated by the insulin-regulated **p70**[Rsk] kinase. Insulin thus promotes protein synthesis by triggering the release of eIFs from phosphorylated ribosomal constituents.

Gigantism and glucose tolerance

The diabetogenic effects of GH form the basis of a test for autonomous GH production in suspected adult **acromegaly** or juvenile **gigantism**. An oral glucose load (glucose tolerance test) usually causes insulin release and GH suppression, but in acromegalics and giants GH suppression is defective. Impaired glucose tolerance (as distinct from frank **diabetes mellitus**) is also characteristic of the diagnosis, though less sensitive than GH nonsuppressibility. Hence, GH and insulin have antagonistic effects on fat and carbohydrate homeostasis, with GH being rather more catabolic and insulin mainly anabolic.

Protein metabolism is a different story, however, with both hormones having anabolic effects. These actions of GH on protein metabolism are due to GH-dependent synthesis of insulin-like growth factors (IGFs, formerly somatomedins). Unlike most peptide signaling molecules, IGFs and GH circulate bound to large carrier proteins which regulate free hormone levels.

Insulin-like growth factors (IGFs) and their binding proteins (IGFBPs)

GH exerts its growth-promoting effect mainly by inducing the hepatic synthesis of **insulin-like growth factor-1** (**IGF1**), a 70-amino-acid anabolic hormone which – similar to its congener IGF2 – structurally resembles proinsulin. Unlike proinsulin, however, the C-peptide of the IGFs is not cleaved. Like insulin, IGF1 activates pre-dimerized receptor tyrosine kinases; but unlike insulin, IGF1 does not suppress hepatic gluconeogenesis.

Insulin-like growth factor-2 (**IGF2**) binds two receptors: an insulin receptor-like tyrosine kinase which also binds IGF1 (the **IGF1 receptor**) and the catalytically inert **mannose-6-phosphate receptor**. The latter receptor also acts as a lysosome-targeting signal, and its IGF2-binding epitope is distinct from that which binds mannose-6-phosphate. Of note, the growth-inhibitory effects of retinoids may also be mediated via this receptor.

There are several **IGF-binding proteins** or **IGFBPs** which maintain total plasma concentrations of IGF1 at levels 1000-fold higher than those of (free) insulin. Synthesis of IGFBPs, like that of IGFs, depends on GH; both IGF1 and GH induce IGFBP expression, whereas insulin reduces it. By reducing the bioavailability of IGF1, IGFBPs may modulate the activity of the (free) circulating growth factor. The most abundant IGFBP isoform in human serum is **IGFBP3**. Enzymes produced by human cancers – such as the serine protease prostate-specific antigen in prostate cancer – may cleave IGFBPs (e.g., within metastatic lesions), thereby enhancing the local bioavailability of growth factors.

GH binding proteins (GHBPs) are circulating GH receptor ectodomains that are bound and dimerized by a single GH molecule with a stoichiometry of 1:2.

IGFs mediate the anabolic effects of growth hormone

The metabolic split of GH action into insulin-like and anti-insulin effects reflects the structure of GH as a prohormone that is proteolyzed to yield two active fragments – a carboxy-terminal catabolic fragment (residues 44–191) mediating the diabetogenic effects, and an amino-terminal anabolic fragment (residues 1–43). The anabolic effects of GH also appear subclassifiable:

1. IGF1-independent (direct, insulin-potentiating) GH effects
   • e.g., Bone elongation due to stimulation of epiphyseal plate cells.

- Adipocytes may be primed by GH to become insulin-sensitive.
2. IGF1-dependent (indirect, insulin-like) GH effects
    - e.g., Promotion of muscle and cartilage synthesis by IGF1.

Muscle is a major site of IGF1 receptor (IGF1R) expression. Hence, the anabolic effects of IGF1 on muscle are consistent with selective IGF1-inducible enhancement of muscle glucose utilization. Ligand binding to IGF1R activates at least two signaling cascades. The first promotes cell survival via the sequential signaling of PI3K, PKB, GSK3β, β-catenin, and the *Myc*-regulatory transcriptional activator TCF4 (p. 214). In human pancreatic cancer cells, activation of PKB may further upregulate IGF1R expression and thus create a positive feedback loop which increases cell survival. In contrast, the second pathway promotes cell proliferation by triggering the Ras-Raf-MAPK cascade. Hence, the different effects of IGF1 in various cell systems may be determined in part by differences in the activation of these pathways.

Whereas IGF1 expression is inducible by GH, IGF2 expression is induced by the GH homolog human placental lactogen. This is particularly so during fetal life, during which expression of IGF2 and its receptor are reciprocally modulated by genomic imprinting (p. 407). Both IGF1 and IGF2 contribute to embryonic growth, whereas IGF2 alone is responsible for placental growth.

The pathogenetic involvement of IGF1 in acromegaly is an illustrative but rare example of a polypeptide growth factor being directly implicated in the phenotype of a human disease. IGF1 plasma levels may be of diagnostic use in acromegaly, and also provide measures of therapeutic response. Low IGF1 levels, on the other hand, are of value in the differential diagnosis of pituitary gland secretory insufficiency or **hypopituitarism.**

CLINICAL KEYNOTE

Growth hormone and IGFs in disease

Since the growth of GH-secreting cells within the pituitary depends upon G-protein-mediated synthesis of cAMP, G-protein mutations causing cAMP overproduction (with consequent overgrowth of pituitary GH-secreting cells) may be associated with pituitary tumors causing **acromegaly.** Knockout of the Jak-STAT suppressor, **SOCS-2,** causes an acromegaly-like syndrome in mice. The IGF-dependent pathogenesis of gigantism in the **Beckwith–Wiedemann syndrome** is considered elsewhere (p. 408).

Dwarfism may result from a variety of causes. Patients with isolated GH deficiencies may have *GH-1* gene abnormalities, whereas those with GH deficiencies combined with other pituitary hormone underproduction (e.g., prolactin, thyrotropin) may have mutations affecting the pituitary-specific transcription factor **Pit-1.** Mutations (e.g., exon deletions) affecting the **GH receptor** are responsible for most cases of **Laron dwarfism,** which is characterized by high immunoreactive GH levels, absent GH-binding proteins, and defective hepatic GH receptors leading to end-organ GH resistance. **Familial pituitary dwarfism** arises due to mutations affecting the POU-domain transactivator GHF1 (PIT1). African **pygmies** are deficient in GH-binding proteins.

Tumor overproduction of IGF2 (e.g., by retroperitoneal fibrosarcomas) may cause **paraneoplastic hypoglycemia** by activating the insulin receptor. Such IGF2 tends to be incorrectly processed: this prevents normal ligand sequestration by IGF-binding proteins in serum.

Low plasma IGF1 levels may be associated with GH resistance in hypercatabolic (autocannibalistic) states such as trauma and sepsis. Free amino acids (for wound healing and new protein synthesis) may thus be derived from muscle protein breakdown.

High serum IGF1 levels have been implicated as a risk factor for cancer (prostate, breast, colorectal). The mammographic density of young breasts, which may lead to diagnostic insensitivity in women aged less than 50, also correlates with tissue IGF1 expression levels.

PHARMACOLOGIC FOOTNOTE

Therapeutic use of growth agonists and antagonists
Infusions of IGF1 may be of therapeutic value in Laron dwarfs, since this maneuver effectively bypasses their end-organ resistance to GH.

Recombinant GH holds promise for the prevention of catabolic wasting induced by illness, drug therapy or old age. GH is now being used investigationally to augment cardiac performance in selected cases of **heart failure** – dilated cardiomyopathy or postinfarction – with promising results. The recombinant protein is also abused by athletes, and is virtually impossible to detect in this context.

The reported efficacy of **octreotide** therapy (a long-acting somatostatin analog) in improving the extrathyroidal manifestations of **Graves disease** is consistent with reports linking IGF1 to extraocular muscle enlargement in this endocrinopathy.

Growth hormone receptor overactivity in **acromegaly** can now be specifically antagonized using pharmacologic antagonists that interfere with the 1:2 receptor dimerization normally induced by ligand. Such receptor antagonists (e.g., **pegvisomant**) can normalize both serum IGF1 levels and symptoms.

Tissue growth factors are local effectors of hormone signaling

Traditional signaling models propose that distant intercellular communication is mediated by hormones whereas local intercellular communication is mediated by growth factors. However, this paradigm is too simple: hormones such as insulin may have local effects (e.g., lipohypertrophy at injection sites) whereas circulating growth factors such as the IGFs and erythropoietin may act distantly. Some of the functional differences between hormones and growth factors relate to the identity of their usual target receptors:

1. Nuclear hormone receptors are usually activated by steroid hormones
   • Exceptions: retinoic acid, calcitriol, thyroid hormone.
2. Peptide hormones usually activate G-protein-coupled receptors
   • Exceptions: insulin, prolactin, growth hormone.
3. Growth factors usually activate receptor tyrosine kinases
   • Exceptions: erythropoietin, granulocyte colony-stimulating factor (G-CSF), transforming growth factor-β.

Whether a hormone affects a given organ depends first and foremost on the tissue-specificity of hormone receptor expression. For example, estrogen selectively affects the breast and endometrium because these organs express estrogen receptors (ER). Once tissue hormone receptors are activated, however, the effects of the hormone may depend upon the pattern of hormone-inducible growth factor release. In the case of estrogen, the main downstream pathways are those involving epidermal growth factor receptors (see below) and IGF1 signaling.

An interplay between hormones and growth factors mediates the effects of the prostatic serine protease **prostate-specific antigen (PSA)**. The dihydrotestos-

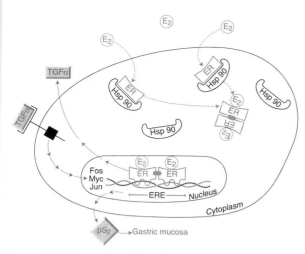

Figure 13.10 Estrogen-dependent cell growth stimulation by growth factor release depends on the estrogen receptor (ER). Estrogen displaces cytoplasmic ER from its complex with Hsp90, leading to dimerization and DNA binding. The activated ER transactivates the transforming growth factor α (TGFα) gene (among others such as pS2), leading to secretion of this growth factor followed by epidermal growth factor (EGF) receptor activation on the same or neighboring cells. ERE, estrogen-response element.

terone-activated androgen receptor binds three response elements upstream of the *PSA* gene, leading to secretion of PSA into the extracellular space. PSA-secreting bone metastases exhibit selective depletion of the PSA substrate *IGFBP3*. Since this loss of IGFBP3 may increase IGF1 bioavailability – and given that IGFs are prime activators of osteoblast function – this hormone-dependent pathway is likely to underlie the distinctive radiosclerotic appearance of **prostate cancer** metastases. Moroever, since IGFBP3 is an activating ligand for the type V transforming growth factor-beta receptor (see below), intralesional PSA could also promote prostate cancer cell growth by attenuating this growth-inhibitory signalling pathway.

An example of crosstalk relevant to **breast cancer** is the signaling interaction between the female sex hormone estradiol (E$_2$) and the downstream mitogens 16f1 and **transforming growth factor α** (TGFα). One of the response elements bound by the E$_2$-transformed ER lies upstream of the TGFα gene; hence, distant E$_2$ release causes ER-positive cells to secrete TGFα (Figure 13.10), leading to ambient activation of epidermal growth factor receptors.

SUPERFAMILY SPOTLIGHT

Epidermal growth factor (EGF)-like ligands

One of the smallest growth factors is **epidermal growth factor** (EGF), a 33-amino-acid (5.5-kDa) secreted peptide that is cleaved from a large membrane-bound precursor. EGF-like domains are a common feature of extracellular molecules, and are characterized by six conserved cysteine residues that form three disulfide bonds. Polypeptides containing EGF-like domains include selectin cell-adhesion molecules, the matrix proteins laminin and tenascin, the cartilaginous proteoglycan aggrecan, thrombomodulin, fibrillin, and vitamin-K-dependent coagulation factors. Some EGF-like domains in these molecules may bind calcium. EGF itself regulates epithelial and mesenchymal cell growth; the only cells consistently lacking EGF receptors (EGFR) are erythroid cell precursors.

The EGF-like growth factor superfamily consists of:

1. **EGF** (acid-stable).
2. **Transforming growth factor α** (TGFα; acid-labile).
3. **Amphiregulin**, **epiregulin**, **betacellulin**, **heparin-binding EGF-like growth factor** (HB-EGF).
   - Epiregulin, betacellulin and HB-EGF also bind ErbB4 (see below). HB-EGF is a membrane-anchored ligand with an EGF-like domain that doubles up as the human receptor for **diphtheria toxin**.
4. **Heregulins** (neuregulins)
   - These ligands cause dimerization of ErbB3 or ErbB4.
   - Normally expressed at high levels in neural tissues.
   - Include heregulins α2, β1-3; and glial growth factors (GGF) 1–3.

EGF was discovered in male salivary glands, consistent with (1) a role in healing wounds inflicted during fighting among animals that lick their wounds, and with (2) its identification as an acid-resistant anti-ulcerogenic activity (urogastrone) in the urine of pregnant women. Once swallowed, the action of EGF is that of a luminal surveillance factor that assists repair of mucosal damage. The importance of EGF signaling in maintaining gut integrity is further illustrated by the efficacy of EGFR antibodies in reversing the clinical phenotype of **Ménétrier disease**, a hypoproteinemic hypertrophic gastropathy. Pharmacologic EGFR kinase inhibitors can likewise cause the regression of intestinal polyps, albeit at the expense of significant gastrointestinal (diarrheal) toxicity.

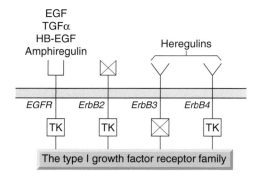

EGF
TGFα
HB-EGF
Amphiregulin

Heregulins

| EGFR | ErbB2 | ErbB3 | ErbB4 |

The type I growth factor receptor family

Figure 13.11 The type I growth factor receptor family and its ligands. Mutations (marked by crosses) in the ErbB2 extracellular domain and the ErbB3 intracellular domain lead to failure of ligand binding and kinase activation respectively.

ErbB2 amplifies ambient growth factor function

The apparent redundancy of EGF-like ligands contributes to the signaling diversity of the type I receptor tyrosine kinase family (Figure 13.11). This growth factor receptor family consists of four proteins:

1. **EGFR**
   - Is bound by multiple ligands, excluding heregulins.
   - Has normal catalytic activity.
2. **ErbB2**
   - Is an orphan receptor with no known ligand.
   - Has normal catalytic activity.
3. **ErbB3**
   - Is bound exclusively by heregulin ligands.
   - Has negligible catalytic activity.
4. **ErbB4**
   - Is bound exclusively by heregulin ligands.
   - Has normal catalytic activity.

Amplification of the *EGFR* gene is often seen in brain tumors and squamous cell carcinomas, whereas the **ErbB2** oncoprotein is commonly overexpressed in adenocarcinomas. Discovered in carcinogen-induced neuroectodermal tumors as a rat mutant (*neu*) with an abnormal transmembrane domain causing spontaneous dimerization, the human EGFR homolog (HER2) tends to be overexpressed only in the wild-type form. An avid heterodimerizer of ligand-activated receptors (particularly EGFR), the wild-type ErbB2 protein lacks critical structural determinants for receptor internalization and downregulation within its intracellular domain. ErbB2 overexpression thus impairs the downregulation of heterodimerized growth factor receptors, thereby amplifying ambient growth factor signaling. Constitutive DNA replication results, leading to selection for subclones capable of resisting normal growth constraints (see Figure 13.12).

ErbB2 can transform cells in vitro when point-mutated to a constitutively activated form, but in human tumors the oncoprotein is rarely if ever mutated. This implies that upregulation of the protein occurs secondary to other mutational events. Indeed, overexpression of ErbB2 in normal cells may lead to cell death, functioning in effect as a growth control protein, whereas knockout of the growth control protein p53 permits acceleration of cell growth in this context. This may explain why most ErbB2-overexpressing tumors are associ-

Figure 13.12 Inhibition of normal EGF receptor downregulation (at left) by heterodimerization with ErbB2 (at right), leading to constitutive signaling.

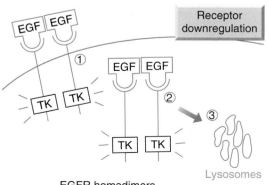

EGFR homodimers

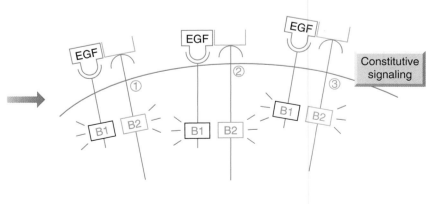

EGFR/ErbB2 heterodimers

ated with p53 mutations, and suggests that cell-cycle control defects may be prerequisites for ErbB2 overexpression.

Just as ErbB2 is distinguished by a ligand-defective extracellular domain, so **ErbB3** is distinguished by an intracellular kinase domain that has been rendered catalytically inert by multiple mutations. Although this structure immediately suggests a dominant negative function, ErbB3 fails to bind the ubiquitin ligase **Cbl**, and therefore fails to be downregulated even in the presence of ligand. Moreover, heterodimerized ErbB3 is readily tyrosine-phosphorylated by heterodimerized receptors such as ErbB2 and EGFR, and thus becomes a rich docking site for SH2-containing PI3K molecules which promote cell survival, tissue invasion and motility.

Different type I receptor oligomers are implicated in different physiologic contexts. Breast development involves EGFR:ErbB2 and ErbB2:ErbB3 complexes, for example, whereas cardiac development is associated with expression of heregulin-dependent ErbB2:ErbB4 heterodimers. Given the latter, the problematic cardiotoxicity of ErbB2 extracellular domain monoclonal antibodies (**trastuzumab**) in breast cancer patients suggests that downregulation of this receptor complex may predispose to cardiac myocyte death.

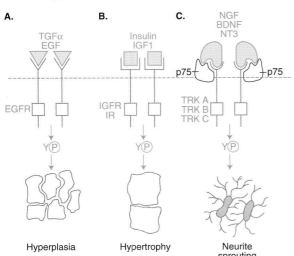

Figure 13.13 Multiple growth factor actions. *A,* Growth proliferation induced by the epidermal growth factor (EGF) system. *B,* Cell hypertrophy induced by the insulin-like growth factor (IGF1)/insulin system. *C,* Neurite extension induced by neurotropins. TGFα, transforming growth factor α.

MOLECULAR MINIREVIEW

Nongrowth functions of growth factors

Growth factors are multifunctional. For example, **hepatocyte growth factor** (HGF, scatter factor) – a large (92-kDa) heterodimeric ligand for the *Met* gene product – enhances motility in epithelial and endothelial cells whereas its mitogenic action is largely restricted to liver cells (e.g., after partial hepatectomy or fulminant liver failure) and kidney cells (e.g., following nephrectomy). Activated Met receptors are expressed in cells bordering ductal gland lumens, suggesting a role for HGF in gland differentiation. Normal renal development also requires normal Met and HGF function; consistent with this, activating *Met* mutations contribute to development of both familial and sporadic **renal cancer**.

Many other so-called growth factor signaling pathways can contribute to cell growth arrest, differentiation or death. For example, receptor tyrosine kinases of the **nerve growth factor receptor** family are expressed in nonproliferating adult neurons. Similarly, growth-hormone-dependent activation of the IGF1 signaling system can trigger hypertrophy (rather than hyperplasia; Figure 13.13) of target myocytes.

Mutations that constitutively activate one of the receptors for fibroblast growth factors may cause a form of dwarfism called **achondroplasia** which arises due to early developmental arrest of bone growth secondary to premature activation of cartilage growth (p. 345). Hence, this disorder begins with growth acceleration but terminates as growth retardation.

Wound healing involves stromal-epithelial crosstalk

The ability to heal wounds is a key evolutionary selection pressure, since deficiencies in this pathway – e.g., inability to arrest bleeding or contain local sepsis – could be fatal (see over).

Cells in culture respond to the addition of serum (=growth factors) by activating an array of genes that mediate aspects of wound healing: extracellular matrix remodeling, clot formation and lysis, chemotaxis, vasoconstriction and immune activation. Many growth factors have thus been implicated in the regulation of wound healing, including epidermal growth factor (EGF), platelet-derived growth factor (PDGF-A, PDGF-B), fibroblast growth factors and transforming growth factor β (TGFβ). EGF stimulates the growth of keratinocytes and other epithelial cells, whereas acidic (aFGF) and basic (bFGF) fibroblast growth factors enhance wound healing by stimulating blood vessel formation.

Platelet-derived growth factor (PDGF) is a 32-kDa homo- or heterodimeric ligand originally isolated as a wound-healing agent present in serum but not platelet-poor plasma. PDGF is encoded at two chromosomal loci, the *PDGF-A* and *PDGF-B* genes, which may be co-expressed to generate the three dimeric ligand isoforms, PDGF-AA, -AB and -BB. These ligands bind either of two receptor tyrosine kinases, PDGF receptor-α and PDGF receptor-β, which have distinct cellular effects. The *Sis* proto-oncogene (encoding the cellular homolog of the retroviral transforming gene product, v-sis) encodes the PDGF-BB homodimer, which is the universal ligand since it binds both α- and β-receptors; the PDGF receptor-α, on the other hand, is the universal receptor, as it binds all PDGF isoforms (p. 260). Moreover, a chromosomal translocation event leads to formation of a PDGF-telomerase fusion protein in **chronic myelomonocytic leukemia**. Bleeding wounds are normally accompanied by PDGF release from platelets and endothelial cells, leading to fibroblast chemotaxis, synthesis of extracellular matrix proteins, and vasoconstriction. PDGF also functions as a mesenchymal mitogen in wound healing, and its recombinant form has been used as a topical treatment for skin ulcers.

The phenotypic effects of growth factors can be mediated by either secreted (soluble) or membrane-bound isoforms. Membrane-bound growth factors activate receptors on neighboring cells – perhaps contributing to contact inhibition of cell growth – whereas soluble growth factors modulate the behavior of cells in the vicinity. Such intercellular signals between epithelial and mesenchymal cell lineages are well illustrated by the *Notch–Delta* cell fate control system in embryogenesis (p. 404).

Crosstalk between stromal and epithelial lineages can thus take place via differential expression of growth factors and their receptors. This gives rise to **paracrine**, **juxtacrine** or **autocrine** growth loops, all of which have been implicated as tumor growth mechanisms in vivo (Figure 13.14). Epithelial cell release of PDGF, for example, can cause fibroblasts (which express PDGF receptors) to secrete IGF1, thereby creating a paracrine loop. Consistent with this, release of PDGF by cancer cells is associated with the scirrhous (fibrotic) phenotype sometimes seen in **primary breast cancer**. In general, tissues that respond to wounding with a strong regenerative response – such as the liver, which regrows following partial hepatectomy – provide a good "soil" for **cancer metastasis**, whereas nonregenerative tissues such as muscle and nerve are rarely metastatic sites.

Figure 13.14 Models of paracrine growth loops operating in normal or malignant cell systems. *A,* Stromal cells may activate insulin-like growth factor-1 (IGF1) receptors on epithelial cells, which respond by activating platelet-derived growth factor (PDGF) receptors on stromal cells. *B,* Tumor cells may release proteases (e.g., prostate-specific antigen, PSA) which cleave growth factor-binding proteins (e.g., IGFBP3), thus making growth factors (e.g., IGFs) bioavailable to activate stromal cells; consequent release of growth factor (transforming growth factor α, TGFα) from the latter may further upregulate tumor cell protease transcription.

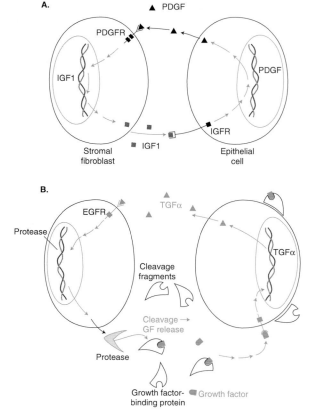

MOLECULAR MINIREVIEW

Trefoil peptides
The integrity of gut mucosa is maintained not only by acid-stable EGF (pp. 261, 329), but also by a group of acid-resistant trophic ligands termed **trefoil peptides** (due to their three-leaf shape). These ligands, which are released by mucus-secreting epithelia into the lumen of the gastrointestinal tract, include:
1. Estrogen-inducible **pS2**
   – Secreted from the gastric fundus
2. Spasmolytic peptide
   – Secreted from the gastric antrum
3. Intestinal trefoil factor (ITF)
   – Secreted from the intestine.
The trophic effects of the tightly folded mucin-associated ITF are apparent from murine knockouts exhibiting fragile gut tissues. In contrast, pS2 knockout mice develop gut adenomas and multifocal carcinomas.

CLINICAL KEYNOTE

Transforming growth factor β in tissue fibrosis
The flip side of wound healing is fibrosis. Overzealous or repetitive attempts at wound healing may result in chronic fibrotic disorders such as pulmonary fibrosis, atherosclerosis, scleroderma, myelofibrosis, chronic pericarditis, and chronic glomerulosclerosis. Fibrosing disorders are mediated by the same growth factors that effect normal wound repair, making these growth factors and their receptors attractive therapeutic drug targets for these disorders.

Reduction of scarring (e.g., in facial laceration repairs) may be achieved by slowing the rate of wound healing with growth factor antagonists, thus permitting more time for correct fibril orientation. This unexpected benefit of growth factor inhibition reflects the fact that cosmesis has not been an evolutionary imperative – at least, not until recently – whereas rapid wound healing has always been so.

The archetypal sclerosing growth factor is **transforming growth factor β** (TGFβ), which promotes the formation of granulation tissue during wound healing by enhancing the synthesis of extracellular matrix proteins (such as collagen, fibronectin, and integrins) while simultaneously inhibiting proteases (such as stromelysins and collagenases). Excessive activity of TGFβ may contribute to the pathogenesis of fibrotic disorders such as **liver cirrhosis, atherosclerosis, iatrogenic lung fibrosis**, and **keloid** scars (Figure 13.15) – with the latter complication being particularly common in blacks, Hispanics and Orientals. Keloid fibroblasts secrete excessive collagen in response to TGFβ, but administration of IFNγ may reduce keloid thickness by 30%.

Iatrogenic pulmonary fibrosis due to prolonged treatment with the radiomimetic anticancer drug **bleomycin** has been linked to increased TGFβ secretion by alveolar macrophages. Purified **decorin**, an extracellular matrix glycoprotein that prevents TGFβ binding to its signaling receptor (see below), has been used to inhibit the fibrotic sequelae of TGFβ. Conversely, impaired wound healing due to **steroid therapy** may be prevented or reversed by TFGβ administration.

Extracellular binding proteins modulate TGFβ signaling

An excellent example of growth factor multifunctionality is that of **transforming growth factor β** (TGFβ) – a ligand with the remarkable dual ability to promote or suppress cell growth. TGFβ is the molecular front man for a growth factor superfamily containing molecules as diverse as **Müllerian-inhibitory**

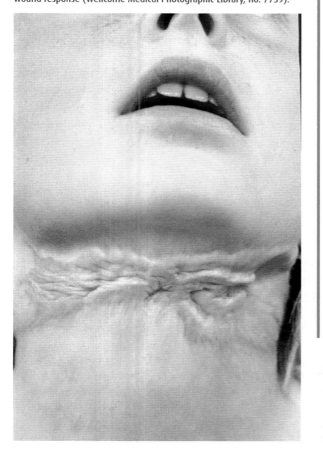

Figure 13.15 Keloid scars, showing the hypertrophy accompanying the wound response (Wellcome Medical Photographic Library, no. 7759).

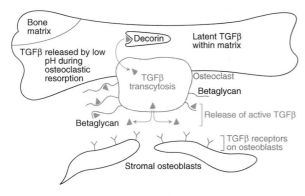

Figure 13.16 Activation of latent transforming growth factor β (TGFβ) in bone matrix. During osteoclastic resorption, a drop in matrix pH releases TGFβ from its binding site to decorin, permitting transcytosis through the osteoclast and presentation by other growth factor binding proteins to TGFβ receptors on osteoblasts. In this way bone resorption and formation are coupled during processes such as repair and remodeling.

substance (MIS: anti-Müllerian hormone), **activins**, **inhibin**, and the **bone morphogenetic proteins** (BMPs; p. 421). The growth-inhibitory potency of this family is illustrated by the induction of male sex characteristics by MIS release from testicular Sertoli cells: activation of MIS receptors in Müllerian ducts represses the development of uterine tubes and uterus in the male fetus.

Three 25-kDa homodimeric human TGFβ isoforms (β1–β3) are initially secreted in latent (inactive) forms covalently bound to one of four **latent TGFβ-binding proteins** or LTBPs. This complex is proteolytically disrupted either by plasmin or thrombospondin, leading to the release of active TGFβ in endothelial and hemopoietic cells (TGFβ1), neuronal and epithelial cells (TGFβ2), or mesenchymal cells (TGFβ3). This process of TGFβ bioactivation represents an integral mechanism of stromal–epithelial crosstalk, for example within bone (Figure 13.16).

A molecular misnomer, TGFβ was originally co-purified with TGFα from the conditioned medium of tumor cells grown in vitro. Unlike TGFα, however, TGFβ differentially regulates embryogenesis, inflammation and tissue repair in mesenchymal and epithelial cells. Consistent with this, knockout of wild-type TGFβ expression causes widespread inflammation, necrosis and wasting in adult transgenic mice. TGFβ has potent immunosuppressant effects on T cell growth and B cell function, and its expression may be induced by certain parasites to help evade immune surveillance. Although often suppressing tumor growth during the early phases of cancer development, some tumors (e.g., prostate cancer) appear to be promoted by TGFβ during the later stages of cancer progression. Growth-regulatory actions of TGFβ include:

1. Growth stimulation of mesenchymal cells
   - e.g., Estrogen-inducible new bone formation is mediated via increases in osteoblast TGFβ expression.
2. Growth inhibition of epithelial (and some carcinoma) cells
   - Associated with TGFβ-induced hypophosphorylation of the cell-cycle tumor-suppressive retinoblastoma protein (p. 371).

TGFβ signals via a heterotetrameric complex of type I and type II receptor serine-threonine kinases: the ligand binds and homodimerizes type II receptors, which transphosphorylate hetero-oligomerized type I receptors. This initiates the kinase activity of type I receptors, which then phosphorylate downstream effectors termed Smads which enter the nucleus and bind DNA.

CLINICAL KEYNOTE

Diseases of the TGFβ receptor superfamily

Approximately 25% of **colorectal cancers** (and as many as 90% of those exhibiting **microsatellite instability**, which make up 20% of the total; p. 81) are associated with type II TGFβ receptor mutations. Many of the remainder exhibit methylation of the same gene locus. Of potential clinical importance, tumors harboring mutations of this receptor are associated with improved survival following adjuvant chemotherapy.

Mutations affecting type II TGFβ receptors likewise appear critical in **hereditary nonpolyposis colorectal cancer** kindreds, which is a potent cause of microsatellite instability (p. 80), as well as in the evolution of some sporadic **gastric cancers**.

In contrast to type I and II receptors, the widely expressed type III TGFβ receptor family does not have a signaling function. Rather, this receptor family (which comprises the extracellular matrix proteins **endoglin**, **decorin** and **betaglycan**) sequesters extracellular TGFβ during wound repair. Genetic defects of endoglin give rise to type I **hereditary hemorrhagic telangiectasia** (**HHT**), whereas loss-of-function mutations of the activin receptor-like kinase gene (*ALK-1*) cause type II HHT associated with **pulmonary hypertension**. This is because the loss of *ALK1* leads to unopposed TGFβ signaling via **ALK5**, leading to selective pulmonary endothelial cell proliferation. Mutations affecting another receptor of the TGFβ receptor superfamily, the type II receptor for bone morphogenetic proteins (**BMPR2**), causes **familial pulmonary hypertension**.

MOLECULAR MINIREVIEW

Smads

Ligand activation of the type I TGFβ receptor leads to phosphorylation of cytoplasmic second messengers termed **Smads**, which in due course form homo- or heterodimers, translocate to the nucleus, and transactivate TGFβ target gene expression. [Smads are so-called because of homology to *Drosophila* proteins termed either *Sma* or *Mad* that transduce signals initiated by a ligand called *decapentaplegic* which is closely related to bone morphogenetic proteins BMP2 and BMP4, p. 421]. The ten or so known Smads can be functionally divided into:

1. **Receptor-regulated Smads**
   - BMP receptor-1 substrates
     - Smads 1/5/8.
   - TGFβ type I and activin type I receptor substrates
     - Smads 2/3.
2. **Co-Smads**
     - Smad 4.
3. **Antagonist Smads**
     - Smads 6 and 7.

The first two of these groups contain *Mad* homology (MH) domains termed MH1 and MH2, but antagonist Smads (e.g., Smad 6, which regulates cardiac development) lack most of MH1 and differ in sequence to the MH2 domain. MH1 and MH2 domains autoinhibit each other in the basal state by mediating homo-oligomerization of receptor-regulated Smads (2/3); once phosphorylated by type I TGFβ receptors (e.g., on $Ser^{465/467}$ in Smad 2), receptor-regulated Smads bind the unphosphorylated co-Smad, Smad 4, which targets them to the nucleus. On approaching DNA, receptor-regulated Smads associate with specific DNA-binding proteins such as **Fast-1** to induce gene transcription (Figure 13.17).

Figure 13.17 The TGFβ-dependent downstream Smad effector signaling system (see text). BMPs, bone morphogenetic proteins; TGF, transforming growth factor.

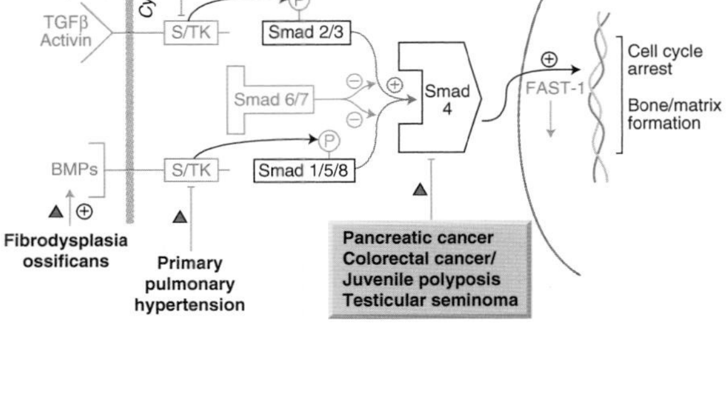

CLINICAL KEYNOTE

Cancer correlates of Smads

Cancer progression may be driven by Smad mutations: 18q21 deletions of Smad 4 in **pancreatic cancer** (50%) and **colorectal cancer** (15%), for example, in which abnormalities of the TGFβ signaling pathway are detectable in over 95% and 80% of cases respectively. Similarly, loss-of-function *Smad 2* mutations occur in colorectal and lung cancer, and aggressive colorectal cancers occur in *Smad3* knockout mice. Smad mutations occur later in tumor development than do *APC* (adenomatous polyposis coli) gene mutations (pp. 214–15): *Smad 4* knockout mice develop few if any polyps, whereas *APC* knockouts incur many. *APC/Smad 4* double-knockouts sustain fewer polyps than do *APC* single-knockouts, but malignant degeneration seems more common in compound heterozygotes. This is analogous to the effects of TGFβ overexpression in keratinocytes, which suppresses papilloma formation but accelerates the progression of papillomas to carcinomas.

In humans, loss-of-function germline *Smad 4* mutations give rise to **juvenile polyposis** prone to malignant degeneration, rather than to adenomatous polyps; a similar syndrome is caused by mutation of the growth-regulatory tyrosine phosphatase PTEN (p. 364). Smad 4 mutations are also reported in approximately 10% of **testicular seminomas**, confirming its status as a key control protein in human tissues. Consistent with this, elevated Smad 4 protein expression in primary **gastric cancer** correlates with improved patient survival.

Summary

Hormones are derived from cholesterol or amino acids. Inactive precursors may be converted to active hormones.

Steroid hormones are synthesized by metabolic interconversion. Transformed steroid receptors translocate to the nucleus. Hormone blockade may cause or revert disease. Receptor–DNA interactions determine gene expression.

Most brain hormones activate G-protein-coupled receptors. Brain and gut hormones may be identical. Inhibitory hormones regulate hypothalamo-pituitary function.

Body size is controlled by circulating factors. Insulin-like growth factors (IGFs) mediate the anabolic effects of growth hormone. Tissue growth factors are local effectors of hormone signaling. ErbB2 amplifies ambient growth factor function. Wound healing involves stromal-epithelial crosstalk. Extracellular binding proteins modulate TGFβ signaling.

Enrichment reading

Bedtime reading

Foulds LM. *Neoplastic development*. Academic Press, New York, 1969

Library reference

Litwack G. *Hormones*. Academic Press, New York, 1997

Rosenfeld RG, Roberts CT (eds). *The IGF system: molecular biology, physiology and clinical applications*. Humana Press, Champaign, IL, 1999

Rumsby G, Farrow SM. *Molecular endocrinology: genetic analysis of hormones and their receptors*. Academic Press, New York, 1999

QUIZ QUESTIONS

1. Name four members of the steroid receptor superfamily, and describe the basic features of their domain structure.
2. Explain how steroid hormone receptors are activated, and how they modulate gene expression.
3. Name three ligands that activate nuclear receptors, and briefly describe any structural differences between them.
4. How are the following signaling molecules transported to target cells: (a) thyroxine, (b) estrogen, (c) insulin, and (d) insulin-like growth factor?
5. Describe three examples of a hormone being activated from an inactive precursor state.
6. Which steroid hormones are produced by (a) the adrenal gland, and (b) the ovary?
7. Explain how estrogens are synthesized.
8. Describe the domain structure of a steroid hormone receptor.
9. What is the pathogenesis of end-organ resistance to hormones? Name two examples.
10. How does growth hormone act? Which other hormones resemble it structurally?
11. What is melatonin, and what does it do?
12. Explain the mechanism of action of somatostatin.
13. Give an example of how a hormone can affect growth factor release.
14. Discuss why the epidermal growth factor receptor has multiple ligands.
15. Describe the effects and regulation of transforming growth factor β (TGFβ) signaling.

Hemopoietins, angiogenins, and vasoactive mediators

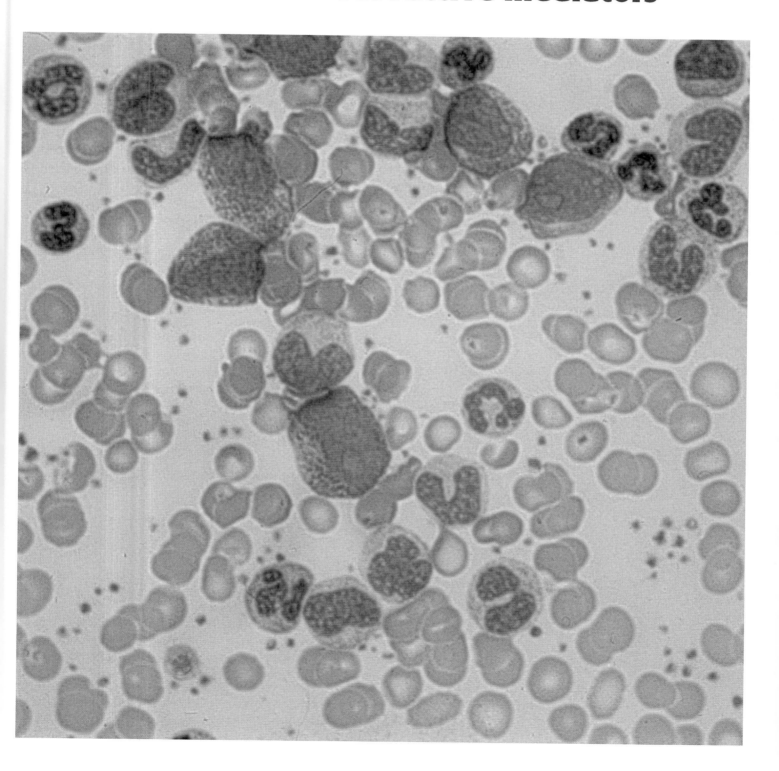

Hemopoietic growth factors

Blood production depends on pluripotential stem cells

All human tissues arise from the division and differentiation of ancestral **stem cells**. Approximately 20 distinct varieties of somatic stem cell are found in humans. The defining characteristics of stem cells are:

1. **Clonogenicity**
   - The stem cell gives rise to viable clones of dividing cell progeny.
2. **Pluripotentiality**
   - The stem cell is able to give rise to a variety of cell lineages, each of which is a committed progenitor for a differentiated cell type.
3. **Self-renewal**
   - The stem cell clone survives and replicates, rather than undergoing irreversible terminal differentiation as do other cell types.

Pluripotential stem cells constitute 0.01% of human bone marrow cells. Such cells express the hemopoietic stem cell marker **CD34** – which signals the capacity for cell renewal – but do not express the lineage-commitment marker **CD38**. Coexpression of CD34 and CD38 occurs in cells that are lineage-committed and hence incapable of extensive self-renewal. However, somatic stem cells may differentiate into unexpected lineages; for example, neural cells may give rise to myeloid cells, while hemopoietic bone marrow cells may yield hepatic or myocardial cells, indicating significant stem cell plasticity despite early differentiation. The prospect of using stem cells to repopulate human tissues requiring replacement (e.g., infarcted hearts, failed livers or kidneys) is therefore an enticing one.

CD34$^+$ CD38$^-$ cells that express HLA-DR can differentiate into all hemopoietic cell lineages including bone-resorbing osteoclasts. However, a more primitive CD34$^+$ CD38$^-$ HLA-DR$^-$ stem cell subpopulation may give rise not only to hemopoietic precursors but also to bone marrow stromal cells, including bone-forming osteoblasts. The latter suggests that a single bone marrow stem cell can reconstitute the entire hemopoietic microenvironment. The growth and survival of hemopoietic stem cells is promoted by the receptor tyrosine kinase ligand **stem cell factor** (SCF).

MOLECULAR MINIREVIEW

Spotty mice, *Steel*, and piebaldism

Stem cell factor (SCF; *Steel* factor, mast cell growth factor) is the ligand for the **Kit** receptor tyrosine kinase. Activity of Kit is required not only for hemopoiesis, however, but also for melanogenesis and gametogenesis.

The SCF mRNA is alternatively spliced to yield either soluble or membrane-bound isoforms. SCF stimulates mainly mast cells and erythrocyte progenitors, but also early myeloid cells and megakaryocytes. In addition, SCF improves the harvest of peripheral blood stem cells in patients scheduled to undergo autologous marrow reinfusion, and promotes the ex vivo survival of human bone marrow cultures.

The effects of SCF on pigmentation result from Kit-dependent activation of MAP kinase, which phosphorylates the transcription factor *Microphthalmia* (**Mi**). Phosphorylated Mi then induces the tyrosinase gene promoter, which causes melanin synthesis. Hypofunctional Kit may therefore lead to the prenatal death of melanocyte clones, and thus to depigmentation.

Male spermatogenesis depends upon Kit activation of the survival-promoting effector phosphatidylinositol-3′-kinase, without which sterility is induced by spermatogonial cell death.

SCF is secreted by bone marrow stromal cell lines from *W* (dominant *White-spotting*) mutant mice expressing defective Kit receptor tyrosine kinases. The secreted stromal factor from these cells, which causes Kit-expressing murine mast cells to proliferate, is encoded by a gene mapping to the site of another mouse coat color mutation, the *Steel* locus. Hence, the mast cell growth factor produced by Kit-defective *W* mice turned out to be the sought-after *Steel* factor. Heterozygous *W* mice exhibit mild anemia and mast cell deficiency, whereas homozygotes are severely anemic and infertile.

CLINICAL KEYNOTE

Germline and somatic *Kit* mutants

Heterozygous deletions affecting the human *Kit* gene are responsible for **piebaldism**, the human phenotype homologous to *W*. While no association with anemia has been reported, mental retardation has been anecdotally linked to piebaldism. This raises the possibility of a common *Kit*-related defect mediating abnormal melanocyte migration (white spotting) and other developmental anomalies affecting cells derived from the neural crest. The apparent lack of hematologic sequelae in *Kit* heterozygotes is consistent with a model of blood cell maturation in which multiple factors share overlapping functions in early hemopoiesis. Piebaldism may be associated with chronic constipation, and *W* mice may develop a paralytic ileus in the postnatal period despite apparently normal intestinal ganglion cell development.

Gain-of-function *Kit* mutations give rise to mesenchymal tumors of the gastrointestinal tract due to constitutive SCF-independent receptor signaling. Relevant to this, the pharmacologic Abl tyrosine kinase inhibitor **imatinib** (STI-571) cross-inhibits Kit, and hence is usually efficacious in the treatment of Kit-dependent **gastrointestinal stromal-cell tumors** (GIST). In contrast to GIST, imatinib is usually ineffective in treating the hematologic disorder **systemic mastocytosis**; this reflects the common presence in this disorder of an activating mutation at the ATP-binding site of *Kit* which prevents drug binding (pp. 268–9).

Bone marrow function is driven by growth factors

Blood is a dynamic organ system with a high cell turnover rate. The proliferation and maturation of the constituent cell lineages are determined by **hemopoietic growth factors** – originally called colony-stimulating factors (CSFs) because of their abilities to promote clonogenic blood cell growth in vitro. Bone marrow stromal cells (such as fibroblasts or adipocytes) produce many of these growth factors in vivo. Hemopoietic growth factors do not form a single molecular superfamily, but consist of two broad groups defined by the structure and signaling of their receptors:

1. Ligands for receptor tyrosine kinases
   - Stem cell factor (SCF).
   - Macrophage colony-stimulating factor (M-CSF).
2. Ligands for cytokine receptors
   - Erythropoietin.
   - Granulocyte colony-stimulating factor (G-CSF).
   - Granulocyte-macrophage colony-stimulating factor (GM-CSF).
   - Interleukins 2–7, especially IL-3 (multi-CSF).

Hemopoietic growth factor receptors are expressed at low levels relative to other receptor classes, typically approximating 100 molecules per cell in vivo.

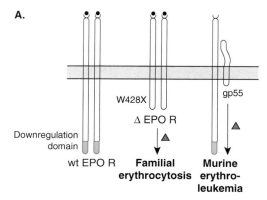

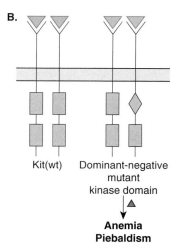

Figure 14.3 Wild-type and mutant cytokine receptors. *A*, The wild-type erythropoietin receptor (wt EPO R) and the constitutively activated mutant counterpart: the intracellular domain stop codon in familial erythrocytosis, and the gp55 transforming product of Friend erythroleukemia virus. *B*, The wild-type stem cell factor receptor (c-Kit), and the dominant negative mutant receptor in piebaldism.

the **Mpl** gene product on megakaryocytes (and other cell lineages including CD34$^+$ bone marrow progenitors). In one syndrome of platelet overproduction, the myeloproliferative disorder **polycythemia vera**, Mpl expression in megakaryocytes is reduced. Recombinant IL-11 can improve thrombocytopenia that is not induced by chemotherapy, whereas TPO is used to maximize platelet yields from apheresis donors.

Erythropoietin in health and disease

The 39-kDa glycoprotein **erythropoietin** is synthesized by the kidney and stimulates erythrocyte proliferation. The maximum activity of this blood hormone requires correct glycosylation and, in particular, sialylation of oligosaccharides. Expression of the erythropoietin gene is inducible by blood loss or hypoxia. This adaptation is mediated by an oxygen-sensing heme protein that activates the 3′ enhancer binding of a hypoxia-inducible transactivator (pp. 450–1).

An activating mutation of its receptor has been implicated in some cases of **familial erythrocytosis** (Figure 14.3). The gp55 membrane glycoprotein of **Friend erythroleukemia virus** induces activation of the erythropoietin receptor, accounting for the transforming activity of this murine retrovirus (Figure 14.3).

Inappropriately high erythropoietin levels occur in some malignancies, whereas abnormally low levels are seen in **chronic renal failure**. Treatment of uremic patients with **recombinant erythropoietin** is effective in relieving symptoms due to anemia, but may occasionally precipitate acute hypertensive episodes.

Leukemia inhibitory factor (LIF)

Like many hemopoietic cytokines, most of the apparent molecular weight of **leukemia inhibitory factor** (**LIF**) is due to glycosylation, which prevents the molecule from being degraded. LIF activity is inhibited by circulating receptor proteins similar to those that regulate the bioavailability of growth hormone. Like the structurally related cytokines G-CSF, IL-6 and oncostatin M, LIF causes in vitro cell differentiation of the morphologic M1 subclass of **acute myeloid leukemia** (hence the name). In addition to this antileukemic effect, LIF exerts pleiotropic effects on many other cellular processes:

1. It enhances the growth of megakaryocytes, monocytes, and myeloid cells.
2. It inhibits differentiation and enhances the survival of stem cells.
3. It stimulates bone resorption and remodeling due to osteoblast proliferation (excessive amounts may be associated with hypercalcemia or dystrophic tissue calcification).
4. It inhibits lipoprotein lipase, leading to cachexia and weight loss.
5. It induces a switch to the cholinergic phenotype in adrenergic neurons.
6. It inhibits vascular endothelial cell growth in the aorta (not capillaries).

Transgenic mice overexpressing LIF exhibit irritability, pylorospasm, weight loss, reduced spermatogenesis, thymic and adrenocortical atrophy, and increased hepatocyte production of acute phase reactants. LIF underexpression, on the other hand, leads to the failure of mammalian blastocyst implantation.

Angiogenic factors

Endothelial cell mitogens stimulate blood vessel formation

Processes such as embryogenesis, endometrial growth, and wound healing all require the formation of new blood vessels. There are two broad varieties of new blood vessel formation: the developmental formation of blood vessels from scratch (**vasculogenesis**), and the remodeling of a mature circulatory network from pre-existing vessels (**angiogenesis**, or arteriogenesis). Such neovascularization is stimulated by **angiogenic factors** including:

1. **Vascular endothelial growth factors** (VEGF A–D).
2. **Fibroblast growth factors**, especially **basic FGF** (bFGF; see below).
3. **Angiopoietins** (Ang 1–4).
4. **Angiogenin** (induces macrophages to release mitogens).
5. **Angiotropin** (stimulates endothelial cell migration).

Numerous other "part-time" angiogenic factors exist. These include platelet-derived endothelial cell growth factor (PD-ECGF), platelet-derived growth factors (PDGF A and B), insulin-like growth factors (IGFs), transforming growth factors (TGFα and β), tumor necrosis factor α (TNFα), interleukin-8 (IL-8), hepatocyte growth factor (HGF), monocyte chemotactic protein-1 (MCP-1), and leptin.

VEGF is a vascular endothelial mitogen that also increases blood vessel permeability. VEGF and bFGF mediate angiogenesis in a synergistic manner by crosstalking with different integrins: VEGF receptors exert angiogenic activity via the $\alpha_v\beta_5$ integrin (and also via Src, which inhibits VEGF-dependent vascular leakage) whereas FGF receptors act via $\alpha_v\beta_3$. Embryonic vasculogenesis requires hemangioblast activation by VEGF, bFGF, PDGF-BB and TGFβ. Vascular progenitor cells exposed to VEGF tend to differentiate into arterial endothelial cells, whereas stimulation of such cells with PDGF-BB redirects the differentiation pathway towards smooth muscle cells and pericytes. Smooth muscle cells in the developing cardiac valves, on the other hand, originate under the influence of $TGF\beta_3$.

Later phases of vessel remodeling require the transcription factor **gridlock**, the TGFβ-binding protein endoglin (null mutations of which cause **hereditary hemorrhagic telangiectasia**), smooth muscle cell recruitment by PDGF-BB, and vessel sealing by angiopoietins. These latter cytokines activate **Tie** receptor tyrosine kinases (Tie1 and Tie2), thereby reducing vascular permeability and opposing VEGF during the maturational phase of circulatory development. One of the most potent stimuli for VEGF gene transcription is hypoxia, which induces a panel of adaptive genes (p. 451).

Lymphatic vessel development is promoted by a member of the VEGF ligand family, **VEGF-C**, which activates the type 2 and 3 VEGF receptors. **Angiogenin** is an RNase-like molecule that stimulates the production of phospholipases within the vessel wall.

CLINICAL KEYNOTE

VEGF in diabetic retinopathy

Uncontrolled angiogenesis plays a role in many disease processes, including **tumor progression**, proliferative **diabetic retinopathy**, and **rheumatoid arthritis**. The defective vasculature in these conditions may lead to the recruitment of angiogenic factors from macrophages by simulating nonhealing wounds.

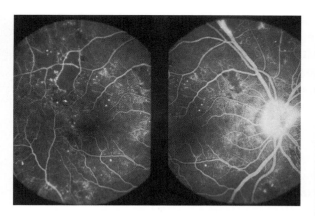

Figure 14.4 Diabetic retinopathy (Wellcome Medical Photographic Library, no. N00022282C).

Figure 14.5 Fibroblast growth factors (FGFs). Following release from extracellular heparin-like extracellular matrix components, FGFs bind their cell-surface receptors, internalize together with the activated receptors, and then – apparently – dissociate from the receptor and migrate to the nucleus. Similar nuclear localization has been reported for other ligands, as well as for various growth factor receptors; but no mechanism to explain nuclear trafficking of the latter is known.

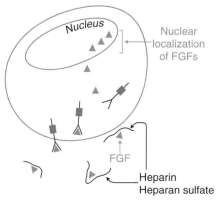

VEGF is linked with pathologic angiogenesis, especially in diabetic retinopathy (Figure 14.4). Diabetic patients have abnormally high VEGF levels in the vitreous humor of the eye, adjacent to the site of retinal new vessels, and in the retina itself. The causality of this association is supported by the finding that experimental retinal neovascularization is inhibited by dominant negative VEGF receptors.

The ability of VEGF to activate MAP kinases depends in part on IGF1 receptor signaling. Consistent with this, the retinopathic effects of VEGF depend upon downstream co-activation of the **IGF1 receptor**, blockade of which inhibits neovascularization. This latter interaction may explain why initiation of insulin treatment can lead to the transient progression of diabetic retinopathy.

The precise mechanism by which diabetes triggers neovascularization remains uncertain. VEGF is induced not only by hypoxia but also by oxygen free radicals and by another stress stimulus – hypoglycemia – rather than by hyperglycemia.

Therapeutic approaches to inhibit VEGF include antisense oligonucleotides (p. 594) and antibody or peptidomimetic therapies. However, at present laser photocoagulation remains the standard for diabetic eye disease.

Tissue vascularity is regulated by fibroblast growth factors

Fibroblast growth factors (**FGFs**) are pleiotropic mitogenic activators that structurally resemble the IL-1 family of inflammatory cytokines. Acidic FGF (aFGF) and basic FGF (bFGF) bind negatively charged heparin-like molecules, as does VEGF. Hence, these molecules are collectively termed **heparin-binding growth factors** (Figure 14.5).

Heparin and **heparan sulfate** are glycosaminoglycans (GAGs; p. 226), i.e., polysaccharide components of proteoglycans such as **syndecan** (-1 or -4), **perlecan**, **decorin**, **glypican** and **versican**. Since aFGFs and bFGFs lack the secretory leader sequence found in most other growth factors, they are not secreted but rather stored as matrix-bound growth factors, which are protected from enzymatic attack by proteoglycans. FGF-binding proteoglycans thus regulate the tissue availability of FGFs: for example, the release of **dermatan sulfate** after injury potentiates the subsequent action of FGF2. Moreover, the LasA virulence factor of *Pseudomonas aeruginosa* enhances host epithelial cell shedding of syndecan, and the liberated syndecan ectodomains directly enhance infectivity via their heparan sulfate chains.

There are at least eight different FGF-family molecules: FGF1 (aFGF), FGF2 (bFGF), FGF3 (the *Int2* gene product), FGF4 (also known as Hst1), FGF5, FGF6, FGF7 (keratinocyte growth factor) and FGF8. Cell types stimulated by FGFs include endothelial cells, vascular smooth muscle cells, and fibroblasts. Consistent with these multiple targets, FGFs play multiple roles as embryonic inducers, endothelial mitogens, and stimulators of protease activity. FGFs may also be trophic for glial cells and neurons, and can facilitate hemopoiesis. Keratinocyte growth factor is distinguished from other FGFs by its target specificity for epithelial cells and lack of mitogenicity for fibroblasts.

Each FGF activates at least one receptor tyrosine kinase, four of which (FGFR1 to -4) are characterized. Alternative splicing of these receptors alters extracellular domain structure and thus ligand affinity, creating defined patterns of ligand action. FGF4 is specifically implicated in trophoblast stem cell proliferation, for example, providing a mechanism for the first-trimester maternal anemia associated with placental hypervascularity (Figure 14.6). Similarly, the release of bFGF by tumors induces $\alpha_v\beta_3$ integrin overexpression in neighboring capillary endothelium, leading to endothelial cell invasion and new blood vessel formation.

FGFs have been implicated in the pathogenesis of several human diseases

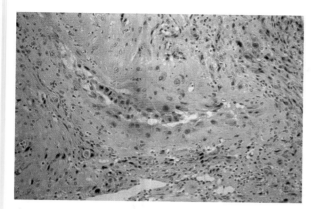

Figure 14.6 Invasion of the trophoblast by new blood vessels under the influence of vascular endothelial growth factor (VEGF) and other pro-angiogenic molecules (Wellcome Medical Photographic Library, no. N0011601C).

occurring at mucosal and endothelial interfaces. For example, long-term hyperglycemic damage to basement membrane glycosaminoglycans may reduce bFGF binding, and thus contribute to diabetic peripheral vascular disease. Intramyocardial FGF injection, on the other hand, can help to revascularize and strengthen chronically ischemic ventricular muscle.

CLINICAL KEYNOTE

Fibroblast growth factor receptor mutations

Germline mutations affecting FGF receptors (FGFRs) are mainly expressed not as disorders of angiogenesis but rather as disorders of developmental bone growth:

1. *FGFR1* (8p11) mutations
   - **Pfeiffer syndrome**[1] (craniosynostosis with interphalangeal ankylosis).
2. *FGFR2* (10q25-26) mutations
   - **Crouzon syndrome** (autosomal dominant craniosynostosis).
   - **Apert syndrome** (craniosynostosis with syndactyly).
   - **Jackson–Weiss syndrome** (craniosynostosis with tarsal-metatarsal coalescence).
3. *FGFR3* mutations (on chromosome 4p)
   - **Achondroplastic dwarfism** (long bone shortening, macrocephaly; complications include dental malocclusion, chronic middle-ear infections, and cervical cord compression due to foramen magnum maldevelopment).
   - **Thanatophoric dysplasia** (similar, but lethal in neonates).

Most of these syndromes result from point mutations affecting the extracellular or transmembrane domains, and thus constitutively activate the mutant receptors – in other words, these disorders result from gain-of-function mutations. For example, 90% of achondroplasia results from an FGFR3 transmembrane domain point mutation ($Gly_{380} \rightarrow Arg$ due to either G1138A or G1138C), which leads to ligand-independent receptor oligomerization and hence kinase activation. Milder forms (hypochondroplasia) occur because of mutations affecting the FGFR3 tyrosine kinase domain ($Asn_{540} \rightarrow Lys$). These phenotypes imply that FGFR3 is a de facto negative regulator of bone growth through its effects on the premature maturation of growing epiphyses and cartilage. New mutations are responsible for 80% of cases, and these mutations usually occur on the paternal allele. As in **Marfan syndrome**, increasing paternal age is a major risk factor for such mutations. Of note, bFGF treatment has also been noted to cause regression of **Ewing tumor**, a malignant bone tumor of childhood.

Vascular proliferation is constrained by angioinhibitors

In healthy (nonwounded) adults the only physiologic site of angiogenesis is the endometrium; sprouting angiogenesis does not occur in the brain, for example, even when wounded. Tumor growth to a diameter greater than 3 mm requires either the co-opting of host blood vessels or new vessel formation, such as may be induced by pro-angiogenic oncogenes like those of **Kaposi sarcoma herpesviruses** (**KSHV**). Blood vessel formation is thus tightly controlled. **Angioinhibins**, or inhibitors of angiogenesis, include:

1. **Endostatin, angiostatin, vasostatin.**
2. **Platelet factor 4, interleukin 4.**
3. **Interferons** (α and β).
4. **Thrombospondin** (an anti-adhesive matrix protein).

---

[1] May also occur as a result of *FGFR2* mutations.

plasma renin activity (PRA). Despite salt deprivation, affected subjects fail to elevate their PRA, consistent with hyperaldosteronism, but plasma aldosterone levels are also normal. The competitive inhibitor of aldosterone spironolactone (which is often used to treat heart failure) fails to abolish the hypertension, unlike the renal tubular sodium reabsorption inhibitor amiloride, which does. Mutations affecting the WW domain of the β-subunit of the amiloride-sensitive epithelial **sodium channel** underlie this syndrome. These mutations trigger the constitutive activation of sodium transport without the need for aldosterone. Interestingly, volume-expanded hypertensive states may be associated with a plasma digitalis-like or ouabain-like activity, suggesting the secretion of an endogenous Na^+/K^+-ATPase inhibitor.

MOLECULAR MINIREVIEW

Hypertension genes

Chronically elevated blood pressure of unknown cause, termed **essential hypertension**, affects over 25% of the population aged over 50. The word "essential" here is instructive: what it implies is that such hypertension is most often induced by a relatively large number of genes, each one of which may have only a small or indirect effect, and that interactions with environmental factors may also be important. However, the familial aggregation of essential hypertension supports a key contribution for genetic variables. To illustrate the indirect nature of such interactions, consider the *apolipoprotein E4* allele which is associated with higher plasma cholesterol levels than *apoE2* and also with **Alzheimer disease** (pp. 169–70) – a disorder which is in turn more common in those with pre-existing hypertension (and hence, presumably, some degree of cerebral microvascular disease).

Linkage studies (p. 568) are less useful for identifying genes of subtle effect, so progress in this field has been gradual. Nonetheless, some of the molecules implicated in the genetic architecture of hypertension include those involved in the renin-angiotensin system (see below), cation transporters (see above), vascular endothelial system (e.g., endothelins; see below), and the sympathetic nervous system. The latter includes molecules such as the β_2-**adrenergic receptor**, in which the Glu^{27} polymorphism is associated with reduced desensitization in response to beta-blockade, leading to greater therapeutic responsiveness.

Renin and ACE activate aldosterone and angiotensin synthesis

Pressure reductions in the arterial (high-pressure) side of the circulation – as sensed by carotid sinus baroreceptors – cause the release of **prorenin** and **renin** from the macula densa in the renal juxtaglomerular apparatus. Such increases may be suppressed in the early stages of cardiac failure by ANP release, which maintains renal blood flow and urine output. Primary increases in arterial pressure can be classified into high-renin (hyper-reninemic) and low-renin (hyporeninemic) varieties of hypertension. Renin is an acid protease that proteolyzes **angiotensinogen** to the decapeptide **angiotensin I** which is in turn converted by **angiotensin-converting enzyme** (**ACE**) to the active octapeptide angiotensin II (Figure 14.7).

Skeletal muscle contains a renin-angiotensin-ACE system similar to that of the circulatory system: a low-activity ACE insertion (*I*) polymorphism is linked to high-performance endurance and weightlifting relative to homozygotes with a high-activity ACE deletion (*DD*) polymorphism, consistent with enhanced muscle efficiency in the presence of low tissue ACE activity. "High-ACE" *DD* individuals, who have excess activation of the renin-angiotensin

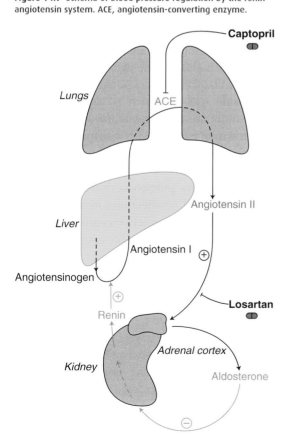

Figure 14.7 Schema of blood pressure regulation by the renin-angiotensin system. ACE, angiotensin-converting enzyme.

system, have a worse outlook in heart failure, but this subgroup gains a proportionately greater therapeutic advantage from the use of **beta-adrenergic blockers** (which cross-inhibit the renin-angiotensin system).

Angiotensin II activates phospholipase C in vascular smooth muscle cells via a G-protein-dependent mechanism. In addition to its peripheral pressor effects, angiotensin II stimulates thirst and salt-craving via a central effect on angiotensin receptors. The autocrine release of angiotensin II may induce cardiac myocyte hypertrophy in response to pressure loading. Other molecules implicated in the pathogenesis of ventricular hypertrophy include the myocardial G-protein G_q – an effector of angiotensin II – and the transcription factor **GATA4** (p. 454), which turns on cardiac muscle hypertrophy genes.

Diabetic kidneys may hypersecrete prorenin, leading to high efferent arteriolar angiotensin II concentrations, elevated glomerular pressures and nephropathy. Angiotensin II and potassium stimulate the synthesis of **aldosterone** by the zona glomerulosa cells of the adrenal cortex. Constitutive aldosterone secretion by an adrenocortical adenoma gives rise to **Conn syndrome**, or **primary hyperaldosteronism**. Secondary aldosterone elevations (up to 20 times the normal range) are seen in **heart failure**, accounting in part for the characteristic salt and fluid retention, and such hyperaldosteronism is exacerbated by reduced hepatic metabolism of aldosterone due to hypoperfusion. A Ser^{810} →Leu point mutation affecting the hormone-binding domain of the mineralocorticoid (aldosterone) receptor confers progesterone-responsiveness upon the receptor, thereby predisposing to **pregnancy-associated hypertension**. The latter syndrome (a.k.a. pre-eclampsia) is also characterized by hypersensitivity to the pressor effects of angiotensin II.

CLINICAL KEYNOTE

Glucocorticoid-suppressible hypertension

The **aldosterone synthase** gene lies adjacent to a homologous ACTH-regulated gene on chromosome 8, **11-β-hydroxylase**, which is involved in both cortisol and aldosterone biosynthesis. Abnormal recombination between these two loci may result in a chimeric 11-hydroxylase-aldosterone synthase gene, which remains under the control of an ACTH-sensitive promoter. This leads to the rare autosomal dominant hypertensive syndrome of **familial hyperaldosteronism type I** (also known as **glucocorticoid-suppressible hyperaldosteronism**), in which the phenotype is highly variable, with many kindred members being normokalemic and/or normotensive.

A distinct hypertensive syndrome termed **apparent mineralocorticoid excess** invariably causes hyperkalemia: null mutations affect the renal cortisol-inactivating enzyme **11β-hydroxysteroid dehydrogenase type 2**. In both syndromes, prescription of **dexamethasone** may paradoxically elevate (low) plasma potassium levels and improve blood pressure via negative feedback on the ACTH-cortisol-aldosterone pathway.

PHARMACOLOGIC FOOTNOTE

ACE inhibitors

ACE is critical to the regulation of systemic blood pressure. Overexpression of ACE secondary to deletion polymorphisms is associated with **coronary atherosclerosis**, and ACE variants have been linked to **hypertension**. Both aldosterone-mediated

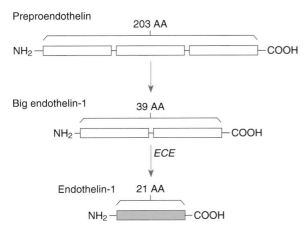

Preproendothelin

Big endothelin-1

ECE

Endothelin-1

Figure 14.8 The formation of mature endothelin-1 from big endothelin-1. Endothelin-converting enzyme (ECE) drives this reaction; the formation of big endothelin derives from domain cleavage of preproendothelin.

sodium/fluid retention and the direct vasoconstrictive effects of angiotensin II may be inhibited by antagonizing angiotensin II production using **ACE inhibitors** such as **captopril**, **enalapril** or **lisinopril**. These drugs, which profoundly reduce cardiac afterload, have revolutionized the therapy of conditions such as heart failure and hypertension. Aldosterone synthesis is transiently inhibited by ACE inhibition, but escape occurs.

The beneficial effects of ACE inhibitors in renal disease exceed their hypotensive effects, particularly in **diabetes mellitus** associated with early proteinuria. This raises the possibility that these serine protease inhibitors may act in part by affecting the bioavailability of extracellular molecules other than angiotensin I. In contrast, low-activity *DD* homozygotes gain little renoprotection from ACE inhibitors; the same is true of patients with **polycystic kidney disease**. Of note, insulin-dependent *DD* diabetics may be more prone to hypoglycemia. ACE genotyping could thus become a useful predictor of therapeutic outcomes.

Angiotensin II inhibitors such as **losartan** have more restricted clinical benefits than do ACE inhibitors. Kinin-dependent side-effects of ACE inhibitors, such as cough, can be avoided by switching to this drug class.

Endothelins are potent vasoconstrictors and inotropes

Reducing intravascular volume leads not only to activation of the renin-angiotensin system, but also to compensatory endothelial production of potent vasoconstrictors termed **endothelins** – 21-amino-acid peptides structurally related to **sarafotoxin snake venom**. **Endothelin-1** (ET-1) is synthesized in endothelial cells from a 38-residue inactive precursor termed **big endothelin**, which is proteolyzed by a membrane-bound protease termed **endothelin-converting enzyme** (ECE), an investigative target for antihypertensive drug development (Figure 14.8).

ET-1 is the most powerful pressor known, being five- to tenfold more potent on a molar basis than angiotensin II. Like angiotensin II, ET-1 may worsen atherosclerosis and myocardial ischemia by acting, respectively, as a vascular smooth muscle mitogen and positive inotrope. ET-1 activates a G-protein-coupled receptor (in this case, the ET_A **receptor**) as do most other vasoconstrictors, including thromboxane A_2 and angiotensin II. Platelet activation releases thrombin and TGFβ, both of which enhance ET-1 synthesis by vascular endothelial cells. In contrast, the synthesis and secretion of ET-1 are inhibited by ANP, while endothelins in turn antagonize the volume-repleting effects of ADH. The ET_A receptor antagonist **tezosentan** has proven useful in managing **heart failure**, in which context ET-1 has a vasoconstrictive effect.

Two other endothelins, **ET-2** and **ET-3**, are expressed in nonendothelial tissues such as neurons and renal epithelia where they activate the ET_B **receptor**. Hence, the endothelin signaling family comprises at least three ligands and two receptors.

Endothelins in human disease
ET-1 has been implicated in the pathogenesis of numerous disorders, including cardiovascular disease (some forms of **hypertension, atherosclerosis, coronary artery disease, congestive heart failure, variant angina,** vasospasm following **subarachnoid hemorrhage, pulmonary hypertension,** and **Raynaud disease**), renal disease (**end-stage renal failure,** renal vasoconstriction in **hepatorenal syndrome,** and **ciclosporin**

nephrotoxicity), bronchial hyperreactivity in **asthma, idiopathic pulmonary fibrosis,** vasculitic ischemia in **inflammatory bowel disease,** and **migraine.**

The nonselective endothelin receptor antagonist **bosentan** appears capable of lowering blood pressure in patients with essential hypertension, and may be useful in other settings including subarachnoid hemorrhage and ciclosporin-induced renal hypoperfusion. The selective ET_A receptor antagonist **BQ123** may prove useful in heart failure.

Endothelins play a key role in neural crest cell migration during embryonic development. For example, knockout of endothelin-1 gene expression during mouse development results in craniofacial and pharyngeal arch syndromes reminiscent of congenital human syndromes such as **Treacher–Collins syndrome** and **Pierre–Robin syndrome,** as well as congenital heart defects. In contrast, knockout of either endothelin-3 or the ET_B receptor causes an aganglionic megacolon syndrome in mice, and mutations of the latter receptor have been detected in kindreds with **Hirschprung disease.**

Endothelins function as neurotransmitters in the central and peripheral nervous system in addition to their vasoactive and intrarenal effects. Other vasoactive molecules that share neurotransmitter roles include the endothelin-like pressor angiotensin II and the physiologic endothelin antagonist **nitric oxide.**

Nitric oxide

Nitric oxide enhances blood flow

In addition to regulating blood pressure by altering blood volume, cytokines may regulate blood pressure by altering blood vessel caliber through their effects on arteriolar smooth muscle. Pressor-regulatory cytokines of this kind include:

1. Vasoconstrictors
   - **Endothelins.**
   - **Angiotensin II.**
   - **Thromboxane A$_2$.**
2. Vasodilators
   - **Calcitonin gene-related peptide** (CGRP).
   - **Atrial natriuretic peptide** (ANP).
   - **Prostaglandins E$_2$ and I$_2$** (PGE$_2$ and PGI$_2$; p. 293).
   - **Bradykinin.**
   - **Potassium ions** (endothelium-derived hyperpolarizing factor).

Endothelial cells synthesize many molecules that maintain vessel patency in the face of vasoconstrictive and thrombogenic stimuli. These molecules include the antithrombotic and antiplatelet cytokines, tissue plasminogen activator and prostacyclin (PGI$_2$), as well as vasoactive endothelial metabolites such as adenosine and platelet-activating factor (PAF).

Vasoconstrictive stimuli are opposed by a potent vasodilatory effector termed **nitric oxide** (NO•; formerly designated endothelium-derived relaxing factor, EDRF). This multifunctional nitrogen monoxide metabolite is a diffusible free radical that circulates bound to albumin via a sulfhydryl linkage. NO• has a half-life of a few seconds and is bioactive within cells at concentrations as low as 10^{-20} M. It activates heme-iron enzyme moieties, particularly soluble **guanylate cyclase** which is, in effect, the NO• receptor. In this way NO• increases platelet cGMP and inhibits platelet aggregation, thereby synergizing with prostacyclin-dependent increases in platelet cAMP. NO• also has antihypertensive effects, which may relate in part to inhibition of vascular smooth

decapeptide **kallidin** (lysine-bradykinin). **Tachykinins** ("fast moving") include sensory neuropeptides such as **substance P** and **neurokinin**. Kinins have been implicated in the pathogenesis of numerous clinical presentations, including:

1. Pain associated with **angina, migraine** and inflammatory conditions such as **arthritis** and **pancreatitis**.
2. **Postgastrectomy dumping syndrome**.
3. Flushing associated with **carcinoid syndrome**.
4. Skin lesions in **psoriasis**.
5. **Pre-eclampsia**.

Impaired peripheral venodilatation following bradykinin (but not sodium nitroprusside) infusions is characteristic of **Raynaud disease**; since bradykinin mediates endothelium-dependent venodilatation whereas nitroprusside causes direct release of NO•, defective kinin-induced endothelial release of nitric oxide may contribute to this disorder. Aberrant placental blood flow during early pregnancy may trigger **neurokinin B** secretion by the outer syncytiotrophoblast in **pre-eclampsia**, raising the prospect of developing receptor antagonists to prevent this disorder.

In an unusual reciprocal relationship, bradykinin is directly inactivated by angiotensin-converting enzyme (ACE), which catalyzes the production of its vasoactive antagonist. Hence, ACE inhibitors act not only by inhibiting angiotensin II and aldosterone production, but also by stabilizing bradykinin; this accounts for the common ACE inhibitor side-effect of cough.

Kinin receptor antagonists have been used with therapeutic benefit in **asthma**, whereas competitive kinin antagonists have been synthesized by modifying the bioactive parent peptide. Like most bioactive peptides, however, these proteolytically vulnerable molecules have proven too shortlived for clinical use.

PHARMACOLOGIC FOOTNOTE

Sildenafil (Viagra™)

Parasympathetic postsynaptic nerves supplying cavernous (erectile) tissue in the genital organs activate soluble guanylyl cyclases in vascular smooth muscle cells by releasing nitric oxide. This leads to increased cGMP within the erectile tissues, causing smooth muscle relaxation and vasodilatation. Erection thus occurs due to increased cGMP levels. Breakdown of cGMP in the corpora cavernosum is mediated by **phosphodiesterase type 5** (PDE5; Figure 14.9), which is the inhibitory target of the potency-enhancing drug sildenafil citrate (Viagra™). In the systemic circulation cGMP levels are also elevated by nitrates (e.g., isosorbide dinitrate). Co-prescription is therefore contraindicated due to the risk of synergistic vasodilatation and hypotension. Of note, sildenafil was first developed (unsuccessfully) as an antianginal drug, an indication which now ranks as a contraindication to the intended use. By restoring neuronal NOS production, sildenafil may improve the pylorospasm (gastric outlet obstruction) of **diabetic gastroparesis**.

Cut flowers also respond to cGMP by standing up straight, creating an additional market for sildenafil among florists.

Summary

Blood production depends on pluripotential stem cells. Bone marrow function is driven by growth factors. Hemopoietic growth factors vary in target cell specificity.

Endothelial cell mitogens stimulate new blood vessel formation. Tissue vas-

Enrichment reading

Library reference

Garland JM (ed). *Colony-stimulating factors*. Marcel Dekker, New York, 1997

Highsmith RF (ed). *Endothelin: molecular biology, physiology and pathology*. Humana Press, Champaign, IL, 1998

Laskin JD, Laskin DL. *Cellular and molecular biology of nitric oxide*. Marcel Dekker, New York, 1999

Rubanyi GM (ed). *Angiogenesis in health and disease: basic mechanisms and clinical applications*. Marcel Dekker, New York, 1999

cularity is regulated by fibroblast growth factors (FGFs). Vascular proliferation is constrained by angioinhibitors.

Pressor molecules may act in part by increasing blood volume. Renin and angiotensin-converting enzyme (ACE) activate aldosterone and angiotensin synthesis. Endothelins are potent vasoconstrictors and inotropes.

Nitric oxide enhances blood flow. Extravascular tissues respond to nitric oxide.

QUIZ QUESTIONS

1. Which characteristics distinguish hemopoietic stem cells from differentiated cells?
2. Name some of the functions of stem-cell factor and its receptor Kit.
3. Explain how hemopoietic growth factors influence bone marrow stem cell maturation.
4. What are some of the clinical indications for specific recombinant bone marrow growth factors?
5. Explain the pathogenesis of anemia in: (1) chronic renal failure, and (2) chronic rheumatoid arthritis.
6. How is new blood vessel growth regulated at the molecular level?
7. Explain what is known of the molecular pathogenesis of diabetic retinopathy.
8. Name some different molecules that affect blood pressure, and explain how they differ in functional terms.
9. What is ACE, and why is it clinically useful to inhibit it in certain clinical scenarios?
10. Describe how endothelins function. What effects can they cause?
11. What is the mechanism of action of nitric oxide? Which disease states is it implicated in?
12. Explain how impotence can be treated with pharmacologic agents.

15

Cell cycle control, apoptosis, and ageing

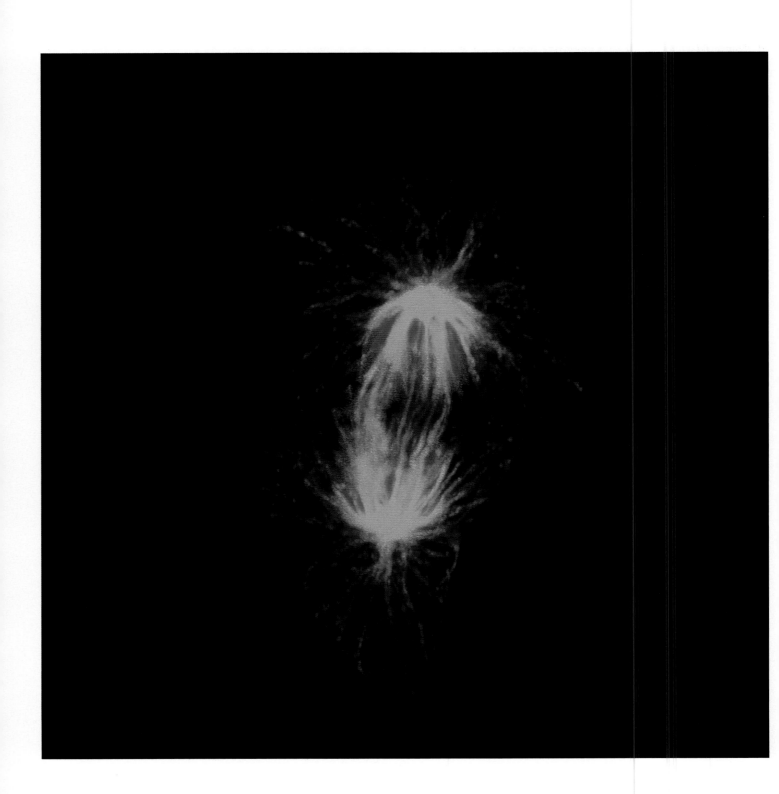

Figure 15.1 (*previous page*) A confocal micrograph of a dividing cell showing the mitotic spindle (Wellcome Medical Photographic Library, no. B0001062C03, credit Dr D. Becker and L. Erskine.

Most cells grow throughout their lifespan. Intestinal crypt cells or bone marrow precursors proliferate continuously, for example, whereas hepatocytes divide intermittently and spend the intervening periods at rest. In contrast, normal adult neurons do not divide to any significant extent. Mature red blood cells and platelets can also be characterized as postmitotic, since neither contain nuclei. Such cells are said to be terminally differentiated. The framework used for considering how cells make decisions about growth, differentiation, senescence, and death is termed the cell cycle.

Cell cycle control genes

Chromosomes separate and rejoin in a cyclical fashion

As detailed earlier, proliferating cells contain chromosomes that undergo recurring structural changes termed interphase, prophase, metaphase, anaphase, and telophase. The last four (mitotic) phases of this **chromosomal cycle** account for only a small percentage of the time involved for a cell to reproduce. Mitosis lasts about an hour in humans, whereas the time between mitoses (interphase) lasts 18–24 hours. In contrast, certain bacteria spend as little as ten minutes between successive divisions.

Though microscopically unremarkable, the interphase period of chromosomal dispersion conceals many of the key molecular events that define the **cell cycle**. The cell (division) cycle represents a set of controls to ensure that one round of division follows one round of DNA replication just as one round of DNA replication follows one of cell division. The only exception to this in human cells is meiosis, where two rounds of cell division follow one of DNA replication. The **phases** of the cell cycle comprise (Figure 15.2*A*):

1. G_1 (gap phase 1)
   - Duration ~10–14 hours in dividing cells.
2. **S** (DNA synthesis)
   - Duration ~three to six hours.
3. G_2 (gap phase 2)
   - Duration ~two to four hours.
4. **M** (mitosis)
   - Duration ~one hour.

G_1 phase can be further subdivided into a metabolically quiescent G_0 phase – lasting from eight hours to years – in which cells are not committed to progress through the cycle. Non-G_0 cells with late G_1-phase DNA content commit to S phase by becoming transcriptionally active. Following completion of S phase, G_2 is reserved for checking the integrity of replication, repairing any mismatches, and thus ensuring readiness of the cell for M phase.

The most direct way to visualize the cell cycle is by measuring changes in cell DNA content using flow cytometry (fluorescence-activated cell sorting; Figure 15.2*B*). Two major cell cycle transitions are revealed by such studies: that for initiation of DNA replication (the **G_1–S** transition), and that for chromosomal segregation (the **G_2–M** transition).

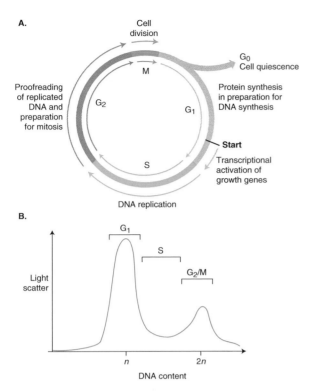

Figure 15.2 The cell cycle as represented by schema and by flow cytometry. *A*, At the time of mitosis, or M-phase, each cell temporarily contains two fully replicated diploid genomes – that is, it exhibits tetraploid (4*n*) DNA content. Following cell division, the daughter cells again contain diploid (2*n*) genomes and are thus definable as having G_1-phase DNA content, where G_1 indicates the first gap in the DNA-based cell cycle. *B*, Flow cytometric measurement of changing cell DNA content and light scatter in the different functional phases of the cell cycle. Cells may enlarge during G_1 phase due to active protein synthesis, although some cell subsets with this DNA content may be metabolically dormant (G_0 phase cells). The G_1 gap ends with the beginning of DNA synthesis, or S-phase, which is characterized by a DNA content intermediate between G_1-phase diploidy and M-phase tetraploidy. This phase involves not only chromosomal replication but also that of the entire chromatin/histone complex, necessitating induction of at least 20 phase-specific genes. S-phase does not terminate in M-phase but in a second gap designated G_2-phase. Cells recovering from cytotoxic insults (e.g., following irradiation) often enter G_2 arrest, presumably to repair DNA lesions; whether this subphase represents a G_2 version of G_0 is unclear. It is during G_2 that the cell decides it is fit to enter mitosis – rather like pilots deciding whether their planes are fit for take-off. This transition involves nuclear envelope dissolution and chromosome condensation.

MOLECULAR MINIREVIEW

Replicative quiescence

DNA content is only a crude measure of cell behavior. Functional cell subsets exist within groups of cells with quantitatively similar DNA contents: one such subset is that of G_0-phase cells which are characterized by G_1-phase DNA content. Such cells are functionally quiescent, exhibiting low rates of RNA and protein synthesis as well as low enzymatic activity. Even so-called **housekeeping genes** undergo sizable inductions (e.g., a 40-fold enhancement of thymidine kinase activity) relative to G_0 on entering S-phase.

G_0 cells respond sluggishly to mitogenic stimuli, taking up to six hours longer to reach S-phase than do cycling G_1-phase cells. Of therapeutic relevance, G_0 cells may form a drug-resistant subpopulation during cancer chemotherapy because of increased time available for DNA repair prior to critical decision points, such as whether or not to traverse a cell cycle **checkpoint**.

Cell cycle checkpoints restrain cell growth

Speaking functionally, the cell cycle contains molecular tripwires for cycling cells. A damaged cell must decide whether to pause at such tripwires or to press on regardless; whereas a cell that progresses and trips must decide when (and whether) to get up again. Such decision points between cell repair and cell death represent a proof-reading mechanism for preventing the replication of unrepaired genomes. The major **cell cycle checkpoints** of this kind are:

1. The **G_1–S transition**
   - Question: is the cell ready to replicate its DNA?
2. The **G_2–M transition**
   - Question: has the DNA been correctly and fully replicated?
3. Exit from mitosis (**M**) back to **G_1**
   - Question: has a functional mitotic spindle been formed?

The cell cycle checkpoint determining the onset of genomic duplication is termed the G_1–S transition. This decision of G_1-phase cells to proceed to S-phase is a critical regulatory step (designated **Start** or the **restriction point** in late G_1 cells) in both normal and neoplastic cell growth. Once a cell reaches S-phase, progression to G_2 becomes independent of extracellular influences – that is, the cell becomes **committed** to completing DNA synthesis (S–G_2 traverse).

Termination of DNA synthesis does not ensure cell division since the **G_2–M transition** remains to be negotiated. S- and M-phases of the cell cycle are tightly coupled, with cells proceeding on to mitosis as soon as G_2 certification of DNA synthesis is complete. Such phase-coupling prevents the division of cells containing incompletely replicated DNA, indicating that misreplicated DNA inhibits the cell cycle machinery.

The **Chfr** (checkpoint with forkhead and ring finger motifs) mitotic stress protein, which delays entry from prophase into metaphase, is often mutated in cancer cells and may thus predict sensitivity to mitosis-disrupting drugs such as the **taxanes**.

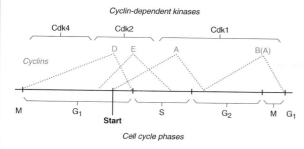

Figure 15.3 Variations in G_1 and G_2 cyclin abundance during the cell cycle. Cyclin D (D1, D2, D3) is the main G_1 cyclin family, cyclin E is G_1–S, cyclin A mainly S, and cyclin B, G_2/M (with a contribution also from A). Certain of the corresponding cyclin-dependent kinases (Cdk) are shown above.

MOLECULAR MINIREVIEW

The G_0–G_1 transition
A major determinant of cell growth is efficiency of the **G_0–G_1 transition**. Net tissue growth rates thus depend on the activation of cells with unduplicated DNA content from quiescence. Such a switch may be associated with the expression of immediate-early gene products such as Fos and Myc in response to mitogenic stimuli such as antigen exposure (B-cell activation), pregnancy (breast ductal hyperplasia), or partial hepatectomy (hepatocyte proliferation).

Immediate-early gene expression is necessary but not sufficient to ensure cell cycle progression. One growth factor might enable a cell to become **competent** to enter the cell cycle, whereas a second growth factor may be needed for cell cycle **progression**.

Cyclins are molecular timers for cell cycle progression

The timing of DNA replication within the cell cycle is determined by a family of enzyme co-factors termed **cyclins** which exhibit cyclical ('sawtooth'; Figure 15.3) oscillations in abundance. These molecular egg-timers activate kinase-active complexes that phosphorylate nuclear control proteins. Cyclins are classified into **A, B, D,** or **E** cyclin groups, reflecting the order in which they were discovered. Cyclins undergo sequential binding to kinase complexes throughout the cell cycle and hence are associated with different checkpoints:

1. **G_1 cyclins**
   - Cyclin D1 (D2, D3).
2. **G_1/S cyclins**
   - Cyclin E.
3. **S-phase** (or late G_1/S) **cyclins**
   - Cyclin A.
4. **M-phase** (mitotic) **cyclins**
   - Cyclins A and B.

D and E cyclins are sometimes called **start** (G_1) **cyclins**. The expression of these cyclins is tissue-specific, and loss of one or more cyclins may signify a shift of cell purpose from proliferation to differentiation. D-group cyclins are responsible for cell cycle traverse through G_1, and thus need to be environmentally aware. Hence, these molecules function not only as nuclear regulatory molecules but also, indirectly, as growth factor sensors and extracellular matrix protein detectors.

B-group cyclins (which contribute to a mitosis-inducing complex called maturation-promoting factor, or MPF) undergo ubiquitin-dependent proteolysis immediately prior to anaphase. Such proteolysis reflects the presence of an amino-terminal **destruction box** within mitotic cyclins, and of a carboxy-terminal **PEST sequence** (p. 138) in G_1 cyclins. The most stringently conserved motif in this protein family, however, is the 100-amino-acid **cyclin box**, which is the binding site for **cyclin-dependent kinases**.

CLINICAL KEYNOTE

Cyclins and cancer
The expression of G_1 cyclins is inducible by growth factors and suppressible by antiproliferative agents such as **interferon-γ** and **tumor necrosis factor**. Conversely, the overexpression of D-type cyclins causes cell hypersensitivity to

growth factor action, which may culminate in tumor formation. It is thus not surprising that cyclins are implicated in human tumorigenesis:

1. Cyclin D1 is often overexpressed in **parathyroid adenomas** because of chromosomal translocations that put the *cyclin D1* gene under control of the parathyroid hormone (*PTH*) gene enhancer.
2. **Liver cancers** may be initiated by insertional mutagenesis of the *cyclin A* gene because of **hepatitis B virus** integration.
3. **Lymphoproliferative disorders** in transplant patients infected with **Epstein–Barr virus** may arise due to viral-dependent overexpression of a D-type cyclin.

Overexpression of cyclin E leads to the shortening of G_1, reduced growth factor requirements, and decreased cell size. These phenotypic changes are also characteristic of malignant transformation.

Cyclin-dependent kinases drive cell growth transitions

Cell nuclei contain molecular timers and dominoes which govern checkpoints and phase transitions respectively. Many of these molecules have been characterized during studies of cell division cycle (*cdc*) mutants in fission yeast. The human homologs of these effectors – the cyclin-dependent kinases or **Cdks** – are constitutively expressed intranuclear protein kinases which are activated in a cell cycle-dependent manner by cyclins. Each set of cyclins has its own distinct preference for Cdk binding:

1. D-type cyclins (G_1 cyclins)
   • Bind **Cdk4** (>Cdk6, Cdk5).
2. Cyclin E (G_1/S cyclin) and A
   • Binds **Cdk2**.
3. Cyclin A and B (mitotic cyclins)
   • Bind **Cdk1** (homologous to yeast cdc2).

The cell cycle may thus be regarded as a recurring **Cdk cycle** in which specific patterns of cyclin–Cdk interaction control the different cell cycle checkpoints:

1. Essential for G_0–G_1 switching
   • **Cyclin D1** (D2, D3).
   • **Cdk4, Cdk2** (Cdk5/6).
2. Essential for (early) G_1–S traverse alone.
   • **Cyclin E**.
   • **Cdk2** (phosphorylates cyclins A and E).
   • **Cdc25A**.
3. Essential for G_2–M traverse alone.
   • **Cyclin B**.
   • **Cdc25B**.
4. Essential for both (late) G_1–S and G_2–M traverse
   • **Cyclin A**.
   • **Cdk1**.

Cdk proteins can thus be considered as the engines of the cell cycle. Unreplicated DNA prevents Cdk1 dephosphorylation, preventing activation of the cyclin B–Cdk1 complex and hence (see below) delaying mitosis. Human cells normally terminate DNA replication as soon as the diploid genome has been reduplicated, preventing aneuploidy.

Figure 15.4 Actions of cyclin-dependent kinases (Cdks) during the cell cycle, showing their phosphorylation substrates. HDAC, histone deacetylase; pRb, retinoblastoma susceptibility gene product.

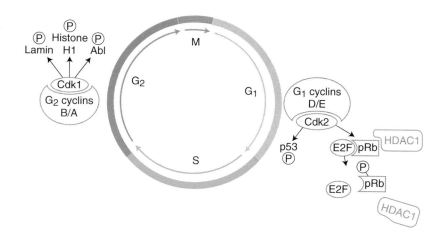

MOLECULAR MINIREVIEW

Cdk1 brakes and accelerators

A master cell cycle serine/threonine kinase is **Cdk1** – the mammalian Cdk homologous to the famous yeast p34^{cdc2}. As shown in Figure 15.4, mitotic Cdk1 substrates include **histone H1** (phosphorylation of which is required for DNA replication and for mitotic chromosome condensation), **lamins** (phosphorylation of which leads to mitotic nuclear envelope dissolution), **myosin** (phosphorylation of which enables spindle polarization during anaphase) and **vimentin** (phosphorylation of which is needed for cytoskeletal reorganization).

The Cdk1 protein kinase is inactivated by Thr^{14}/Tyr^{15} phosphorylation. Although expressed throughout the cycle, the phosphorylation state of Cdk1 varies with the net activity of ambient kinases and phosphatases within the nucleus. Two key molecules responsible for the dephosphorylation (activation) and phosphorylation (inactivation) respectively of Cdk1 are:

1. The cell cycle accelerator **Cdc25B**
   - A nuclear tyrosine phosphatase which dephosphorylates and thus activates Cdk1 (Figure 15.5*A*).
   - Enters the nucleus together with cyclin B1 at the G$_2$/M transition.
   - Promotes mitosis by antagonizing Wee1
2. The cell cycle brake **Wee1** (p107)
   - A dual-specificity tyrosine/threonine kinase and pocket protein (p. ***) that phosphorylates and inactivates Cdk1 (Figure 15.5*B*).
   - Null mutants produce "wee" (Kiwi for "small") daughter cells.
   - Inhibits mitosis by antagonizing Cdc25B.
   - Fine-tunes cell cycle timing by delaying nuclear localization of Cdk1.
   - Increases in response to radiation damage.

Cdc25A mimics the effects of Cdc25B, but at the G$_1$–S transition instead of mitosis. Hence, Cdc25A tyrosine-dephosphorylates Cdk2, thereby triggering G$_1$-phase cell entry to S-phase. Conversely, DNA damage induces rapid ubiquitin-dependent Cdc25A degradation, leading to sustained Cdk2 tyrosine phosphorylation and G$_1$–S arrest. Cell cycle control thus requires a complex mix of positive and negative

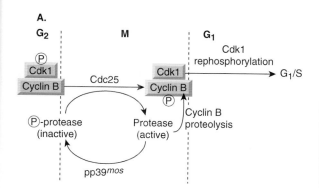

Figure 15.5 Interaction between cyclin-dependent kinases (Cdks) and the phosphatase Cdc25. *A*, Cdc25-dependent activation of Cdk1 at the G$_2$–M interface. Cdk1 is maintained in an inactive state immediately prior to mitosis via phosphorylation at tyrosine-15 and threonine-14 (by Wee1; see below). Dephosphorylation at this site is effected by the phosphatase Cdc 25B, abruptly activating Cdk1. This is associated with phosphorylation of cyclin B and its consequent proteolysis; the responsible protease is rephosphorylated by the meiotic serine-threonine kinase Mos. Proteolysis of cyclin B permits exit from M, followed by rephosphorylation of Cdk1 and re-entry into active G$_1$-phase. *B*, Rephosphorylation of Cdk1 (or 2) by p107^{Wee1}, permitting cell entry into G$_2$ (or G$_1$) and thence into M (or S).

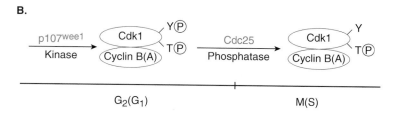

regulatory molecules to regulate Cdk activity. An additional set of control proteins are the **Cdk inhibitors**.

Cdk inhibitors can convert growth to differentiation

Activation of Cdks by cyclins leads to a wave of phosphorylation, which drives the cell through the relevant cell cycle checkpoint. However, the function of Cdks is further regulated by **Cdk-inhibitory proteins** designated by their differing molecular weights:

1. INK4 (**in**hibitor of Cd**k4**) proteins:
   - **p14**^{ARF} (human homolog of mouse p19^{ARF}).
   - **p15** (INK4B, encoded by the *CDKN2B* gene).
   - **p16** (INK4A, encoded by the *CDKN2A* gene).
   - **p18** (INK4C).
2. Cip/Kip (**C**dk2 **i**nhibitor **p**rotein) family
   - **p21** (Cip1, Waf1, Sdi1).
   - **p27** (Kip1).
   - **p57** (Kip2).

The **Cip/Kip** family of Cdk inhibitors inactivates **Cdk2** (i.e., cyclin E and cyclin A complexes), whereas **INK4** proteins inhibit cyclin D1-dependent Cdks (**Cdk4** >**Cdk6**). Hence, the main action of INK4 proteins occurs before the restriction point, whereas Cip/Kips act subsequently (Figure 15.6). Note, however, that the expression of INK4 proteins may also inhibit Cdk2 activity via intracellular redistribution of Cip/Kip proteins.

Cdk inhibitors bind to Cdks, cyclins or cyclin–Cdk complexes. Such binding inhibits the catalytic activity of Cdks, preventing cell cycle progression: transcriptional upregulation of p27^{Kip1} causes cell growth arrest, for example, whereas haploinsufficiency of p27^{Kip1} can predispose to tumor development. Similarly, high levels of p27 immunoreactivity herald a good prognosis in many tumor types, whereas low levels correlate with chemoresistance and rapid demise. Interestingly, mice that do not express p57^{Kip2} resemble the human **Beckwith–Wiedemann syndrome** (gigantism, renal/adrenal malformations, and tumors).

In normal tissues the p53-inducible Cdk inhibitor p21^{Cip1} exemplifies how Cdk inhibitors effect the switch from proliferation to differentiation. This is consistent with the frequent allelic loss or methylation of the encoding genes in human tumors. A different pathologic expression of Cdk overactivity is seen in the neurodegeneration of **Alzheimer disease**, where increased **Cdk5** activity (which causes pathologic hyperphosphorylation of tau and the PKA inhibitor DARPP-32; see Figure 20.20) arises due to constitutive association with its cleaved regulatory subunit p25.

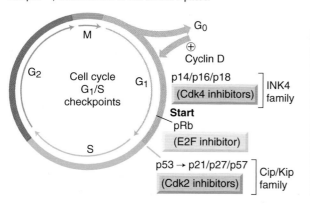

Figure 15.6 Cyclin-dependent kinases (Cdk) inhibitors. Inhibitors of Cdk4 (INK4) include p14^{ARF} and p16 (INK4A, CDKN2A), and are active in early- to mid-G$_1$; Cip/Kip-family Cdk inhibitors include p21^{Cip}, p27^{Kip1} and p57^{Kip2}, and are active in and around S-phase.

MOLECULAR MINIREVIEW

The CDKN2 (p16^{INK4A}/p14^{ARF}) two-gene locus

Human tumors often disrupt the second exon of the *CDKN2A* gene locus encoding the **p16**^{INK4A} protein. The latter molecule normally binds and inhibits the mitogenic **Cdk4–cyclin D1** interaction, thereby preventing cells from progressing through G$_1$- to S-phase (Figure 15.6). In disease, p16^{INK4A} mutation (or silencing by hypermethylation) is implicated most clearly in the pathogenesis of **familial melanoma**, but also **pancreatic**, **hepatobiliary** and **breast cancers**, **glioblastoma**, and **mesothelioma**. Mutations affecting the central portion of the protein (ankyrin repeats II and

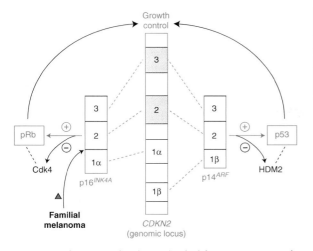

Figure 15.7 Alternate reading frames (ARF) of the *CDKN2A* gene, and their role in linking growth control via the pRb and p53 systems. The designated exons of *CDKN2* are transcribed in different reading frames to yield two distinct growth-control proteins, p16^{INK4A} and p14^{ARF} which respectively inhibit the Cdk4 and Cdk2 mitogenic pathways as shown.

III in the Cdk-binding cleft) are more potently oncogenic. Importantly, familial melanoma-associated *CDKN2A* mutations may also occur in the 5′ noncoding region (G→T, 34 bp upstream of the initiator codon) associated with a 9p21 haplotype of suspected Celtic origin, and additional linked polymorphisms occur in the 3′ untranslated region. More rarely, familial melanoma mutations may directly activate the *Cdk4* gene on 12q13, though pancreatic cancer is not linked to this genotype.

A remarkable feature of the *CDKN2* locus in humans is that it encodes not one but two gene products: p16^{INK4A} and a second overlapping product in an alternate reading frame termed p14^{ARF}, or p19^{ARF} in mice (Figure 15.7). The former interacts with the retinoblastoma susceptibility product, whereas the latter interacts with the p53 protein (see below). Since exons 2 and 3 (but not 1) are common to both genes, the question arises as to which loss of protein function gives rise to tumors in patients with exon 2 deletions. Point mutations in p16^{INK4A} are more heavily implicated in melanoma (as well as in atypical moles, also known as **dysplastic nevi**), whereas deletions affecting both genes (as well as p15^{INK4B}) are common in glioblastoma.

Growth and growth-control genes

Proto-oncogenes encode proteins that activate cell growth

Genes that cause the morphological transformation of cells are termed **oncogenes**, or cancer-causing genes. Transforming oncogenes in human tumors are constitutively activated by gain-of-function mutations, and thus act in a dominant (heterozygous) fashion. The wild-type versions of these genes, termed **cellular oncogenes** or **proto-oncogenes**, encode normal proteins involved in cell signaling and growth regulation. With respect to nomenclature, human cellular oncogenes are denoted by **c-** (e.g., *c-Raf*), whereas transforming viral homologs are designated by **v-** (e.g., *v-Src*). Examples of such molecules include:

1. Growth factors
   - e.g., Platelet-derived growth factor (PDGF) encoded by *c-Sis*.
   - c-Sis overexpression has been implicated in fibrotic disorders such as **myeloid metaplasia (myelofibrosis)** and **pulmonary fibrosis**.
2. Receptor tyrosine kinases
   - e.g., The **Ret** oncoprotein (p. 261).
   - Gain-of-function mutations result in **thyroid cancer** and other cancers.
3. Nonreceptor tyrosine kinases
   - e.g., Chromosomal translocations constitutively activate the nuclear tyrosine kinase **Abl** in **chronic myeloid leukemia** (p. 268).
4. G-proteins
   - **Gsp** and **Gip2** stimulatory and inhibitory α-subunit mutants are implicated in **pituitary adenoma** growth (p. 277).
5. Small GTP-binding proteins
   - e.g., Activating **Ras** mutations are found in many solid tumors, including **colorectal cancer**.

Transforming genes from tumor viruses and human malignancies may be derived from any part of the signal transduction pathway. More than one oncogene may require activation to transform a normal cell, however, and constitutive expression of an oncogene may only be possible following the acquisition of defects in cell cycle control.

The **Myc** family of transcription factors includes the immediate-early proto-oncogene products **c-Myc**, **L-Myc**, and **N-Myc**, any of which can trigger cell proliferation or cell death. Either gene may be amplified in human tumors: N-*Myc* amplification, which sensitizes normal cells to cell death, is characteristic of poor-prognosis **neuroblastomas**, a childhood tumor type that occasionally undergoes spontaneous (i.e., unexpected) regression. L-*Myc* amplification is likewise common in **small-cell lung cancer**, whereas c-*Myc* amplification (as well as fusion gene formation) occurs in **Burkitt lymphoma**. These tumors may escape normal cell death via Myc-dependent overexpression of the mitogenic **Id** protein Id2, which is a dominant negative antagonist of the cell cycle control protein pRb (see below).

MOLECULAR MINIREVIEW

Survival factors

Life is more than a matter of growth and death. At any one time many of your cells are not actively progressing through the cell cycle: such cells are either **differentiated** (postmitotic) or **surviving** (premitotic). Transcription is quiescent in survival-mode cells, even if chromatin structure remains in the open-and-ready position (see Figure 3.13). The partial withdrawal of growth factors can convert cells from growth to survival, whereas cell death may ensue from total withdrawal.

Surviving cells are thus precariously balanced between growth and death. Cells threatened with cell death may be rescued by **survival factors** such as epidermal growth factor (EGF) and insulin-like growth factor-1 (IGF1), which activate a survival pathway. These latter ligands activate receptor tyrosine kinases that can promote cell survival by heterodimerizing and transphosphorylating two large docking proteins: the kinase-inactive transmembrane receptor **ErbB3**, and the cytoplasmic metabolic intermediary **insulin receptor substrate-1** (**IRS1**), respectively. The common structural feature of these two proteins is a plethora of Y*XX*M amino acid motifs which, when tyrosine-phosphorylated, bind the SH2-containing lipid kinase phosphatidylinositol 3′-kinase (**PI3K**).

PI3K phosphorylates membrane PIP_2 to PIP_3, which in turn activates a phosphoinositide-dependent kinase (**PDK**) required for activation of protein kinase B (**PKB**, Akt). Activated PKB then phosphorylates and inactivates **glycogen synthase kinase-3**, leading to dissociation of **β-catenin** from the **APC** protein (p. 397). Nuclear translocation of β-catenin (and perhaps also of PKB) triggers formation of a transactivating complex with **TCF4** and consequent induction of survival genes. Note that this is but one of several survival pathways (Figure 15.8).

PI3K can also activate the PKC-MAP kinase signaling pathway, thus promoting cell growth as well as survival. Moreover, PI3K-dependent depletion of PIP_2 triggers activation of the membrane-ruffling protein **Rac**, thereby predisposing to tissue invasion. As a negative feedback mechanism, the lipid kinase activity of PI3K is inhibited by the lipid phosphatase **PTEN**.

CLINICAL KEYNOTE

PTEN and polyps

Certain molecules act by inhibiting oncogene action. Examples include GTPase-activating proteins such as **Ras-GAP**, which inhibits Ras activity, and the dual-specificity lipid phosphatase **PTEN** (phosphatase and tensin homolog deleted on chromosome **ten**) which functionally opposes:

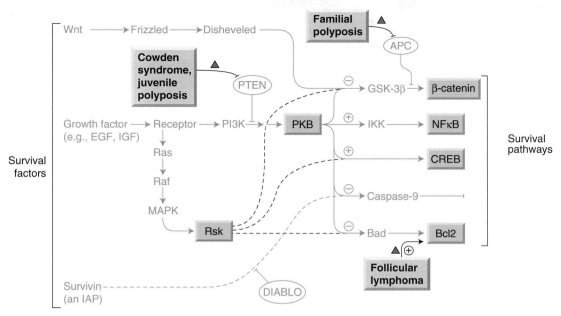

Figure 15.8 Signaling pathways favoring cell survival. Growth-factor-dependent activation of phosphatidylinositol 3'-kinase (PI3K) leads to increased PIP$_3$ levels which permit kinase (PDK1/2) activation of protein kinase B (PKB, Akt). PKB has several actions, including activation of p90^{Rsk} and subsequent protein synthesis; phosphorylation of glycogen synthase kinase-3β (GSK-3β), leading to dissociation of APC from β-catenin; phosphorylation of Bad, leading to its sequestration by 14-3-3 proteins and thus permitting Bcl2 action; and inactivation of caspase 9.

1. The survival-promoting lipid kinase **PI3K**.
2. Tyrosine kinases such as **Fak**.

In papillomavirus-induced **laryngeal papillomas**, PI3K-dependent activation of the survival kinase PKB is increased even though PTEN is overexpressed. This is reminiscent of the familial cancer disorder, **Cowden syndrome** – multiple intestinal hamartomas, as well as some thyroid and breast cancers – in which the lipid phosphatase activity of mutated PTEN is lost but the tyrosine phosphatase activity is retained. PTEN loss-of-function mutations may also occur in the premalignant syndrome of **juvenile polyposis**, as well as in sporadic glioblastoma, melanoma, and cancers of the kidney, uterus, breast and prostate.

The growth-suppressive activity of PTEN thus seems likely to reflect its ability to inactivate the PKB pathway via its effects on PIP$_3$ production, consistent with the abundance of phosphorylated PKB in thymic lymphomas from *PTEN* knockout mice. Note that expression of the checkpoint protein p27^{Kip1} is a prerequisite for PTEN-dependent G$_1$-phase growth arrest. PTEN-mediated Fak and PI3K inhibition is also associated with reduced focal adhesions and cell motility, suggesting a role for PTEN in regulating cell interactions with the extracellular matrix.

Tumor suppressor genes control cell cycle progression

The functionality of cell cycle control governs the maintenance and integrity of the genome. Cell cycle checkpoints have both short- and long-term roles:
1. Short-term: prevention of inappropriate cell cycle progression
   - i.e., Permitting DNA repair by arresting viable damaged cycling cells.
2. Long-term: maintenance of gene and chromosomal integrity
   - i.e., Ensuring genomic stability between cell generations.

Accordingly, loss of checkpoint control causes both uncontrolled cell growth and loss of genetic stability – an ideal recipe for tumor progression. For this reason genes encoding checkpoints are termed **tumor suppressors**, though not all tumor suppressor genes encode checkpoint proteins (the GAP family, for example). Activation of tumor suppressor genes by damaging stimuli may trigger cell death, thereby preventing the propagation of dangerous genetic errors, whereas loss-of-function mutations may disrupt the proofreading process with resultant tumor outgrowth. Consistent with this, proteins synthesized by DNA tumor viruses (e.g., **human papillomavirus**, **adenovirus**, and **Epstein–Barr virus**) may directly inhibit cell cycle control proteins.

The existence of tumor suppressor genes was first suggested by **somatic cell fusion** studies showing that the malignant phenotype is recessive – that is, that transfer of genetic material from normal cells can restore growth control to transformed cells. Examples of such genes – sometimes termed **recessive oncogenes** because it is necessary to lose both alleles for cell transformation – include:

1. The *Rb* retinoblastoma susceptibility gene
   - **Retinoblastoma** (bilateral if familial), **osteosarcoma**.
2. The *p53* cell cycle control gene
   - Numerous sporadic and familial cancers (pp. 375–6).
3. The *CDKN2A* (*p16 ^{INK4A}*) cell cycle control gene
   - **Melanoma, pancreatic cancer, mesothelioma, glioblastoma.**
4. The familial breast cancer susceptibility genes (*BRCA1, BRCA2*)
   - **Female breast cancer, ovarian cancer** (*BRCA1*).
   - **Breast cancer** (including male), **prostate cancer** (*BRCA2*).
5. Wilms tumor gene (*WT1, WT2*)
   - **Nephroblastoma** (Wilms tumor).
   - Associated also with **rhabdomyosarcoma** and **adrenal tumors** (p. 408).
6. The adenomatous polyposis coli (*APC*) gene
   - **Colorectal cancer; periampullary carcinomas, adrenal adenomas.**
   - **Brain tumors, osteomas, desmoids, gastroduodenal polyps.**

Many tumor suppressors can be characterized as either genomic **guardians** (also known as **caretakers**), which maintain genetic integrity and stability, or cell cycle **gatekeepers**, which regulate cell growth and death decisions (Table 15.1). In this model, the mutation of a guardian gene predisposes to additional downstream (gatekeeper) mutations. Guardian gene mutations thus tend to be found in tumors of affected kindreds, together with (say) p53 mutations. In contrast, sporadic (nonfamilial) tumors rarely contain guardian gene mutations, but may be full of gatekeeper mutations.

Most tumor suppressor genes have been isolated using labor-intensive positional cloning strategies (p. 570) based on rare cancer families harboring instructive chromosomal microdeletions: 13q14 for **familial retinoblastoma**, 17q13 for p53 (**Li-Fraumeni syndrome**), 11p13 for **Wilms tumor**, and 9q21 for p16 (**familial melanoma**). Chromosome 22 and the Y chromosome are noteworthy for the apparent absence of tumor suppressor genes and oncogenes.

Patterns of tumorigenesis in cancer families suggest a **two-hit** model of recessive oncogenesis. In this model, the germline mutation inactivating the protein represents the first hit, and a second (stochastic) somatic mutation affecting the remaining allele triggers tumor initiation. **Loss of heterozygosity** for marker DNA sequences (restriction fragment length polymorphisms; p. 536) close to the genomic region of interest may therefore be pathogenetically informative in this context, as also in sporadic carcinogenesis.

CLINICAL KEYNOTE

The phakomatoses

There are about a dozen rare autosomal dominant conditions that present as "spotty" neurocutaneous syndromes associated with tumors – often benign (hamartomas) but sometimes malignant. These syndromes, historically termed **phakomatoses**, mainly involve the skin, eye, kidney, and nervous system. All are due to an inherited loss-of-function mutation affecting a single gatekeeper-type tumor

Table 15.1. Tumor suppressors: guardians or gatekeepers?

Guardian (caretaker) gene	Guardian-preventable tumors	Gatekeeper gene	Gatekeeper-preventable tumors
BRCA1/2	Breast (ductal), ovarian	p53	Breast, sarcoma, glioma, adrenal, melanoma
MLH1, MSH2, MSH6, PMS1, PMS2	HNPCC: Colorectal, endometrial, ureteric, gastric, small-bowel carcinoma, hepatobiliary, ovarian, glioma	Rb	Retinoblastoma, osteosarcoma, bladder
		VHL	Renal cell (clear cell) carcinoma
ATM	Leukemia, lymphoma, breast	E-cadherin	Breast (lobular), gastric (diffuse)
DNA-PK	Lymphomas	APC	FAP: colorectal cancer (CRC)
XRCC	Squamous cell skin cancer		Gardner syndrome: CRC, osteomas, desmoid tumors
BLM	Leukemias		Turcot syndrome: CRC, brain tumors
		PTEN	Cowden syndrome: glioma, thyroid, head and neck cancers; Juvenile polyposis
		Smad4	Pancreatic cancer Colorectal cancer Juvenile polyps
		STK11	Gut hamartomas and adenocarcinomas
		PTCH	Basal cell carcinomas

Notes:
APC, adenomatous polyposis coli; ATM, ataxia-telangiectasia protein; FAP, familial adenomatous polyposis; HNPCC, hereditary nonpolyposis colorectal cancer; PTEN, phosphatase and tensin homolog deleted on chromosome ten.

suppressor gene. These latter genes tend to be very large, explaining the variable severity and manifestations of the clinical disorders unmasked by the second (somatic mutational) hit. The resultant phakomatoses include:

1. **Neurofibromatosis 1** and **2**
   - Due to mutations of *NF1* and *NF2* gene loci, respectively (p. 285).
2. **Tuberous sclerosis 1** and **2** (*TSC1* and *TSC2*; p. 286)
   - Due to mutations affecting **hamartin** and **tuberin**, respectively.
3. **Von Hippel–Lindau disease**
   - Due to mutations affecting the elongin-binding **VHL** protein (p. 100).
4. **Peutz–Jeghers syndrome**
   - Due to mutations affecting the *STK11* gene, which encodes a serine-threonine kinase (**LKB1**) with homologies to Rsk and PKA.
5. **Juvenile polyposis** and **Cowden syndrome**
   - Due to mutations affecting the **PTEN** lipid phosphatase.
6. **Gardner syndrome**
   - Due to mutations affecting the **APC** signaling regulator.
7. **Gorlin (nevoid basal cell carcinoma) syndrome**
   - Due to mutations affecting the **Patched** ion channel (p. 399).
8. **Multiple endocrine neoplasia type 1**
   - Due to mutations affecting the *MEN1* gene (p. 262).

Note that mutations of *NF1*, *PTEN*, *TSC2* and *VHL* all reduce expression of the **p27**^{Kip} cell cycle control protein, suggesting a common final pathway of tumor formation in these syndromes. This hypothesis is supported by homozygous *p27* knockout mice which develop adrenal and pituitary gland tumors.

BRCA proteins are sensors of DNA damage

Among the most famous of tumor suppressors are the breast (and ovarian) cancer susceptibility genes *BRCA1* (pron. "bracker-1") and *BRCA2*. Hundreds of different *BRCA1* and *BRCA2* mutations affect index families, indicating a high de novo mutation rate. Since the genes are large, many disease mutations can be suspected on the basis of a reduction in protein molecular weight (protein truncation testing; p. 553).

The 81-kb *BRCA1* gene locus on chromosome 17q21 comprises 24 exons, of which the largest (and most often mutated) is exon 11. The 7-kb *BRCA1* mRNA encodes a 220-kDa nuclear RING finger phosphoprotein (p. 138) which is expressed in a cycle-dependent manner and binds histone deacetylase, suggesting a role in local chromatin remodeling. The nuclear checkpoint kinase **Chk2** (pronounced "check-2"), the ataxia-telangiectasia protein **ATM** (p. 379), and another enzyme called **ATR** (ATM-Rad3-related kinase) phosphorylate BRCA1 in response to DNA damage, thereby triggering its translocation to subnuclear foci. Phosphorylated BRCA1 fixes double-strand DNA breaks by homologous recombination with the aid of radiation repair enzymes such as **Rad51** – a human homolog of the bacterial RecA protein – and also activates the p53-inducible cell cycle growth arrest genes *p21*^{Cip} and *GADD45* (see below). Mutational inactivation of *BRCA1* is usually associated with destabilizing *p53* mutations which arise secondary to defective BRCA1-dependent transcription-coupled DNA repair.

The very large 3418-amino-acid (384-kDa) **BRCA2** protein is encoded by a 27-exon gene at 13q12-13, and the 12-kb mRNA is expressed in thymus, testis, ovary, and mammary epithelium. Although in structural terms BRCA2 exhibits little homology to other known proteins, it resembles BRCA1 in functional terms, being highly expressed in dividing cells (particularly at the G_1/S cell cycle checkpoint) and interacting with Rad51. The two BRCA proteins thus cooperate in homologous recombination, perhaps regulating meiotic sister chromatid interactions and/or transcription-coupled repair.

Unlike most other tumor suppressor genes, *BRCA* gene mutations are not characteristic of sporadic breast tumors. This supports the impression that such mutations play an early (guardian or caretaker) role in breast cancer predisposition rather than being part of a final (gatekeeper; Table 15.1) common pathway. Moreover, it is consistent with the failure of *BRCA* gene re-expression to abolish the transformed phenotype of *BRCA*-null tumor cells, which usually have accumulated other mutations such as those affecting *p53*. The BRCA1 and estrogen receptor (ER) proteins are also functionally related: estrogens activate *BRCA1*, which in turn blocks the ER-dependent signaling required for mammary cell proliferation, and *BRCA1*-mutant tumors are typically ER-negative.

CLINICAL KEYNOTE

Hereditary breast cancer

Genetic susceptibility accounts for about 5% of all breast cancer. Approximately 3% of breast cancer patients younger than 40 will have a germline *BRCA1* mutant allele, as will up to 15% of such patients with high-risk family histories. Inheritance of one of these rare but highly penetrant mutant alleles increases the lifetime risk of breast cancer by about 20-fold. Moreover, such mutations account for about 50% of all breast cancer families and about 80% of families with both breast and ovarian cancer. Heterogeneous loss-of-function *BRCA1* mutations have a population frequency of 1 in 800, except amongst Icelanders and Ashkenazi Jews (in whom the 185delAG mutation affects 1 in 100). Interestingly, Ashkenazis have a similar incidence of *BRCA2* – 6174delT – mutations. Unlike *BRCA1*, *BRCA2* is not linked to **ovarian cancer**, but loss-of-function mutations predispose more strongly to **male breast cancer** and **prostate cancer** as well as to female breast cancer.

Cancers accumulate dozens of genetic errors

Common cancers are common because they involve the progressive acquisition of common genetic effects. Lung cancers, for example, have been found on average to contain 20–25 tumor suppressor gene defects. Hence, the clinical distinction between cancers behaving as "tigers" or "pussycats" may relate in part to the number of accumulated growth-control defects. The polyp-cancer sequence of colorectal cancer provides an illustrative model of multi-stage carcinogenesis. Adenomas (5% risk of malignancy) and sporadic colorectal cancers often contain *APC* gene truncations; consistent with a gatekeeper role for *apc* in growth control, overexpression leads to G_1–S arrest. However, many other genetic changes are implicated in sporadic colon tumors (Figure 15.9), including:

1. Genomic hypomethylation.
2. Point mutational activation of the proto-oncogene K-*Ras*.
3. Tumor suppressor gene loss:
   • *p53* and/or *Smad4*.

Note that colorectal cancers only occur in homozygous *p53* knockout mice in the presence of intestinal microflora, suggesting a contributory role for bacteria in colorectal carcinogenesis.

The **DCC** (**d**eleted in **c**olon **c**ancer) gene product is a member of the immunoglobulin superfamily that acts as a receptor for a family of neuronal guidance proteins termed **netrins**, which are related to extracellular matrix laminin proteins. Although the absence of DCC expression in stage II or III colorectal cancers correlates with a poorer survival outcome, no pathogenetic relationship of DCC to colorectal tumorigenesis is proven. Moreover, transgenic knockout of *DCC* fails to cause tumors, and DCC can induce cell death in vitro. The *DCC* gene is located close to the *Smad4* gene, suggesting that co-deletion of *Smad4* may underlie the association of *DCC* deletion with prognostic disadvantage.

CLINICAL KEYNOTE

Gatekeepers and guardians in hereditary colonic neoplasms

Colorectal cancer is the commonest malignancy of Western nonsmokers (though 20% of its incidence is now attributed to smoking). Inherited predispositions to colorectal cancer include:

1. *APC* gene mutations
   • **Familial adenomatous polyposis coli** (**FAP**; 95% cancer risk).
   • A disorder of cell growth and death control (gatekeeper defect).
   • Presents with numerous benign polyps, each of which is prone to malignant degeneration.

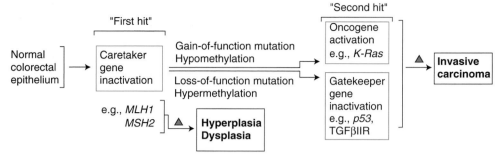

Figure 15.9 Guardian-and-gatekeeper model of colorectal carcinogenesis in HNPCC.

- Also associated with gastroduodenal polyps (premalignant) and benign retinal, skin, and bone anomalies.
- The APC protein defect permits cytoplasmic β-catenin to translocate freely to the nucleus.

2. Mismatch repair (especially **MLH1, MSH**) gene mutations (Figure 15.9)
- **Hereditary nonpolyposis colorectal cancer** (**HNPCC**; 70% cancer risk).
- A disorder of genetic stability (guardian defect).
- The responsible gene product (usually MLH1) repairs base mismatches, i.e., it acts like a computer spellcheck program.
- Tends not to present with florid polyposis like FAP, but rather with colonic (especially ascending colon, or multiple) and extracolonic (endometrial, ovarian, ureteric, or other gastrointestinal) carcinomas.
- Mismatch repair gene mutations affect about 1:200 individuals, and account for about 1% of all colorectal cancer.

3. Mutations affecting either **Smad4** or **PTEN** gatekeeper genes
- Give rise to hamartomatous **juvenile polyposis** (15% cancer risk).

A mutant pocket protein predisposes to retinoblastoma

Many proteins are involved in cell cycle regulation in addition to the cyclins and Cdks. Some of these are DNA-binding phosphoproteins that not only modulate cell cycle traverse but also prevent uncontrolled (neoplastic) growth. These growth-regulatory proteins include the Cdk4-binding protein p16^{INK4}, the DNA damage-inducible transactivator p53, and the **retinoblastoma (Rb) susceptibility** gene product.

The latter – also referred to as the **retinoblastoma protein** or **pRb** – is a 105-110 kDa nuclear phosphoprotein that is expressed throughout the normal cell cycle. pRb is a **master brake** protein which controls cell activation events within G$_1$ (particularly at the G$_1$–S transition) by sequestering transcription factors of the **E2F** family. Serine phosphorylation events regulate pRb function (Figure 15.10):

1. **Hypophosphorylated pRb** (p105)
- Detected in G$_0$/early G$_1$.
- Binds (and thus prevents DNA binding) of E2F.
2. **Hyperphosphorylated pRb** (p110)
- Releases E2F.
- Permits G$_1$–S transition.
- Detected in S, G$_2$ and M.

Figure 15.10 Modulation of pRb function by phosphorylation and dephosphorylation. The inhibitory pRb/E2F complex dissociates following pRb phosphorylation by Cdk4 (and later Cdk2), leading to E2F-dependent gene expression, ongoing DNA synthesis, and cell cycle progression.

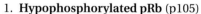
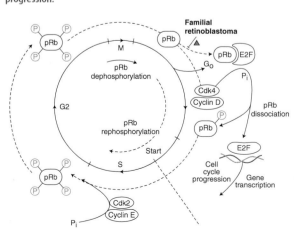

Rb phosphorylation by Cdk1 occurs from mid-G$_1$ onwards. Regulation of growth-suppressive transcriptional events by hypophosphorylated pRb, on the other hand, involves the formation of inhibitory complexes with E2F. Like its homologs pRb2^{p130} and Wee1^{p107} (p. 361), pRb is a **pocket protein** that binds E2F and converts it from a transactivator to a silencer. This process occurs via masking of the E2F transactivation domain by the pRb pocket, and also through Rb-dependent recruitment of a **histone deacetylase** (**HDAC1**) to the E2F/Rb-containing transcription complex, leading to local chromatin condensation (Figure 15.4). Conversely, the transforming human papillomavirus (HPV) E7 protein displaces HDAC1 from the pRb pocket, thus promoting cell growth.

Formation of the inhibitory pRb/E2F complex is antagonized by cyclin E/Cdk2-dependent pRb phosphorylation which causes complex dissociation (Figure 15.10). Conversely, E2F overexpression drives arrested cells into S-phase, mimicking the transforming effects of viral oncogenes. Cells lacking functional pRb may thus inappropriately activate E2F-responsive genes – namely, **cyclin E, thymidine kinase, thymidine synthase, DNA polymerase-α** and **dihydrofolate reductase** – and enter S-phase. Dysregulation of this type can also lead to cell death and, thus, to selection for additional mutagenic events that permit tumor formation.

The growth-controlling cytokine **transforming growth factor beta** (**TGFβ**) upregulates p27^{Kip1} expression, preventing activation of the cyclin D-Cdk4 complex. This leads to the persistence of hypophosphorylated pRb with consequent G$_1$ arrest. A similar antiproliferative mechanism is seen with other growth-inhibitory cytokines such as **interferon-α**. Overexpression of Cdk4 renders cells resistant to growth arrest by TGFβ, on the other hand, promoting tumor formation. TGFβ also stimulates recruitment of HDAC1 by pRb2^{p130}.

Figure 15.11 Retinoblastoma – an unusually advanced case (Wellcome Medical Photographic Library, N0011054C).

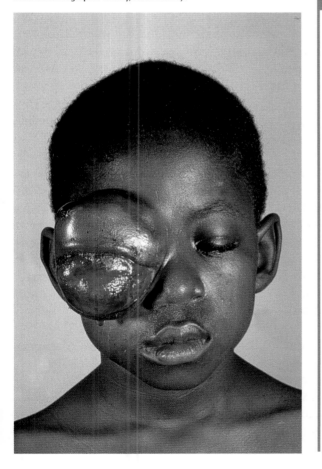

MOLECULAR MINIREVIEW

Rb and tumor suppression

The pRb pocket is bound by several DNA tumor virus transforming proteins, including:

1. **Human papillomavirus** (p. 376) **E7** protein.
2. **Adenovirus E1A** proteins.
3. **SV40 large T antigen**.
4. **Epstein–Barr virus** (p. 385) **EBNA-5** protein.

The transforming ability of these viral oncoproteins can be destroyed by mutating their pRb binding domains, indicating that their mode of action involves sequestering pRb. Hence, these viruses can mimic the oncogenic effects of Rb null (homozygous) mutations, disrupting complexes of pRb with human D-type cyclins and (thus) constitutively activating G$_1$ transit.

Germline Rb mutations cause a syndrome of **hereditary retinoblastoma** in which tumors of the retina occur bilaterally (Figure 15.11). In addition, ectopic intracranial retinoblastomas (**pineoblastomas**) occur in about 10%, whereas other tumors including **osteosarcoma** also occur at increased frequency. In contrast, mice with these mutations develop only pituitary tumors. Why should defects in a general cell cycle control protein yield such organ-specific neoplasms? The answer may lie in different tissue-specific cell development programs. For example, the developing retinal cell (retinoblast) contains no pRb, whereas mature retinocytes express abundant pRb – suggesting that a null mutation of Rb may preferentially disrupt growth regulation in mature retinal cells. Compare this with the situation in colonic cells: like retinal cells, migrating colonic cells express little pRb at the base of the intestinal crypt but a lot at the tip of the villus; unlike retinal cells, however, colonic cells are rapidly sloughed into the intestinal lumen, making colonic Rb mutations relatively benign in this context.

Many human tumor types acquire Rb mutations by somatic mutation. This

A.

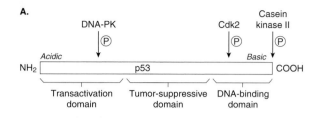

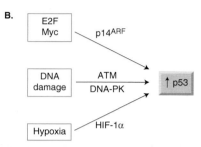

Figure 15.12 Structure and function of the p53 gene product. *A,* The amino-terminal transactivation region contains many serine phosphorylation sites, some of which are phosphorylated by DNA-PK in response to damage-dependent strand-breaks. The basic carboxy-terminal region contains the DNA-binding region, and target serine residues for casein kinase II and Cdk2. *B,* Trans-activation by tetramerized p53 is stimulated by a variety of exposures, including DNA damage, hypoxia, and the pRb-E2F-p14^{ARF} pathway. Note, however, that p53 protein levels may also be increased by loss-of-function mutations which impair its normal cytoplasmic degradation (see text). ATM, ataxia-telangiectasia protein; HIF, hypoxia-inducible factors.

secondary genetic change provides a further growth advantage for subclone selection in genetically unstable tumor cell populations. Indeed, mutation or methylation of either Rb, cyclin D1 or p16^{INK4A} may be a prerequisite for human tumorigenesis.

Of note, **SV40-like DNA** has been identified in human **osteosarcomas**. Since up to 30% of Salk polio vaccine batches may have been contaminated with SV40 virus, it is not quite inconceivable that viral inhibition of pRb function could contribute to the pathogenesis of some of these tumors.

DNA damage induces p53 expression and G₁–S arrest

A central molecule underlying human tumorigenesis is the multidomain 53-kDa transactivating phosphoprotein **p53** (Figure 15.12*A*). Like its cell cycle cousin pRb, p53 suppresses tumor cell growth in gatekeeper style by providing a molecular "passport control" for the G₁–S checkpoint. Hence, transit is normally denied if DNA damage, hypoxia, or pRb signaling defects are detected (Figure 15.12*B*). Wild-type p53 shares many other behavioral characteristics with pRb: it co-localizes to intranuclear DNA replication sites, is selectively phosphorylated on serine residues, and is inhibited by the viral oncoprotein SV40 large T antigen (via a different binding site to that which binds pRb).

The p53 homologs **p63** and **p73** may mimic the pro-apoptotic effects of p53. However, truncated p73 variants may also inhibit p53-dependent apoptosis in developing cells, perhaps by forming p53 heterotetramers. Note that the mitogenic transcription factor E2F can induce apoptosis in the presence of p73, creating a p73-dependent decision fork for cell growth and death.

Unlike pRb, p53 does not interact with the transforming proteins adenovirus E1A or HPV E7, but rather with **adenovirus E1B** and **HPV E6**. Cell transformation by E1B and E6 mimics that seen in cells expressing mutant p53 molecules that exert a dominant negative influence over wild-type protein. Relevant to this, it was the characterization of a point-mutated dominant negative *p53* gene which led early investigators to believe that p53 was an oncogene rather than a tumor suppressor.

Induction of wild-type p53 by DNA damage is followed by palindromic DNA binding (GGACATGTCC . . .) leading to the expression of p53-responsive proteins, including:

1. **HDM2**
   - Encoded by the so-called **h**uman **d**ouble **m**inute gene (named after the murine homolog MDM2 that was found in extrachromosomal DNA) which is amplified in 30% of human **sarcomas**.
   - Is a 90-kDa RING finger protein which complexes with p53 (and also with E2F), promoting rapid ubiquitin-dependent p53 degradation and thus permitting G₁/S traverse without apoptosis.
   - Negatively feeds back on p53 transactivation (i.e., it is an oncogene).
   - Is antagonized by p14^{ARF} binding to the complex (see below) which opposes the p53-degradative of HDM2.

2. **p21**^{Cip1}
   - **C**dk-**i**nteracting **p**rotein (also known as WAF-1, **w**ild-type p53-**a**ctivated **f**ragment; SDI-1, **s**enescence cell-**d**erived **i**nhibitor, and PIC-1, **p**53-regulated **i**nhibitor of **C**dks).
   - Decides whether a cell divides or differentiates.
   - Inhibits Cdk2, thus halting cell cycle progression and giving the damaged cell an opportunity to repair prior to S-phase (Figure 15.13).
   - May exert anti-tumor activity similar to that of p53 itself.

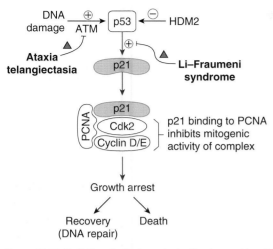

Figure 15.13 Mediation of p53-dependent cell cycle arrest by p21. Following DNA damage induction and DNA-PK activation, p53 binds to DNA and transactivates p21, leading to Cdk2 inhibition. HDM2 antagonizes this p53-initiated pathway. PCNA, proliferating cell nuclear antigen.

Many proteins other than HDM2 bind p53, including **WT1** (the **Wilms tumor** suppressor), **EBNA5** (EB virus nuclear antigen 5), the **LANA** protein of **Kaposi sarcoma** herpesvirus, Hsp70 and the general transcription factor **Sp1**. Binding of TATA-binding protein (p. 86) by p53 causes the transcription complex to arrest, which may in turn contribute to p53-dependent growth arrest.

Binding of p53 to the promoter of p21^{Cip1} requires initial dephosphorylation of Ser[376], permitting the binding of 14-3-3 transcriptional co-factors (p. 266) and thus allowing p53 tetramerization. This pathway may be defective in some human **melanomas** which, despite expressing wild-type p53, exhibit resistance to the cell-killing effects of radiation and drugs due to impaired damage-inducible Ser[376] dephosphorylation. Together with another damage-inducible p53-dependent protein, **GADD45**, p21^{Cip1} halts G_1/S cell cycle progression by interacting with the DNA-replicating protein **PCNA** (proliferating cell nuclear antigen; Figure 15.13). De novo *p21* mutations on 6p21.2 may occur in **prostate cancer**, but do not otherwise appear common.

MOLECULAR MINIREVIEW

p53 overexpression or p53 mutation?
Increased nuclear p53 levels accompany the exposure of cells to DNA-damaging agents such as X-rays and ultraviolet light. This stabilization comes about because HDM2 is released following p53 phosphorylation by ATM, Chk2 and DNA-PK at the amino-terminal Ser[15], Ser[20] and Ser[37] sites respectively (Jnk may also phosphorylate these residues). Moreover, phosphorylation at these sites masks the p53 nuclear export signal, thereby preventing p53 cytoplasmic degradation and prolonging its half-life from less than 30 minutes to over 3 hours. Such p53 stabilization causes G_1-phase prolongation, allowing the cell to repair genomic damage prior to DNA synthesis. Tumor overexpression of immunoreactive p53 is often, but not always, associated with an underlying p53 mutation which prolongs the molecule's half-life.

Stabilization of p53 by hypoxia, another common trigger of p53 upregulation, is mediated by the direct binding of **hypoxia-inducible factor-1α** (**HIF-1α**). This interaction may cause apoptosis or, in tumors, induce erythropoiesis and angiogenesis. Insults such as hypoxia can also downregulate *HDM2* expression and thereby induce p53 accumulation.

CLINICAL KEYNOTE

Germline p53 mutations and cancer
Damaged DNA that is permitted to replicate despite the presence of a checkpoint – as in the chromosomal fragility syndrome ataxia telangiectasia in which ionizing radiation fails to induce cell cycle delay (see below) – predisposes to mutations and, thus, malignancy. Approximately half of all human tumors (including breast, lung, gastrointestinal, mesenchymal, and hemopoietic neoplasms) contain somatic mutations in p53. Such mutations promote tumor progression by permitting the replication of damaged DNA (thereby enhancing growth; Figure 15.14) and by increasing genomic instability (thus accelerating the selection of growth-advantaged clones). p53 function may be lost in human tumors via a variety of mechanisms, including:

1. Heterologous molecular derangements, e.g.:
   - *HDM2* amplification.
   - HPV E6 expression.
   - p14^{ARF} deletion.
   - *Chk2* mutation.
2. Loss-of-function *p53* gene mutations, e.g.:
   - DNA-binding domain (prevent transactivation).
   - Tetramerization domain.

As with pRb, germline *p53* mutations (**Li–Fraumeni syndrome**) predispose to a relatively small number of tumor types: **breast cancer** (in 25%), **brain tumors** (10–15%), **soft-tissue sarcomas** (10–15%), **osteosarcomas** (5–10%), **leukemias** (5–10%), and **adrenocortical carcinomas** (~1%). This selectivity may relate to tissue-specific requirements for the antimutagenic proofreading function of p53. Transgenic mice

Figure 15.14 The molecular biology of cancer progression: effects on the balance between cell growth, survival, differentiation, and death. In this model, neoplastic cell selection occurs via a variable sequence of cell cycle checkpoint loss (favoring selection by increased growth) and signal amplification (causing selection by cell death). EGFR, epidermal growth factor receptor; HDAC, histone deacetylase; TGF, transforming growth factor.

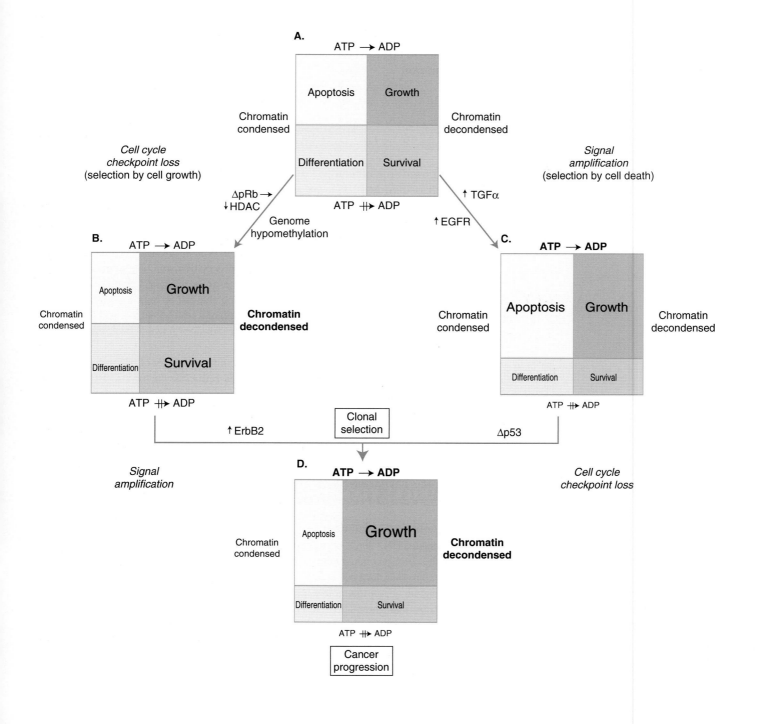

in which both p53 alleles have been disrupted are also unusually prone to neoplasms in early life. Germline mutations affecting the p53 kinase Chk2 may be responsible for occasional cases of Li–Fraumeni syndrome in which p53 is not mutated. Polymorphisms affecting the *p53* gene at codon 72 of exon 4 are frequent, leading to either arginine-containing (CGC) or proline-containing (CCC) forms: Arg/Arg homozygotes have been reported to be more susceptible to **cervix cancer** than are heterozygotes, whereas Pro/Pro homozygotes may be more susceptible to certain varieties of **lung cancer** and **bladder cancer**.

Loss of p53 function causes genetic instability

Wild-type p53 prevents damaged DNA from attempting replication. This failsafe mechanism for preventing the cell cycle progression of genetically damaged cells involves an interplay between the p53 and pRb systems. Deregulation of E2F-dependent gene induction – due, for example, to *Rb* allelic loss or oncogene activation – induces expression of the Cdk4 inhibitor p14^{ARF} which then binds and stabilizes the HDM2–p53 complex, preventing p53 degradation. This link between the Rb–E2F system and the p14^{ARF}–p53 system provides a set of controls for growth arrest and apoptosis in the event of a single pre-p53 mutation, ensuring that at least two critical mutations are needed to destabilize the replicating genome. If the Rb-E2F-p14^{ARF} pathway is dysregulated, the vast majority of cells expressing p53 mutations will fail to heed the G$_1$/S cell cycle checkpoint. For this reason p14^{ARF} gene therapy has been used experimentally to arrest growth of the asbestos-related malignancy **mesothelioma**.

In a damage-prone environment, mutant p53 acts like a corrupt genomic traffic cop who offers illicit S-phase passage to unrepaired DNA. Premature crossing of the G$_1$/S checkpoint due to p53 mutations increases tumor cell replicative errors and thus promotes genetic instability. This culminates in the characteristic genetic stigmata of tumors: **gene amplification** and **aneuploidy**. The term aneuploidy indicates that the average cellular DNA content of the tumor no longer matches that of normal somatic cells – consistent with abnormal cell cycle checkpoint control and/or mitotic chromosomal disjunction. Aneuploidy is thus also associated with abnormalities of chromosome number and morphology, and may be used to predict the risk of cancer in premalignant conditions such as oral **leukoplakia**.

Somatic mutations of *p53* are detectable in about 50% of adult human tumors, but affect up to 90% of some cancer types. These mutations mainly affect exons 3–5 encoding the DNA-binding region of p53, and contribute to disease progression (via genetic instability) and drug resistance. Tumors select for specific patterns of *p53* mutation, with codons 175, 248 and 273 being most often affected. Since each one of these hotspots centers on a CpG dinucleotide – and since the usual mutations at these sites are GC→AT transitions – methylation-dependent deamination seems the most likely mechanism of mutation (p. 58). Ultraviolet light induces characteristic C→T transversions affecting *p53* codon 248 in sunburnt skin, for example, whereas the liver carcinogen **aflatoxin** causes **hepatocellular carcinomas** distinguished by codon 249 (GC→TA transversion, Arg→Ser) mutations. **Benzpyrene** (a cigarette smoke carcinogen) also leaves a recognizable mutational footprint in **small-cell lung cancers**, which contain a high frequency of p53 GC→TA transversions. Tumors lacking *p53* mutations may nonetheless be defective in p53-dependent signaling because of either loss-of-function mutations affecting p14^{ARF} or the amplification of *HDM2* (Figure 15.15).

In summary, many functional p53 defects contribute to human cancer

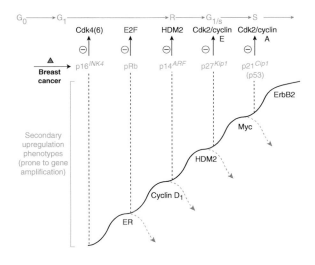

Figure 15.15 Model of breast cancer progression due to sequential selection for cell cycle null mutations. Compensatory overexpression and/or amplification of growth-promoting genes may be permitted by the progressive accumulation of null mutants, with the pattern changing depending upon the order and severity of checkpoint loss.

development. These include prevention of p53 tetramerization by carboxy-terminal domain deletions; the failure of p53-dependent transactivation due to mutations of the DNA-binding domain; mutational loss of the p53 nuclear localization signal, leading to its cytoplasmic sequestration (e.g., in **neuroblastomas**); deletion of the *p14^{ARF}* gene, leading to excessive HDM2-dependent p53 degradation (in tumors without *p53* mutations); *HDM2* amplification; and infection with oncogenic viruses that synthesize p53-inactivating proteins.

CLINICAL KEYNOTE

Human papillomavirus (HPV)

As noted above, two HPV gene products are custom-made to inhibit human tumor suppressor gene function and thus to promote the survival and proliferation of infected cells:

1. The **E7** protein of HPV binds the pRb pocket, inactivating pRb (and p21^{Cip}/p27^{Kip}) while activating cyclins E and A.
2. The **E6** protein of HPV triggers p53 degradation – suppressing p16^{INK4A} expression, inhibiting apoptosis, activating telomerase, and destabilizing chromosomes.

Immortalization of infected cells requires not only E6 and/or E7, however, but also additional genetic events such as the p14^{ARF} (*CDKN2*) or *FHIT* (*fragile histidine triad*; p. 67) mutations. Relevant to this, HPV expresses an **E5** protein which complexes with cell-surface receptors for EGF, PDGF or M-CSF, and which suppresses p21^{Cip} function. Note, however, that E5 is not consistently expressed in HPV-transformed cells. Since **genital warts** caused by HPV6 or HPV11 do not express E6 or E7, such lesions are not prone to cancer development.

Certain HPV serotypes – especially 16, but also 18, 69, and some others – predispose to **squamous cell carcinomas** of the cervix (and other anogenital tissues: penis, vulva, anus) via p53 inactivation. Up to 25% of squamous cell cancers of the head and neck are also HPV16-positive: only 10% of these tumors harbor *p53* mutations (compared with two-thirds of HPV-negative tumors), consistent with E6 expression sufficing for p53 inhibition. Of note, these HPV-induced cancers (which often continue to express wild-type p53) have a better prognosis than common cigarette-and-alcohol-induced head and neck cancers, perhaps indicating a smaller number of pathogenetic steps and hence greater genetic stability. Interestingly, whereas HPV-16 is associated with the induction of squamous cell carcinomas (often well-differentiated), HPV-18 is also linked to the occurrence of **adenocarcinomas** in the cervix and elsewhere.

PHARMACOLOGIC FOOTNOTE

p53 mutations and tumor chemosensitivity

Malignancies such as **germ cell tumors** (e.g., testicular teratomas) rarely contain *p53* mutations, and are characterized by exquisite chemosensitivity and curability even when widespread. Similarly, cell lines displaying hormone-sensitivity (such as the ER-positive human breast cancer cell line, MCF7) are usually characterized by a wild-type *p53* gene, consistent with their ability to stop growing following exposure to a hormone antagonist. In contrast, breast cancer cells overexpressing **ErbB2** are usually characterized by *p53* mutations and relative chemoresistance. Hence, human breast tumor progression could occur via a form of punctuated evolution involving: (1) sequential loss of cell cycle checkpoints accompanied by increased resistance to cell death, permitting (2) the upregulation of oncogene product activity, leading to (3) compensatory overexpression of cell cycle control proteins, duly complicated by (4) selection for further cell cycle control gene mutations (see Figure 15.15).

Inactivation of p53 is associated with induction of the **Mdr** multidrug efflux pump which contributes to chemoresistance. Cytotoxic drugs may promote the selection of resistant tumor cell subclones, thus accelerating tumor progression. An illustrative example is that of **cisplatin** drug treatment, which efficiently selects for methylation or allelic loss of the *MLH1* mismatch repair gene. Taxane cytotoxic drugs (**paclitaxel, docetaxel**) appear to act via a p53-independent pathway, and may thus remain active in malignancies with *p53* mutations.

Cellular radioresistance is also linked to p53 status in many experimental systems, but the relationship appears complex. Full sequencing of the *p53* genotype is a good (albeit labor-intensive) predictor of tumor response to both cytotoxic and radiation therapy.

Apoptosis and ageing

Genetically damaged cells undergo repair or apoptosis

With the exception of the immune response, cell proliferation and differentiation tend to be inversely related. Numerous constraints govern cell growth, and cells that violate these constraints undergo one of two catastrophic outcomes (Figure 15.16):

1. Programmed cell death
    • **Apoptosis**.
2. Cell transformation and tumorigenesis
    • **Neoplasia**.

Damaged cells or tissues may undergo **necrosis** – a mode of cell death that occurs via swelling and bursting of the cytoplasmic contents into the extracellular space, often giving rise to an inflammatory response. Genetically damaged cells, on the other hand, either temporarily arrest growth (the repair/survival track) or die in a noninflammatory process of shrinkage and fragmentation (the apoptosis track). Unlike necrosis, apoptosis is an energy-dependent process of self-immolation that lasts approximately 30 minutes. Illustrative examples of normal apoptosis include:

1. Embryonic sculpting of body shape (e.g., the formation of digits; p. 391).

Figure 15.16 Potential consequences of DNA damage, including cancer and (cell) death.

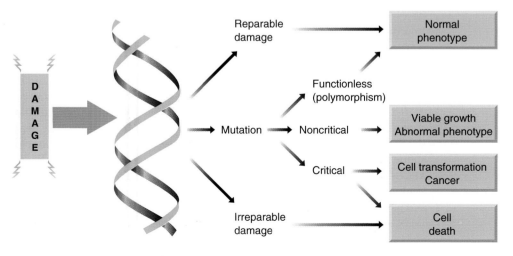
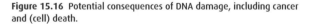

2. Autoreactive thymocyte deletion during acquisition of tolerance (p. 485).
3. Synapse formation in the central nervous system during development.
4. Organ involution in response to hormonal flux, for example:
   - Menstrual or post-partum uterine epithelial sloughing.
   - Breast involution following full-term pregnancy.
5. Hair follicle regression (**catagen**) in the outer root sheath, which follows active regeneration of the proliferating hair follicle (**anagen**) and precedes resting of the follicle (**telogen**) prior to stem cell reactivation.
6. Turnover of colorectal epithelial cells as they migrate from the (proliferative) base of the intestinal crypt to the (apoptotic) top.

Transgenic knockout of *p53* may be associated with secondary upregulation of growth factor receptors (such as the IGF1 receptor and ErbB2). This illustrates how apoptosis suppression enhances survival in preneoplastic states. Conversely, the growth-inhibitory effect of transforming growth factor β (TGFβ) in epithelial cells may depend upon the presence of wild-type p53.

Growth factors are only one input into cell cycle control, however. Extracellular matrix proteins also signal to the nucleus via the integrin-Fak pathway, creating a requirement for cell adhesion to sustain growth. Indeed, the growth of most human cell types depends on anchorage; basically, this means that cells like to have a good stretch. Cell anchorage to a substratum activates integrins, inducing the phosphorylation of pRb and p107, permitting accumulation of cyclin A, and thus driving progression through the cell cycle. Cyclin A overexpression eliminates anchorage dependence and allows cells to proliferate without the usual control signals provided by neighboring cells. Conversely, cell detachment from the substratum leads to loss of integrin signaling, failure of cyclin A accumulation, and cell death.

In epithelial, endothelial and muscle cells, loss of adhesion to extracellular matrix initiates the membrane damage→ceramide→Jnk signaling pathway, resulting in cell death which in this context is termed **anoikis** (Gr. "homelessness"). Anoikis plays a role in embryonic development, breast involution, and in the prevention of cancer cell metastasis. Overexpression of adhesion molecules such as carcinoembryonic antigen (p. 211) inhibits normal anoikis, on the other hand, thereby promoting malignant transformation.

MOLECULAR MINIREVIEW

DNA-PK

How do cells sense and respond to DNA damage? A key molecule in this process is **DNA-dependent protein kinase** (DNA-PK), a member of the PI3K superfamily. DNA-PK requires binding to the free ends of double-strand DNA breaks for its activation. Two functional subunits contribute to the structure of DNA-PK: a 350-kDa catalytic domain, and the DNA-binding **Ku** domain, which in turn consists of 70- and 80-kDa heterodimeric proteins (Ku is an autoimmune antigen in other contexts; p. 71). Activation of DNA-PK by the stress-inducible transactivator **heat-shock factor** and/or by the nuclear tyrosine kinase **Abl**, combined with double-strand break binding of Ku, stimulates the DNA-PK homologs **DNA ligase IV** and **XRCC4** (mutated in **xeroderma pigmentosum**). This leads to nonhomologous end-joining of DNA free ends and phosphorylation of transcription factors such as Jun and p53.

DNA-PK is mutated in one variety of **severe combined immunodeficiency** (**SCID**), and DNA-PK mutations can predispose to **lymphoma** development. Another PI3K-like protein involved in the response to DNA damage is that encoded by the *ATM* gene which is mutated in ataxia telangiectasia.

ATM is needed for p53-dependent growth arrest

The *ATM* (ataxia telangiectosia mutated) gene on 11q22 encodes a massive 12kb transcript and a DNA damage-inducible 370-kDa protein kinase which, like DNA-PK, is a member of a PI3K subfamily involved in DNA repair, cell cycle control, meiotic recombination, and telomere length monitoring. Approximately 2% of the human population are *ATM* heterozygotes, and most mutations are truncations or point mutations (of which more than 50 are described). However, the gene is extremely large, and mutations may not be detected in up to 20% of clinical ataxia telangiectasia (AT) presentations.

Ionizing radiation (in addition to other noxious stimuli, e.g., the radiomimetic drug bleomycin) activates ATM, causing it to phosphorylate the p53 kinase **Chk2** which in turn phosphorylates p53 on Ser[15] while also triggering Cdc25A degradation (via serine 123 phosphorylation) and, thus, Cdk2 inhibition. In AT homozygotes irradiation causes subnormal activation and stabilization of p53, manifesting as a failure of G_1/S cell cycle arrest and reduced p53 accumulation respectively. In contrast, DNA-PK phosphorylates p53 on Ser[15] and Ser[37], thus preventing HDM2 interaction and stabilizing p53. Nonetheless, cells with DNA-PK deficiency exhibit a normal response to irradiation in terms of arrest and p53 accumulation.

The initial (rapid) phase of radiation repair proceeds normally in AT cells but fails to be completed, leaving unrepaired double-strand breaks. This repair defect persists in noncycling cells, which remain hypersensitive to radiation damage (as defined by residual damage burden) even while appearing damage-insensitive as defined by their failure to undergo normal p53-dependent arrest or apoptosis.

In addition to p53, ATM normally activates the nuclear tyrosine kinase **Abl** – which uses its SH3 domain to bind ATM – in response to radiation damage, leading in turn to Abl-dependent p53 stabilization. The tumor suppressor protein **BRCA1** is another ATM phosphorylation target, as is the germline homozygous **Nijmegen break syndrome** double-strand break repair protein **Nbs1**.

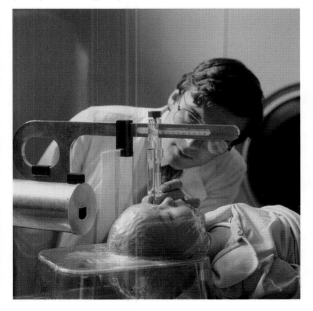

Figure 15.17 Killing of cancer cells by radiotherapy (Wellcome Medical Photographic Library, no. N0017118C). Both normal cells and cancer cells will die from radiation-induced strand-breaks; hence, the dose to normal tissue is minimized by shielding and field placement. Cells from patients with ataxia telangiectasia fail to undergo cell cycle arrest due to radiogenic strand-breakage, leading to a high mutation and (hence) second malignancy rate.

CLINICAL KEYNOTE

Ataxia telangiectasia

Ataxia telangiectasia (AT) is an autosomal recessive disorder manifesting with ataxia, telangiectasia, and a variety of additional features including immune deficiency and predisposition to certain cancers – particularly **lymphoma, leukemia** (T cell acute lymphoblastic leukemia in children, T cell prolymphocytic leukemia or B cell chronic lymphocytic leukemia in adults) and **breast cancer**. A striking feature of the disease is hypersensitivity to ionizing radiation (Figure 15.17), which is associated with both the failure of damaged cells to undergo cell cycle arrest – particularly at the p53-dependent G_1/S checkpoint (but also at G_2/M) – and resistance to apoptosis. Premature ageing and neuronal degeneration are presumed to result from this failure of DNA repair surveillance. AT cells in vitro are short-lived,

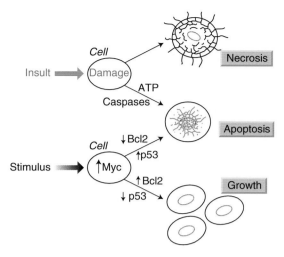

Figure 15.18 Role of Bcl2 in determining cellular outcomes: high Bcl2 levels permit cell growth, whereas Bcl2 repression permits p53-dependent growth arrest and/or cell death.

prone to spontaneous (as opposed to inducible) apoptosis, chromosomally unstable, and have shortened telomeres. The resultant genetic instability leads to defective V(D)J recombination in B and T cells, leading to **immune defects** in addition to the other phenotypes. This "p53 booster" ability of wild-type *ATM* to ensure correct DNA repair and genetic stability marks it as a guardian-style (caretaker) tumor suppressor gene – as is DNA-PK. Of note, however, *ATM* expression is often reduced in sporadic breast cancers.

Life and death are decided by the Bcl2/Bax balance

Death is a normal process and its prevention is not necessarily a good thing. An instructive example is the 14:18 chromosomal translocation of **follicular lymphomas** which juxtaposes the 5′ immunoglobulin heavy chain region (constitutively transcribed in B cells) to the 3′ anti-apoptotic *Bcl2* (B cell lymphoma) gene. Other chromosomal translocations such as that producing the *Bcr/Abl* fusion gene in **chronic myeloid leukemia** may induce constitutive expression of Bcl2 by an indirect mechanism. The Bcl2 protein family regulates cell survival and death via a p53-dependent heterodimeric interplay (Figure 15.18) between its members, which include:

1. Anti-apoptotic (pro-survival) proteins
   - **Bcl2**.
   - **Bcl-X$_L$, Bcl-w, Mcl-1**.
2. Pro-apoptotic proteins
   - **Bax**.
   - **Bak, Bad, Bid, Bcl-X$_S$, Noxa**.

Membrane-spanning (BH1, BH2) domains in Bcl2, Bcl-X$_L$ and Bax contain α-helices that contribute to the formation and patency of membrane permeability-transition pores. For example, Bcl-X$_L$ contains seven such helices in a bundle comprising two central hydrophobic helices forming a 3-nm (30-Å) "dagger" surrounded by five amphipathic helices. Given the resemblance to bacterial toxins (e.g., **colicin, diphtheria toxin**), this structure suggests an umbrella-like mechanism for piercing mitchondrial membranes. The megachannels so formed comprise both a voltage-dependent anion channel in the outer mitochondrial membrane and an adenine-nucleotide translocator in the inner mitochondrial membrane. Interaction of **Bax** with these proteins triggers a mitochondrial permeability transition in which **cytochrome *c*** is leaked to the cytosol, activating a pro-apoptotic pathway (Figure 15.19*A*).

The **Bcl2:Bax ratio** can thus determine critical cell decisions, with a high ratio favoring life and a low ratio favoring death. This reflects the stoichiometry of Bax–Bcl2 heterodimers to Bax–Bax homodimers. An illustrative example occurs in the intestinal crypt, wherein basal proliferative cells overexpress Bcl2, while apical (dying) cells express abundant Bax, Bak, and APC. The recruitment of Bcl2 opposes the lethal action of Bax by blocking translocation of cytochrome *c* across the mitochondrial membrane.

The pro-apoptotic effect of the **Myc** protein depends on its ability to transactivate Bax (Figure 15.19*B*). Consistent with this, loss of Myc-dependent apoptosis in **Burkitt lymphoma** is invariably associated with Bc12 upregulation and disruption of the p14^{ARF} – HDM2–p53 pathway. Similarly, the chemopreventive apoptotic effect of aspirin depends upon reduced expression of Bcl-X$_L$, thus elevating the Bax:Bcl-X$_L$ ratio. By restricting mitochondrial release of cytochrome *c*, tumor overexpression of Bcl2 prevents activation of critical death enzymes termed **caspases**.

A.

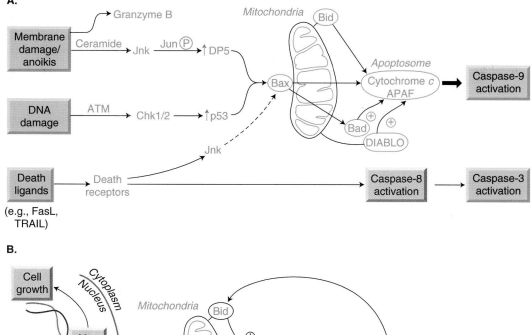

B.

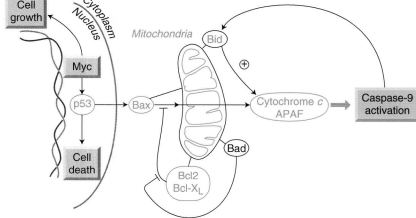

Figure 15.19 The role of Bcl2 family members in cell death. *A*, Overview of cell death pathways, showing its activation by the p53 and Jnk pathways. *B*, Functional interactions between Bcl2 family members.

CLINICAL KEYNOTE

Bcl-family proteins in disease

Many disease processes involve accelerated cell death. Progressive myocardial dysfunction due to **cardiomyopathies** may reflect apoptosis-induced loss of myocytes, for example, whereas **osteoporosis** may be prevented by using estrogen to inhibit the apoptosis of ageing osteoblasts. Increased expression of pro-apoptotic proteins is typically associated with organ involution (e.g., postlactational breast involution), neurodegenerative diseases (including **AIDS dementia**), and antitumor activity. In contrast, Bcl2 immortalizes memory B cells when activated, and inappropriate activation of Bcl2 is implicated in the pathogenesis of both lymphoproliferative and autoimmune disorders. **Colorectal tumors** characterized by microsatellite instability select for frameshift mutations of Bax. In contrast, immortalized erythroid cells in **polycythemia vera** overexpress Bcl-X$_L$.

The survival-promoting effect of Bcl2 does not appear to be simply a mitogenic effect. To illustrate this, consider that myocytes from **heart failure** patients exhibit a twofold increase in Bcl2 with normal Bax expression; Bcl2 overexpression is associated with an improved neuronal phenotype in transgenic models of **motor neuron disease**; and elevated Bcl2 expression in **breast cancer** has a favorable prognostic significance. Interestingly, an antisense oligonucleotide targeted against Bcl2, **augmerosen**, has been reported to show activity in **melanoma** patients.

A killer enzyme cascade triggers DNA fragmentation

The process of programmed cell death includes cytoskeletal alterations, the formation of apoptotic bodies, cell-surface changes (e.g., blebbing) that target the dying cell for phagocytosis, and chromatin condensation. These processes are initiated by cysteine-dependent aspartate-specific **cysteine proteases** or **caspases**. The first of these enzymes to be characterized in lymphocytes was **ICE** (**interleukin-1β-converting enzyme**, or **caspase 1**), a proinflammatory regulator of interferon-γ production. Of the remaining caspases, most (except caspases 4 and 5, which are implicated in cytokine activation) are primarily involved in cell death induction. These include (Figure 15.20):

1. **Initiator caspases**
   - **Caspase-8** (FLICE) Initiates the cell death pathway following activation of membrane death receptors. Viral inhibitors (**FLIPs**) protect infected cells and intracellular herpesviruses from apoptosis.
   - **Caspase-9** Initiates the cell death pathway in response to leaching of mitochondrial cytochrome c into the cytoplasm, which triggers ATP-dependent polymerization of the adaptor protein **APAF-1**. The latter complex then binds pro-caspase-9, forming an **apoptosome** which autocatalytically activates itself, then activates caspase-3. Caspase-9 is inactivated by PKB-dependent phosphorylation.
   - **Caspase-12** Initiates cell death in response to endoplasmic reticulum stress, and is also implicated in β-amyloid-dependent **amyloid precursor protein** (**APP**) cleavage and neuronal death in **Alzheimer disease**.

2. **Executor caspases**
   - **Caspase-3** (apoptosis-inducible cysteine protease, CPP32) is a key apoptotic executioner which recognizes DEVD sequences. Caspase-3 knockout mice are brain-damaged due to hyperplasias.
   - **Caspase-6, caspase-7.**

Figure 15.20 Activation of caspase-family enzymes in the genesis of cell death.

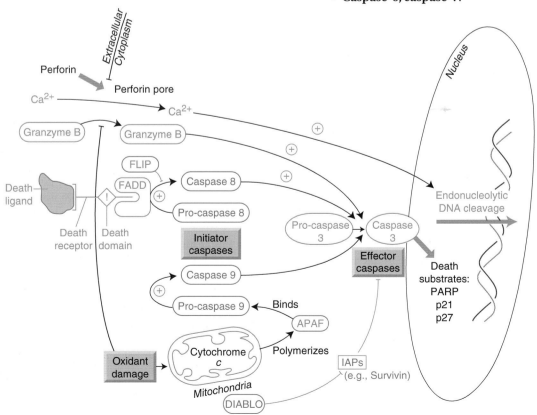

All caspases are proteolytically activated to yield heterodimeric enzymes. Initiator caspases such as caspase-8 and -9 induce downstream caspases, whereas executor caspases such as caspase-6 and -7 proteolyze target proteins (for example, cleavage of APP by caspase-3 following initiation by caspase-12). Caspase expression is normally transactivated in response to DNA binding by p53. Conversely, caspases-3 and -7 are inhibited during mitosis by the Bcl2-linked anti-apoptotic spindle protein **survivin** in fetal and cancer tissues. Survivin is one member of a conserved family of proteins termed **IAPs** (inhibitors of apoptosis) which are in turn inhibited either by anti-apoptotic proteins such as *Grim* and *Reaper* (in fruitflies) or by human homologs like the mitochondrial protein **DIABLO**. IAPs like survivin suppress apoptosis by using their zinc-binding domains to inhibit caspase function. Proteins such as DIABLO in turn inhibit IAPs by sterically interacting with the zinc-binding domain, thereby activating caspases by default. Since certain cancers overexpress IAPs, small-molecule drugs that simulate DIABLO binding could prove useful.

CLINICAL KEYNOTE

Caspases and APAFs as disease determinants

Aggressive **neuroblastomas** suppress expression of caspase-8, preventing initiation of the cell suicide cascade despite upregulation of the apoptotic sensitizer N-Myc. High plasma levels of caspase-3, on the other hand, are associated with increased chemocurability of **acute leukemia**. Caspase-3 is also a target of the ceramide-Jnk pathway (p. 291) which is activated by **steroids**, **radiation** and **chemotherapy**.

Malignant **melanomas** may methylate the *APAF1* gene, thereby disabling the normal apoptotic response. In contrast, loss-of-function mutations (e.g., frameshifts) affecting the pericentromeric chromosome 16 locus *NOD2* – a member of the *APAF* gene family that normally activates the transcription factor NFκB in response to bacterial lipopolysaccharide – predispose to the inflammatory bowel disorder **Crohn disease**.

Proteases and nucleases autodigest doomed cells

Granzyme B is an enzyme released by neighboring cells that gains entry to target cells via perforin-dependent membrane defects. Once inside, granzyme B coactivates caspase-3 (as well as caspases-7 and -2), which in turn cleaves the DNA-protecting enzyme **poly(ADP-ribosyl) polymerase-1** (**PARP1**; pp. 136–7) into hallmark 85- and 29-kDa fragments that are often used for experimental confirmation of apoptosis. PARP1 permits damage-inducible p53 nuclear accumulation and target gene transactivation, thereby shielding the human genome from wear and tear and improving genetic stability. Repair of radical-induced base damage is also enhanced by PARP1, reducing the propensity of such damage to induce cell transformation.

Functional loss of PARP1 sets the scene for internucleosomal DNA scission. The latter is mediated not by caspases, but by caspase-dependent cleavage of cytoplasmic DNase chaperone proteins that allows DNase to slip through the nuclear envelope. Endonuclease activity within the nucleus manifests electrophoretically as the **DNA laddering** of apoptosis – an agarose gel finding which denotes DNA fragmentation. Apoptotic destruction of the cytoplasmic architecture is triggered by calcium-dependent activation of **transglutaminase** and **calpain** (Figure 15.21).

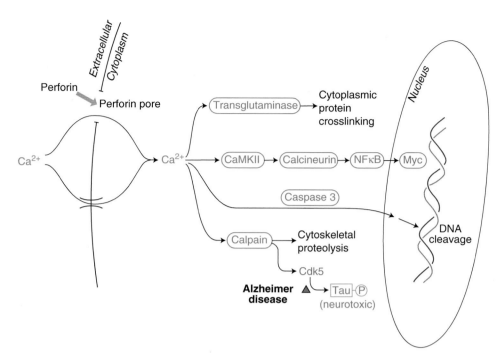

Figure 15.21 Calcium-dependent enzymatic cell death pathways.

Key proteins that are caspase cleavage substrates include not only **Bcl2** and **PARP**, but also the cytoskeletal proteins **lamin** and **gelsolin** which effect apoptotic cell morphologic changes such as rounding up, membrane blebbing, and nuclear envelope dissolution; the survival-promoting kinase **PKB** (Akt); the protein synthesis initiation factor **eIF4**; the integrin transducer focal adhesion kinase (**Fak**); the pro-apoptotic netrin receptor **DCC**; **p21**^{Cip}**1** and **p27**^{Kip}**1**; and the p53-inhibitory **HDM2**. Neuronal caspase substrates other than **APP** include **tau**, **presenilin**, and **huntingtin**, suggesting the centrality of this pathway in neurodegenerative disease.

MOLECULAR MINIREVIEW

Fas and the Death Receptors
T cells need both to kill target cells at the appropriate time, and also to reduce their own number following termination of an immune response. These cytocidal tasks are achieved partly via a membrane-bound TNFα homolog on lymphoid cells termed **Fas ligand** (**FasL**) which binds the lymphocytic **Fas** surface receptor (**CD95**). Homologous **death receptors** of the TNFα/NGF receptor family include **TRAIL receptor** (DR4) and **TRAMP** (DR3). All such receptors contain 80-amino-acid **death domains** necessary for inducing apoptosis, and a variety of death-modifying proteins congregate around this domain (Figures 15.19A and 15.20). The ability of all-*trans*-retinoic acid (ATRA) to induce cell death in **acute promyelocytic leukemia** (p. 55) depends on an ATRA-induced increase in TRAIL expression which in turn activates caspase-8. This leads in turn to cytochrome *c* release, caspase-3 activation, Bid cleavage, and DNA fragmentation.

Fas activation mimics the TNF-dependent stress response pathway mediated by sphingomyelinase and ceramide signaling, and activates caspase-3 both by proteolytic zymogen cleavage and by denitrosylation. Subsequent activation of Jnk signaling is linked to cell death. Any resulting apoptotic cells are vacuumed up by CD14-expressing macrophages. The physiologic importance of CD95-dependent cell death is illustrated by the consequences of *Pseudomonas aeruginosa* exposure of wild-type and CD95/CD95 ligand-null mice: the normal mice incur widespread lung epithelial cell apoptosis but do not become septic, whereas the CD95-null (ligand) mice incur no apoptosis and rapidly succumb to sepsis.

Alcoholic hepatitis may be associated with abnormally high plasma levels of soluble FasL. Of possible relevance to this, anticancer trials of the pro-apoptotic TNF-like TRAIL ligand have been complicated by massive liver and brain cell death. **Decoy receptors** for FasL and TRAIL may be expressed by **colon cancers** and **lung cancers**, thereby promoting tumor cell escape from immune attack.

Null mutations of Fas cause the rare autoimmune lymphoproliferative disorder, **Canale–Smith syndrome**. Allografts from certain sites (the testis, and the anterior chamber of the eye) are not efficiently rejected by transplant recipients despite HLA mismatch. As these immunologically privileged sites express abundant Fas, functioning testicular allografts may release a factor that causes the apoptosis of cytotoxic (CD8$^+$) T cells and thus prevents rejection. Anti-rejection therapies based on this insight could help maintain the viability of animal-derived (xenografted) tissues. Conversely, certain tumors that overexpress FasL (e.g., **melanoma**) may facilitate metastatic tumor growth by compromising lymphocyte-dependent immune surveillance within lesions.

CLINICAL KEYNOTE

EBV in human cancer

Like other herpesviruses, **Epstein–Barr virus** (EBV) bears a symbiotic relationship to human cells, having already infected about 90% of the world's population as we speak. Though usually subclinical, primary EBV infection most often manifests in developed countries as **infectious mononucleosis** associated with atypical lymphocytosis in adolescents. EBV activates and immortalizes hitherto resting human B lymphocytes, and is linked to the pathogenesis of B cell malignancies in several contexts:

1. **Burkitt lymphoma**
   - 99% (endemic), 15% (sporadic).
2. **Hodgkin disease** (HD)
   - 80% (developing world), 40% (developed world).
   - Commoner after infectious mononucleosis.
3. Immunosuppressive lymphoproliferative disease (**non-Hodgkin lymphoma**)
   - AIDS or post-transplant (may be polyclonal).
   - X-linked lymphoproliferative disease (XLP).

The B cell tropism of EBV reflects the affinity of the major EBV envelope glycoprotein **gp350** for the **C3d complement receptor** (CD21) on the B cell membrane. However, EBV can also immortalize epithelial cells of the nasopharynx (particularly in Chinese populations), thereby predisposing to the development of **nasopharyngeal carcinoma** (NPC). Other EBV-inducible neoplasms include **T cell lymphomas**, and **oral hairy leukoplakia** in HIV patients.

EBV expresses close to 100 genes, of which EBV-infected cells express 11:

1. **EBNA**1, -2, -3A, -3B, -3C, -LP (**EB n**uclear **a**ntigens).
2. **LMP**1, -2A, -2B (**l**atent **m**embrane **p**roteins).
3. **EBER**1, -2 (**EB-e**xpressed **RNA**s).

EBNA1 is a viral episomal genome maintenance protein. In contrast, EBNA2 upregulates the oncogenic LMP1 protein (which encodes a six-transmembrane-domain functional homolog of the TNF receptor) while interacting with the *Notch* signaling pathway (p. 404). Five EBV genes are required for B cell immortalization: *EBNA1, -2, -3A, -3C,* and *LMP-1.* The intracellular domain of LMP-1 acts as a nidus for the aggregation of TRAFs (TNF receptor-associated factors 1 and 3 in particular) which activate IKK (IκB kinase), NFκB and B lymphocytes, and thus mimic the effects of CD40 ligation. LMP1 also activates Jnk, leading to AP1 induction. B cells that are transformed by this LMP-driven constitutive signaling pathway may acquire an additional chromosomal translocation that activates Myc, unleashing Burkitt lymphoma.

LMP2 inhibits host cell tyrosine phosphorylation and thus blocks EBV reactivation, thereby making latent infections lifelong. Healthy EBV carriers express only *LMP2* and *EBER1/2* of the latent viral genes. In contrast, only EBER1/2 and EBNA1 are expressed in Burkitt lymphoma, whereas both of these and both LMP proteins are expressed in nasopharyngeal carcinoma and Hodgkin disease. All latency genes are expressed during infectious mononucleosis, as well as in immunosuppression-linked lymphoproliferation.

Ageing is the p53-dependent play-off of apoptosis and cancer

Age is a terminal disease. Living organisms can be genetically successful either by reproducing quickly (e.g., bacteria) or by repairing well (e.g., elephants), but only in the latter case is it possible to evolve nonrenewable multicellular organs such as the brain. The postmitotic nature of neurons is an advantage in early life since it permits stable retention of complex synaptic transmission patterns, but it is disadvantageous in old age since degeneration is inevitable in the absence of a capacity for self-renewal.

The miracle of life lies in the germline. Germ cells age within an individual, manifesting as an increased risk of chromosomal defects in progeny from older parents, but the germline lineage itself does not age between generations. Quantifiable measures of ageing in somatic tissues include the extent of collagen crosslinking and of DNA methylation.

Somatic human cells have a lifespan measured in divisions (say, 50–60). With each division about 50 bp of telomeric shortening ensues. If a large number of division cycles is exceeded, the cell undergoes a telomere crisis, which is usually resolved by apoptosis, but occasionally by immortalization. Coincident loss of p53 function extends the number of cell divisions required to bring the cell to crisis. More importantly, p53 loss increases the subsequent probability of immortalization, an event that is often associated with an increase in **telomerase** expression. The latter development allows telomere repair (prevention of further shortening) and indefinite proliferation.

The wild-type *p53* gene can act as a **senescence gene** in addition to its other roles, as illustrated by the rapid ageing of transgenic mice expressing hyperfunctional *p53* mutants. Increased p53 activity in senescing cells results from dwindling HDM2 activity. The consequent enhancement of p53 function – manifested as increased DNA-binding and transcriptional activity in the absence of increased expression – causes increased p21^{Cip} synthesis, leading to Cdk inhibition and cell cycle arrest (which may manifest as senescence) or cell death. Expression of p21^{Cip} is also upregulated in differentiating cells by the differentiation factor **C/EBPα** which stabilizes the p21^{Cip} protein. The *C/EBPα* gene is often mutated in the M2 subtype of **acute myeloid leukemia**, leading to the loss of p21^{Cip} expression and leukemic cell immortalization. Activation of Ras can accelerate the senescence of untransformed cells by causing CBP/p300-dependent acetylation of the p53 protein at lysine 382.

Approximately 25% of interindividual differences in longevity appear genetic in origin. The **apoE2** genotype increases the probability of living longer than 100 years, for example, whereas **apoE4** militates against this. Hence, these traits represent age-of-onset modifiers of senescence. Of all environmental variables, **caloric restriction** is the only one that extends lifespan in lab-

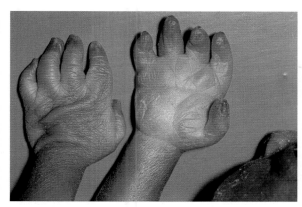

Figure 15.22 Werner syndrome (progeria), showing accelerated degeneration of the skin in a young child. (Wellcome Medical Photographic Library, N0007280C).

Enrichment reading

Bedtime reading

Clark WR. *A means to an end: the biological basis of aging and death.* Oxford University Press, Oxford, 1999

Holliday R. *Understanding ageing.* Cambridge University Press, Cambridge, 1995

Cheap'n'cheerful

Cooper GM. *Oncogenes.* Jones & Bartlett, 1995

Hesketh R. *The oncogene and tumor suppressor gene factsbook.* Academic Press, New York, 1997

Library reference

Gutkind JS (ed). *Signalling networks and cell cycle control: the molecular basis of cancer and other diseases.* Humana Press, Champaign, IL, 2000

Kaufman SH (ed). *Apoptosis: pharmacological implications and therapeutic opportunities.* Academic Press, New York, 1999

Stein GS et al (eds). *The molecular basis of cell cycle and growth control.* Wiley, New York, 1998

Wilson JW et al (eds). *Apoptosis genes.* Kluwer, Dordrecht, 1998

oratory mice. Studies using this system have identified an ageing-suppressor gene, *klotho*, which inhibits ceramide-dependent apoptosis.

CLINICAL KEYNOTE

Progerias

There exist several rare inherited conditions in which features normally associated with ageing are evident during childhood. Such disorders have been labeled **progerias**, though their causes are heterogeneous and largely unrelated to true cellular ageing as defined above. Note that mutations affecting DNA repair or connective tissue may also be involved. These disorders include:

1. **Hutchinson–Gilford syndrome** (autosomal dominant.)
2. **Werner syndrome** (autosomal recessive.)
3. **Wiedemann–Rautenstrach syndrome** (autosomal recessive.)

Hutchinson–Gilford syndrome (**HGS**) occurs with increased frequency if paternal age is advanced, and is associated with accelerated atherosclerosis (often terminating in death from myocardial infarction prior to age 20), aged appearance of skin and face reflecting a lack of subcutaneous fat, alopecia, and short stature.

Werner syndrome (**WS**) is a mutator (genomic instability) syndrome which is associated with many of the external features of accelerated ageing, including scleroderma-like skin changes such as wizened facies (Figure 15.22), premature atherosclerosis and diabetes, osteoporosis, hypogonadism, and cataracts. Skin fibroblasts from WS individuals exhibit abnormally high levels of collagenase, accounting for the accelerated loss of skin elasticity. The wild-type *WRN* gene encodes a 1432-amino-acid DNA helicase (with added exonuclease activity) that interacts with p53 to promote genetic stability. Other mutator disorders include **ataxia telangiectasia** (AT), **Cockayne syndrome**, **Nijmegen break syndrome** (a variant of AT; p. 379) and **Rothmund–Thomson syndrome**. Like Bloom syndrome and WS, Cockayne and Rothmund–Thomson syndromes arise because of helicase mutations leading to abnormal recombination.

The aged phenotype of Wiedemann–Rautenstrach syndrome (**WRS**) is evident at birth, and generally terminates in death during childhood. Absent subcutaneous fat is invariable in WRS, and an associated leukodystrophy (leading to cerebral demyelination) is common.

Summary

Chromosomes separate and rejoin in a cyclical fashion. Cell cycle checkpoints restrain cell growth. Cyclins are molecular timers for cell cycle progression. Cyclin-dependent kinases drive cell growth transitions. Cdk inhibitors can convert growth to differentiation.

Proto-oncogenes encode proteins that activate cell growth. Tumor suppressor genes control cell cycle progression. BRCA proteins are sensors of DNA damage. Cancers accumulate dozens of genetic errors. A mutant pocket protein predisposes to retinoblastoma. DNA damage induces p53 expression and G_1–S arrest. Loss of p53 function causes genetic instability.

Genetically damaged cells undergo repair or apoptosis. ATM is needed for p53-dependent growth arrest. Life and death are decided by the Bcl2/Bax balance. A killer enzyme cascade triggers DNA fragmentation. Proteases and nucleases autodigest doomed cells Ageing is the p53-dependent play-off of apoptosis and carcinogenesis.

QUIZ QUESTIONS

1. Describe the temporal relationship between the morphologic changes of chromosomal structure and the phases of the cell cycle.
2. What are the major cell cycle checkpoints, and how does their significance differ?
3. Explain how cyclins regulate the periodicity of the cell cycle.
4. Describe the function and effects of Cdks. Which molecules modify their effects?
5. What is an oncogene? Give some examples.
6. Name three tumor suppressor genes, and explain how they function.
7. What is the significance of loss of heterozygosity for a given gene locus in cancer?
8. Explain how the pRb and p53 proteins prevent tumor formation.
9. Why do p53 protein levels rise following DNA damage induction?
10. Describe the consequences of progressive genetic instability in a cell.
11. What are the differences between necrotic and apoptotic cell death?
12. Name some of the processes involved in cellular ageing and senescence.

IV

From molecular cell biology to human physiology

16

Development

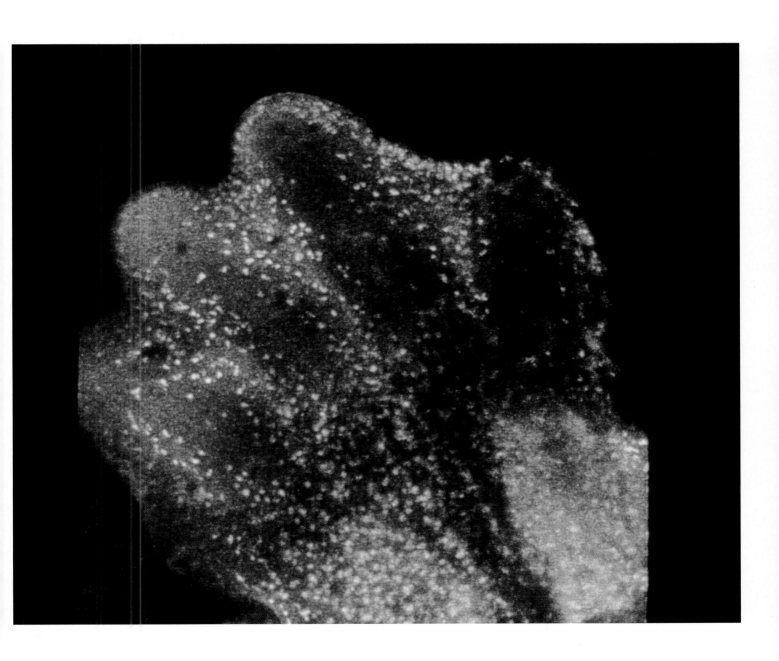

Figure 16.1 (*previous page*) Apoptosis giving rise to the beginnings of the interdigital web-spaces during embryogenesis (Wellcome Medical Photographic Library, no. B0001006C06).

The molecular narrative of how life begins is one of the most fascinating in biology. How does a multifaceted organism arise from an amorphous cell mass? How are patterns imposed on tissues arising from a common cellular progenitor? And what genetic constellations determine phenotypes as diverse as blue eyes, a left-sided heart, or an artistic temperament?

Embryonic induction

Life begins when egg integrins meet sperm ADAMs

Embryogenesis is initiated by a five-step process: chemoattraction of sperm to the egg; sperm–egg surface binding; discharge of sperm vesicle contents onto the egg surface (acrosome reaction); sperm penetration of the egg-coat; and fusion of sperm-egg membranes, permitting restoration of the diploid genome.

Mature ova attract sperm by releasing subpicomolar chemotactic factors within the female genital tract. Spermatozoa lured to the egg by species-specific chemoattractants are first made hypermotile by bicarbonate-induced cAMP signaling, then activated by egg-coat extracellular matrix **ZP3** (zona pellucida) oligosaccharides that bind human-specific galactosyltransferases on the sperm surface. Membrane clustering of these enzymes activates sperm sensor G-protein-coupled receptors, causing transmembrane influx of sodium ions; this is followed by tyrosine phosphorylation of the ZP3 receptor, leading in turn to sperm pronuclear binding of the ZP2 receptor in the inner membrane leaflet (Figure 16.2). Nitric oxide synthase from activated sperm stimulates a wave of egg nitrosation within seconds of fertilization, thereby activating egg development. Mobilization of calcium follows diffusion of the sperm calcium-regulatory protein **oscillin** into the ovum.

Sperm–egg fusion proceeds via the interaction of sperm membrane **fertilins** (homologous to **meltrins**, which mediate the fusion of myoblasts to multinucleate muscle fibers). These ~100-kDa gamete-fusion proteins belong to the **ADAM** (**a d**isintegrin **a**nd **m**etalloprotease) structural superfamily. ADAM proteins – which resemble snake venom metalloproteases, but remain membrane-anchored – mediate neurogenesis, myogenesis and inflammation in addition to fertilization. Human sperm express at least six ADAMs, including ADAMs 1 and 2 (fertilins α and β): the latter binds the egg via $\alpha_6\beta_1$ integrins, whereas the former mediates subsequent membrane fusion. ADAM-dependent egg activation induces calcium waves, blocks polyspermy, modifies cytoskeletal proteins and maternal mRNAs, and triggers the resumption of oocyte cell cycle progression. Sperm fertility defects have been associated with fertilin-β (ADAM-2) mutations in mice.

Figure 16.2 The molecular phases of sperm–egg fusion, mediated via interactions between egg-binding proteins in the sperm head and receptors in the zona pellucida.

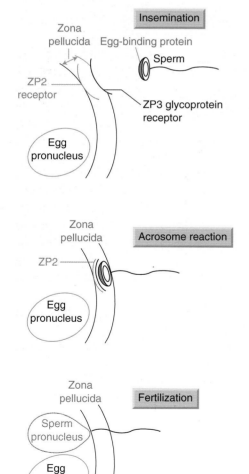

MOLECULAR MINIREVIEW

Anteroposterior axis formation in the embryo
There are certain decisions in life you do not want to get wrong – one of these is which end of your body will be your head and which your tail. How does an embryo develop a sense of direction – up/down, front/back, left/right – and how does it decide to move some of its cells in one direction but not in others?

The sperm–egg acrosome reaction is followed by a sequence of embryogenetic events, beginning with **cytoplasmic rotation** that leads to specification of the dorsoventral axis (Figure 16.3). Cytoplasmic rotation is followed by mesoderm

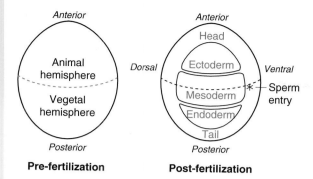

Animal
hemisphere

Vegetal
hemisphere

Anterior

Posterior

Pre-fertilization

Anterior

Head

Ectoderm

Dorsal — Mesoderm — *Ventral*

Endoderm

Tail

Posterior

Sperm
entry

Post-fertilization

Figure 16.3 Formation of the embryonic poles. Oocyte asymmetry gives rise to animal and vegetal hemispheres (the anteroposterior axis), whereas fertilization-dependent cytoplasmic rotation gives rise to the dorsoventral axis. The ectoderm, mesoderm, and endoderm are also specified following fertilization.

induction, blastula invagination (gastrulation), and the development of organ systems. These latter events depend upon asymmetric cell divisions that are accompanied by intracellular segregation of gene-regulatory molecules. The transcriptional induction of embryonic axes via zygotic segmentation is complex. In insects this process involves several groups of genes: (1) **segment-polarity** genes, (2) **gap** genes that regulate **pair-rule** genes (which in turn imprint segment-polarity genes), and (3) **homeotic** genes (p. 401). Human homologs of these genes – probably about 100 in all – interact in a hierarchical fashion to determine the position of specialized (differentiated) cells along the anteroposterior embryonic axis.

Maternal messages control early embryonic development

Human oocytes slumber undisturbed within the ovarian follicle for decades, hibernating at the G_2/M cell cycle checkpoint. Under ordinary circumstances oocyte meiosis is arrested by high intracellular levels of cAMP. In response to ovulation, however, rising gonadotrophin levels cause surrounding follicle cells to release progesterone, which competitively inhibits oxytocin receptors on the oocyte membrane (p. 317). This reduces adenyl cyclase activity, intra-oocyte cAMP levels, and protein kinase A signaling, thus permitting meiotic fusion of gametocyte genomes and initiating embryogenesis.

A second pathway regulating oocyte maturation is that controlled by the meiosis-specific serine-threonine kinase **Mos** (cytostatic factor) which is also present in sperm. Rising progesterone levels trigger polyadenylation of Mos transcripts, permitting translation; the p39^{Mos} so produced prevents meiotic maturation until fertilization-dependent activation of calcium/calmodulin-dependent protein kinase II removes this constraint.

Fertilization causes widespread alterations in chromatin structure – e.g., gene methylation, chromatin decondensation – as well as altered activity of gene products that regulate transcriptional activity. However, many of the earliest phases of development proceed in the absence of transcription.

Most oocyte mRNAs remain untranslated prior to fertilization. These stockpiled mRNAs have short poly(A) tails which distinguish them from mRNAs in somatic cells. Unlike oocytes, sperm contribute no cytoplasm (and hence no RNA or mitochondrial DNA) to the zygote. Following fertilization, oocyte-derived mRNAs are responsible for vital developmental functions such as body axis specification and cell cycle control; for example, the embryonic body axis is indicated by the polarity of localized maternal mRNAs containing conserved motifs in their 3′ untranslated sequences. Translational control of maternal messages is regulated by two main mechanisms:

1. **Masking**, or reversible repression, of mRNA translation by the binding of phosphoproteins to 3′ untranslated sequences
   - When a predetermined developmental stage is reached, the critical sequence is unmasked and translation initiated.
2. Polyadenylation and deadenylation of maternal mRNAs
   - Polyadenylation is associated with message recruitment,
   - Deadenylation is associated with mRNA-polysome dissociation.

Modifications of mRNA poly(A) tail length regulate the translational efficiency of maternal messages. Such alterations may enhance the postconceptional translation of mRNAs such as those for histone H1 and fibronectin. Maternally inherited mRNAs may be masked (dormant) during oocyte maturation, yet translationally active following fertilization. Alternatively, messages that are active during meiotic maturation may be removed from polysomes at later developmental stages.

Loss-of-function mutations affecting the RNA-processing enzyme **MRP** (**m**itochondrial **R**NA **p**rocessing) – a predominantly nucleolar RNA–protein complex that cleaves 5.8S ribosomal RNA – cause the recessively inherited syndrome of **cartilage-hair hypoplasia**. Seen in the Amish and Finnish kindreds, this syndrome manifests with short stature, abnormalities of cartilage and hair, and a tendency to develop **lymphomas**.

MOLECULAR MINIREVIEW

Experimental analysis of embryogenesis

There are several strategies for assessing the developmental significance of specific genes using experimental animals:

1. **Chimeric** animals created by injecting recipient embryos with pluripotential cells – blastomeres, teratocarcinoma cells, or (most commonly) genetically engineered embryonic stem (ES) cells (p. 581).
2. **Transgenic** animals created by injecting recipient zygotes with a gene of interest linked to a strong (perhaps tissue-specific) promoter.
3. A variation of the latter is to target dysfunctional genes for genomic insertion via homologous recombination – a strategy termed gene knockout (p. 585).

The resulting phenotypes may not be predictable from known effects of gene expression/mutation in adult life. Murine knockout of the tumor suppressor retinoblastoma gene causes intrauterine fetal death associated with major hematopoietic and nerve defects, for example, whereas targeting of the endogenous transforming growth factor α gene causes curly hair.

Embryonic induction determines body patterns

Is embryogenesis programmed – the Aristotelian "master builder" model of a preformed homunculus – or are body parts successively induced in response to epigenetic stimuli?

The book of life consists of recipes rather than blueprints. Embryos do not form simply by shaking a cocktail of biomolecules, nor on the other hand can development be reduced to a domino-like process. Rather, external signals interact with information encoded within; so life goes on within you and without you. Certain features of embryonic cells underlie this complexity:

1. **Automaticity** of embryonic cell growth
   - e.g., Cell growth following in vitro fertilization.
2. **Plasticity** of embryonic cell phenotype
   - i.e., Phenotypic interconvertibility of stem cells transplanted into embryonic regions with different ambient growth factors.

Since error accumulation could easily be lethal in embryogenesis, there are evolutionary advantages in developing systems with functional redundancy. Embryos tolerate this looseness of gene control by building in microenvironmental controls and temporal cues. Embryonic cells adopt their specialized functions via sequential rather than random processes: such cells await timed signals from other cells to specify their fate. This process of one embryonic cell mass telling another cell mass what to do is termed **embryonic induction**. The notochord in paraxial mesoderm – which forms somites – induces the differentiation of sclerotomes, for example (Figure 16.4), whereas forebrain structures in the anterior neural tube are induced by the prechordal plate.

Figure 16.4 Embryonic induction of neural crest tissue to yield (*A*) somites, and (*B*) spinal nerves (Wellcome Medical Photographic Library, B0001054C06 and B0001056C06, respectively).

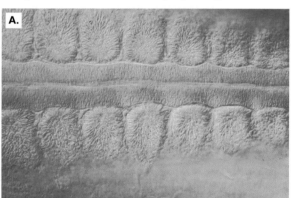

A.

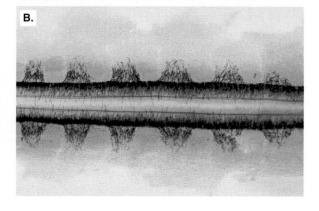

B.

Embryonic inducing factors thus act as pattern-determining factors or **morphogens**. These morphogens include inducers such as growth factors, which send short-lived signals across small distances within the embryo – perhaps as little as a few cell diameters. In this way inducers convert the early embryo from a clump of similar cells (the blastula) to a diversified organism.

Activins and **inhibins** are mutually antagonistic members of the transforming growth factor β (TGFβ) superfamily of peptide signaling molecules. First identified as a pituitary FSH-releasing peptide (and subsequently as an erythroid differentiation factor), activin exists as homo- or heterodimers of β_A and β_B subunits. In contrast, **inhibins** are obligate heterodimers containing either of these subunits complexed to a distinct α polypeptide; the type III TGFβ receptor betaglycan functions as an inhibin co-receptor. Another activin antagonist is **follistatin**, which binds stoichiometrically to activin β-chain monomers, thus preventing receptor binding. Like fibroblast growth factors and TGFβ, activins are mesoderm-inducing factors which stimulate the formation of axial mesodermal structures (segmental myotomes and notochord) from ectoderm, giving rise to neural and muscle tissue. In contrast, hepatocyte growth factor induces gland formation (Figure 16.5A).

Morphogenetic fields

Morphogenetic gradients specify embryo spatial organization

Why does a human embryo not become a mouse? Phenotypic differences between species arise in part from the spatial organization of the 300 or so different mammalian cell lineages. Such spatial organization is specified by positional information within embryonic cells which, when known, can be summarized as a **fate map**. Cell memory of embryonic position enables differentiated cells from one compartment to retain their phenotype despite being transplanted to a different developmental location. Shape changes such as gastrulation reflect aggregate embryonic effects of this positional information, and lead to embryonic asymmetry.

Three axial polarities are conferred upon the human embryo: anteroposterior, left–right and dorsal–ventral. TGFβ-family signaling molecules – including the active ventral signal, BMP4, which is bound and inactivated by dorsal signals – are implicated in these processes. Activin is released from vegetal cells, for example, inducing mesoderm in cells expressing appropriate receptors; over a period of hours the activin signal may passively diffuse over about ten cell diameters, leading to differential patterns of target gene expression. Dorsal–ventral patterning is thus imposed upon the three embryonic germ layers: the ventral derivative of the ectoderm is the skin (epidermis), for example, whereas the dorsal derivative is the nervous system. Similarly, the ventral derivative of the mesoderm is the blood and mesenchyme, whereas the dorsal derivative includes muscle, notochord, and head mesoderm. Endoderm gives rise to gut.

Fetal asymmetry reflects the existence of diffusible morphogens within the embryo. These include inducers such as retinoic acid that create functional **morphogenetic gradients** defining structural **morphogenetic fields**. The first

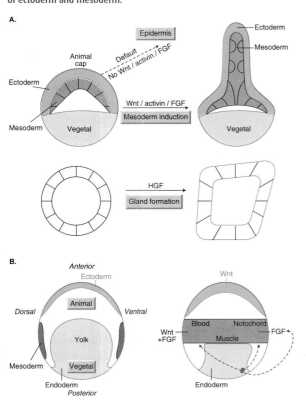

Figure 16.5 Specification of embryonic cell fates by growth factors and Wnts. *A*, Induction of mesoderm (giving rise to muscle and nerves) by activin, and of gland formation by hepatocyte growth factor (HGF). In the absence of activin, epidermis is formed instead of mesoderm. *B*, Wnt-dependent specification of embryonic cell fate. Cross-talk between Wnt and fibroblast growth factors (FGFs) differentially affects the fate of ectoderm and mesoderm.

morphogenetic gradient arises de novo due to oocyte asymmetry, whereas subsequent gradients are formed by secretion from embryonic polarizing regions (Figure 16.5B). When a small concentration gradient is exceeded, a threshold-activated switch induces a transcriptional cascade resulting in the specification of embryonic positional coordinates and the division of the embryo into body-part domains. An example relates to liver induction from foregut endoderm expressing FGF receptors 1 and 4: adjacent cardiac mesoderm secretes FGFs 1, 2 and 8, of which the first two induce the initial hepatogenic response, whereas the last promotes liver outgrowth.

MOLECULAR MINIREVIEW

Left–right asymmetry

Of the three axial polarities conferred upon the embryo – antero–posterior, dorsal–ventral and left–right – the latter is least understood. Indeed, left and right cannot even be defined until the antero–posterior and dorsal–ventral axes have been specified. A cup-shaped depression in the embryonic midline, called the **node**, is a key patterning center: the ventral side of the node is composed of cells with a single cilium. Factors implicated in the genesis of left–right asymmetry include:

1. The gene **Inv** (inversion of embryonic turning) controls early postimplantation embryonic turning, which is one of the first manifestations of visceral right–left polarity. Transgenic knockout of *Inv* causes invariant (as opposed to random; see below) situs inversus, as well as cystic kidneys.
2. **N-cadherin** is asymmetrically expressed prior to gastrulation, whereas the activin receptor **ActRII** is expressed on the right side of the primitive streak following gastrulation.
3. **Sonic hedgehog**, the TGFβ family member **Nodal**, and the transcription factor **Snail** localize expression in the lateral mesoderm to the left side of the node.

The direction of rotation (clockwise or anticlockwise) of nodal cilia is critical for determining left–right symmetry. One of the first signs of correct left–right body patterning is that the heart tube veers to the right. However, ciliary dysfunction due to mutations of axonemal **dyneins** gives rise to **random visceral orientation** (i.e., a 50% incidence of **situs inversus** – having the heart and liver on the wrong sides) in the autosomal recessive disorder **Kartagener syndrome**. Individuals with complete situs inversus are usually OK, but those with partial left–right disorganization may find themselves in deep trouble. Random left–right orientation may also be caused by mutations affecting activin, Sonic hedgehog, and **Wnt**.

Developmental cell fate is specified by *Wnts*

The fate of embryonic cells is specified by similar (paralogous) pathways in flies, worms, frogs, and humans. This is unfortunate, since it means that human developmental signaling pathways can only be discussed using the bizarre molecular nomenclature developed by fruitfly-and-frog scientists. Nonetheless, **Wnt** (*wingless* in flies; Figure 16.6A) is a critical family of extracellular ligands that activates these cell fate pathways. Each of the 40- to 45-kDa Wnt (pronounced "wint") ligands bind either G-protein-coupled receptors of the **Frizzled** (Fz) family, or else receptors of the single transmembrane domain **LDL receptor-related protein** (LRP) family. Activation of Frizzled recruits the multifunctional signaling protein **Disheveled** (Dsh) – which regulates cell polarity during gastrulation – to the plasma membrane. This leads to inhibition of glycogen synthase kinase 3β (GSK-3β) which nor-

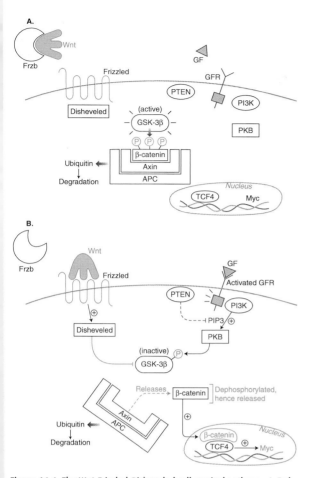

Figure 16.6 The Wnt-Frizzled-Disheveled cell survival pathway. *A*, Frzb sequesters Wnt, thereby opposing activation of its homolog Frizzled. This permits continued activation of glycogen synthase kinase-3β (GSK-3β), thus specifying the phosphorylated β-catenin–axin–APC complex for degradation. *B*, Activation of Frizzled and Disheveled leads to inhibition of GSK-3β, releasing β-catenin to the nucleus.

mally phosphorylates β-catenin and thus promotes its ubiquitin-dependent proteolysis (p. 138).

Wnt-dependent GSK-3β inhibition triggers dissociation of the APC/Axin complex (p. 214), thus releasing free dephosphorylated β-catenin into the cytosol. This leads in turn to the nuclear translocation of β-catenin, followed by its binding to the HMG-box transcription factor TCF4 that induces Wnt target genes (Figure 16.6*B*). *Wnt* knockouts exhibit abnormalities of the central nervous system, kidney, hair and pigmentation.

TCF4 is a transcriptional repressor when bound to **Groucho**, but the binding of β-catenin reveals a transactivation domain that triggers the TCF4-dependent induction of Myc. This initiates a symmetry-breaking pathway during development which results in tissue differentiation (e.g., myogenesis) via genes such as *Pax3*, *Myf5* and *MyoD*. A secreted protein with homology to the ligand-binding domain of Frizzled, **Frzb** (pronounced "frisbee"), antagonizes Wnt and Frizzled signaling by competitively binding Wnts (Figure 16.6*A*). In mice *Wnt* functions as an oncogene, but human *Wnt* appears to be only indirectly involved in tumor formation (e.g., in colorectal cancer, desmoid tumors, hepatoblastoma, or melanoma) via the β-catenin-dependent activation of *Myc*. Since Wnt requires downstream β-catenin signaling for its activity, β-catenin is considered a proto-oncogene.

In knockout models β-catenin loss causes anterior cells in the embryo to become posterior. Inhibition of the β-catenin signaling pathway also prevents Wnt signaling, leading to differentiation of adipocytes. Wnt signaling thus mediates inductive interactions that are critical for the normal development of the body axis, limbs, adipose tissue, and breast. Graphic examples include *headless* zebrafish induced by a loss-of-function TCF3 mutant which fails to inhibit Wnt signaling; and ectopic head formation in frog embryos triggered by **Dickkopf** (Dkk-1; German *kopf*, head; *dick*, fat), which inhibits Wnt signaling by competitively binding its "second receptor" **LRP5/6**. The latter model system was the first to demonstrate Wnt-dependent formation of master signaling centers termed organizers.

MOLECULAR MINIREVIEW

Organizers

Together with the TGFβ signaling pathway, the Wnt signaling system governs the establishment of primordial signaling centers within the gastrula. Two master cell clumps called **organizers** trigger the cascade of inductive signals that specify embryonic pattern formation:

1. The **head organizer**
   - Located in the anterior visceral endoderm.
2. The **trunk organizer**
   - Found in the distal primitive streak within dorsal mesoderm.

By specifying the head and trunk, the proximal–distal asymmetry of these organizers is translated into the antero–posterior **polarity** of the embryo. This process is mediated in part by **Cripto** ligands of the epidermal growth factor family. Transplantation of organizers to heterologous gastrulas results in the formation of a second embryonic body axis.

Organizer cells are richly endowed with inhibitory ligands. These include the TGFβ-superfamily **bone morphogenetic proteins**, or **BMPs**, which mediate developmental bone growth (p. 421). Crosstalk between the Wnt and TGFβ signaling pathways within organizers is illustrated by the formation of an intranuclear complex involving β-catenin, TCF4 and Smad4. Moreover, BMP and Wnt signaling determines the formation of the heart and blood from the anterior and posterior mesoderm, respectively: BMP availability plays a permissive role in both processes, whereas Wnts (e.g., Wnt3a, Wnt8) promote blood development while repressing cardiogenesis. Heart development may also be repressed by BMP antagonists (e.g., Chordin, Noggin; p. 421), or else stimulated by the secretion of Wnt antagonists (e.g., Crescent, Dkk-1 or Frzb). Hence, heart and blood formation appear to be opposite developmental choices, both of which are regulated by GATA-family transcription factors (p. 454).

Patched inhibits Smoothened in the absence of Hedgehogs

Unlike intracellular signaling in adult tissues, developmental signaling often occurs via sequential inhibitory interactions. This is well illustrated by the Hedgehog-Patched-Smoothened signaling pathway which, like the Notch signaling pathway (p. 404), is central to embryonic pattern formation. **Patched** (PTCH) is a 12-transmembrane domain ion channel with segment-polarity activity which structurally resembles the proton-dependent lipid translocator mutated in type C1 **Niemann-Pick disease**. Signaling from the mitogenic G-protein-coupled receptor **Smoothened** (Smo) – a Frizzled homolog – is inhibited by Patched (Figure 16.7A). **Sonic hedgehog** (Shh) in turn antagonizes the negative effect of Patched. By facilitating Smo signaling in this manner, Shh triggers activation of the serine-threonine kinase **Fused** and the zinc finger transactivator **Gli** (Figure 16.7B). The latter (so named for being first detected in mutant form in gliomas) induces Wnt signaling, and is thus repressed by

Figure 16.7 The Patched–Smoothened–Wnt–Hedgehog signaling pathways during development. *A*, Inhibition of the Smoothened proto-oncogene by unligated Patched. This inhibition is abolished by loss-of-function *Patched* mutations, as shown. *B*, Activation of Smoothened (by loss-of-function mutations or ligation by Sonic) leads to activation of the Fused–Gli–Wnt signaling pathway, thus promoting cell survival. BCC, Basal cell carcinoma.

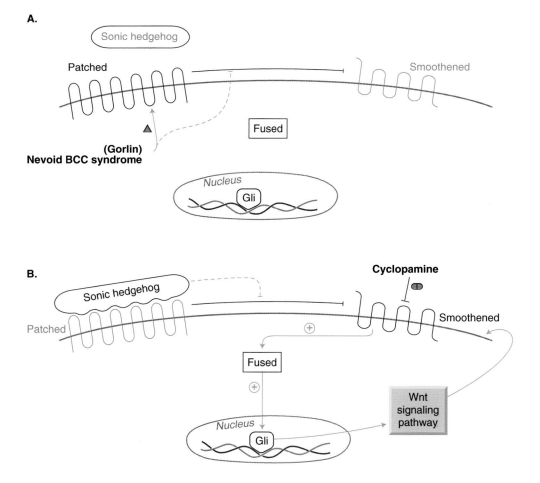

Patched and derepressed by Shh. The tumor suppressor activity of Patched (see below) is thus attributable to its inhibitory effects on Wnt and Smo signaling. For similar reasons, Smo and Gli are proto-oncogenes.

Signals initiated by Shh are required for an embryonic hand to distinguish, say, its thumb from its fifth finger. This process is initiated by induction of the dHAND transactivator in the posterior limb bud, triggering local Shh release. Murine knockout of Shh leads to **cyclopia** (fusion of two eyes into one), **holoprosencephaly** and other drastic central nervous system defects. Still other lesions occur in tissues where Shh is not transcribed, however, confirming that Hedgehog pattern-forming ligands (which include Echidna, Desert, and Tiggy-Winkle in addition to Shh) are diffusible. Relevant to this, the carboxy-terminal domain of Hedgehog exhibits both autoproteolytic activity and cholesterol transferase activity: extracellular release of the bioactive amino-terminal Hedgehog fragment (HhN) is thus accompanied by the addition of cholesterol to the cleavage site of the processed ligand. This modification makes HhN bind more tightly to Patched, impairing ligand diffusion within the extracellular space. Short- and long-range signaling by Hedgehogs can thus be modulated by autoprocessing.

CLINICAL KEYNOTE

Basal cell carcinomas and *Patched*

Monoallelic knockout of *Patched* gives rise to large transgenic mice prone to hindlimb defects and/or cerebellar **medulloblastomas**. In humans, the rare hereditary **Gorlin syndrome** of **multiple nevoid basal cell carcinomas** (BCCs) of the skin associated with medulloblastomas and ovarian fibromas also arises because of truncation mutants of *Patched* that activate the Smoothened signaling pathway (Figure 16.7).

Parallels have been drawn between the occurrence of BCCs in Gorlin syndrome and of colonic polyps in **familial adenomatous polyposis** (FAP). Aneuploidy is lacking in both lesion sets, indicating that both *APC* and *Patched* act as gatekeeper-style tumor suppressor genes. Consistent with this, 40% of sporadic (sun-induced) BCCs and 20% of sporadic medulloblastomas harbor biallelic *Patched* mutations. Basal cell carcinomas are inducible in transgenic mice by Shh overexpression while Gli is overexpressed in sporadic BCCs even when Shh is not. Approximately 20% of nonhereditary BCCs contain activating mutations of *Smo* (especially 1604 G→T, Trp→Leu) in the absence of loss-of-function *Patched* mutations. Similarly, *Gli* is amplified in some brain tumors and sarcomas.

Pregnant sheep deliver offspring with cyclops deformities after eating lilies (*Veratrum californicum*) containing the aptly-named chemical **cyclopamine**. It turns out that cyclopamine is a Hedgehog pathway inhibitor – acting downstream of Patched but upstream of Gli, making Smo the likely target – that also arrests BCC cell growth in vitro, indicating a therapeutic significance.

Hair follicle formation is mediated by β-catenin and Hedgehog. Epithelial morphogenesis is also regulated by the TNF-family **ectodermal dysplasia and anhidrosis** – or *EDA* – gene. Human *EDA* loss-of-function mutants exhibit alopecia, anhidrosis, and edentulousness (i.e., no hair, sweat or teeth).

Retinoids are potent morphogens and teratogens

Retinoic acid (RA) is one member of the retinoid family – a molecular group not only important for retinal vision but also for the spatial "vision" of

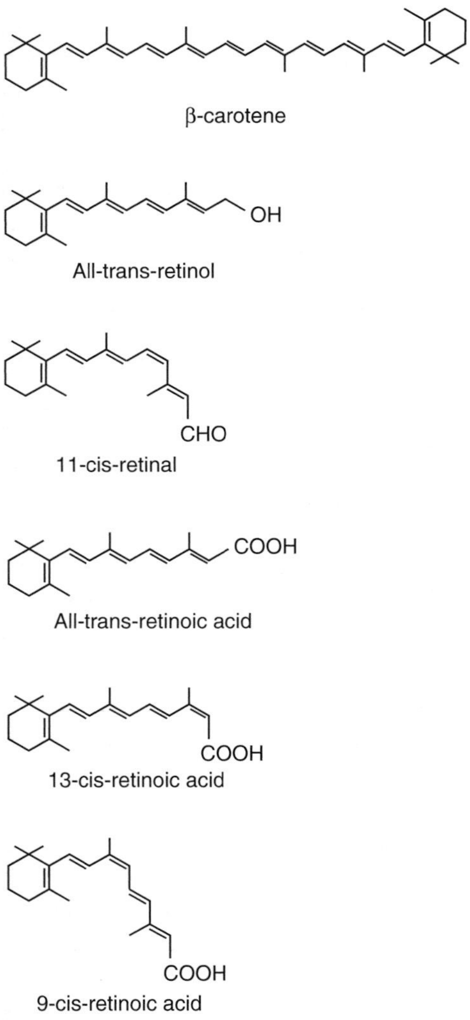

β-carotene

All-trans-retinol

11-cis-retinal

All-trans-retinoic acid

13-cis-retinoic acid

9-cis-retinoic acid

Figure 16.8 Chemical structures of the retinoid family.

Figure 16.9 Diverse effects of retinoic acid on gene expression and embryonic development.

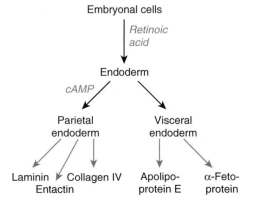

developing cells (Figure 16.8). Retinoids induce the expression of embryonic pattern-forming genes that regulate formation of the central nervous system, limbs, face, and digits. Note that the same ligand can have distinct effects in different tissues (Figure 16.9), consistent with the variety of retinoid receptor dimers.

The differentiating effects of retinoids may be related to the histone acetylation of target genes. The hypoxia-inducible **CBP/p300** transcriptional co-regulator – a histone acetyltransferase required for p53-dependent apoptosis – is required for RA-induced differentiation, suggesting that the latter process may require p53-dependent growth arrest. Increased expression of the Cdk inhibitor p27^{Kip1} and reduced *Myc* expression is also implicated as part of the RA differentiation pathway. These effects may be relevant to the antitumor effects of retinoids, such as those implicated in the chemoprevention of skin and mouth cancers. Of note, however, dietary supplementation with the retinol precursor β-**carotene** has been associated with more (rather than fewer) lung cancer deaths.

Exogenous retinoids are powerful **teratogens** that predispose to congenital limb malformations (such as syndactyly and phocomelia), cranial defects, and neural tube deformities. A notorious retinoid in this respect is the drug **13-cis-retinoic acid (isotretinoin)** which is prescribed for **cystic (conglobate) acne**. The therapeutic effects of this drug are mediated via retinoic acid γ receptors (**RAR**γ) in skin; transgenic knockout of RARγ is associated with skin fragility. In contrast, the teratogenic effects of isotretinoin affect the central nervous system (especially the hindbrain), craniofacial mesenchyme, branchial arches, and limb buds (Figure 16.10). These latter tissues are distinguished by high levels of cellular retinoic-acid-binding proteins or **CRABPs** which – like cellular retinol-binding proteins (**CRBPs**), fatty acid-binding proteins, and myelin P2 protein – sequester hydrophobic ligands and transfer them to the nucleus. In general, the tissue abundance of CRABPs varies inversely with that of RARs.

CLINICAL KEYNOTE

Waardenburg syndromes

Gene products that regulate the embryo's spatial organization fall into two main groups: (1) diffusible morphogens (especially activin, TGFβ, bFGF, and retinoic acid), and (2) transcriptional regulators. The latter include **Hox** (homeobox; see below) proteins, **Pax** (paired-box) proteins, and **Sox** (SRY-box; p. 413) proteins.

Pax1 mediates thymus and vertebral disc development, whereas **Pax2** is involved in renal and optic development and **Pax3** in neural crest maturation. Mutations affecting *Pax3* underlie the dominant white spotting (white forelock and deafness) disorder **Waardenburg syndrome type I** (*splotch* in mice; p. 580). The occurrence of neural tube defects in *splotch* mice reflects abnormal folate metabolism such as is also implicated in **spina bifida** in humans (Figure 16.11).

Waardenburg syndrome type II arises because of mutations of the basic helix-loop-helix transcription factor **Microphthalmia** (**Mi**). Activation of *Kit* leads to phosphorylation of Mi, which (under normal circumstances) transactivates the *tyrosinase* gene promoter responsible for melanin production and pigmentation. Hence, melanocyte dysfunction appears the common thread underlying this phenotype, and explains why mutations affecting c-Kit also cause the dominant white spotting phenotype (**piebaldism**; p. 338).

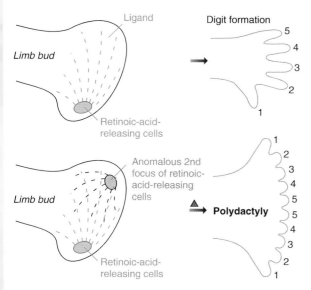

Figure 16.10 Experimental demonstration of retinoid patterning effects. Injection of retinoic acid into a second site on the limb bud (lower diagrams) causes polydactyly.

Figure 16.11 Spina bifida occulta (Wellcome Medical Photographic Library, no. N0004643C).

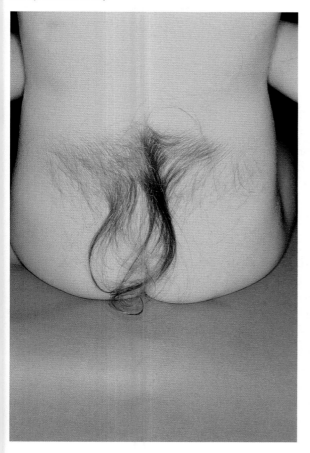

Homeobox gene clusters are activated in sequence

As a rule of thumb, any gene whose name ends in X probably has something to do with development. This is because conserved gene sequence similarities between species are termed **boxes** (e.g., paired box, SRY box; see above), and such conservation in turn suggests a developmental role. **Homeobox (*Hox*) genes** are ancient genes that specify cell fate in the antero–posterior embryonic axis and thus determine body plan. By activating the expression of subsidiary transcription factors, *Hox* genes encode positional information critical to the maturation of body parts such as limb buds.

As many as 40 *Hox* genes are responsible for limb formation alone. Each digit is specified by a separate gene; digital identity is conferred by BMP signaling from interdigital mesoderm prior to its regression into the web space. DNA-binding proteins encoded by *Hox* genes regulate the expression of other genes in a hierarchical fashion. For example, body-part-determining (**homeotic**; i.e., resemblance-causing) genes may regulate the activity of tissue-determining genes which may in turn control the activity of enzymes, adhesion molecules, and structural genes. At least 20 such genes may be controlled by a master *Hox* gene during the formation of any body part; examples of downstream transcription factors required for such normal pattern development are listed in Table 6.1.

Despite the vast phylogenetic distance separating humans and invertebrates, homologies between human *Hox* genes and those of insects (e.g., *Drosophila*) have been maintained. Such evolutionary conservation illuminates morphogenetic history, suggesting as it does that heads have evolved (for example) via the lower spinal segments of headless ancestors.

The common 61-amino-acid motif encoded by the 183-bp *Hox* gene sequence is termed a **homeodomain** (Figure 16.12*A*), an α-helical protein domain that binds specific DNA consensus sequences. Intraembryonic gradients of homeodomain-containing proteins convey positional information necessary for normal development. Mutations of *Hox* genes may thus cause **homeotic transformation** with visible deformity such as the replacement of one body part with another. Conversely, potent morphogens such as retinoic acid co-operate with fibroblast growth factors in limb bud development by simulating the action of *HoxB*. Of note, not all homeodomain-containing proteins are *Hox* gene products: examples of non-Hox homeoproteins include Msx2, Hesx1, Emx2, and SHOX (see Table 16.1).

Like all mammals, humans have four major *Hox* gene clusters – **A** to **D** – on separate chromosomes (Figure 16.12*B*), with each cluster containing about ten genes (39 in all). These gene clusters evolved through duplication of the primordial invertebrate homeotic gene complex. Developmental activation of *Hox* genes occurs in a 5′ to 3′ chromosomal sequence which exhibits co-linearity with posterior-to-anterior patterns of body axis expression (Figure 16.13). Domains of these genes overlap like Russian dolls, structurally interlinking the order of their expression within developing limbs. Hence, the spacing of mammalian *Hox* gene clusters correlates with the developmental timing of body part formation, suggesting upstream regulatory mechanisms similar to those mediating embryonic switching of the hemoglobin genes (p. 453). These upstream cis-regulatory elements have been conserved throughout phylogeny (similar to the *Hox* gene clusters themselves).

Hox gene activity may regulate cell proliferation and/or survival, and is implicated in neoplasia: examples include *HoxA5* in **breast cancer**; *HoxA9* and

A.

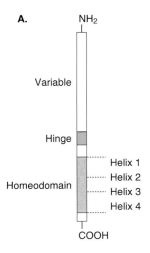

B.

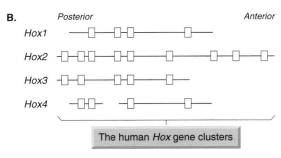

Figure 16.12 Homeobox genes and proteins. *A*, Homeobox (Hox) protein, showing the position of the homeodomain and its constituent helices. *B*, Relative chromosomal alignments of the *Hox* gene clusters, showing the common antero–posterior directionality of the developing anatomic regions so regulated.

Mutated transcription factor	Congenital malformation or syndrome
Sox9	**Campomelic dysplasia** (testicular maldevelopment with feminization, cleft palate, tibial bowing)
SHOX	**Leri–Weill dyschondrosteosis** (short stature and short mesomelic limbs)
HoxD13	Synpolydactyly, hypospadias (severity depends upon the size of the trinucleotide insert encoding polyalanine)
Msx2	Craniosynostosis, short first metatarsal (due to gain-of-function mutations)
Hesx1	**Septo-optic dysplasia**
Emx2	**Schizencephaly**
Pax 2	Vesicoureteric reflux, renal dysplasia, optic colobomas (heterozygotes)
Pax 3	**Waardenburg syndromes I and III** (pigmentary abnormalities, deafness, and dystopia canthorum, i.e., wide-spaced eyes)
Pax 6	Aniridia (heterozygotes), anophthalmia (homozygotes)
MITF (microphthalmia-associated transcription factor)	**Waardenburg syndrome II** (like WSI, plus hand, limb and craniofacial anomalies, but no dystopia canthorum)
POU3F4	**X-linked deafness**
WT1	**Denys–Drash syndrome** (Wilms tumor, renal failure, hermaphroditism)
Treacle	**Treacher–Collins syndrome** (mandibulofacial dysostosis)
CBP	**Rubinstein–Taybi syndrome**
Gli3	**Greig syndrome** (polydactyly of hands and feet, macrocephaly)

Table 16.1. Transcription factor mutations in birth defects

Figure 16.13 Illustration of overlapping *Hox* gene sequences correlating with the developing embryonic anatomy.

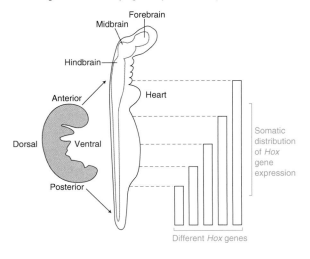

HoxA10 in **acute myeloid leukemia**; and *Hox11* in T cell acute lymphoblastic leukemia. Of note, *Hox11* also controls spleen formation.

Differentiation

Cell growth and differentiation are often inversely related

Only about 10–20% of the average cell's 30 000 genes are active, and the majority of these active genes are non-tissue-specific housekeeping genes. Cell differentiation is the process by which a cell restricts the function of most of its genome to match the specialized needs of its tissue or organ system. This involves long-term changes in transcription factor availability, which may be accompanied by genomic alterations such as chromatin condensation, cytosine methylation, and histone deacetylation. Differentiating neurons of the central nervous system increase their nuclear diameters to as large as 25 μm. Specialized genes are amplified in a few cell types, but this is exceptional; most of an individual's cells contain identical genomic DNA despite tissue-specific differences in gene expression.

Some differentiated cells are capable of proliferation while others are not. Certain studies indicate that neurons, formerly regarded as nondividing, may be capable of replicating in adults. Of note, neuronal differentiation is actively inducible via cytokines such as BMP9 which induces the cholinergic phenotype by triggering the coordinated expression of acetylcholine, choline acetyltransferase, and the vesicular acetylcholine transporter.

In cell types which normally proliferate, the in vitro induction of differentiation is often associated with repression of genes mediating cell growth – just as continuous growth induction may prevent differentiation. A graphic illustration of the reciprocal relationship between growth and differentiation is seen in cancer, where uncontrolled cell growth is typically accompanied by progressive loss of the differentiated phenotype. Rare tumors such as pediatric **neuroblastoma** may spontaneously regress in vivo. Similarly, residual radiographic masses following the chemotherapy of germ cell tumors may prove to be **differentiated teratomas** rather than viable tumors.

Embryogenesis is a period of massive cell growth, but is also characterized by widespread cell death or apoptosis. Body patterns are sculpted from viable tissues, rather than being lain down in exact sequence; for example, embryonic fingers are heavily webbed, but this webbing normally disappears as the fetus grows. Similar apoptotic cascades underlie the healthy maturation of the cerebral circuitry, but chronic ethanol ingestion may impair neural cell adhesion and thus precipitate the cerebral neuronal apoptosis characteristic of **fetal alcohol syndrome**.

MOLECULAR MINIREVIEW

In vitro models of cell differentiation

Cell culture models of inducible differentiation include:
1. Retinoic acid→embryonal carcinoma (EC) cell differentiation.
2. Leukemia inhibitory factor→embryonal stem (ES) cell differentiation.
3. 5-azacytidine→mouse erythroleukemia (MEL) cell differentiation.
4. Nerve growth factor→pheochromocytoma (PC12) cell differentiation.

Retinoic acid (RA) is a powerful inducer of cell differentiation, in which context it may modulate extracellular matrix protein synthesis and MHC gene expression. Retinoids are used in the clinic as differentiation therapy for adult-onset neoplastic and preneoplastic conditions: for example, the malignancy **acute promyelocytic leukemia**, and the premalignant oral condition **leukoplakia**, may be responsive to RA.

The short-chain fatty acid **sodium butyrate** inhibits histone deacetylases – presumably by competing with acetyl groups at the substrate level – and hence increases histone hyperacetylation. The resultant chromatin decondensation leads to cell differentiation via activation of the $p21^{Cip1}$ gene. High luminal concentrations (10–20 mM) of butyrate derived from the fermentation of ingested carbohydrates ("fiber") by symbiotic intestinal microflora may trigger colorectal epithelial cell apoptosis either via this route, or else via the ceramide-Jnk pathway (p. 291), and thereby contribute to dietary prevention of **colorectal cancer**. Topical butyrate enemas increase mucosal vascularity and oxygen uptake in damaged colorectal epithelium, and may be used with therapeutic benefit in inflammatory conditions such as **acute radiation proctitis**.

Nonspecific inducers of in vitro differentiation include polar solvents such as **dimethylsulfoxide** (DMSO) that act by altering cell membrane potential.

Differentiation is inducible by tissue-specific gene silencing

Despite the frequent reciprocal relationship between growth and differentiation, a few physiologic stimuli trigger both pathways. These include:

1. Antigen binding by surface immunoglobulin on B cells
   - Leads to clonal expansion *and* plasmacyte differentiation (pp. 475–7).
2. Hemopoietic cytokine stimulation of bone marrow precursors
   - Causes lineage determination *and* cell proliferation.

During erythropoiesis there is a progressive reduction in nuclear size (late-stage normoblasts are only 5 μm in diameter) accompanied by an increase in compacted chromatin and reduced transcriptional activity. Unlike pluripotential stem cells – undifferentiated cell progenitors capable of unlimited self-renewal – most cells become committed to a terminally differentiated lineage. Pathologic insults may cause **retrodifferentiation** of such cells to a less specialized phenotype.

Tissue-specific phenotypes may be induced by microenvironmental crosstalk between cells, extracellular matrix proteins, and soluble signaling molecules. Much of this crosstalk arises from contiguous cells expressing tissue-specific cell-surface or soluble ligands.

MOLECULAR MINIREVIEW

Notch, Delta, and lateral inhibition

Molecular studies of *Drosophila* have clarified how embryonic neurons develop within a field of non-neuronal cells. Impaired signaling from the transmembrane receptor **Notch** may result in conversion of the entire cell field to neurons, reflecting overcommitment of ectodermal cells to the neural (rather than epidermal) lineage. The extracellular domain of Notch contains 36 EGF-like repeats, whereas the intracellular domain contains 6 ankyrin repeats. Notch signaling in non-neuronal cells is activated by extracellular binding of other transmembrane molecules – either **Delta** or **Serrate** – expressed on nascent neurons. The interaction of Delta or Serrate with Notch is modified in the Golgi by Fringe-family glycosyltransferases (e.g., **Lunatic Fringe**, **Manic Fringe**, **Radical Fringe**) which elongate fucosyl residues attached to EGF-like repeats near the Notch ligand-binding domain.

The intracellular domain of Notch binds a transcriptional regulator termed **CSL**. Proteolytic CSL cleavage by ADAM disintegrin metalloproteases (e.g., **Kuzbanian**) releases bioactive ligand fragments that diffuse into the extracellular space until binding Notch receptors on nearby cells. Ligand binding in turn activates juxtamembrane domain cleavage of Notch by γ-**secretase** (the same protease that cleaves amyloid precursor protein in **Alzheimer disease**), triggering nuclear translocation of CSL and Notch-dependent gene induction. This activation of Notch on adjacent cells triggers an inhibitory signaling pathway, with such **lateral inhibition** preventing neighboring non-neuronal cells from undergoing neural morphogenesis. Mutations of Notch3 cause accumulation of the defective protein within the vasculature, leading to the syndrome of **CADASIL** (cerebral autosomal dominant arteriopathy with subcortical infarcts and leukoencephalopathy).

Muscles develop in response to the master gene *MyoD*

Skeletal muscle development is controlled by a family of proteins that are expressed at different times during embryogenesis (Figure 16.14). Fibroblast-to-myoblast conversion is inducible in vitro by demethylation of a single locus containing the critical developmental gene *MyoD* (myogenic determi-

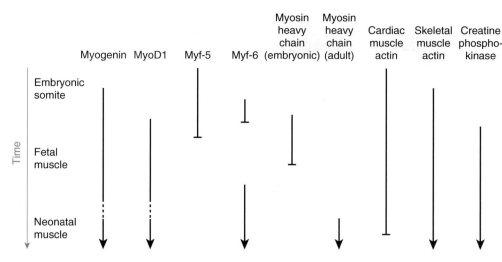

Figure 16.14 Relative timing of gene expression involved in muscle development.

nation factor). *MyoD* encodes a basic helix-loop-helix (bHLH) transcription factor that orchestrates the myogenic program by binding to E-box sequences (CACCTG) in the promoters of muscle-specific genes; other members of this master gene family have been identified in cardiac myocytes and in osteoblasts. The bHLH transcription factor family is divided into three groups:

1. Tissue-specific inducers (e.g., MyoD).
2. Enhancers (e.g., **E12, MEF2**) that heterodimerize with inducers.
3. Repressors (e.g., **Id** – inhibitor of differentiation) that heterodimerize to suppress activation of inducers by preventing enhancer binding.

Myogenic conversion can be induced in differentiated cell lines by expressing MyoD. Antagonism of myodifferentiation by expression of the immediate-early protein Jun may reflect direct association of Jun with the leucine zipper of MyoD. A point mutation affecting the 13-amino-acid DNA-binding domain of MyoD may impart Myc-like properties to the mutant protein; conversely, myogenic capability may be conferred upon the nonspecific E12 bHLH enhancer by substituting as few as three residues from the MyoD basic region. Myoblast differentiation is accompanied by the shuttling of a histone deacetylase (**HDAC5**) from the nucleus to the cytoplasm, permitting dissolution of HDAC5–MEF2 complexes and thus facilitating the transactivation of MEF2-dependent genes by MyoD/MEF2 heterodimers.

MyoD is one of several muscle proteins that are transcriptionally regulated by neuromuscular activity. **Myogenin** and the **Myf** proteins (Myf-5, Myf-6) are also myogenic helix-loop-helix trans-activators; null mutations of MyoD cause compensatory expression of Myf-5. Like MyoD, transgenic knockout of Myf-5 is associated with normal skeletal muscle development despite abnormalities of lateral sclerotome formation. In contrast, transgenic knockout of myogenin leads to muscle dysfunction, indicating that this gene (unlike *MyoD* or *Myf-5*) is indispensable for muscle development.

The differentiating activity of MyoD depends upon the retinoblastoma protein (pRb) that reversibly binds MyoD. Cell growth arrest due to pRb hypophosphorylation accompanies TGFβ-dependent Cdk4 inhibition; consistent with this, Cdk4 inhibitors such as p16^{INK4A} activate muscle-specific gene expression and myoblast differentiation. Such pathways may underlie the TGFβ-dependent **epithelial–mesenchymal transformation** of embryonic cardiac endothelial cells that is needed for the formation of valves and septa.

Molecular pathology of congenital heart disease

Inherited cardiac diseases may exhibit genetic locus heterogeneity: examples include **hypertrophic cardiomyopathy** (over 100 mutations; p. 247) and **long QT syndrome** (at least five mutations; p. 184). Congenital cardiac syndromes include:

1. **Holt–Oram syndrome**: atrial (or ventricular) septal defect + polydactyly (often)
   - Caused by mutations affecting the **TBX5** T-box transcription factor. Of note, 5′ mutations in TBX5 genes tend to cause more cardiac than skeletal lesions, whereas 3′ lesions cause more skeletal than cardiac defects.
2. **Atrial septal defect** with AV conduction defects
   - Caused by mutations affecting the homeobox **NKX2-5** transcription factor (a homolog of the fruitfly *tinman* gene).
3. **Pulmonary stenosis** may be caused by mutations of the genes for **Jagged-1, connexin-43, neurotrophin-3** or the **TrkC receptor**.
4. **Tetralogy of Fallot** may occur with mutations of genes encoding **Jagged-1** or **NKX2-5**.
5. **Dilated cardiomyopathies** may result from mutations affecting the genes for any of several α-actinin-binding proteins; for example, muscle LIM-domain protein (**MLP**), **desmin**, or **titin**.
6. **Patent ductus arteriosus** arises because of mutations affecting the transcription factor **TFAP2B**.
7. **Aortic aneurysms** (p. 236) may be caused by mutations disrupting **fibrillin**
8. Gene mutations affecting **elastin** cause **supravalvar aortic stenosis** (p. 230).

Normal cardiac aortopulmonary valve development depends upon the T cell transcription factor **NF-ATc** which regulates signals contributing to embryonic valvulogenesis. **DiGeorge syndrome** (conotruncal heart defects – truncus arteriosus, tetralogy of Fallot – thymic/parathyroid aplasia, facial dysmorphism) arises because of a heterozygous deletion of chromosome 22q11.2 causing haploinsufficiency of the *Tbx1* gene, which mediates the pharyngeal endoderm–mesenchyme interactions required for normal aortic arch segmentation.

Genomic imprinting

Maternal and paternal alleles are separately imprinted

The human race cannot do without sex. To put it another way, humans have difficulty cloning themselves asexually – in contrast, certain animals can reproduce either by parthenogenesis (virgin birth, i.e., from two sets of haploid female chromosomes) or by having one zygotic female pronucleus removed and substituted by a male-sex pronuclear transplant. Such clones have not yet been forthcoming in human cell systems, which suggests that the genetic contributions of male and female gametes are complementary rather than simply additive.

Notwithstanding the advent of cloning by somatic nuclear transfer (p. 582), unfertilized diploid genomes tend to be bad evolutionary news for mammals. This is probably because uniparental diploid genomes incorporate a double dose of recessive genes and thus predispose to germline extinction. An alternative explanation is that maternal genes have evolved to reduce the nurturing demands of the offspring on the mother, whereas paternal genes are concerned only with maximizing offspring size and hence evolutionary fitness. The degree to which such genes are expressed varies with their parent of origin: these alleles are marked or **imprinted** in the germ line – probably during meiosis – enabling them to remember, as it were, from which parent they came (Figure 16.15). Since imprinting affects whole genomic regions rather than operating on a gene-by-gene basis, this process is termed **genomic imprinting**. Properties of this process include:

1. Imprinting is reversible
   - Unlike mutations or polymorphisms.
2. Imprinting persists through multiple rounds of DNA replication
   - Unlike DNA damage.
3. Imprinting is heritable
   - Unlike microenvironmentally determined patterns of gene expression.

Imprinting (parental allele-specific gene expression) makes the phenotypic contributions of parental alleles unequal: a filly mating with an ass yields a mule, but a stallion servicing a she-ass yields a hinny. However, since the expression of most human genes is identical in maternal and paternal gene copies, this parent-of-origin effect is only relevant to a minority of genes.

The phenomenon of genomic imprinting probably involves differential germline methylation of large GC-rich chromosomal domains. Such domains undergo parent-specific asynchronous DNA replication during S phase from the time of gametogenesis until completion of embryogenesis. Note that **random monoallelic expression** is also characteristic of certain nonimprinted genes, including X-inactivated genes (see below) as well as those encoding IL-2, T cell receptors, and olfactory receptors.

MOLECULAR MINIREVIEW

IGF2 imprinting

The **insulin-like growth factor-2** (*IGF2*) gene undergoes imprinting in both humans and mice (Figure 16.16). Expression of *IGF2* is turned on throughout the embryo in terms of the paternal allele, but off with respect to the maternal allele (except in the choroid plexus and meninges). Conversely, only the maternal allele for the IGF2 receptor is expressed. Because the *IGF2* gene is only expressed from the paternal chromosome during fetal life, the growth factor gene is said to be **maternally imprinted** – that is, the inactivated allele is the imprinted one – whereas the receptor gene is **paternally imprinted**.

Imprinting affects the promoters (especially P2, P3, P4) for *IGF2*. Transgenic mice expressing a dysfunctional mutant copy of the *igf2* gene of maternal origin are thus of normal size; in contrast, paternally transmitted *igf2* mutations result in small offspring as does maternal disomy (see below). Reciprocal imprinting is also seen between the paternal *igf2* (in mesodermal tissues) and maternal *H19* (in endodermal tissues) genes in mice, reflecting promoter competition for identical enhancers. Note that the *H19* mRNA is itself untranslated, but regulates *IGF2* expression.

Figure 16.15 Imprinting. Differential epigenetic modification (here shown in red) of parental genomic regions – for example, by methylation – results in allele-specific differences in gene expression that are independent of gene sequence. Genes are shown in black.

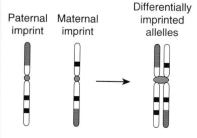

Paternal imprint   Maternal imprint   Differentially imprinted allelles

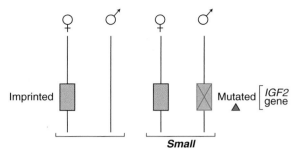

Figure 16.16 Maternal imprinting of the insulin-like growth factor-2 (*IGF2*) gene. Null mutation of the paternal allele alone leads to small body size.

Wilms, WAGR, Denys–Drash and Beckwith–Wiedemann

IGF2 expression is transcriptionally downregulated by the **WT1** repressor protein. Germline mutations of *WT1* (which maps to chromosome 11p13) may deregulate IGF2 production, and such mutations are associated with most cases of **Wilms tumor**. Male Wilms patients with associated aniridia, genitourinary malformations, and mental retardation exhibit the **WAGR syndrome**, whereas Wilms patients with intersex abnormalities and nephropathy exhibit **Denys–Drash syndrome**. These syndromes imply the involvement of additional genes (e.g., *Pax6* mutations causing aniridia) by more extensive chromosomal abnormalities such as deletions. **Hemihypertrophy** is another imprinting-associated phenotype related to this genetic locus (Figure 16.17).

Patients with the congenital overgrowth diathesis **Beckwith–Wiedemann syndrome** exhibit gigantism, macroglossia, exomphalos, neonatal hypoglycemia, and childhood cancers (including Wilms, rhabdomyosarcoma, and adrenal tumors). This condition is mainly transmitted via the female germline at the 11p15.5 locus, in which region approximately ten genes are imprinted. The resultant inappropriate relaxation of imprinting makes the maternal *IGF2* allele look as if it is dressed in male attire, genetically speaking. Some cases of Beckwith–Wiedemann syndrome carry two or three copies of paternal chromosome 11 with consequent overexpression of *IGF2*; that is, they exhibit paternal disomy or trisomy (see below). Unbalanced duplications of this kind are associated with a worse prognosis than are balanced rearrangements of maternal origin.

Chromosomal disomy decouples parental gene expression

Fusion of same-sex human gametes (uniparental chromosomal **disomy**) does not yield viable progeny. Disomy has the following teratogenic expressions:

1. Bimaternal genome (maternal disomy) →**ovarian teratoma**
   - Nonviable due to deficient extraembryonic (trophoblastic) tissues.
   - Can affect virgins (i.e., arises by parthenogenesis).
2. Bipaternal genome (paternal disomy) →**hydatidiform mole** ("water-like droplet")
   - Nonviable due to deficient embryonic (endodermal, mesodermal, ectodermal) tissues.
   - Cannot affect virgins.

When a nonaborted trisomic (triploid-chromosome) fetus loses a chromatid, a uniparental-disomic fetus will be the result in one-third of cases. Indeed, as many as 1% of live births may exhibit some degree of chromosomal disomy. Disomic phenotypes lack the appropriate parental gene contribution, with the relevant genes having been silenced by a nondeletional (cytogenetically normal) mechanism such as imprinting. Uniparental **heterodisomy** (two distinct chromosomes, i.e., from different-sex grandparents, contributed by the same parent) may be as pathogenic as **isodisomy** (two identical chromosome copies contributed by the same parent). Two parental alleles inherited from the index case's grandparents may thus function normally in the parent but not in the affected child – indicating that the abnormal phenotype derives from the transmission of these genes via a single parent rather than from the genes themselves. In contrast, isodisomy alone may lead to uniparental transmission of recessive disorders such as **cystic fibrosis, thalassemias, osteogenesis imperfecta, rod monochromacy** (p. 515) and **retinoblastoma** (Figure 16.18).

Much of what is known about human imprinting has been derived from

Figure 16.17 Hemihypertrophy, a common correlate of aniridia and Wilms' tumor (Wellcome Medical Photographic Library, no. N0004613C).

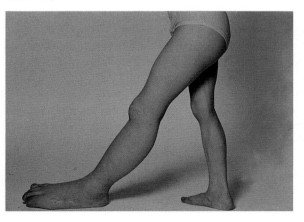

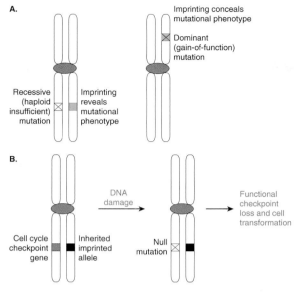

A.

Imprinting conceals mutational phenotype

Dominant (gain-of-function) mutation

Recessive (haploid insufficient) mutation

Imprinting reveals mutational phenotype

B.

DNA damage

Cell cycle checkpoint gene

Inherited imprinted allele

Null mutation

Functional checkpoint loss and cell transformation

Figure 16.18 Differential effects of imprinting. *A*, Imprinting may reveal the presence of a (haploinsufficient) mutation on the other allele, or conceal the presence of a gain-of-function mutation of the same allele. *B*, Damage-inducible mutation of a single checkpoint gene may lead to cell transformation in the presence of allelic imprinting.

sporadic instances of partial uniparental disomy. Studies of patients affected with two distinct congenital syndromes of mental retardation – **Angelman syndrome** ("happy puppet" – inappropriate laughter, ataxia, seizures) and **Präder–Willi syndrome** (obesity, short stature, hypogonadism, hypoactivity) – have provided evidence for genomic imprinting. These disorders may arise either due to errors affecting the postfertilization wave of gene methylation, or else due to deletions. Microdeletions of paternal chromosome 15q11-13 are detectable in Präder–Willi syndrome (indicating paternal disomy), whereas maternal deletions at the same chromosomal locus are associated with Angelman syndrome (indicating maternal disomy). The gene affected in both cases is that encoding the **GABA receptor** for the inhibitory brain neurotransmitter (pp. 497–8). Even in patients without cytogenetically detectable deletions, uniparental chromosomal disomy is often demonstrable.

CLINICAL KEYNOTE

Genomic imprinting in human disease

Imprinting has been implicated in different disease contexts, e.g.:
1. Autosomal dominant inheritance with parental bias
   - **Fragile X syndrome**.
   - **Myotonic dystrophy** (congenital form).
   - **Early-onset epilepsy**.
2. Parental-specific loss of heterozygosity
   - Sporadic **Wilms tumor**, **rhabdomyosarcoma** and **osteosarcoma**.
   - **Beckwith–Wiedemann syndrome**.

The effects of parental origin on other dominant and negative mutations are:
1. Maternal transmission usual (i.e., normal maternal allele not expressed)
   - Fragile X syndrome.
   - Myotonic dystrophy (congenital form).
   - **Neurofibromatosis I** (increased severity).
   - **Neurofibromatosis II** (earlier onset).
   - Early-onset epilepsy.
   - Sporadic Wilms tumor, osteosarcoma (loss of maternal alleles).
   - Beckwith–Wiedemann syndrome.
2. Paternal transmission usual (i.e., normal paternal allele not expressed)
   - **Familial glomus tumor**.
   - **Huntington disease** (early onset).
   - **Spinocerebellar ataxia** (early onset).

Many of the time-honored concepts of clinical genetics – such as **incomplete penetrance** and **variable expressivity** of genotypic changes – may be explained by imprinting. Nonimprinting sex-specific influences on inheritance are also recognized, however, such as maternal mitochondrial DNA transmission (p. 39).

Sex development

Females are mosaics of inactivated X chromosomes

Human females have two X chromosomes per diploid cell, unlike males who are **hemizygous** for the X chromosome. Since most X chromosomal genes are essential for function in both sexes – factor VIII and glucose-6-phosphate dehydrogenase being examples – X-linked **gene dosage compensation** is needed to

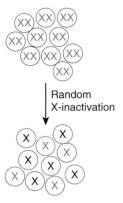

Figure 16.19 Random X chromosomal inactivation in embryonic cells. When postmeiotic paternal (black) and maternal (red) X chromosomes fuse following conception (top), the "choice" of which X is inactivated is random (bottom), leading to functional X chromosomal mosaicism in female offspring.

ensure equivalent expression in both sexes, thus avoiding double-dose X lethality. Certain species achieve dosage compensation by doubling X gene expression in males, whereas *SEX* genes in worms encode nuclear hormone receptors that count X chromosomes. In humans dosage compensation is achieved via a process of chromosomal condensation termed **X chromosome inactivation** (lyonization; Figure 16.19) which can thus be considered a form of whole-chromosomal imprinting for balancing male hemizygosity. Indeed, genomic imprinting may originally have evolved as a sex-chromosomal dosage compensation mechanism. X-inactivation is defined:

1. Functionally, by the presence of one transcriptionally active allele and one silent allele of most X chromosomal genes in a female nucleus.
2. Structurally, by an X-chromosomal **Barr body** of condensed heterochromatin which is cytogenetically visible in interphase nuclei.

Partly feminized XXY males (**Klinefelter syndrome**) exhibit Barr body formation; X chromosome inactivation is thus specified by the number of X chromosomes rather than by sexual phenotype. The Klinefelter sex-chromosome excess results from sperm chromosomal nondisjunction in 50% cases, from oocyte chromosome nondisjunction in 40%, and from postzygotic mitotic errors in the rest. Serum inhibin B levels are low, reflecting Sertoli cell loss due to testicular fibrosis.

Since somatic cells undergoing meiosis to form germ cells reactivate their X chromosomes for several cell cycles, this process is – like imprinting – reversible. Also like imprinting, a potential mechanism for X chromosome inactivation is methylation. Chromosomal methylation may only maintain (rather than initiate) X chromosomal inactivity, however, raising the question as to whether this modification is a cause or consequence of X chromosome inactivation. The hypermethylated X chromosome is replicated with other inactive chromatin towards the end of S phase, several hours after the replication of active genomic regions.

The long-range *cis*-gene regulation signaling of X chromosome inactivation is governed by a unique gene that expresses **X-inactivation-specific transcripts** (**XIST**) from a locus termed the **X-inactivation center** (**XIC**) at Xq13 on the inactivated chromosome (Figure 16.20). The 15-kb XIST transcript, which is not produced by the active X chromosome, does not contain any conserved open reading frames. This exclusively nuclear (untranslated) mRNA may therefore play a structural role by binding to the inactivated X chromosome and acting as a chromatin nucleation site immediately prior to X chromosome inactivation. Inactivated X chromosomes do not require the continued presence of XIC for transcriptional repression, however, suggesting that XIC may only play an initiating role in X chromosomal inactivation.

Figure 16.20 Role of the X-inactivation center (XIC) in X chromosomal condensation: whichever one is randomly inactivated specifies the active X chromosome.

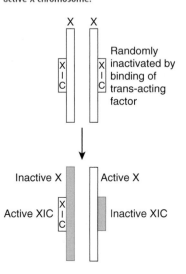

X-inactivation studies and tumor clonality

Inactivation of the 150-megabase X chromosome begins approximately three days after implantation of an XX blastocyst, at which time transcribing paternal X chromosomes (X^p) become selectively inactivated in extraembryonic (trophoblastic) tissues. Within 48 hours of this event, a wave of fetal X chromosome inactivation randomly affects either the paternally derived X chromosome or the maternally derived X chromosome (X^m) in each embryonic cell. This gives rise to distinct

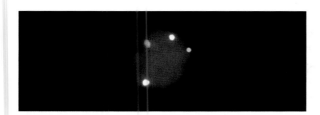

Figure 16.21 Normal male human cell showing the sex chromosomes. FISH probes: X chromosome green, Y chromosome red, chromosome 1 pair white. (Wellcome Medical Photographic Library, B0000355C05, Dr Joyce Harper)

paternal and maternal clones, making somatic female tissues a **mosaic** of parentally X-inactivated (and, thus, functionally hemizygous) cells (Figure 16.21).

Maternal **microchimerism** occurs when cells of maternal origin (i.e., XX) are identified in male individuals. Such microchimerism has been associated with the development in males of **autoimmune disorders** (which are more often seen in females) such as **dermatomyositis**; chimeric cells may initiate a graft-versus-host response directed against nonchimeric (XY) cells.

In females expressing polymorphic parental alleles, the clonality of neoplastic tumors may be assessed by demonstrating the presence (polyclonality) or absence (monoclonality) of such polymorphisms. In the case of the most popularly assayed trait – **glucose-6-phosphate dehydrogenase** – such polymorphisms reach useful frequencies only in African populations. The amplification of point mutant polymorphisms using polymerase chain reaction (PCR) may improve the utility of this approach.

Pseudautosomal regions express homologous X and Y alleles

Few genes besides XIST are expressed on the inactivated X chromosome. Notable exceptions are those genes in the Xp22.3 region adjacent to the **pseudautosomal region** common to both sex chromosomes (Figure 16.22).

Mammalian X and Y chromosomes probably originated from a homologous chromosome (autosome) pair that underwent rearrangement during the evolution of sex. The ancestry of this process is indicated by the presence of identical (>95% homologous) sequences in the subtelomeric (Xp22-Xpter, pseudautosomal) regions of Xp and the Y chromosome; these sequences undergo obligatory X-Y recombination during male meiosis. Of note, however, the **steroid sulfatase** and **amelogenin** (tooth bud protein) genes are located centromeric to the pseudautosomal region yet continue to be expressed in X-inactivated (Xi) chromosomes, as does the gene encoding the **granulocyte-macrophage colony-stimulating factor receptor**.

Another pseudautosomal-like gene in this region is that responsible for **Kallmann syndrome** (p. 211 and Figure 9.3). Before the responsible KAL gene product – an adhesion molecule guiding neuronal pathfinding (Figure 16.23) – was identified, a sixfold excess of affected males had suggested Kallmann syndrome to be X-linked. Deletion mapping and linkage analysis of affected families localized the putative *KAL* gene to Xp22.3; a cognate allele exists at Yq11.21. Hence, this regional Xp/Yq homology probably originated via displacement of a chromosomal fragment from the pseudautosomal region by Y-chromosomal pericentric inversion during primate evolution. Of note, nonpseudautosomal genes also occur within Xp22.3, giving rise to allelic pairs of activated X (Xa) and inactive Y copies in males; females express such genes from both X chromosomes, though expression of the Xi gene copy may be relatively reduced. A second pseudautosomal region lies near the Xq/Yq telomere.

Figure 16.22 The X chromosome, showing a subset of genes escaping X-inactivation, including the *XIST* gene on Xq.13, and the *ZFX* and *STS* genes in the pseudautosomal region of Xp.

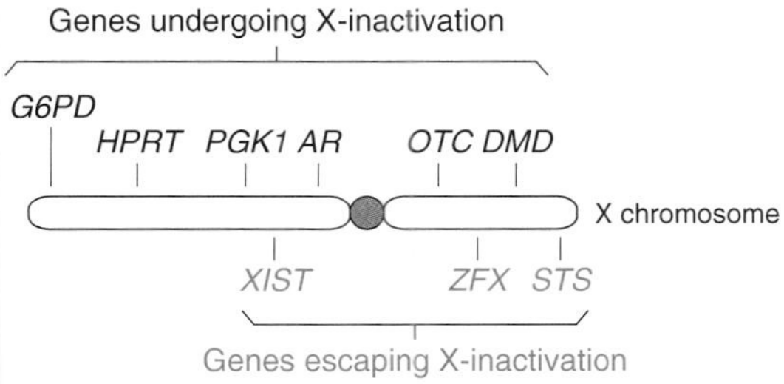

Genes undergoing X-inactivation

G6PD
HPRT PGK1 AR   OTC DMD
X chromosome

XIST   ZFX STS

Genes escaping X-inactivation

CLINICAL KEYNOTE

Turner syndrome

X-chromosomal loss is the only monosomy compatible with postnatal life, consistent with the usual hemizygous state of the X chromosome. Hemizygous 45XO females (**Turner syndrome**; monosomy X) exhibit a diverse phenotype that includes

Enrichment reading

Bedtime reading

Wolpert L. et al. *The principles of development.* Oxford University Press, Oxford, 1998

Cheap'n'cheerful

Ball P. *The self-made tapestry: pattern formation in nature.* Oxford University Press, Oxford, 1999

Library reference

Edelman GM. *Topobiology: an introduction to molecular embryology.* Basic Books, Barcelona, 1993

Strachan T, Lindsay S, Wilson DI (eds). *Molecular genetics of early human development.* Academic Press, New York, 2000

QUIZ QUESTIONS

1. Which molecules are involved in the recognition and fusion of a sperm with an ovum?
2. Why are oocyte mRNAs more important developmentally than sperm mRNAs?
3. Explain what is meant by the term embryonic induction.
4. Discuss how fetal asymmetry occurs during development.
5. What is the relative importance of cell growth and cell death during embryogenesis?
6. Explain the tissue specificity of retinoid-induced teratogenesis.
7. What are homeobox genes, and how do they function in fetal life?
8. What is differentiation and how does it occur?
9. Give an example of a cell lineage that can be stimulated to differentiate and proliferate at the same time.
10. Explain the molecular basis of genomic imprinting, and its clinical consequences.
11. Describe the effects of chromosomal disomy.
12. How does X chromosome inactivation occur? Why has this evolved?
13. Explain what pseudautosomal genes are.
14. How is human sex determined during development?

MOLECULAR MINIREVIEW

Y-linked inheritance

The presence or absence of a Y chromosome dominantly determines sexual phenotype in placental mammals. Y chromosomal genes are essential for male-specific functions such as spermatogenesis, yet not all Y chromosomal genes are male-specific; for example, the GM-CSF receptor gene is expressed on the Y chromosome (as is an identical allele on the X).

Y-linked inheritance characterizes a few clinical phenotypes – hairy ears, porcupine skin, and webbed toes – though the inheritance of such conditions may yet prove to be autosomal dominant, with the sex predilection being indirect in origin. Despite intensive efforts, Y chromosomal genes for many other male traits – repairing gadgets, playing air guitar, hogging the channel changer, reading in the bathroom – have not yet been mapped.

Summary

Life begins when egg integrins meet sperm ADAMs. Maternal messages control early embryonic development. Body patterns form due to embryonic induction.

Morphogenetic gradients specify embryo spatial organization. Developmental cell fate is specified by *Wnts*. *Patched* inhibits *Smoothened* in the absence of *Hedgehogs*. Retinoids are potent morphogens and teratogens. Homeobox gene clusters are activated in sequence.

Cell growth and differentiation are often inversely related. Differentiation is inducible by tissue-specific gene silencing. Muscles develop in response to the master gene *MyoD*.

Maternal and paternal alleles are separately imprinted. Chromosomal disomy decouples parental gene expression.

Females are mosaics of inactivated X chromosomes. Pseudautosomal regions of sex chromosomes express homologous X and Y alleles. Sex is decided by a Y chromosomal transcription factor.

17

Metabolism

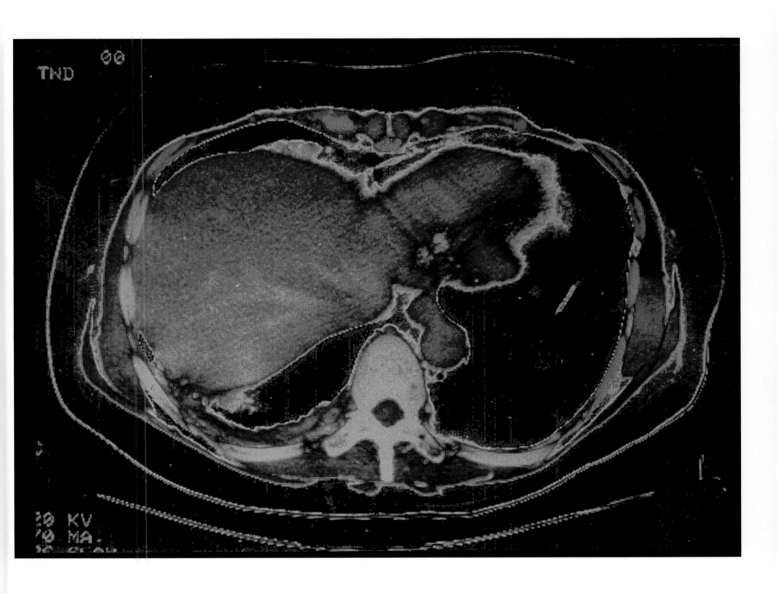

Figure 17.1 (*previous page*) Dynamic CT scan of a liver – a key organ of human metabolism (Wellcome Medical Photographic Library, no. N0013250C).

Figure 17.2 Regulation of calcium metabolism in bone and gut by parathyroid hormone (PTH) and calcitriol (vitamin D). ECF, extracellular fluid.

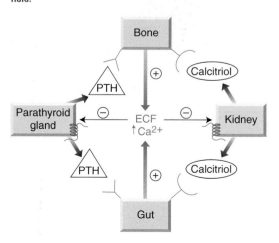

Bone metabolism

Cholecalciferol regulates calcium metabolism

Calcium is a divalent nonmetal that forms stable compounds such as calcium carbonate (chalk and limestone) and bone (calcium phosphate). Within cells calcium is often ionized, expediting its association with nucleophiles. Calcium can thus function equally well as an extracellular structural element or an intracellular signaling molecule (p. 271). Since only 1% of total body calcium circulates in peripheral blood, major alterations in calcium homeostasis usually reflect the action of bone-interactive cytokines.

Vitamin D is a prohormone that may be synthesized in the skin or ingested. Endogenous vitamin D_3 (**cholecalciferol**) is produced in the skin following UV-induced metabolism of the cholesterol precursor 7-dehydrocholesterol – elevated plasma levels of which occur in a lethal inherited disorder of cholesterol biosynthesis termed **Smith–Lemli–Opitz syndrome** (7-dehydrocholesterol reductase deficiency).

Measurement of the 25-hydroxy metabolite (25-OHD) is the best indicator of vitamin D deficiency or intoxication. Conversion of this metabolite to the active $1,25(OH)_2D$ (**calcitriol**) is catalyzed by **renal 1α-hydroxylase**, a P_{450} mixed-function oxidase inducible by **parathyroid hormone** (PTH). PTH inhibits the conversion of 25-OHD to the inactive metabolite $24,25(OH)_2D$, whereas calcium-independent inhibition of PTH gene transcription by $1,25(OH)_2D$ provides a homeostatic negative feedback loop. An unusual feature of vitamin D is its ability to upregulate its own receptor.

$1,25(OH)_2D$ increases intestinal calcium absorption in addition to enhancing both osteoblastic and osteoclastic activity in bone, indicating that its net effect may be to antagonize PTH-mediated bone resorption (Figure 17.2). Calcitriol is involved in bone mineralization, and deficiency leads to increased hydroxylysine incorporation and (hence) soft bones. High serum $1,25(OH)_2D$ levels may be seen in **hereditary hypophosphatemic rickets** with hypercalciuria or in hypercalcemia associated with **sarcoidosis**; case reports of hypercalcemic anephric patients suggest that extrarenal 1α-hydroxylation of 25-OHD occurs in the latter granulomatous disease.

CLINICAL KEYNOTE

Vitamin D deficiency states

Unlike **osteoporosis**, which reflects a deficiency of bone formation relative to resorption, **osteomalacia** is a deficiency of bone mineralization. Bone disease due to **rickets** (in childhood) or osteomalacia (in adulthood) may be inherited or acquired. These syndromes are categorized as either calcium-deficient (**calcipenic**) or phosphate-deficient (**phosphopenic**). Calcipenic vitamin D deficiency states (which may induce compensatory oversecretion of parathyroid hormone, i.e., **secondary hyperparathyroidism**) include:

1. True $1,25(OH)_2D$ (calcitriol) deficiency, caused by inadequate diet, fat malabsorption, or renal disease.
2. Vitamin D resistance, or pseudodeficiency, due to:
   - **Type 1 vitamin-D-dependent rickets** (autosomal recessive reduction of renal 1α-hydroxylase activity; treated with $1,25(OH)_2D$),
   - **Type 2 vitamin-D-dependent rickets** (inactivating point mutations of the $1,25(OH)_2D$ receptor causing intestinal malabsorption of dietary calcium; treated with massive calcium supplementation).

Causes of phosphopenic vitamin D deficiency states (which tend to be associated with normal bone mass) are:

1. Renal phosphate wasting
   - **Fanconi syndrome** (primary/secondary renal tubular "leak"),
2. Familial hypophosphatemic rickets
   - **X-linked hypophosphatemic rickets** (impaired renal phosphate reabsorption and 1α-hydroxylase activity; treated with $1,25(OH)_2D$ and phosphate),
   - **Hereditary hypophosphatemic rickets** with hypercalciuria (associated with weakness and high $1,25(OH)_2D$ levels; treated with phosphate).

Control of parathyroid hormone is driven by CaR

Parathyroid hormone (PTH) is an 84-amino-acid peptide synthesized and released by the parathyroid glands. It is detectable in serum as either a 9.5-kDa intact peptide, a 2.5-kDa metabolically active amino-terminal fragment or, most commonly, a 7-kDa inactive carboxy-terminal fragment. The carboxy-terminal fragment is renally excreted, whereas the active amino-terminal fragment is metabolized in bone. Rare loss-of-function mutations affecting the PTH receptor cause the hypocalcemic syndrome, **Blomstrand lethal chondrodysplasia**. The main target organs for PTH are bone and kidney:

1. In bone PTH stimulates osteoblasts to release cytokines, which activate osteoclast resorptive activity.
2. In the kidney PTH increases the tubular reabsorption of calcium and phosphate and enhances 1α-hydroxylation of 25-OH-vitamin D.

Feedback regulation of PTH secretion depends on the ionized fraction (about 50%) of serum calcium. Parathyroid and renal tubular cells express a 120-kDa G-protein-coupled **calcium-sensing receptor (CaR)** that is activated by extracellular domain conformational changes induced by high divalent cation (calcium or magnesium) levels. Receptor activation leads to the mobilization of intracellular calcium and consequent inhibition of PTH secretion from parathyroid chief cells. Conversely, reducing the extracellular ionized calcium concentration below the set-point for CaR activation removes this inhibitory pathway and thus triggers PTH release. Hypercalcemia-induced release of calcitonin (see below) is stimulated directly by CaR activation.

Loss-of-function CaR mutations may manifest clinically as **familial benign hypocalciuric hypercalcemia (FBHH)**, an autosomal dominant disorder characterized by heterozygous CaR mutations that render the set-point for extracellular calcium abnormally high. Moreover, the common A986S missense polymorphism is associated with significant variations in albumin-corrected (ionized) extracellular calcium levels. FBHH is distinguishable from primary hyperparathyroidism by the higher urinary calcium excretion of the latter disorder. Although FBHH is a relatively benign disorder, serious complications such as **pancreatitis** and **chondrocalcinosis** occasionally occur. Homozygous CaR null mutations cause **severe neonatal hyperparathyroidism** manifesting with parathyroid hyperplasia, constitutive PTH release, and skeletal fractures.

Rare gain-of-function CaR mutations cause **autosomal dominant hypocalcemia with hypercalciuria (ADHH)** in which the set-point for extracellular calcium (and hence, in addition, the serum PTH level) is low. ADHH patients are usually asymptomatic, but may be at risk of nephrocalcinosis if treated with vitamin D to restore biochemical normocalcemia. In the future, ADHH may be better treated with parenteral PTH.

CLINICAL KEYNOTE

Parathyroidopathies

In **primary hyperparathyroidism** due to parathyroid adenomas, PTH hypersecretion leads to high serum calcium levels, phosphaturia and nonsuppressible nephrogenous cAMP excretion. Note that normal serum PTH levels are compatible with the diagnosis in the presence of inappropriately elevated calcium. **Secondary hyperparathyroidism** most often occurs as a result of renal failure with phosphate retention, and serum calcium levels are normal. Development of a parathyroid adenoma in the latter context leads to **tertiary hyperparathyroidism** with hypercalcemia and severe osteodystrophy.

The *Gcm1/2* master genes for parathyroid development may be mutated in (nonautoimmune) **hypoparathyroidism**. Similarly, the chromosome 21q22.3 *AIRE* (autoimmune regulator) gene is mutated in the rare **polyglandular autoimmune type 1 syndrome** (also known as **APECED**, or autoimmune polyendocrinopathy-candidosis-ectodermal dystrophy).

Inactivating mutations affecting stimulatory G-proteins ($G_s\alpha$) may give rise to either **pseudohypoparathyroidism** (type Ia) or **pseudopseudohypoparathyroidism**. Both of these disorders cause osteodystrophy, but the former is an X-linked dominant syndrome of end-organ PTH resistance, whereas the latter is associated with normal calcium levels plus dwarfism, obesity and retardation.

MOLECULAR MINIREVIEW

PTHrP, Indian hedgehog, and exostoses

Parathyroid hormone-related protein (PTHrP) is a 173-amino-acid 16-kDa polypeptide that shares homology with the 13 amino-terminal residues of PTH. The receptor for PTHrP is identical to that for PTH, and resembles those for the secretin and calcitonin receptors. Synthetic peptides containing the first 34 amino acids of PTHrP produce identical effects on calcium flux in vitro and in vivo as does a similar-sized peptide fragment from PTH. PTHrP is synthesized by amnion and lactating breast tissue, and inhibits uterine muscle contraction prior to parturition by enhancing transplacental calcium transport. PTHrP is also synthesized by human keratinocytes in which it has a growth-inhibitory and pro-alopecia (i.e., promoting baldness) effect.

PTHrP is essential for tooth eruption and chondrocyte growth, and its absence leads to bony shortening. Perichondrial cells secrete PTHrP in response to the developmental pattern-determining ligand **Indian Hedgehog** (Ihh; p. 398), which is released in long-bone growth plates by prehypertrophic chondrocytes. The effect of PTHrP in this context is to stimulate chondrocyte proliferation while preventing hypertrophy and differentiation, delaying cartilage mineralization.

EXT genes encode galactosyltransferases, and loss-of-function *EXT* gene mutations impair the diffusion (and hence signaling) of Hedgehogs. This leads to the familial condition of **hereditary multiple exostoses** (short stature and bony spurs). *EXT-1* controls synthesis of glycosaminoglycans (GAGs) in the endoplasmic reticulum, and could therefore be involved in the production of a GAG that binds Ihh – perhaps promoting its translocation to neighboring cells.

Whereas PTH hypersecretion causes the chronic hypercalcemia of **idiopathic (primary) hyperparathyroidism**, PTHrP hypersecretion is the usual cause of the fulminant hypercalcemia of malignancies such as **squamous cell lung cancer**, **renal carcinoma**, and **breast cancer**. At least in theory, such hypercalcemia may occur in the absence of bone metastases. Interestingly, PTHrP-producing primary breast tumors appear less likely to metastasize to bone than do PTHrP-negative tumors.

Alternative splicing of the *CGRP* gene yields calcitonin

Calcitonin is a 32-amino-acid peptide hormone produced by parafollicular thyroid gland C cells. Like PTH, human calcitonin is located on chromosome 11p15.5; in the mouse, both genes are found on chromosome 7 (p. 579). Unlike PTH, however, calcitonin functions as a neurotransmitter in addition to its bony effects. The elevated levels of plasma calcitonin during growth and pregnancy suggest that it protects skeletal integrity during times of calcium stress.

Although long suspected of being a physiologic PTH antagonist – reducing bone resorption and increasing renal calcium clearance – no homeostatic role for calcitonin in normal calcium metabolism is clear. Plasma levels of calcitonin are used to monitor the rare heritable neoplasm, **medullary carcinoma of the thyroid** (MCT; pp. 261–2).

Calcitonin is expressed in a tissue-specific manner that varies with alternative splicing of the **calcitonin/calcitonin gene-related peptide** (*CGRP*) gene. The standard form of calcitonin is encoded by exons 1–4 of this gene. An alternatively processed variant may be monitored as a tumor marker for patients with MCT, who may remain asymptomatic despite plasma calcitonin levels reaching 10 000-fold above normal.

CGRP is a 37-amino-acid hormone encoded by exons 1–3 and 5–6 (especially 5) of the calcitonin/CGRP gene (Figure 17.3). CGRP functions as a potent vasodilator molecule in the periphery and as a modulator of pancreatic islet function and gastric acid production, and is also abundantly expressed in the central nervous system (especially the locus ceruleus).

PHARMACOLOGIC FOOTNOTE

Calcitonin treatment of Paget disease

Paget disease of bone (not to be confused with Paget disease of the breast) is an irregular bony overgrowth affecting primarily the lower limbs, pelvis, and spine of older individuals. Its etiology is uncertain but may be viral. Although often asymptomatic, Paget disease can cause pain due to bony expansion or compression. Less common manifestations are deafness (due to involvement of the ossicles in the ear), high-output cardiac failure (due to shunting of blood through extensively vascularized bone), and **osteosarcoma** (a bony malignancy that occurs at increased rates in pagetic bone).

Calcitonin has been used to treat Paget disease, though its expense and requirement for parenteral administration have reduced its popularity. The neurotransmitter function of calcitonin produces central nervous system analgesia via a pathway distinct from that triggered by opiate receptors. This helps to explain the molecule's potent analgesic properties which, in the setting of Paget disease, may be distinct from its effects on bone.

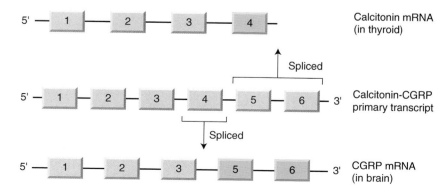

Figure 17.3 Alternative splicing of the calcitonin-CGRP transcript to yield either hormone. CGRP, calcitonin/calcitonin gene-related peptide.

Bone growth is controlled by growth factors and cytokines

The skeleton provides structural support for life and locomotion, but also functions as a metabolic organ that participates in mineral homeostasis and hemopoiesis. Bone formation is initiated by stromally derived osteoblasts that synthesize bony matrix from collagen, noncollagenous proteins such as **osteocalcin** and **osteonectin**, and proteoglycans such as **decorin**. The synthesis of these osteoblast products is followed by incorporation of calcium phosphate into the matrix as hydroxyapatite, a process termed mineralization in which osteoblasts differentiate into mature osteocytes (bone cells).

Resorption of intact bone is executed by osteoclasts, which are macrophage-derived collagenase-secreting multinucleate giant cells. Like blood cells, osteoclasts arise from bone marrow stem cells and are driven to differentiate by marrow stroma. Osteoclasts are cellular proton pumps (rather like renal collecting duct epithelial cells), which use membrane-bound vacuolar H^+ATPases to secrete hydrogen ions into the extracellular space, thus dissolving hydroxyapatite and liberating bicarbonate and calcium phosphate into the bloodstream. Bone density is maintained by a balance of osteoblastic and osteoclastic activity in turn regulated by:

1. **Osteoclast-activating factors**
   - Promote increased resorptive activity of mature osteoclasts
     - PTH and PTHrP.
     - IL-1 and IL-6.
     - TNFα (tumor necrosis factor α.
     - TGFα (transforming growth factor α.
2. **Osteoclast-recruiting factors**
   - Promote the proliferation and maturation of osteoclast progenitors.
     - M-CSF (macrophage colony-stimulating factor).
     - GM-CSF (granulocyte-macrophage colony-stimulating factor).
3. **Osteoblast-stimulating factors**
   - TGFβ.
   - PDGF (platelet-derived growth factor).
   - IGF1 (insulin-like growth factor-1).

Normal bone participates in an ongoing cycle of formation and resorption. This flux is most dramatic during bone remodeling in childhood and adolescence.

Excessive conversion of calcium phosphate to hydroxyapatite crystals around articular surfaces leads to loss of joint mobility, erosion of cartilage, and ectopic formation of bony outgrowths or osteophytes. Of potential clinical relevance to this, **pyrophosphates** – inhibitors of calcium phosphate crystal formation which are also used in toothpaste to inhibit the accumulation of calcific deposits found in tartar – are normally transported out of cells by the product of the human *Ank* gene on chromosome 5p. Null mutations of this multidomain transporter give rise to mice with an arthritic phenotype resembling the HLA B27-linked disease **ankylosing spondylitis**. Similarly, the murine *tiptoe walking* phenotype results from defects in a surface ectoenzyme that produces extracellular pyrophosphate, and resembles the human syndrome of **ectopic paraspinal ligament ossification** (i.e., **Forestier disease**, or **DISH**: diffuse idiopathic skeletal hyperostosis).

BMPs in bone metabolism

The **bone morphogenetic proteins** (BMPs), or osteogenins, are extractable components of demineralized collagenous bone matrix that interact with osteoblasts and basement membranes to induce endochondral bone formation and bony transformation of soft tissues in vivo. Unlike the rest of the BMP family, which has seven canonical cysteine residues, BMP1 is a procollagen-C protease. Approximately 20 other BMPs are known, including those of the BMP2/4 family, the BMP3 (osteogenin) family, the BMP7 (osteogenic protein-1 or OP-1) family, which comprises BMPs 5–11, and the GDF (growth/differentiation factor) family which includes BMPs 12–15.

BMPs belong to the transforming growth factor (TGF) β superfamily, and may stimulate expression of $TGF\beta_1$ – enhancing bony matrix generation during chondrogenesis while promoting ectopic bone formation induced by matrix proteins such as collagen. Other members of this superfamily (such as **activin, inhibin,** and **Müllerian inhibitory substance**) determine cell fate during embryogenesis. Indeed, the process by which bone repairs itself after a fracture closely resembles embryonic growth, and BMP mutations have been associated with birth deformities in experimental animals.

Different varieties of mammalian dentition are induced by BMP signaling. Inhibition of BMP signaling by the BMP antagonist **Noggin**, for example, results in incisors becoming molars. Similarly, release of Noggin from organizer cells (p. 397) modulates BMP4 signaling during cartilage formation: overexpression of the latter ligand during embryonic life causes the congenital syndrome of abnormal bone buildup known as **fibrodysplasia ossificans progressiva** in which repeated minor trauma culminates in widespread joint ankylosis (loss of mobility).

Runt domain mutations in bone and blood diseases

Conversion of uncommitted precursor bone stem cells to osteoblasts is dictated by the heterodimeric transcription factor **CBFA1**, whose gene is a master gene for bone development and osteoblast differentiation. Germline *CBFA1* mutations affecting the so-called **Runt domain** (named after a *Drosophila* developmental gene product) prevent DNA binding, thereby causing the devastating human congenital skeletal abnormality **cleidocranial dysplasia**. *CBFA1* gene expression may be affected by a variety of bone-regulatory growth factors including TGFβ, fibroblast growth factors (FGFs), Indian Hedgehog, PTHrP, and leptin.

The structure of the Runt domain resembles that of the p53 DNA-binding domain, and Runt domain-containing transcription factors appear critical for the normal development of blood as well as bone. This link between bone and blood extends to many other molecules, including the TNF-like osteoprotegerin ligand (see below), which regulates both osteoclast and lymphocyte development. Two blood disorders associated with Runt domain point mutations are: (1) **acute myeloid leukemia** (AML) and (2) **familial platelet disorder** (familial thrombocytopenia with predisposition to leukemia), both of which affect the *AML1/CBFA2* (CBFβ) gene.

Estrogen inhibits osteoporosis by modulating cytokine release

Both osteoclasts and osteoblasts express estrogen receptors, and estrogen stimulation of osteoblasts directly induces gene expression. Consistent with this, postmenopausal women with low serum estradiol and high **sex-hormone binding globulin** (SHBG) levels are prone to osteoporotic fractures. Estrogen inhibits bone resorption by:

1. Inhibiting osteoblast release of the osteoclast-activating cytokine interleukin-6 (**IL-6**).
2. Stimulating osteoblast expression of procollagen and matrix via:
   - **TGFβ** (synthesis requires vitamin D),
   - **IGF1** (also induced by PTH).

Noncollagenous protein components of bone include osteonectin and sialoprotein, but the most abundant such component is the γ-carboxylated 6-kDa polypeptide **osteocalcin** (or bone Gla-protein). Osteocalcin is produced by osteoblasts in response to calcitriol, and is then bound to hydroxyapatite. The small amount of osteocalcin detectable in the blood serves as an index of new bone formation, and these levels tend to be highest during puberty when they parallel elevations of IGF1. Raised osteocalcin levels in postmenopausal osteoporosis may indicate high bone turnover and thus predict benefit from estrogen. The uterotrophic effects of estrogen pose a risk of **endometrial cancer**, however, which is reduced by administration of progestins.

Postmenopausal estradiol deficiency leads to a reduction of bone TGFβ and rapid serum elevation of the bone-resorbing cytokines **IL-1**, **TNFα** and **GM-CSF**, both of these processes being reversible by estrogen replacement. IL-1 regulates proteases involved in cartilage proteoglycan matrix degradation and bone remodeling, and has been implicated in the pathogenesis of osteoporosis.

Selective estrogen receptor modulators or SERMs are pharmacologic agents that bind estrogen receptors (ERα and/or ERβ, p. 317): these include triphenylethylenes (tamoxifen, clomiphene), benzothiophenes (raloxifene), napthalenes, and benzpyrans. The divergent end-organ effects of these SERMs could reflect differential interactions with ER isoforms: raloxifene acts as an estrogen agonist in bone but an antagonist in the breast and uterus, for example, suggesting an attractive therapeutic ratio for osteoporosis prophylaxis.

CLINICAL KEYNOTE

Osteopetrosis

Marble bone disease or **osteopetrosis** is a congenital disorder of skeletal formation in which bones are abnormally dense. This condition is mimicked by **op** mice, which express a deleterious mutation of the gene encoding colony-stimulating factor 1 (CSF1: murine homolog of human **M-CSF**) and thus fail to form osteoclasts. Murine osteopetrosis may also be caused by null mutations or transgenic knockouts affecting the following osteoclast activators:

1. The cytosolic tyrosine kinase **Src**
2. The immediate-early gene product Fos.
3. The immuno-/hemopoietic transcription factor NFκB.
4. The enzyme **carbonic anhydrase H**.

This impressive degree of genetic locus heterogeneity attests to the complexity of molecular pathways which regulate development and maintenance of bone density.

Making RANK RANKL

Normal bone resorption is regulated by the interplay of: (1) a TNF-like transmembrane ligand on osteoblasts termed either **RANKL** (*r*eceptor *a*ctivator of *N*FκB *l*igand) or osteoprotegerin ligand (OPGL; see above), which stimulates osteoclast differentiation; (2) its osteoclast-based receptor **RANK**; and (3) the decoy receptor **osteoprotegerin** (OPG, a TNF receptor homolog), which inhibits osteoclastic differentiation and/or activity. Activated T cells release RANKL in response to antigen, activating RANK on chondrocytes and thereby triggering osteoclastogenesis and bone loss. RANK activation is competitively inhibited by OPG. Production of interferon-γ by activated T cells inhibits osteoclastogenesis by inducing ubiquitin-dependent degradation of the RANK adaptor protein TRAF6, thus impairing RANKL-dependent downstream activation of Fos, Src (both of which activate osteoclasts), NFκB, and Jnk.

Estrogen promotes the maintenance of bone density by inhibiting RANKL synthesis whereas another class of anti-osteoporotic drugs – the biphosphonates (see below) – act in part by upregulating OPG. In contrast, calcitriol and PTH stimulate osteoclastic activity by enhancing RANKL production while inhibiting OPG expression.

Bone-forming and bone-resorbing activities are coupled

Most human metabolic bone disorders involve an imbalance of bone formation and resorption. Assays for analyzing the relative contribution of these processes to such disorders include:

1. Indicators of bone formation
   - Serum **alkaline phosphatase**.
   - Serum **osteocalcin**.
   - Serum **procollagen type 1**.
2. Indicators of bone resorption
   - Serum **acid phosphatase** (tartrate-resistant: TRAP).
   - Urinary **hydroxyproline** excretion.
   - Urinary **galactosyl hydroxylysine**.
   - Urinary **pyridinoline crosslinks**.

The principal constituent of bone matrix is type 1 collagen, the precursor of which is **procollagen type 1**. Elevations of this circulating precursor correlate with new bone formation in disorders such as **Paget disease**. An increased risk of postmenopausal osteoporotic fractures has been associated with intronic polymorphisms of the gene encoding collagen type Iα1.

Bone resorption by osteoclasts results in the liberation and urinary excretion of the collagen-specific amino acid **hydroxyproline**. Hydroxyproline excretion lacks specificity and sensitivity, however, and has been superseded by measurements of **urinary pyridinium crosslinks**, which provide quantitative indices of collagen 1 and 2 breakdown. These crosslinks arise from **pyridinoline** derivatives formed during lysyl-oxidase-mediated collagen fibril maturation from hydroxylysine. Crosslink excretion is elevated in bone-resorptive conditions such as **osteoporosis, osteomalacia, hyperparathyroidism, hyperthyroidism, Paget disease**, and **metastatic bone disease**, and declines with effective therapy. Conversely, malnourished growth-stunted children exhibit abnormally low cross-link excretion which increases with proper nutrition.

Osteoclasts lyse and remodel bone by secreting **tartrate-resistant acid phosphatase (TRAP)** into resorbing bone fields. Serum acid phosphatase levels often rise as a secondary response to bony involvement from **metastatic prostate cancer,** which typically causes osteoblastic (radiosclerotic) lesions. Conversely, diseases such as metastatic breast cancer that cause predominantly lytic bone lesions are often associated with compensatory increases of serum alkaline phosphatase. Elevations of resorption markers (such as hydroxyproline excretion and acid phosphatase) often coincide with those of bone synthesis markers such as alkaline phosphatase, indicating that the two processes occur together. Indeed, some osteoinductive factors (including PTH and vitamin D) stimulate both new bone formation and bone resorption.

The plasma cell dyscrasia **multiple myeloma** causes widespread lytic bone disease by decoupling these processes, as illustrated by the minimal elevations of alkaline phosphatase characteristic of this disorder. IL-6 is a promoter of bone resorption in this disorder, and may also play an autocrine role.

CLINICAL KEYNOTE

Hereditary hyperphosphatasia
Osteoblasts synthesize a bone-specific isoform of alkaline phosphatase (AP), a glycosylphosphatidylinositol-anchored ectoenzyme that promotes mineralization by removing pyrophosphates and hence promoting calcium phosphate crystallization. Serum elevations of AP are therefore a hallmark of osteoblastic activity, and may be induced by many ligands including osteogenin and vitamin D_3. Distinct isoforms of AP are synthesized by other organs such as liver and placenta. Elevations of serum AP may be useful markers of therapeutic response in metastatic malignancies involving bone or liver.

Hereditary hyperphosphatasia is an autosomal recessive disorder characterized by massive elevations of serum AP. This is a calcitonin-responsive condition that presents with pagetoid deformities in childhood, fractures, and deafness due to auditory nerve compression.

PHARMACOLOGIC FOOTNOTE

Antiosteoclastic drugs
Patients with malignant disease may develop hypercalcemia as a result of lytic bone metastases or the paraneoplastic secretion of cytokines such as PTHrP. Such complications may be reversed by drugs that inhibit osteoclastic activity. These drugs include:
1. Biphosphonates (e.g., **pamidronate, alendronate, clodronate).**
2. **Calcitonin** (also antagonizes renal tubular reabsorption of calcium).

Biphosphonates are pyrophosphate analogs in which various side-chains (often nitrogenous) replace the central oxygen. Following absorption into bone, the osteoclast enzyme **farnesyl diphosphate synthase** is inhibited, leading to inhibition of the small GTP-binding proteins Rho and Rab and thus to osteoclast apoptosis. These drugs are now a mainstay of prophylactic treatment for senile or postmenopausal **osteoporosis;** they are also used in **Paget disease,** and for symptomatic therapy of **bone metastases** and/or **hypercalcemia.**

The mild hypocalcemic effects of **glucocorticoids** in hemopoietic malignancies such as **myeloma** are probably direct antitumor actions, since chronic use of these drugs induces bone loss. Steroids may also revert the hypercalcemia caused by excess vitamin D effect as in **sarcoidosis**; this vitamin-D-inhibitory action may contribute to the osteopenic sequelae of long-term corticosteroid therapy.

Carbohydrate metabolism

Hypothalamic neuropeptides regulate appetite

Unlike plants, animals require appetitive behaviors to regulate their changing nutritional and energy needs. These changing needs include alterations in ionic balance, protein degradation, cholesterol biosynthesis, mineral absorption, sugar utilization, and co-factor (vitamin) requirements. The feeding behavior of humans therefore requires tight molecular regulation in the same way as intracellular biochemical reactions. Neuroanatomic stimulation studies have revealed that the lateral hypothalamic area is a **hunger center** whereas the ventromedial nucleus of the hypothalamus is a **satiety center**. Two key hypothalamic neuropeptides implicated in the control of feeding are:

1. **Orexigenic peptides**
   - Anabolic hormones which stimulate appetite.
2. **Anorexigenic peptides**
   - Catabolic hormones which reduce appetite.

Neuropeptide Y (NPY) is the classic orexigenic peptide. NPY exerts its hyperphagic and anabolic effects by activating hypothalamic **feeding receptors** (termed Y1 and Y5) of the G-protein-coupled receptor superfamily. Administration of NPY to animals increases feeding and reduces energy expenditure, resulting in obesity, but may also improve memory, inhibit sexual activity, relieve anxiety, enhance seizure control, precipitate hypothermia, and re-set circadian rhythms. Moreover, brain levels of NPY correlate with the effects of alcohol, with higher NPY expression being associated with greater sedation and reduced alcohol ingestion, and vice versa.

Suppression of NPY expression (with loss of appetite) is inducible by pharmacologic inhibitors of fatty acid synthase such as cerulenin: such inhibition increases malonyl CoA levels, leading to negative feedback of both NPY and the feeding-inducible **acetyl CoA carboxylase** (**ACC1/2**) enzymes. Since *ACC2*-knockout mice exhibit a higher fatty acid oxidation rate, less adipose tissue, and a normal lifespan, therapeutic ACC2 inhibitors could be used to induce fat loss without reducing caloric intake.

Surprisingly, NPY knockouts may exhibit normal feeding patterns. Other hypothalamic appetite-stimulating neuropeptides including **Agouti-related protein** (AGRP; see below), **melanin-concentrating hormone** and the **hypocretins** (also known as orexins) could thus contribute to feeding maintenance. The most potent short-term orexigenic peptide is NPY, whereas AGRP is the most long-lived: both are expressed in the arcuate nucleus of the hypothalamus, and are released by fasting.

The circulating peptide hormone **ghrelin**, which activates pituitary growth hormone secretion via its binding to hypothalamic receptors, is synthesized and secreted by gastric mucosal cells in response to fasting. Hence, the signaled requirement for metabolic efficiency also leads to an increase in feeding.

Anorexigenic neuropeptides mediate catabolic effects and reduce food intake. These weight-losing chemicals include the melanocortin **α-melanocyte-stimulating hormone** (α-MSH), **thryotropin-releasing hormone** (TRH), **corticotropin-releasing hormone** (CRH) and **cocaine- and amphetamine-regulated transcript** (CART). Cleaved from **pro-opiomelanocortin** (POMC; see Figure 13.4), α-MSH regulates energy output by binding melanocortin receptors 3 and 4 (**MC3**, **MC4**). **Agouti** is the murine homolog of α-MSH; human AGRP is also a structural melanocortin homolog but a functional antagonist, since it exerts its anabolic effects by competitively blocking α-MSH binding to MC4. Illustrative of this interaction, MC4 knockout mice are hyperphagic and obese. Hypocretin deficiency is responsible for the disabling daytime somnolence syndrome of **narcolepsy**.

Feeding behavior is more than simply a matter of appetite. Meal size (when to stop eating), meal frequency (how soon to recommence eating) and the availability of long-term energy stores (when to consider doing without) are all variables that require distinct signaling pathways for their regulation, as discussed below.

MOLECULAR MINIREVIEW

Satiety and adiposity signals

Most of us stop eating on sensing that familiar sense of gastric distension we refer to as "full". If you thought this was just a physicospatial sensation related to having no further space in your stomach for storing food, think again; the sense of being replete requires a complex signaling pathway that is initiated by molecules termed **satiety signals**. Unlike other aspects of feeding behavior, meal termination is not mediated by the hypothalamus but rather by vagus nerve afferents linking the stomach to an area of the caudal brainstem (viz., nucleus of the solitary tract).

The best characterized satiety signal is **cholecystokinin** (CCK). From the beginning of a meal, ingested nutrients stimulate the release of CCK from neuroendocrine cells in the proximal small bowel, leading to CCK-dependent activation of the above-mentioned brainstem satiety tracts. However, another key effect of CCK is to enhance the postprandial release of two hormones:

1. **Insulin**.
2. **Leptin**.

Both of these hormones bind receptors in the hypothalamus, leading to reduced food intake, and circulate in peripheral blood at levels that are proportional to body fat. The so-called **lipostatic** effect of these two hormones on feeding has led to their being dubbed **adiposity signals**: i.e., stimuli that increase fat will also trigger release of these hormones. Unlike insulin which is released by pancreatic islets, however, leptin (Greek *leptos*, thin) is produced mainly by fat cells.

Leptin increases energy expenditure and reduces feeding

The differences between leptin and insulin become clear when considering their respective deficiency phenotypes. The human **leptin** (Lep) gene product is encoded in mice by the *ob* gene – so-called because homozygous mutant *ob/ob* mice (which express no leptin) are gluttonous and hence obese. Restoration of *ob* gene expression in these mice reduces both appetite and weight; starvation reduces serum leptin levels whereas refeeding restores them.

Similar effects are seen with hypothalamic **leptin receptor** mutations. Mutant diabetic (*db*) mice express a splice variant of the leptin receptor

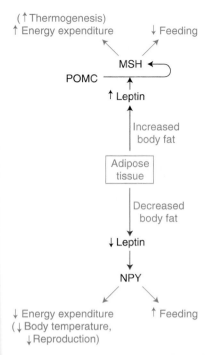

Figure 17.4 Regulation of appetitive behavior (feeding) and catabolism (energy expenditure) by the adipose-derived hormone leptin. Increases in body fat enhance leptin release, reducing feeding and increasing thermogenesis via the melanocortin signaling system. Loss of body fat, on the other hand, reduces leptin, increasing feeding while stimulating a hibernation mode of energy homeostasis. MSH, melanocyte-stimulating hormone; NPY, neuropeptide Y; POMC, pro-opiomelanocortin.

which results in a truncated cytoplasmic domain with absent signaling, whereas the obese *fatty* rat expresses a leptin receptor with a point-mutated (Gln269Pro) extracellular domain. The *db/db* mouse also has a sweet tooth, consistent with the finding that leptin suppresses the desire for sweet substances.

Unlike the insulin receptor tyrosine kinase, the leptin receptor belongs to the type 1 cytokine receptor family and signals via the Jak-STAT system. In humans, null mutations of the leptin receptor are associated not only with obesity but also with failure to undergo puberty, suggesting a broader role for leptin in regulating the hypothalamo–pituitary–gonadal axis. Rare kindreds with hyperphagia and obesity have leptin deficiency due to null mutations of the leptin gene. Hence, via its primary effects on energy regulation, leptin appears to confer secondary insulin sensitivity.

Postprandial hyperglycemia or hyperlipidemia normally triggers leptin synthesis by adipose cells, with the strength of the signal varying with adipose mass (Figure 17.4). Plasma leptin levels may be linked to satiety via a hypothalamic interaction with NPY. Obese animals such as *ob/ob* mice have high brain NPY levels; in normal animals, intraventricular injection of NPY stimulates hyperphagia followed by insulin release and leptin induction. High leptin levels lower cerebral NPY levels, and also block NPY-induced feeding by stimulating the release of CART from the arcuate nucleus. Since leptin deficiency causes massive obesity – whereas insulin deficiency does not – leptin appears more closely entwined with bodyweight homeostasis than is insulin.

PHARMACOLOGIC FOOTNOTE

Antiobesity drugs
At first glance the mutant phenotypes mentioned above suggest that diabetic and/or obese individuals might benefit from leptin treatment. Unfortunately, evidence so far suggests that most obese individuals will not lose weight by taking leptin pills. Plasma leptin levels in obese individuals already tend to be elevated (~4 times normal), suggesting a secondary rise in leptin levels due to end-organ resistance; this is reminiscent of the hyperinsulinemia seen in non-insulin-dependent **diabetes mellitus**. There are four main categories of candidate antiobesity drugs:

1. Appetite (food intake) suppressants.
2. Stimulators of fat mobilization.
3. Enhancers of energy expenditure.
4. Fat absorption blockers.

Appetite suppressants include **sibutramine**, a serotonin and noradrenaline reuptake inhibitor; **dexenfluramine**, which triggers the release of serotonin from nerve endings, was discontinued following reports of heart valve damage. NPY receptor antagonists, fatty acid synthase inhibitors, or CCK agonists might also be useful. Stimulators of fat mobilization may eventually include agonists affecting thermogenic proteins such as **uncoupling enzymes** (pp. 433–4) as well as growth hormone. **Caffeine** increases energy expenditure, as does **ephedrine**. The synthetic dietary additive **orlistat** blocks pancreatic lipases, leading to malabsorption of triglycerides and consequent weight loss.

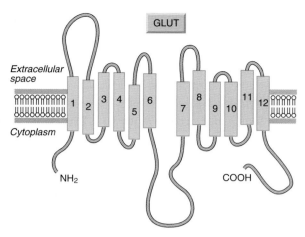

Figure 17.5 Cartoon of a glucose transporter (GLUT), showing the 12-transmembrane-domain structure. The structure is similar to that of the multidrug transporter family (p. 191).

Sugars require transport across membranes

Feeding involves the ingestion of food as a prelude to digestion. Hydrolysis of dietary polysaccharides by gut mucosal digestive enzymes yields the monosaccharides glucose and galactose which, on presentation to the intestinal microvilli, undergo ATP-dependent active transport against a concentration gradient. This process – similar to that mediating renal tubular glucose/galactose reabsorption – is driven by a transmembrane sodium ion electrochemical gradient. The membrane protein responsible for this coupled transport, the **sodium-glucose co-transporter**, contains 12 transmembrane domains which make up the base of a pore-forming homotetramer.

These molecular transport mechanisms are clinically relevant. Missense mutations affecting the co-transporter (such as $Asp^{28} \rightarrow Asn^{28}$ at the transmembrane junction) may cause autosomal recessive **glucose-galactose malabsorption**. Moreover, oral rehydration therapy for severe diarrhea (such as **cholera**) uses glucose solutions to activate the sodium-glucose co-transporter, thereby enhancing Na^+/H_2O absorption. Unlike glucose and galactose, fructose is absorbed by the gut via facilitated transport (p. 182).

Facilitated transport is also used to transport glucose into cells following its absorption into the bloodstream, thus distinguishing this phase of glucose transport from that noted above for gut absorption. On exiting the bloodstream and entering the extracellular space, glucose travels back across the plasma membrane and into the cytosol via valve-like protein channels known as **glucose transporters** or **GLUTs** (Figure 17.5). These molecules resemble the sodium-glucose co-transporter in that they contain 12 transmembrane domains and form membrane pores (pentagonal, rather than tetrameric).

Under resting circumstances the human brain – which, unlike muscle, cannot utilize free fatty acids for energy – consumes 80% of circulating glucose; in contrast, 60% of insulin-inducible glucose transport into tissues occurs in muscle. The brain requires a constant (rather than fluctuating) supply of glucose, and has therefore evolved its own high-affinity glucose transporter (GLUT3; see below). Key regulators of GLUT, function include the ambient glucose concentration, muscle contractile activity, hypoxia, and the peptide hormone insulin.

MOLECULAR MINIREVIEW

GLUTs

Because glucose utilization occurs mainly within skeletal muscle, the rate-limiting step of glucose metabolism is that of glucose transport into muscle cells. Glucose transporters – all of which exhibit 40–65% amino acid homology – include:

1. **GLUT1** (erythrocyte transporter)
   - Most widely expressed transporter; caters for basal glucose requirements of most resting cells (including muscle),
   - Highly expressed in endothelial cells lining the **blood–brain barrier**, thus ensuring cerebral glucose homeostasis,
   - Hypoglycemia enhances expression.
2. **GLUT2** (liver transporter)
   - Expressed in liver, small intestine, kidney (all deliver glucose to the blood), and pancreatic β-cells,
   - High K_m for glucose (about 25 mM; cf. GLUTs 1 and 4, ~5 mM); hence, the rate of transmembrane glucose transport parallels alterations in ambient glucose

levels, enabling accurate sensing of glucose availability such as is required by pancreatic islet cells or liver cells delivering glucose to the bloodstream.

3. **GLUT3** (brain transporter)
   - Like GLUT1, expressed ubiquitously but especially in the brain.
   - Higher glucose affinity than GLUT1, thus ensuring smooth intracerebral glycemia when operating together.
4. **GLUT4** (muscle/fat transporter)
   - Principal transporter in insulin-sensitive tissues; quantitatively responsible for most glucose transport in the body.
   - Insulin and exercise cause membrane translocation (activation) of pooled intracellular GLUT4 in fat and muscle cells respectively, increasing glucose uptake approximately 20-fold.

In addition to these major GLUTs, GLUT5 is expressed in the jejunum, *GLUT6* is a pseudogene, and GLUT7 is active in hepatic microsomes. Insulin stimulation of glucose transport occurs especially in muscle and fat cells following mobilization of cytoplasmic GLUT4 to the cell surface. A smaller insulin-dependent enhancement of glucose transport is mediated by the catalytic activation of GLUT1. Defective glucose transport may contribute to the pathogenesis of: **benign renal glycosuria**; certain instances of **hypoglycorrhachia** (low cerebrospinal fluid glucose) associated with neuroglycopenic childhood seizure disorders, **bacterial meningitis** or **meningeal carcinomatosis**; and diabetes mellitus (especially non-insulin-dependent; see below).

Insulin prevents oxidant damage to microvascular endothelium

Affecting almost 5% of the adult population – and up to 30% of some cohorts – diabetes mellitus is one of the commonest chronic human diseases. The hallmark of the disorder, hyperglycemia due to ineffective insulin signaling, is directly or indirectly responsible for most of the acute and long-term sequelae.

Insulin activates its receptor tyrosine kinase, leading to heavy transphosphorylation of the 160-kDa insulin receptor substrate 1 (IRS-1) – a YXXM-rich protein which accordingly recruits numerous phosphatidylinositol-3′-kinase (**PI3K**) molecules. PI3K is a critical downstream insulin effector that is essential for glucose transport (via stimulation of glucose transporter vesicle fusion), glycogen synthesis (via stimulation of the **glycogen synthase kinase-3** pathway) and **phosphoenolpyruvate carboxykinase** induction (leading to gluconeogenesis). Activated PI3K induces the protein kinase B (**PKB**, Akt) signaling pathway, which is essential for insulin-dependent stimulation of glucose uptake into adipocytes. Since the pro-apoptotic lipid ceramide antagonizes the latter process, the metabolic action of insulin (and IGF1) appears tightly linked to its PKB-dependent effects on cell survival. The importance of this pathway for glucose homeostasis is emphasized by gene knockout experiments targeting the PI3K effector **S6 kinase** (**Rsk**): the resultant signaling deficit produces pancreatic islet cell atrophy and hypoinsulinemic glucose intolerance reminiscent of **type 2 diabetes**. Insulin receptor activation further enhances cell glucose uptake by causing the **Cbl** ubiquitin ligase (p. 260) to bind **flotillin**, a caveolin-associated lipid raft protein (p. 180).

In the absence of effective insulin signaling, glucose intolerance or frank hyperglycemia (diabetes) ensues, leading to complications such as osmotic polyuria, dehydration, ketoacidosis, lactic acidosis, and coma. Mechanisms of long-term hyperglycemic target tissue damage include:

1. Endothelial deposition of **advanced glycation end-products** (AGE; p. 130).
2. Glucose-inducible activation of protein kinase C and NFκB.
3. Aldose-reductase-dependent **sorbitol** accumulation.

Each of these pathogenetic pathways is associated with increased mitochondrial superoxide production. Diabetic microvascular damage thus arises secondary to hyperglycemic induction of reactive oxygen species. However, reports suggesting that insulin confers cognitive benefit may reflect a direct effect of insulin on neurons.

MOLECULAR MINIREVIEW

GAD: stiff men with diabetes

The 64-kDa pancreatic β-cell enzyme **glutamic acid decarboxylase** (GAD) is a trigger of type 1 (juvenile-onset) diabetes. Early cases of insulin-dependent diabetes may be associated with the presence of GAD autoantibodies, perhaps arising via molecular mimicry following infection with coxsackievirus P2-C. There are two GAD isoforms: GAD65, which predominates in islet cells, and GAD67 which is present in GABA-ergic nerve terminals. Relevant to this distinction, GAD autoantibodies are also detectable in 50% of cases of **stiff-man syndrome** – a clinical rarity (1 per million) consisting of rigidity and gait disturbance ("tin soldier" phenotype).

Type 1 diabetes is exclusively associated with GAD65 autoantibodies, whereas stiff-man syndrome is characterized by GAD65 and/or GAD67 antibodies. The latter syndrome may also feature IgG4 or IgE autoantibodies, unlike type 1 diabetes in which anti-GAD is consistently IgG1. Moreover, the antigenic epitopes of the GAD antibodies appear distinct in diabetes (regions 161–243 and 473–555) and stiff-man syndrome (regions 81–171 and 313–403), though occasional overlap cases with both phenotypes are reported. T_H1 immune responses dominate in type 1 diabetes, whereas T_H2 immunity seems more important in stiff-man syndrome.

CLINICAL KEYNOTE

Type 1 vs. type 2 diabetes

Diabetes mellitus is a heterogeneous disorder. **Type 1 diabetes** is a T-lymphocyte-mediated autoimmune disease which usually arises in childhood; destruction of pancreatic islet β cells by T_H1 cells leads to insulin deficiency. The pathogenetic importance of environmental factors (such as viral infections) is suggested by the low concordance (30%) in identical twins. Since concordance is higher in dizygotic twins than in other siblings, but lower than in monozygotic twins, both genetic and environmental factors are likely to be important. Two major histocompatibility complex (MHC) class II genes, *HLA-DQA1* and *HLA-DQB1*, are associated with the disease, but do not account for the concordance in monozygotic twins.

Type 2 diabetes differs from type 1 disease with respect to the older onset of presentation, high concordance of the disease in identical twins (almost 100%), and milder phenotype. Patients tend to be obese and exhibit peripheral insulin resistance rather than insulin deficiency; indeed, the chronic hyperinsulinism may itself exacerbate (rather than reflect) the obesity. Type 2 diabetics are unable to push plasma glucose into muscle and fat, even with high insulin levels: the high glucose level tells the pancreas to keep pumping out insulin, leading to the pathology. In pathogenetic terms this is a far more complex disorder than type 1 diabetes (insulin deficiency), and one which has reached epidemic proportions in developed countries.

Diabetes results from the interplay of genes and environment

Numerous molecules involved in insulin signaling are implicated in the pathogenesis of diabetes. For example, there are four insulin receptor substrate proteins (IRS1–IRS4), all of which contain PH and PTB domains in addition to carboxy-terminal tyrosine sites that are phosphorylated by insulin receptor activation. Murine knockout of **IRS1** (which recruits numerous PI3K molecules to its carboxy-terminal YXXM sites when phosphorylated) causes growth retardation and insulin resistance but not clinical diabetes, reflecting a compensatory increase in insulin secretion. In contrast, knockout of **IRS2** causes type 2 (insulin-resistant) diabetes, while **IRS3** knockout has no phenotype and **IRS4** knockout causes hypoglycemia. IRS2 knockout also causes obesity and infertility, thus linking bodyweight with fertility in females – a complex association, since both **anorexia nervosa** (thin) and **polycystic ovary disease** (obese) are associated with amenorrhea. Murine knockout of the protein kinase B homolog *Akt2* also causes profound insulin resistance.

In addition to the mutations underlying maturity-onset diabetes of the young (MODY; see below), other candidate gene mutations in type 2 diabetes include insulin (rare), insulin receptor (rare), and **mitochondrial leucine tRNA synthase** (also associated with type 1 diabetes). Missense mutations of the nuclear envelope **lamin A/C** protein are associated with insulin resistance in the syndrome of autosomal dominant **familial partial lipodystrophy**. The genetic basis of other lipodystrophy syndromes – **generalized congenital lipodystrophy** (Berardinelli-Seip syndrome) or **partial lipodystrophy** (Dunnigan syndrome) – remains uncertain, but could involve the C/EBP family of adipocyte transcriptional regulators. The neutral cysteine protease **calpain-10** is also implicated in type 2 diabetes, reflecting its effects on insulin secretion and gluconeogenesis. Insulin resistance in animal models is inducible by heterozygous knockout of **GLUT4**.

Knockout of protein tyrosine phosphatase activity can remove the normal inhibition of insulin receptor function. This is the case for at least two phosphatases: **PTP1B** and the SH2-containing lipid phosphatase **SHIP2**. Both knockouts are ultrasensitive to the hypoglycemic effects of insulin, exhibit enhanced GLUT4 recruitment, and are resistant to weight gain despite a high-fat diet. Drugs that inhibit the activity of either PTP1B or SHIP2 could therefore prove useful in the treatment of diabetes. Note, however, that autoantibodies to the pancreatic islet cell tyrosine phosphatase **IA-2** have been associated with type 1 diabetes in conjunction with increased growth.

Insulin resistance is also associated with genetic deficiency of **CD36** – a common phenotype in African and Asian populations in which this membrane glycoprotein is a high-affinity receptor for the malarial parasite *Plasmodium falciparum*. CD36 functions as a transmembrane transporter of long-chain fatty acids and oxidized low-density lipoproteins (LDL). Murine CD36 knockouts exhibit reduced atherogenesis, however, suggesting that LDL requires CD36 to be taken up by endothelial macrophages. CD36 is transcriptionally induced by the adipocyte nuclear receptor **peroxisome proliferator-activated receptor-γ (PPARγ)**; as detailed below, the latter protein may be disabled by mutations in certain diabetic kindreds, and is also a target of **thiazolidinedione** ("glitazone") oral hypoglycemic drugs (p. 442). A related molecule in the pathogenesis of diabetes is a secreted insulin-antagonizing hormone, regulated by PPARγ and inhibited by thiazolidinediones, termed **resistin**.

Resistin

The association of type 2 diabetes with obesity has spawned the hypothesis that fat cells release a molecule that impairs glucose tolerance. Progressive accumulation of lipid droplets by adipocytes is accompanied by the release of molecules such as free fatty acids and TNFα which confer insulin resistance. Moreover – as noted above and described in detail later – differentiated fat cells express the receptor PPARγ in abundance, and insulin resistance can be lowered by thiazolidinedione drugs that inhibit PPARγ function (p. 442).

This reflects the fact that PPARγ induces the adipocyte synthesis and secretion of a circulating insulin hormonal antagonist termed **resistin**. Plasma resistin levels are high in type 2 diabetics and also in genetic forms of obesity. Treatment of such individuals with PPARγ inhibitors lowers circulating resistin levels, with consequent improvement of glucose tolerance and insulin action. Resistin signaling may thus explain the link between obesity and type 2 diabetes.

Maturity-onset diabetes of the young (MODY)

There exists an important type 2 diabetes subtype termed **maturity-onset diabetes of youth (MODY)** which accounts for 2% of all diabetes. MODY should be suspected if there is an autosomal dominant pattern of diabetes in a young non-obese patient, including teenagers. Since the penetrance of MODY is 85% (as contrasted with the 20% penetrance of non-MODY type 2 diabetes), diagnosis of this genetic diathesis mandates presymptomatic family testing. Early use of conservative interventions such as diet, exercise, and sulfonylureas may obviate the need for insulin.

All MODY subtypes are single-gene disorders of pancreatic β-cell endocrine regulation. Prototypical of MODY are mutations affecting the glycolytic enzyme **glucokinase**, which catalyzes a rate-limiting step in glucose metabolism. Glucokinase thus acts as a glucose sensor that regulates insulin secretion, and loss-of-function mutation causes the clinical **MODY2** syndrome which is mimicked by glucokinase knockout mice. Conversely, a rare autosomal dominant syndrome of **familial hyperinsulinism** has been associated with a gain-of-function V455M glucokinase mutation that increases the affinity of the enzyme for glucose. Glucokinase expression is regulated by the upstream homeobox protein **insulin promoter factor-1 (IPF1)**; **MODY4** arises due to heterozygous mutations affecting this molecule, whereas homozygosity causes pancreatic agenesis.

MODY2 and MODY4 rank among the milder of these syndromes, but the other subtypes may lead to insulin dependence and vascular complications such as retinopathy. The commonest subtype is **MODY 3** which is caused by mutations affecting the **hepatocyte nuclear factor-1α** (*HNF1α*) gene, though mutations affecting *HNF4α*, *HNF1β*, and *HNF6* also cause MODY (Table 17.1). **Fanconi-Bieckel syndrome** is an uncommon MODY subtype caused by mutational defects of *GLUT2*. **Insulin receptor** loss-of-function mutations are a rare non-MODY single-gene cause of diabetes.

Lipid metabolism

Mobilization of fat varies with metabolic rate

The rate at which a resting human being converts food energy to heat – the basal metabolic rate – varies between individuals. Two key hormone signaling

Table 17.1. Maturity-onset diabetes of the young (MODY) molecules

MODY subtype	% of all MODY	Mutant gene	Age of onset (years)	Characteristics
3	70	HNF1α	12–35	Sensitive to sulfonylureas
2	15	Glucokinase	0–35	Mild; may only require treatment during pregnancy
1	5	HNF4α	12–35	
5	2	HNF1β	12–35	Associated with renal cystic disease
4	1	IPF1	12–35	

systems regulate metabolic rates: the **thyroid** (p. 159) and **adrenergic hormone** systems. Adrenergic hormone family members – **epinephrine** (formerly, adrenaline), **norepinephrine** (noradrenaline), and **dopamine** – are tyrosine derivatives collectively termed **catecholamines**. These biogenic amines act distantly as hormones and locally as neurotransmitters.

Adrenergic regulation of metabolism involves the release of norepinephrine from sympathetic nerve endings, leading to stimulation of G-protein-coupled **β-adrenoceptors**. These receptors are expressed on the surface of brown fat adipose cells and, when stimulated, trigger intracellular increases in cAMP. This activates protein kinase A (PKA) which in turn phosphorylates the transcription factor CREB (cAMP response element binding protein). Transgenic mice with increased PKA expression remain thin despite high-calorie diets, raising the possibility that β-adrenoceptor agonist drugs could be developed to treat obesity. PKA activates two downstream targets that affect fat metabolism:

1. **Hormone-sensitive lipase**, a lipolytic enzyme activated by phosphorylation of perilipin (a protein which sits on triglyceride droplets).
2. **Thyroxine deiodinase**, an enzyme that catalyzes the formation of active thyroid hormone (triiodothyronine, T_3) which in turn affects the uncoupling of mitochondrial respiration from ATP generation.

Hormone-sensitive lipase releases energy by hydrolyzing triacylglycerols in adipose tissue, a process termed lipolysis. In contrast, **pancreatic lipase** functions in digestion. This latter process involves the solubilization by bile acids of dietary fatty acids and glycerol within gut luminal complexes termed micelles. Ingested fatty acids are incorporated into triacylglycerols in adipose tissues for energy storage, whereas ingested triacylglycerols are broken down to fatty acids and glycerol for intestinal absorption.

The differential distribution of fat around the body reflects the distribution of lipid-regulatory cytokines. Insulin-dependent lipolysis targets mainly subcutaneous fat, whereas the principal target of catecholamine-dependent lipolysis is visceral fat. Leptin is predominantly expressed in subcutaneous fat, whereas glucocorticoid receptors and peroxisome proliferator-activated receptors are mainly expressed in visceral fat.

MOLECULAR MINIREVIEW

Uncoupling proteins

Body heat is generated in the brown fat of hibernating animals by inner mitochondrial membrane **uncoupling proteins** (UCPs). These proteins uncouple oxidative phosphorylation, thereby effecting a proton leak which reduces the

electrophoretic HDL subspecies termed pre-β HDL may bind directly to cells, thus stimulating receptor-mediated translocation of intracellular cholesterol to the plasma membrane. On binding HDL, cholesterol molecules are esterified by the apoA1-dependent enzyme **lecithin:cholesterol acyltransferase** (**LCAT**). The resultant hydrophobic cholesteryl esters enter the HDL core and are transported via an apoA1-binding ATP-binding cassette protein, the **ABCA1 transporter** (p. 189). This cholesterol efflux protein directs cholesteryl esters to the liver where they are metabolized without catabolic HDL loss; for this reason, HDL-cholesterol turns over 25 times more rapidly than do HDL apolipoproteins.

The apoB:apoA1 thus ratio thus reflects the status of cholesterol transport to tissues. High apoB:apoA1 ratios are strongly predictive of cardiovascular disease, and may be even more accurate in this regard than the HDL:LDL-cholesterol ratio.

HDL-cholesterol may also be transported by a nonlipolytic route involving cholesteryl ester transfer between lipoproteins that have docked onto cell-surface proteins in the liver, ovary, and adrenal gland. Transfer of HDL-cholesterol to VLDL is catalyzed by an enzyme called **cholesteryl ester transfer protein** (**CETP**) which exchanges HDL-cholesterol for VLDL-triglyceride. Cholesterol-rich VLDL particles are then catabolized to potentially atherogenic LDL molecules. Ingestion of dietary cholesterol induces *CETP* gene expression, thus increasing the risk of cardiovascular disease. The atherogenicity of CETP is indicated by its inverse relationship with HDL-cholesterol levels, the association of high CETP levels with atherosclerosis, and the successful inhibition of atherogenesis in animals by pharmacologic CETP inhibitors. Homozygotes for the CETP-upregulating *B1* allele (as well as individuals with pro-atherogenic polymorphisms of β-fibrinogen and lipoprotein lipase) may benefit to a greater extent from pravastatin therapy.

Figure 17.8 Palmar xanthomata in a patient with hypercholesterolemia (Wellcome Medical Photographic Library, N0010106C).

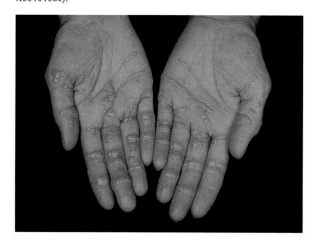

CLINICAL KEYNOTE

Lipoprotein deficiencies and human disease

More is known about the function of LDL-cholesterol than HDL-cholesterol. Although reverse transport of HDL-cholesterol is often assumed to underlie the antiatherogenic effects of high plasma HDL, several anomalies cloud this observation:

1. Certain disorders unassociated with vascular disease may be associated with reduced HDL-cholesterol. These include **LCAT deficiency** and **fish-eye disease.**
2. Patients with low HDL levels due to inherited **apo AI** and **AII polymorphisms** incur no excess cardiovascular morbidity.
3. Hypolipidemic drugs such as probucol may reduce HDL-cholesterol levels while causing regression of xanthomata (Figure 17.8).

Low HDL levels may also reflect reduced **lipoprotein lipase** activity: overexpression of lipoprotein lipase protects transgenic mice from diet-induced hyperlipidemias, suggesting a mechanism for the protective effects of high HDL.

Null mutations affecting another lipid transfer protein, **microsomal triglyceride transfer protein** (MTP), may be responsible for the clinical syndrome of **abetalipoproteinemia** (Bassen–Kornzweig syndrome) in which LDL-cholesterol levels are low, causing neuropathy, retinopathy, spur cell anemia, and malabsorption.

Inherited HDL deficiency – **analphalipoproteinemia** or **Tangier disease** – presents with massive reticuloendothelial accumulation of cholesteryl ester due to loss-of-

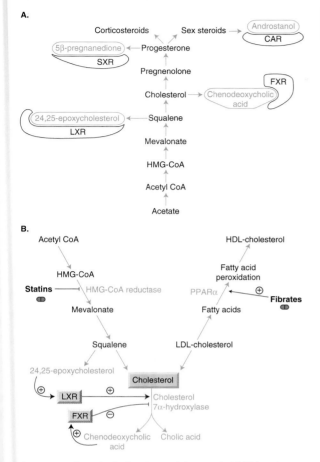

Figure 17.9 Biosynthesis, function, and therapeutic inhibition of orphan receptor ligands. *A*, Synthesis of rexinoid receptor ligands from cholesterol. *B*, Activation of FXR and LXR by their ligands, with downstream effects on enzyme signaling pathways. Enzyme and receptor inhibition by hypolipidemic drugs is also shown, contrasting the mechanism of fibrates with that of statins. CAR, constitutive androstane receptor; FXR, farnesoid X receptor; LXR, liver X receptor; PPARα peroxisome proliferator-activated receptor α; SXR steroid and xenobiotic receptors.

function *ABCA1* mutations. Pharmacologic upregulation of ABCA1 could thus prove an attractive atheroprotective strategy.

Orphan nuclear receptors

Rexinoid receptors regulate cytochrome P450 genes

Metabolism of carbohydrates and lipids depends upon a variety of transactivating nuclear receptors. There are about 80 such receptors in all, approximately half of which are termed **orphan receptors** because high-affinity (nanomolar) endogenous ligands have not yet been identified. Paradoxically, such receptors may be associated with numerous low-affinity endogenous or exogenous ligands: the former include steroids, retinoids and prostaglandins (Figure 17.9*A*) whereas the latter (termed **xenobiotics**) include drugs, toxins, poisons, and solvents. A common effector target for these ligand-activated DNA-binding nuclear receptors is the **cytochrome P450** (*CYP*) gene superfamily which encodes hepatic microsomal enzymes. The intimate link between this enzyme family and the steroid hormone signaling system is illustrated by the P450 enzyme **aromatase** (estrogen synthetase) which converts testosterone to estrogen in both gonadal and peripheral tissues.

Liver X receptors (**LXRs**) are nuclear hormone receptors that heterodimerize with retinoid X receptors (RXRs) following LXR activation by oxycholesterol (hydroxycholesterol and epoxycholesterol) – that is, LXRs are oxysterol receptors. LXR–RXR heterodimers transactivate the cytochrome P450 *CYP7A1* gene promoter which encodes the enzyme **cholesterol 7α-hydroxylase** (Figure 17.9*B*). This enzyme controls the rate-limiting step involved in the conversion of plasma cholesterol to hydrophilic bile acids.

Farnesoid X receptors (**FXRs**) are nuclear bile acid receptors activated by the endogenous gallstone-dissolving biomolecule **chenodeoxycholic acid** (CDCA; Figure 17.9*B*). Transcription of both the *CYP7A1* gene and the *ABCA1* reverse cholesterol transporter gene are repressed by CDCA-dependent FXR activation in liver and intestinal cells, creating negative feedback loops between bile acid availability and synthesis on the one hand, and between cholesterol production and excretion on the other. Bile acid synthesis is thus upregulated by LXR and downregulated by FXR.

RXR agonist ligands (**rexinoids**; p. 320) may alter cholesterol absorption, bile acid synthesis and reverse cholesterol transport by triggering RXR heterodimerization of FXRs and/or LXRs. This raises the possibility that certain rexinoids (or LXR-interactive drugs) could prove useful as hypolipidemic agents. Yet another family of orphan receptors – the **steroid and xenobiotic receptors** or **SXRs** (homologous to murine pregnane X receptors or PXRs) – heterodimerize with RXRs in response to drugs. SXR–RXR heterodimers bind to a xenobiotic response element in the promoter for the *CYP3A4* gene, thereby upregulating the enzyme (p. 444). SXRs are endogenously activated not only by C21 steroids (pregnanes) but also by estrogens and glucocorticoids, which are in turn catabolized via SXR-dependent *CYP3A4* induction.

Constitutive androstane receptors or **CARs** are antagonized by testosterone metabolites termed androstanes which, when removed, permit CAR signaling and *CYP2B* gene induction. Expressed in the liver, CAR is a key mediator of xenobiotic-dependent *CYP2B10* induction by **phenobarbital-like drugs** (though SXR is also activated by phenobarbital).

CLINICAL KEYNOTE

The ABC of LXRs

The autosomal recessive hyperlipidemia **sitosterolemia** arises from mutations affecting LXR-inducible *ABC G5* (encoded on chromosome 2p21) and *ABC G8* cholesterol half-transporters, which transfer enterocyte cholesterol to the gut lumen. This disorder can be distinguised from **familial hypercholesterolemia** via its features of hemolytic anemia and exquisite diet-responsiveness; the diagnostic distinction is important because pharmacologic LXR agonists can increase jejunal ABCG5 expression by greater than three-fold. Other LXR-regulated gene products include CETP and **ABC A1** – the **Tangier disease** transporter which transfers dietary sterols to gut lymphatics and thence to the liver. The connective tissue disorder **pseudoxanthoma elasticum** – which, as the name suggests, presents with xanthoma-like lesions – also results from an ABC transporter gene mutation.

MOLECULAR MINIREVIEW

Peroxisome proliferator-activated receptor (PPAR) ligands

Many xenobiotics are classifiable as **peroxisome proliferators** (i.e., they trigger an increase in cellular organelles containing detoxifying peroxidative enzymes; p. 131), as are several endogenous steroid and fatty acid ligands. Receptors that bind such ligands have been assigned the tongue-twisting title of **peroxisome proliferator-activated receptors** (PPARs), another family of rexinoid-dimerizing nuclear receptors. As shown by reverse endocrinology, ligands activating PPARs include the fatty acids **phenylacetate** and **phenylbutyrate** as well as:

1. PPARα ligands
   - Fatty acids: **linoleic acid, linolenic acid, phytanic acid.**
   - Eicosanoids: **leukotriene B$_4$, 8S-hydroxyeicosatetraenoic acid (8S-HETE).**
2. PPARγ ligands
   - Eicosanoids: **prostaglandin J$_2$, 15-HETE.**
3. PPARβ/δ ligands
   - Eicosanoids: **prostaglandin I$_2$** (prostacyclin).

PPAR ligand-binding regions tend to be about three-fold larger than those of other steroid hormone receptors, consisting of a double-domain pocket involving both the amino-terminal regulatory A/B domain and the usual carboxy-terminal ligand-binding domain. This structure is consistent with the notion that PPARs have evolved as sensor molecules for intracrine signaling via bulky endogenous lipids. As with other orphan nuclear receptors, ligand-activated PPARs heterodimerize RXRs prior to the interaction of their central DNA-binding domains with response elements (PPREs) in target genomes.

The 8-HETE PPARα ligand is a major product of arachidonic acid metabolism via the 8S-lipoxygenase pathway. 8-HETE induces epidermal differentiation via activation of PPARα. Other HETE ligands have distinct molecular targets: for example, 12-HETE binds and activates protein kinase C. Muscle catabolism in **cancer cachexia** is induced by myocyte release of 15-HETE in response to a circulating **proteolysis-inducing factor** (PIF).

A.

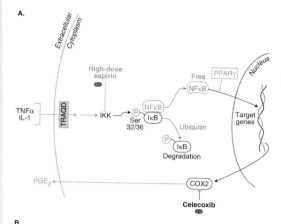

B.

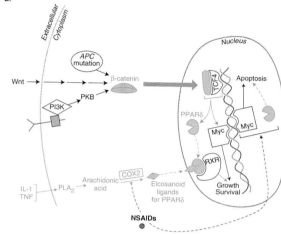

Figure 17.10 Actions of peroxisome proliferator-activated receptors PPARγ and PPARδ. *A*, Anti-inflammatory action of PPARγ, which resembles that of PPARα. Induction of NFκB-dependent target genes such as cyclooxygenase-2 (COX2) (p. 296) is inhibited by PPARγ, thus preventing eicosanoid release; the same pathway is more proximally interrupted by aspirin-dependent inhibition of IKK (IκB kinase). *B*, The putative tumor-promoting role of PPARδ in colorectal carcinogenesis, showing the proposed chemopreventive mechanism of nonsteroidal anti-inflammatory drugs (NSAIDs) such as aspirin or sulindac. Ligand-activated PPARδ mediates the survival signaling of β-catenin, but this growth loop is inhibited by NSAID-induced COX2 blockade which prevents synthesis of eicosanoid ligands for PPARδ.

PPARs direct lipid and glucose metabolism

Three subtypes of the PPAR family – PPARα, PPARβ/δ and PPARγ – have the following features:

1. **PPARα**
   - Promotes hepatic oxidation of fatty acids during fasting (catabolism).
   - May have antiatherogenic effects.
2. **PPARβ/δ**
   - Regulates cell growth and differentiation via its effects on lipid metabolism and signaling in gut epithelium, brain, and placenta.
   - May have tumor-promoting effects.
3. **PPARγ**
   - Enhances the storage of fatty acids in adipose tissue (lipogenesis) under anabolic (nonfasting) conditions.
   - May have antidiabetic, antiatherogenic, and antitumor effects (Figure 17.10*A*).

PPARα is expressed primarily in liver, fat, and muscle where it catabolizes fatty acids by β-oxidation, lowering both total and HDL-cholesterol levels. Once activated by its ligand leukotriene B$_4$, activated PPARα transcriptionally inhibits NFκB signaling and (thus) cyclooxygenase-2 (COX2) expression. PPARα also inhibits aortic smooth muscle cell activation, suggesting that pharmacologic agonists may reduce postangioplasty restenosis. Fibrate hypolipidemics (**clofibrate, gemfibrozil, bezafibrate, fenofibrate**) bind and activate PPARα, thereby upregulating HDL-cholesterol and apoAI/AII while downregulating apoCIII and plasma triglyceride levels (Figure 17.9*B*). Although nongenotoxic hepatocarcinogenesis in mice (which have higher PPARα levels than humans) is PPARα-mediated, long-term clinical use of fibrates has not so far been associated with increased cancer. **Clofibrate-induced myopathies** are mediated via PPARα activation in muscle.

The anti-inflammatory (and perhaps antiatherogenic) actions of PPARα and PPARγ receptor families are similar, but the adipogenic and energy-storing actions of PPARγ contrast sharply with those of PPARα. PPARγ is one of two key adipogenic transcription factors – the other is CCAAT/enhancer binding protein-α (C/EBPα), a member of the **C/EBP** family of adipocyte differentiation proteins. Adipocyte target genes induced by these transactivators include lipoprotein lipase, acyl CoA synthase, fatty acid transport protein, and adipocyte fatty acid binding protein. Leptin gene expression in adipose tissue, on the other hand, is suppressed by PPARγ. Lipogenesis is positively regulated by PPARγ-dependent induction of the gluconeogenic (and glyceroneogenic) enzyme **phosphoenolpyruvate carboxykinase** (PEPCK; p. 164).

PPARγ1 is expressed mainly in the liver, whereas PPARγ2 primarily regulates the differentiation of adipose tissue. These PPARγ subtypes inhibit macrophage function in response to prostaglandin D$_2$ release from activated mononuclear cells; both receptor subtypes are also activated by endogenous prostaglandin J$_2$ derivatives (see above) and by thiazolidinedione antidiabetic drugs (e.g., **rosiglitazone**). Endogenous PPARγ-activating ligands can inhibit aromatase activity (hence, estrogen biosynthesis; p. 316) in human breast adipose tissue. Rosiglitazone has antitumor activity in adipose-derived mesenchymal tumors termed **liposarcomas**.

PHARMACOLOGIC FOOTNOTE

PPARγ, thiazolidinediones, and familial diabetes

Ligand-activated PPARγ heterodimerizes with retinoid X receptors (RXRs) to induce adipocyte differentiation. PPARγ receptors are activated by insulin-sensitizing thiazolidinedione antidiabetic drugs (including the discontinued hepatotoxic drug troglitazone in addition to pioglitazone and rosiglitazone). Like the older biguanide drug metformin, thiazolidinediones sensitize muscle, fat, and liver cells to the action of insulin (unlike sulfonylureas such as tolbutamide which act by increasing insulin secretion) and are therefore suitable for treating type 2 diabetes; weight gain is a frequent side-effect.

Insulin resistance can occur because of heterozygous germline mutations in the PPARγ ligand-binding domain that impair transactivation in a dominant-negative manner. Missense mutations preventing the normal insulin-dependent phosphorylation of Ser[114] in PPARγ2, for example, are associated with insulin resistance and obesity. The commonest PPARγ mutation is the amino-terminal Pro[12]→Ala missense substitution. Obesity without apparent alteration of insulin sensitivity has been associated with Pro[115]→Gln mutations. Conversely, null mutations may cause early-onset type 2 diabetes, hypertension and acanthosis nigricans (hyperinsulinemic skin darkening) but no obesity; such mutations may account for 2–5% of severe insulin resistance. In contrast, constitutively activating PPARγ mutations may cause obesity with low insulin levels. Wild-type PPARγ may thus enhance insulin sensitivity and fat deposition.

CLINICAL KEYNOTE

PPARβ/δ and colorectal cancer chemoprevention

PPARβ/δ is expressed in all tissues but especially in the colon, brain, kidney, and heart. This receptor subtype is inducible by β-catenin-dependent activation of the transcription factor TCF4, as occurs constitutively with null mutations of the *APC* tumor suppressor gene (Figure 17.10B). Since wild-type *APC* represses PPARβ/δ gene expression, PPARβ/δ activation could promote colonic neoplasia. Consistent with this, inhibitors of COX2 impair PPARβ/δ ligand release, preventing PPARδ/RXR heterodimers from binding to DNA. Such drugs may trigger colonic epithelial cell apoptosis, as illustrated by the ability of the anti-inflammatory drug sulindac to reduce polyp formation (via ERK1/2 inhibition) in familial polyposis, and by the ability of long-term aspirin administration to prevent colon cancer (Figure 17.10). In contrast, synthetic ligands which activate PPARα or PPARγ reduce colonic tumorigenesis in rodent models of colitis. *COX2* knockout mice crossed with *APC* knockout mice yield a progeny that incur 85% fewer intestinal polyps than do standard *APC* knockout mice.

Xenobiotic metabolism and pharmacogenetics

Toxins are eliminated by hepatic mixed-function oxidases

Unlike foreign antigenic proteins – which elicit a cellular immune response – noxious chemicals undergo inactivation by an array of detoxifying enzymes. The most important classes of detoxifying enzymes include:

1. **CYPs** (cytochrome P450s).
2. **GSTs** (glutathione-*S*-transferases).
3. NATs (*N*-acetyltransferases).

There are at least 30 cytochrome P450 (CYP) enzymes residing in hepatocyte endoplasmic reticulum and mitochondria. These xenobiotic-metabolizing enzymes catalyze the incorporation of an oxygen atom into the substrate of interest, with the remaining atom of the modifying O_2 molecule being reduced (by NADPH-coupled flavoproteins) to water. Cytochromes are heme-containing membrane-anchored proteins that specialize in electron-transfer reactions involving lipophilic substrates. Substrate specificity varies with each P450 isozyme but often overlaps, as might be expected of xenobiotic reactants. For each mono-oxygenase enzyme the initial reaction catalyzed involves transfer of a hydroxyl group from a donor molecule to the substrate, creating a reactive intermediary which can undergo oxidation, epoxidation, dealkylation, desulfuration or deamination. Microsomal P450 enzymes are sometimes termed **mixed-function oxidases** to reflect this functional pleiotropism. A distinct xenobiotic-oxidizing enzyme class is the **peroxidase** family.

P450 enzymes are implicated in a variety of functions in addition to the detoxification of xenobiotics. They play an important role in normal growth and development, especially through their ability to catalyze hydroxylation reactions. This is illustrated by the syndromes of precocious puberty seen in **congenital adrenal hyperplasia** due to abnormalities affecting the *CYP2C11* (testosterone 16α-hydroxylase) and *CYP2C12* (androstenediol disulfate 15β-hydroxylase) gene loci, for example. Of note, the specificity of these steroid-hydroxylating P450 cytochromes tends to be much tighter than for xenobiotic-metabolizing enzymes, indicating that enzymes currently regarded as detoxifiers may prove to have endogenous catalytic roles. Indeed, even processes as natural as regulation of flower color are controlled by CYPs.

Unfortunately, hepatic metabolism does not always detoxify xenobiotics. Immune-mediated tissue damage may be triggered exclusively by xenobiotic metabolites: examples include **autoimmune hepatitis** due to **halothane** or **tienilic acid** (caused by the metabolites trifluoroacetylchloride and thiophene sulfoxide, respectively). Of note, tienilic-acid-induced hepatitis is associated with **CYP2C10** antibodies, and **hydralazine-induced hepatitis** with **CYP1A2** antibodies. *CYP2A6*-null individuals are less able than others to convert nicotine to cotinine, and hence may have a decreased risk of becoming addicted smokers. Other examples of toxigenic metabolic conversions include **practolol-induced oculomucocutaneous syndrome** (due to **practolol epoxide**), **lupus** due to **hydralazine** or **procainamide** (caused by hydralazine radicals and *N*-hydroxyprocainamide, respectively), and the gentle art of boozing.

CLINICAL KEYNOTE

Alcohol metabolism

Intestinal microorganisms produce small quantities of **alcohol** – a classic lipophilic xenobiotic with toxic effects on the liver and neuromuscular system. To combat this hazard the liver expresses the enzyme **alcohol dehydrogenase** (ADH) which converts alcohol to **acetaldehyde** – a pungent metabolite responsible for the aroma of ripening fruits and amontillado sherry – which is in turn converted to acetate by **acetaldehyde dehydrogenase** (ALDH). Acetaldehyde causes the not-unpleasant vasodilatory (flushed) sensation often experienced within minutes of imbibing an alcoholic beverage. It also contributes to the less pleasant hangover symptoms, and may predispose to oral cancers. Ethanol metabolism depletes ATP while increasing the NADH:NAD ratio, leading to hepatocyte necrosis and triglyceride deposition

Table 17.2. CYP3A4 inducers and inhibitors

CYP3A4 inducers (i.e., reduce drug effects)	CYP3A4 inhibitors (i.e., increase drug effects)
Rifampicin	Erythromycin, clarithromycin
Barbiturates	Ciclosporin, tacrolimus
Carbamazepine	Ketoconazole, fluconazole, itraconazole
Phenytoin	Fluoxetine
Nafcillin	Verapamil, nifedipine
Griseofulvin	Indinavir, ritonavir
Dexamethasone	Terfenadine

(fatty liver) respectively. Thiamine is consumed during hepatic metabolism of ethanol: the hypothalamus responds to thiamine deficiency by ordering an increase in hepatic ADH activity, leading to enhanced ethanol degradation.

Methanol itself is not much more toxic than ethanol, but methanol is metabolized by ADH to aldehyde and **formic acid**. These metabolites may cause blindness and lethal metabolic acidosis unless ADH is inhibited by the competitive substrate ethanol or by **fomepizole** (4-methylpyrazole). The latter is also useful for treating ethylene glycol (antifreeze) intoxication.

Two- to three-fold differences in individual tolerance to ethanol may relate to genetic polymorphisms (*ADH2* and *ADH3*) affecting the ADH enzyme. Moreover, approximately 50% of ethnic Chinese individuals lack the **ALDH2** isoenzyme, thereby predisposing to acetaldehyde-induced flushing and tachycardia.

About 15% of ingested alcohol is metabolized not by ADH but by **CYP2E1**. **Disulfiram** (Antabuse™) is a CYP2E1-inhibitory drug used as a preventative in alcoholics: it impairs the conversion of acetaldehyde to acetic acid, leading to accumulation of the toxic metabolite and rapid onset of acetaldehydemic symptoms after alcohol ingestion.

PHARMACOLOGIC FOOTNOTE

CYP3A4

The metabolism of up to 50% of drugs depends on CYP3A4, reflecting the common induction of this enzyme activity by SXR–RXR heterodimers. The induction of CYP3A4 by **rifampicin** may enhance oxidation of the oral contraceptive **ethinylestradiol** (i.e., leading to unplanned pregnancies), for example, whereas grapefruit juice may inhibit CYP3A4 and thus potentiate the effects of co-administered CYP3A4 inhibitors (see Table 17.2). Similarly, the CYP3A4-inhibiting antifungal **ketoconazole** can be prescribed in conjunction with the immunosuppressant **ciclosporin** to permit lower doses of the latter (expensive and toxic) drug. *N*-demethylation of intravenous [^{14}C]erythromycin by CYP3A4 is the basis of the ($^{14}CO_2$) erythromycin breath test for CYP3A4 phenotyping.

A common **CYP3A5** polymorphism resulting in a smaller and less active enzyme is associated with **midazolam** sensitivity.

Xenobiotic-metabolizing enzymes are inducible by drugs

The substrate specificity of enzymes makes them excellent drug targets. Xanthine oxidase regulates purine metabolism (p. 26), for example, and is inhibited by **allopurinol** to prevent gout. **Monoamine oxidase** (MAO) is likewise a target for certain antidepressants, but such inhibition may predispose to catastrophic hypertension if tyramine-containing foodstuffs are ingested (p. 528). Drugs may also be targets for enzymes, and most drugs undergoing enzymatic inactivation do so via oxidative metabolism. The **P450 enzyme** family is the prime mediator of such processing, but many other enzymes detoxify drugs: these include **glutathione-*S*-transferases** (which metabolize halothane), **glucuronyltransferases**, and **sulfotransferases**. Instead of using NADPH as the co-factor, such enzymes use glutathione (which contains a free sulfhydryl group), UDP-glucuronic acid or phosphosulfate respectively as modifying groups. Glucuronidation is a stereoselective process in which only one enantiomer within a racemic mixture is modified.

Acute drug intoxication leads to saturation of enzyme capacity. An example is that of acute **acetaminophen** (paracetamol) poisoning which impairs normal hepatic glucuronidation of bilirubin. Conversely, individuals with *CYP1A2* null mutations may be unable to metabolize the acetaminophen precursor

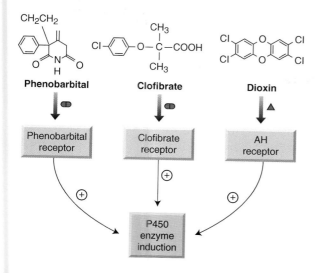

Figure 17.11 Orphan receptors ligated by xenobiotics, leading to hepatic P450 enzyme induction. AH, aryl hydrocarbon (dioxin).

drug **phenacetin**, and thus present with cyanosis due to **methemoglobinemia** (pp. 455–6). Acetaminophen-induced hepatic necrosis may be reduced by administering peroxisome proliferators such as **clofibrate** which minimize glutathione depletion and protein arylation.

Chronic drug exposure can lead to P450 enzyme induction. This substrate-inducibility of xenobiotic-metabolizing enzymes enables the matching of catalytic activity to the severity and/or frequency of a microenvironmental hazard. Chronic smoking (CYP1A2), alcohol ingestion (CYP2E1) or repeated administration of drugs – including phenobarbital (CYP2B) and rifampicin (CYP3A4), for example – may thus alter the body's ability to handle medications.

Mechanisms of P450 enzyme induction vary between drugs. Phenobarbital directly activates transcription of the *CYP2B* gene via its nuclear receptor – as do **clofibrate** (**CYP4A1**), **dexamethasone** (**CYP3A1**), and **dioxin** (**CYP1A1**; Figure 17.11) – whereas ethanol enhances CYP2E1 activity by protein stabilization. P450 enzymes are also responsible for the metabolic activation of certain substrates to reactive compounds or carcinogens. For example, the anticancer drug **cyclophosphamide** does not acquire its alkylation-dependent DNA-damaging ability until activated by **CYP2B1**, and is therefore inactive if applied topically (e.g., into the peritoneal, pleural or intraspinal space). By the same token, the carcinogenicity of cyclophosphamide – that is, its unwanted toxic ability to cause second malignancies of the bladder or bone marrow – depends upon CYP2B1 activation. This carcinogenic toxicity tends to be expressed only in the context of long-term accumulated DNA damage.

MOLECULAR MINIREVIEW

The aryl hydrocarbon (AH, dioxin) receptor

Dioxin (TCDD: tetrachlorodibenzo-*p*-dioxin) is a halogenated chemical used in pesticides. Animal exposure is associated with **hepatotoxicity**, skin lesions (**chloracne**), **endometriosis**, thymic involution, birth defects, **soft tissue sarcomas** and **breast cancer**. Enhanced secretion of transforming growth factor α (TGFα) may contribute to these sequelae of dioxin exposure. Dioxins bind and activate the **aryl hydrocarbon receptor** (AHR) – a ligand-activated transcription factor that regulates xenobiotic metabolism, but in which the DNA-binding motif is the basic helix-loop-helix rather than the zinc finger. Ligand-activated AHR heterodimerizes in the nucleus with the **AH receptor nuclear translocator protein** (**ARNT**) – a common heterodimeric subunit of many transcription factors characterized by basic helix-loop-helix motifs, including hypoxia-inducible factor-1 (HIF-1; p. 450). AHR knockout results in lymphopenia, hepatic hypoplasia and fibrosis, indicating a role for this receptor in normal hepatogenesis and immune development.

Polycyclic aromatic hydrocarbons such as benzpyrene (in cigarette smoke) may also trigger the AHR-dependent pleiotropic response pathway, which includes **glutathione-*S*-transferase** (GST) and **CYP1A1**. Inducible CYP1A1 isoenzymes have been associated with increased susceptibility to **lung cancer**, particularly in light smokers, whereas null GST variants (GSTM1, GSTT1) predispose to **smoking-induced bladder cancer** and also to **aflatoxin-induced liver cancer**. Cruciferous vegetables such as broccoli and cabbage contain dietary **isothiocyanate** precursors which, by providing the requisite donor sulfhydryl groups, assist GST-dependent carcinogen detoxification.

Fatal pharmacogenetic faults

Mutations affecting drug-metabolizing enzymes can have drastic clinical sequelae. The field of predicting drug sensitivity or resistance by assessing the gene structure of metabolizing enzymes is termed **pharmacogenetics**. Well-known examples include:

1. **Malignant hyperthermia**
   - A potentially fatal postanesthetic syndrome sometimes caused by mutations affecting the calcium-regulatory ryanodine receptor (pp. 272–3).
2. **Pseudocholinesterase deficiency**
   - Prolonged postsuccinylcholine paralysis/apnea syndrome.

Polymorphic differences in drug metabolism are common, with about a third of unselected patients failing to respond to statins (HMG CoA reductase inhibitors), β-blockers or antidepressants. The underlying genetic differences are classified as polymorphisms rather than mutations since it is not possible to ascribe wild-type status to one gene sequence.

Genetic polymorphisms determine individual drug sensitivity

The field of molecular epidemiology is expanding on many different fronts in the pharmacogenetic domain. Approximately 90% of the population express high activity of the enzyme **thiopurine methyltransferase** (**TPMT**), whereas about 1% are homozygotes with low activity (9% being heterozygotes with intermediate activity). TPMT metabolizes the antileukemic purine analogs 6-mercaptopurine and 6-thioguanine as well as the immunosuppressive purine analog azathioprine. Hence, poor metabolizers may experience life-threatening myelotoxicity when administered conventional doses of these drugs.

The poor metabolizer *CYP2C19* polymorphism is five times more common in Asians than Caucasians (20% versus 4%), accounting for the differential handling of omeprazole, citalopram, phenytoin, diazepam, and proguanil: omeprazole is more effective in such individuals, whereas diazepam causes prolonged sedation. Polymorphisms associated with reduced **CYP2C9** activity (15% heterozygous, 1% homozygous) reduce the metabolism of warfarin, tolbutamide, glipizide, ibuprofen, fluvastatin, sildenafil, phenytoin, and diazepam, potentiating these agents. In contrast, the angiotensin II antagonist losartan exhibits impaired antihypertensive efficacy in these individuals.

Another pharmacogenetic polymorphism is that affecting the enzyme **dipyrimidine dehydrogenase** (**DPD**) which inactivates the anticancer drug 5-fluorouracil (5-FU). Null mutant DPD homozygotes (0.1% of the population) treated with 5-FU incur major toxicity including prolonged **myelosuppression, panmucositis** and **cerebellar damage**. Another cytotoxic drug used in colorectal cancer, the topoisomerase I inhibitor irinotecan, causes excessive diarrhea and bone marrow toxicity in 10% of the population due to promoter polymorphisms affecting the *UGT1A1* (UDP-glucuronyltransferase) gene. Additional pharmacogenetic interactions relate to polymorphisms affecting the function of the HDL-associated esterase **paraoxonase** (predisposing to **organophosphate-induced nerve damage** and **atherosclerosis**), the porphobilinogen-synthesizing **aminolevulinic acid dehydrase** (predisposing to **lead poisoning)** and the **HLA-DP bet1** marker (predisposing to **lung berylliosis**). Polymorphisms of membrane transporter genes also modify drug handling: reduced insulin response to tolbutamide is seen in sulfonylurea receptor gene (*SUR1*) polymorphisms, sudden death due to antiarrhythmic drugs in *LQT* gene (p. 184) polymorphisms encoding cardiac ion channels, resistance to β-blockers in polymorphisms of the β_2-adrenergic receptor gene, and **digoxin toxicity** in multidrug resistance (*Mdr*) gene polymorphisms.

PHARMACOLOGIC FOOTNOTE

Drug metabolism and CYP2D6 genotyping

The drug-metabolism polymorphism of the cytochrome P450 gene *CYP2D6* (responsible for impaired oxidation of the former antihypertensive **debrisoquine**) is a striking example of a founder mutation. About 6% of Caucasians are **slow metabolizers** of debrisoquine, rising to 15% in Nigerians but falling to less than 1% in the Japanese; in contrast, **ultrarapid** debrisoquine metabolism (reflecting *CYP2D6* gene amplification) is seen in 20% of Ethiopians but only in 1% of Swedish people. For slow metabolizers **codeine** is ineffective (reflecting reduced bioactivation). Parent drug accumulation of **perhexiline maleate** causes neuropathy and hepatotoxicity; on the other hand, **phenformin** causes lactic acidosis, **phenacetin** causes methemoglobinemia, **antidepressants** cause confusion, **propranolol** hypotension and **captopril** agranulocytosis. The opposite is true for ultrarapid metabolizers who (for example) may present with **codeine toxicity** or with **tricyclic-resistant depression**. Indeed, *CYP2D6* genotyping is used routinely in some centers to optimize psychiatric drug dosing. Reduced CYP2D6-dependent metabolism of nitrosamines in tobacco smoke is also linked to increased **lung cancer**.

CLINICAL KEYNOTE

Fast acetylators, slow acetylators, and NAT

Another common pharmacogenetic polymorphism is that relating to xenobiotic **acetylation**. The enzymes implicated here are the **NAT1** and, more especially, the **NAT2** isozymes of *N*-acetyltransferase. These enzymes catalyze both *N*-acetylation and *O*-acetylation; the former reaction usually inactivates, and the latter usually activates, aromatic and heterocyclic amine carcinogens.

Reduced NAT2 protein expression (i.e., the *NAT2* acetylation polymorphism) is often seen in slow acetylators. Approximately 60% of Caucasians (highest among Egyptians) and Africans are slow NAT2 acetylators. Such individuals are more prone to **bladder cancer** induced by arylamine, benzidine, naphthylamine, aminofluorene, and other aromatic amine carcinogens (such as are also present in cigarette smoke). This association implies an equilibrium between carcinogen inactivation by NAT2 acetylation and carcinogen activation by the cytochrome P450 system. In contrast, 85% of Orientals and 95% Inuits express dominant fast NAT2 acetylation alleles. Such individuals are at higher risk for **colorectal cancer**, which arises in part due to acetylation-dependent activation of dietary heterocyclic amine carcinogens (such as are present in charred meats).

In total, over 25 different alleles of both NAT1 and NAT2 have been identified. Phenotyping for NAT2 acetylation status is often performed using urinary measurement of **caffeine**, another acetylation substrate, whereas NAT1 phenotyping can be carried out using *p*-**aminosalicylic acid**. Acetylation status is relevant to the efficacy of drug treatment with **isoniazid**, **hydralazine**, **procainamide**, and **dapsone**. Slow acetylators tend to develop more side-effects (including **drug-induced lupus**), whereas rapid acetylators are more likely to experience therapeutic failure. Of note, the NAT2 slow acetylation phenotype is also associated with **familial Parkinson**

Enrichment reading

Bedtime reading

Salway JG. *Metabolism at a glance*. Blackwell, Oxford, 1999

Cheap'n'cheerful

Brody TM, Larner J, Minneman KP (eds). *Human pharmacology: molecular to clinical*. Mosby, New York, 1998

Favus MJ. *Primer on the metabolic bone diseases and disorders of mineral metabolism*. Lippincott/Williams & Wilkins, Baltimore, 1999

Library reference

Bilezikian JP, Raisz LG, Rodan GA (eds). *Principles of bone biology*. Academic Press, New York, 1996

Josephy DP, De Montellano PO. *Molecular toxicology*. Oxford University Press, Oxford, 1996

Scriver CR, Beaudet AL, Sly WS (eds). *The metabolic and molecular bases of inherited disease*. McGraw Hill, New York, 2000

disease, raising the possibility that heritable susceptibility to environmental neurotoxins (such as methylphenyltetrahydropyridine, MPTP) may be pathogenetic.

Summary

Cholecalciferol regulates calcium metabolism. Control of parathyroid hormone is driven by a 120-kDa calcium-sensing G-protein-coupled receptor (CaR). Alternative splicing of the *CGRP* gene yields calcitonin. Bone growth is controlled by growth factors and cytokines. Estrogen inhibits osteoporosis by modulating cytokine release. Bone-forming and -resorbing molecules are functionally coupled.

Hypothalamic neuropeptides regulate appetite. Leptin increases energy expenditure and reduces feeding. Sugars require transport across membranes. Insulin prevents oxidant damage to microvascular endothelium. Diabetes results from the interplay of genes and environment.

Mobilization of fat varies with metabolic rate. HMG-CoA reductase modulates cholesterol synthesis. Hypercholesterolemia downregulates LDL receptors. HDLs mediate reverse cholesterol transport.

Rexinoid receptors regulate cytochrome p450 (CYP) genes. Peroxisome proliferator-activated receptors (PPARs) direct lipid and glucose metabolism.

Toxins are eliminated by hepatic mixed-function oxidases. Xenobiotic-metabolizing enzymes are differentially induced by drugs. Genetic polymorphisms determine individual drug sensitivity.

QUIZ QUESTIONS

1. How does vitamin D increase bone mineralization?
2. What are the functions of parathyroid hormone?
3. How does the structure and function of calcitonin differ from that of calcitonin/calcitonin gene-related peptide (CGRP)?
4. Explain the molecular basis of postmenopausal bone loss.
5. Name some serum and urinary proteins which vary in amount during bone formation and resorption, respectively.
6. Explain the difference between active transport and facilitated transport of glucose.
7. Name the main glucose transporters and describe their functions.
8. Discuss the etiology and molecular pathophysiology of diabetes mellitus.
9. What is metabolic rate, and how is it regulated?
10. Distinguish the functions of leptin and neuropeptide Y.
11. What is the function of HMG CoA reductase, and what is its therapeutic significance?
12. Compare and contrast the functions of low-density (LDLs) and high-density (HDLs) lipoproteins.
13. Describe some of the clinical sequelae of lipoprotein gene mutations.
14. Briefly describe how P450 enzymes detoxify xenobiotics. What other actions may they have?
15. How is alcohol metabolized?
16. Which nuclear receptors are implicated in xenobiotic metabolism?
17. Briefly explain the clinical significance of the debrisoquine and acetylation pharmacogenetic polymorphisms.

18 Blood

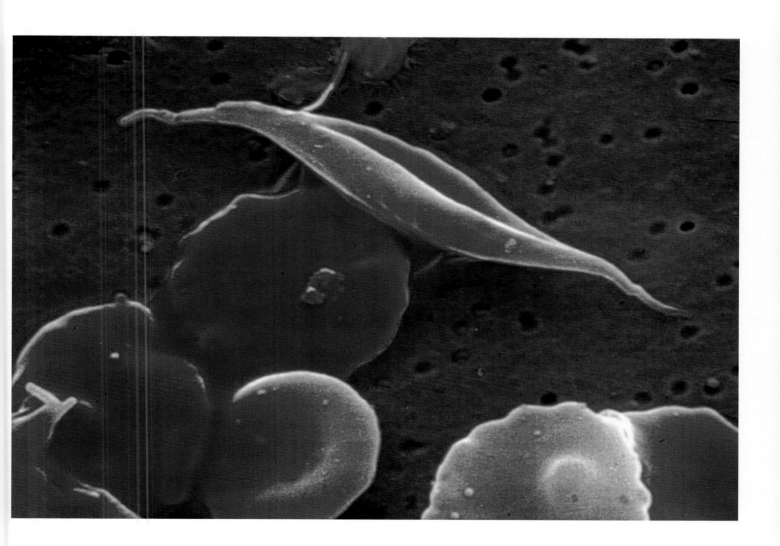

Blood arises in fetal life from reticuloendothelial tissue (liver, spleen, and lymph organs) and in adult life from bone marrow precursors – collectively termed the hemopoietic system. Blood cells are distinguished by their ability to circulate around the body. These circulating cells comprise a variety of lineages including red cells (erythrocytes), white cells (leukocytes: lymphocytes, polymorphs, and mononuclear cells) and platelets (cytoplasmic fragments shed by bone marrow megakaryocytes). The way in which these blood cells grow, signal, adhere to tissue surfaces, and mediate inflammatory responses is considered in detail elsewhere. Here we examine how the blood delivers oxygen to tissues, senses antigenic red cells, and controls injuries by reversible clot formation.

Tissue oxygenation

Oxygen acquires reactivity on entering cells

If carbon represents the structural basis of human life, the functional basis is oxygen. The physiologic importance of oxygen reflects two opposing qualities:

1. Environmental oxygen is stable and hence ubiquitous
   - Photosynthesizing organisms (e.g., plants) use solar energy to activate chlorophyll, which in turn converts the thermodynamically stable oxidation substrate water (H_2O) to atmospheric oxygen (O_2).
   - Atmospheric oxygen is stable because its electronic ground state includes two unpaired electrons which hinder volatile singlet-state reactions.
2. Cellular oxygen is unstable and hence highly reactive
   - Cellular oxygen (O_2^-) provides a thermodynamically reactive substrate for reduction to water.
   - By facilitating the oxidation of biological reductants in this manner, oxygen provides a way to generate cellular energy (Chapter 1).

Cellular oxygen is thus ideal for modulating the catalytic reactivity of enzymes. A disadvantage of oxygen's reactivity relates to the production of tissue-damaging free radicals in certain diseases. However, the generation of cytotoxic oxygen radicals can also be helpful for killing bacteria responsible for tissue inflammation. Since tissue hypoxia reduces free radical generation, the effectiveness of anticancer treatments such as radiotherapy and radical-generating chemotherapies (e.g., the radiomimetic drug **bleomycin**, or the DNA intercalator **doxorubicin**) may be impaired in poorly oxygenated tumors that have outgrown their original blood supply.

MOLECULAR MINIREVIEW

Oxygen-sensing HIFs

A key skill in life involves sensing when you are running out of oxygen. Changes in ambient oxygen concentrations are detected by **oxygen-sensing proteins**. The best characterized subclass of such proteins is made up of the basic helix-loop-helix (bHLH) transactivating **hypoxia-inducible factors** (HIFs) which contain oxygen-binding ferrous groups. Increased DNA binding of oxygen-depleted HIFs depends mainly on HIF protein stabilization by hypoxia. Once activated, HIFs induce a plethora of compensatory genes (see below).

HIF1 is a heterodimer comprising the unique hypoxia-inducible **HIF1α** subunit and a second constitutively expressed protein termed **HIF1β** (also known as the aryl hydrocarbon receptor nuclear translocator or ARNT, p. 445) which heterodimerizes promiscuously to bHLH transcription factors. Hence, the HIF1 complex only forms in response to hypoxia, and is absent under normoxic conditions. The HIF1 heterodimer binds cis-acting hypoxia-response elements containing **E-box motifs** (so-called because they were first described in the 3′ flanking region of the erythropoietin gene). Hypoxia-responsive genes other than erythropoietin include those encoding the pressor molecules **endothelin-1** and **angiotensin-converting enzyme**.

Overexpression of HIF1α accompanies p53 upregulation, angiogenesis and metastatic progression in a variety of human tumors, and may occur secondary to loss-of-function mutations affecting the *VHL* gene in **renal cell carcinomas** (p. 100).

Hypoxia triggers a series of adaptive molecular responses

Ambient oxygen deprivation or **anoxia** induces a rapid reduction of arterial oxygen concentration (**hypoxemia**) which is fatal if prolonged. An exception relates to the submersion of young children in ice-cold waters, under which circumstances tissue utilization of oxygen may be extremely low; **tissue hypoxia** is thus minimized even though respiration (or, more strictly, ventilation) has ceased. Tissue hypoxia induced by vascular insufficiency is termed **ischemia**. Genes induced in response to tissue ischemia include those for:

1. **Vascular endothelial growth factor** (VEGF).
2. Glycolytic (anaerobic) enzymes, including **lactate dehydrogenase, pyruvate kinase, phosphofructokinase**.
3. **Erythropoietin** and **transferrin**.
4. Inducible **nitric oxide synthase** (iNOS).
5. **Glucose transporter-1** (GLUT 1).
6. **Heme oxygenase**.

Stabilization of the mRNAs for these genes occurs via non-HIF hypoxia-inducible proteins which bind AU-rich regions in the 3′ untranslated regions of target mRNAs, thereby masking these destabilizing sequences (p. 106). Chronic reductions of oxygen availability may induce the expression of different subsets of compensatory genes. For example, systemic adaptation to hypoxia is further mediated by erythropoietin gene transcription, which can increase 1000-fold in response to high altitude, anemia or chronic lung disease; this induction is mediated via a hypoxia-sensitive 3′ enhancer sequence. Tissue adaptation to hypoxia is further mediated by angiogenic factors such as VEGF, as well as by induction of anaerobic glycolytic enzymes that supply cells with energy in the absence of oxidative phosphorylation.

Iron deficiency causes heme deficiency, hence anemia, and may also disinhibit HIF-dependent gene transactivation. Reduced expression of the iron storage protein **ferritin** restricts the expression of oxygen-binding proteins, potentially worsening iron-deficiency anemia.

PHARMACOLOGIC FOOTNOTE

Cyanide and carbon monoxide poisoning

Oxygen binding to red blood cells may be mimicked by the binding of **cyanide** (CN^-) to ferric (Fe^{3+}) heme. Cyanide-induced tissue hypoxia is mediated in part by the inactivation of **cytochrome oxidase**, thus blocking the mitochondrial electron transport chain (Figure 18.2).

Carbon monoxide (CO) is also sensed by red cells as an oxygen mimic, binding

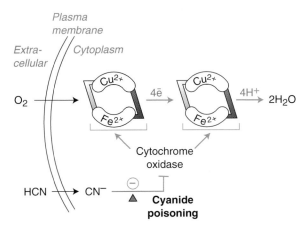

Figure 18.2 Mechanism of cyanide toxicity. Hydrogen cyanide (HCN) dissociates to form intracellular cyanide (CN⁻) ions, which in turn inhibit cytochrome oxidase, thereby poisoning the mitochondrial electron transport chain.

ferrous (Fe^{2+}) heme with 200-fold higher affinity than oxygen. This means that inhaled CO is bound in preference to O_2, whereas O_2 dissociates more readily than CO from red cells during tissue transit. However, CO also impairs O_2 extraction by increasing its heme affinity; the severity of tissue hypoxia is therefore underestimated by blood CO saturations.

The tight but reversible binding of CO occurs via a series of docking interactions in which water is progressively displaced. As with cyanide intoxication, CO-induced tissue hypoxia may be severe in the heart and brain where mitochondrial respiration is critically affected, and where oxidative damage may cause lipid peroxidation. Since CO blocks induction of the usual hypoxic gene cascade, its effects on tissue hypoxia are intensified.

CO is produced not only by car exhausts but also by endogenous metabolism. Heme catabolism by **heme oxygenase** (p. 459) produces CO, which serves an anti-inflammatory function by inhibiting tumor necrosis factor α (TNFα) and interleukin IL-1β expression. Hence, the recognized oxidant-protective effects of heme oxidase may derive in part from its ability to generate CO. In addition, endogenous CO may mimic some of the actions of nitric oxide such as smooth muscle relaxation.

Hemoglobin

Globin proteins transport oxygen to tissues

Molecules that transport oxygen link the environment with the reactive interior of human cells. Such oxygen-binding proteins, termed **globins**, form key subunits of three human oxygen-carrying molecules:

1. **Myoglobin**
   - A single-chain molecule supplying oxygen to muscle.
2. **Hemoglobin**
   - A 64.5-kDa tetrameric molecule, composed of noncovalently linked α dimers, which is expressed solely in red blood cells.
3. **Neuroglobin**
   - A 17-kDa globin expressed mainly in the brain.

Myoglobin has the highest oxygen affinity of these three globins, and hemoglobin the lowest; this means that hemoglobin releases oxygen to tissues more readily than does myoglobin Cerebral hypoxia triggers an increase in brain neuroglobin expression, leading to a neuroprotective effect.

Both myoglobin and hemoglobin contain an oxygen-binding heme prosthetic group consisting of a protoporphyrin ring complexed to a ferrous (Fe^{2+}) ion. Other oxygen-dependent proteins such as the mitochondrial **cytochromes** may use a central copper (Cu^{2+}) atom for oxygen binding and reactive autocatalysis.

Each globin chain folds to form a hydrophobic pocket into which one heme group is inserted. This heme binds a singlet oxygen; hence, the hemoglobin tetramer is able to bind (and release) four oxygen molecules. Each hemoglobin subunit thus encircles oxygen like a glove. Mutations that affect the function of hemoglobin cause syndromes termed **hemoglobinopathies** (Table 18.1).

The transport of oxygen from the lungs to circulating hemoglobin occurs across a pressure gradient that is optimized for oxygen loading and unloading. The difference in oxygen tensions between the lungs and circulation is termed the **alveolar–arterial oxygen (A–a) gradient**. This is normally less than 15 mmHg, but can rise because of (common) ventilation-perfusion mismatching, (occasional) shunting, or (rare) diffusion defects. To maximize the efficiency of oxygen delivery to tissues, hemoglobin releases not only oxygen but also nitric oxide, thus triggering erythrocyte-dependent vasodilatation.

Table 18.1. Hemoglobinopathies

1. Thalassemias (defective globin chain production)
   - α-thalassemias
   - β-thalassemias, including structural variants:
   - Hb E
   - Hb Lepore
2. Sickle cell anemia (Hb S)
3. Hereditary persistence of fetal hemoglobin
4. Mutant hemoglobins with abnormal oxygen affinity
   - High-affinity hemoglobins; e.g., Hb Zürich, Hb Köln
   - Low affinity hemoglobins; e.g., Hb Kansas, Hb Seattle

Figure 18.3 Positions and structures of the α- and β-globin clusters on chromosomes 16 and 11 respectively. HS, hypersensitive site; LCR, locus control region.

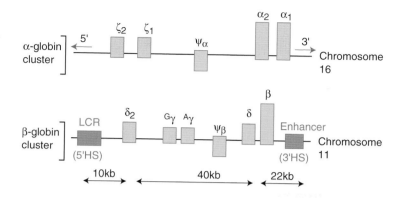

CLINICAL KEYNOTE

Thalassemias: syndromes of globin imbalance

Unlike the hydrophobic heme pocket, hemoglobin's external surfaces are studded with hydrophilic residues that enhance the molecule's solubility. If an imbalance of globin chain synthesis results in the liberation of unpaired globin molecules, this external hydrophilicity is disturbed and solubility reduced. Precipitation of free globin chains is the outcome, leading to the clinical expression of hemoglobinopathies termed **thalassemias**; for example, homozygous β-thalassemia (**β-thalassemia major**) causes a primary reduction in β-chain synthesis, leading to a relative excess of α-globin chains.

In these disorders – which in their heterozygous (either **thalassemia minor** or **thalassemia trait**) forms protect against red cell parasitization by malaria – the nature of the mutation determines the severity of the phenotype. Gene deletions commonly cause **α-thalassemia**, whereas mutations outside the globin gene coding sequence (e.g., in the promoter) are more often responsible for β-thalassemia. These latter lesions may cause reduced β-chain production through the impairment of translation or aberrant mRNA splicing.

Hemoglobin gene clusters are switched on and off in utero

The globin moiety of hemoglobin is encoded not by a single gene but by a family of genes that undergo serial changes of transcriptional expression during development. **Hemoglobin switching** is the name given to this coordinated process. The sequence of this gene activation cascade (embryonic→ fetal→adult) parallels the switching of the primary erythropoietic site from the blood islands of the yolk sac to fetal liver (at 10–12 weeks' gestation) and then to bone marrow (at 36–38 weeks). The structurally divergent proteins synthesized as a result of hemoglobin switching include:

1. **Embryonic hemoglobins**
   - $\zeta_2\varepsilon_2$: Hb Gower I.
   - $\zeta_2\gamma_2$: Hb Portland.
2. **Fetal hemoglobins** (HbF)
   - $\alpha_2 G_{\gamma_2}$.
   - $\alpha_2 A_{\gamma_2}$.
3. **Adult hemoglobins**
   - $\alpha_2\beta_2$: HbA.
   - $\alpha_2\delta_2$: HbA$_2$ (a minor adult Hb, elevated in **β-thalassemia minor**).

The order in which different hemoglobins are expressed during ontogeny is influenced by chromosomal positioning of the single-copy genes in question. For example, the mammalian **β-globin gene cluster** on chromosome 11 arose

Figure 18.4 Hemoglobin switching by the locus control region (LCR). Transcription of embryonic, fetal and adult hemoglobins depends upon sequential 5′ to 3′ gene inactivation through chromatin modification.

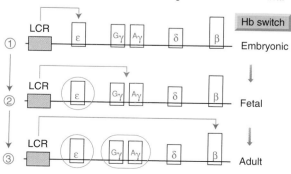

approximately 200 million years ago via a series of tandem duplications, and these genes are developmentally expressed in the $5' \rightarrow 3'$ direction: first the embryonic ε gene, then the fetal G_γ and A_γ genes, and finally the adult δ and β_1/β_2 genes. Globins encoded by these genes contain 146 amino acids, unlike the 141-amino-acid proteins encoded by the **α-globin gene cluster** on chromosome 16; the latter genes are first expressed as the 5′ embryonic $\zeta2$ genes before switching to the 3′ fetal and adult α_2/α_1 genes (Figure 18.3). Since α-globins (but not β-globins) are produced in fetal life, homozygous α-thalassemias may cause symptoms in the neonatal period (or even prenatally, e.g., **hydrops fetalis**) whereas β-thalassemia major rarely causes symptoms before three months of age.

Transcriptional regulation of the α- and β-globin clusters is modulated by an enhancer-like **locus control region** (LCR; Figure 18.4) situated 5–50 kb upstream of the respective embryonic globin genes. The LCR contains five DNase I-hypersensitive sites, which each have a core region of approximately 250 bp: globin gene transactivation is most critically dependent upon sites two to four. These processes may involve wave-like changes in chromatin structure associated with alterations in gene methylation that silence transcription within cytosine-phosphate-guanine (CpG) islands. This flip-flop control mechanism (by which LCR-like regulatory elements "jump over" intervening genes) appears particularly important for regulating fetal (γ) hemoglobin.

MOLECULAR MINIREVIEW

Erythropoiesis and GATA

X-chromosome-encoded **GATA-binding proteins** or **GATA factors** (e.g., GATA1) are key determinants of globin gene expression. These zinc finger proteins activate erythropoiesis and megakaryocyte gene expression (as well as spermatogenesis) by binding GATA nucleotide sequences in upstream regulatory elements. The proto-oncogene product **Myb**, which is also necessary for adult erythropoiesis, is a GATA-binding transactivator that is often dysregulated in **leukemias**.

GATA1 binds and activates the gene promoter regulating transcription of the Duffy antigen receptor for chemokines (**DARC**) on erythrocytes. A GATA-blocking single nucleotide polymorphism in the DARC promoter of many West Africans confers protection against *Plasmodium vivax* infection in these Duffy-negative individuals – though not against other malarial parasites.

Not all GATA genes are restricted to hemopoietic cells. Haploinsufficiency of the **GATA3** gene results in the congenital disorder of hypoparathyroidism, deafness and renal anomalies (**HDR**) which resembles **diGeorge syndrome** (p. 406). Like GATA3, **GATA2** suppresses adipocyte differentiation when expressed, whereas **GATA4** is implicated in the pathogenesis of cardiac hypertrophy. Yet another GATA-like gene product, **hairless**, is deleted in the rare familial syndrome of **alopecia universalis** (total hair loss).

CLINICAL KEYNOTE

Fetal hemoglobin (HbF)

Globin gene mutations affecting upstream regulatory elements may have a variety of consequences, including:

1. Evolution of transcriptionally inert pseudogenes.
2. Unbalanced globin chain production (thalassemias).

Figure 18.5 Normal and abnormal meiotic recombination of parental globin gene alleles. Normal crossing-over results in homologous recombination of the β-globin gene; however, allelic misalignment may lead to anomalous recombination involving β-globin and δ-globin, resulting in formation of Hb Lepore.

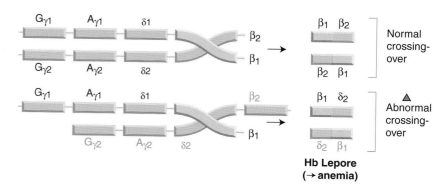

3. Dysregulation of normal hemoglobin switching.

A syndrome that illustrates the latter effect is **hereditary persistence of fetal hemoglobin** (HPFH). This condition arises because of mutations affecting the 5′ regulatory regions of the fetal hemoglobin (HbF, γ-globin) genes.

HbF expression is controlled by the methylation of clustered cytosine residues in nearby DNA sequences. The hypomethylating agent **5-azacytidine** increases γ-globin expression in patients with homozygous hemoglobinopathies such as **β-thalassemia major** and **sickle-cell anemia** (SCA) – thus increasing the formation of HbF, improving oxygen delivery to tissues, and reducing hemolysis. By reducing the need for transfusions, such treatments may prevent the deleterious effects of long-term iron overload (p. 161). However, this approach has so far proven disappointing in the major hemoglobinopathies. In one β-thalassemia variant, **Hb Lepore** – which results from an aberrant recombinational fusion of the homologous δ- and β-globin genes (Figure 18.5) – therapeutic HbF enhancements have been obtained using differentiating agents such as **butyrate** and **hydroxyurea** (p. 403).

Tetramers of hemoglobin allosterically bind and release oxygen

Globin proteins undergo structural transitions between quaternary forms in response to oxygen binding. These shape changes make myoglobin and hemoglobin excellent models of allosteric protein modification (p. 124). Normal hemoglobin alters conformation depending upon its state of ligation:

1. Fully ligated (oxidized, Fe^{2+}) **oxyhemoglobin**.
2. Unligated **deoxyhemoglobin**.
3. Fully reduced (Fe^{3+}) **methemoglobin**

How do structural hemoglobin transitions take place? High-affinity $\alpha_1\beta_1$ and $\alpha_2\beta_2$ dimers tend to be maintained, whereas weak contacts between $\alpha_1\beta_2$, $\alpha_2\beta_1$ and $\alpha_1\alpha_2$ dimers are modified during oxygen-dependent conformational changes. These structural transitions occur continuously, taking only 30 million-millionths of a second (picoseconds) for hemoglobin to open up and release oxygen; such transitions smooth conversion of the free energy of oxygen binding to a useful form.

This inequivalence of hemoglobin α- and β-subunits forms the basis for **cooperativity** of local unfolding reactions involved in oxygen binding by the different heme groups – the further the reaction goes, the easier it gets (p. 124). The globin moieties of deoxyhemoglobin exhibit low oxygen affinity, binding tightly instead to each other in a **tense** (T) conformation stabilized by electrostatic bonds. Initial oxygen binding shatters the latter, laying open the remaining oxygen binding sites in a **relaxed** (R) conformation wherein Hb-oxygen affinity increases 500-fold.

The normal autocatalytic quality of tetrameric heme–heme interactions manifests as the steep S-bend of the **oxyhemoglobin dissociation curve** which implies the presence of multiple identical oxygen-binding sites.

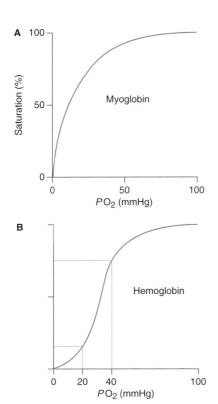

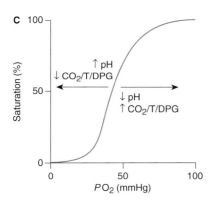

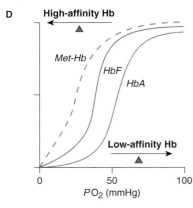

Figure 18.6 The oxygen dissociation curves (ODC) for myoglobin (A) and hemoglobin (B). The monomeric structure of myoglobin results in a nonsigmoid dissociation curve, whereas the tetrameric hemoglobin structure causes cooperative binding. Ambient factors modifying Hb affinity are shown on C; D, both fetal hemoglobin (HbF) and methemoglobin (Met-Hb) cause a leftward shift of the ODC. DPG, 2,3-diphosphoglycerate; HbA, adult hemoglobin; T, temperature.

Mutant proteins composed of identical subunits – such as the β-subunit tetramer hemoglobin H (**HbH**) which accumulates in children who have co-inherited two distinct heterozygous α-thalassemia alleles – fail to display cooperativity, and hence provide poor oxygen transport to tissues.

MOLECULAR MINIREVIEW

The oxyhemoglobin dissociation curve

Heme-oxygen binding is modified by interactions of the complex with competing (heterotropic) ligands such as **carbon dioxide** (CO_2) or **hydrogen ions** (H^+), both of which reduce Hb-O_2 binding affinity and thus promote tissue oxygenation (the Bohr effect). These two ligands stabilize the T conformation of (deoxy)hemoglobin by binding different sites thereon: CO_2 binds the globin amino-terminal to form carbaminohemoglobin, yielding free H^+ which binds specific amino acids elsewhere within the globin molecule. These characteristics of the oxyhemoglobin dissociation curve (**ODC**; Figure 18.6) are illustrated by the behavior of certain hemoglobinopathies:

1. **High-affinity hemoglobin disorders** (often autosomal dominant)
   - Cause asymptomatic polycythemia,
   - Cause a leftward shift of the ODC.
2. **Low-affinity hemoglobin disorders** (rare)
   - Cause cyanosis and pseudoanemia,
   - Cause a rightward shift of the ODC.

Since erythrocytes lack nuclei, they also lack the genomic genes required for mitochondrial function, and are hence wholly dependent upon glycolysis for their energy needs. Accordingly, feedback control of hemoglobin function is supplied by the glycolytic intermediate **2,3-diphosphoglycerate** (DPG). Increased anaerobic energy requirements (e.g., at high altitude, or in chronic lung disease) cause an increase in red cell DPG which binds between the globin β-chains and thus stabilizes deoxyhemoglobin in the T conformation, facilitating oxygen release. As oxygenation improves, sequestration of DPG by deoxyhemoglobin declines in parallel with increased red cell oxyhemoglobin content.

Hemoglobin is also allosterically regulated by **nitrosylation** (addition of an *S*-nitrosothiol group from nitric oxide, NO) at position Cys[93] on the β-globin chain. NO is transferred to red cell membranes from *S*-nitrosohemoglobin: liberated *S*-**nitrosothiol** or **SNO** is then transferred to cysteine residues in the cytoplasmic (hemoglobin-binding) domain of the **anion exchanger protein**, AE1. Hence, deoxygenation of hemoglobin is accompanied by a switch from the relaxed (R) structure to the tight (T) conformation, leading in turn to hemoglobin-dependent release of SNO from AE1 followed by local vasodilatation. Elevated body temperature (as in fever) is yet another mechanism for facilitating oxygen release from hemoglobin.

CLINICAL KEYNOTE

Sickle cell anemia

A point mutation within the β-globin gene (an invariant A→T transversion at codon 6, leading to replacement in HbA of hydrophilic Glu by hydrophobic Val) is responsible for **sickle cell anemia** (SCA). Mutant **HbS** molecules clump together as inflexible rods, leading to sickling and the hemolysis of affected red blood cells in response to oxidant stress: the oxygen affinity of soluble HbS is normal, but

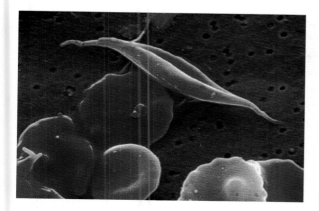

Figure 18.7 Sickle cell anemia, showing sickled erythrocytes. (Wellcome Medical Photographic Library, no. B0000521C14), (E.M. Unit, Royal Free Hospital School of Medicine).

declines dramatically following sickling (Figure 18.7). A vicious cycle can be created when sickled cells obstruct capillaries, worsening tissue deoxygenation and acidosis and precipitating a painful sickling crisis. The adhesion of sickled cells to microvessels may be exacerbated by the following interactions:

1. Red cell $\alpha_4\beta_1$ integrin binds endothelial VCAM-1.
2. Red cell thrombospondin binds either endothelial CD36 (a thromobospondin receptor which is also a *P. falciparum* receptor) or the $\alpha_v\beta_3$ integrin.
3. Red cell von Willebrand factor (VWF; see below) binds the endothelial complex of gp1b, factor IX and factor V.

Either the inhalation or the induction (by **hydroxyurea**) of NO may prove helpful in terminating such crises.

Prenatal diagnosis of SCA can be achieved using labeled sequence-specific oligonucleotides to detect both the mutant and the wild-type gene sequences during Southern blotting of fetal cells obtained at amniocentesis. The homogeneity of this GAG→GTG β^S allelic defect makes the correction or replacement of this defect by a wild-type β^A allele a prime objective for gene therapy (p. 600).

Heme proteins are formed from porphyrin precursors

Normal erythrocyte function depends upon the correct synthesis and incorporation of heme into **hemoproteins**. These proteins – which include catalase, cytochromes, and hemoglobin – oxidize heme to **hemin**, which regulates oxygen-dependent intracellular reactions by modulating the transcription and translation of heme-inducible genes (Figure 18.8). Since these oxygen-dependent reactions are essential for cell respiration, any dysregulation of heme synthesis or utilization is likely to cause a clinically abnormal phenotype.

Sideroblastic anemias are heritable or acquired disorders of heme synthesis in which the iron transported to mitochondria fails to be incorporated into heme. The characteristic ringed sideroblast cellular appearance is due to mitochondrial iron accumulation; treatment with pyridoxine is sometimes useful. Together with the thalassemias, the sideroblastic anemias form a heterogeneous group of iron-loading anemias characterized by ineffective erythropoiesis. Gut hyperabsorption of iron is the result, with potentially serious multiorgan consequences because of parenchymal iron excess (p. 161).

Heme is an intermediary product of vitamin B_{12} metabolism and the citric acid cycle. The key enzymatic steps in hepatic heme biosynthesis involve precursor compounds termed **porphyrins** (Figure 18.9):

1. Conversion of glycine and succinyl CoA to **aminolevulinic acid (ALA)** by **ALA synthetase (ALAS)** – the rate-limiting step.
2. Conversion of ALA to **porphobilinogen (PBG)** by ALA dehydrase.
3. Coalescence of four PBG molecules into a tetrapyrrole that is deaminated to form **uroporphyrinogen**.
4. Decarboxylation of uroporphyrinogen to form **coproporphyrinogen**.
5. Desaturation of coproporphyrinogen to form **protoporphyrin IX**.
6. Metabolism of protoporphyrin IX by **ferrochelatase** to form heme.

ALA is converted to heme in hepatocytes and erythrocytes by separately encoded ALAS isoforms. Approximately two-thirds of liver-derived heme replenishes cytochrome P450 mixed-function oxidases (Figure 18.10). Hepatic heme synthesis is negatively regulated by control loops involving the heme-dependent inhibition of hepatic ALAS (**hALAS**) and heme-inducible expression of heme oxygenase. Other intermediary enzymes such as coproporphyrinogen oxidase are also subject to end-product inhibition by heme.

Unlike hALAS, erythrocyte ALAS (**eALAS**) is not directly inhibited by heme. Like the transferrin receptor and ferritin, eALAS is post-transcriptionally con-

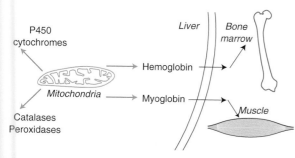

Figure 18.8 Functions of hemoproteins. In addition to hemoglobin and myoglobin, heme is used to make catalases, peroxidases, and hepatic microsomal (P450) enzymes.

trolled by cytoplasmic iron-regulatory proteins, as suggested by the presence of an iron-responsive element (IRE; p. 111) in the 5′ untranslated region of *eALAS* mRNA. The eALAS protein is encoded by an X-chromosomal gene that is a candidate gene for the rare heritable (X-linked) form of sideroblastic anemia. However, most mutations affecting the heme synthetic pathway cause symptoms due to the accumulation of bioactive porphyrin precursors. These phenotypically diverse disorders are termed **porphyrias**.

Figure 18.9 Porphyrin biosynthesis from heme (see text).

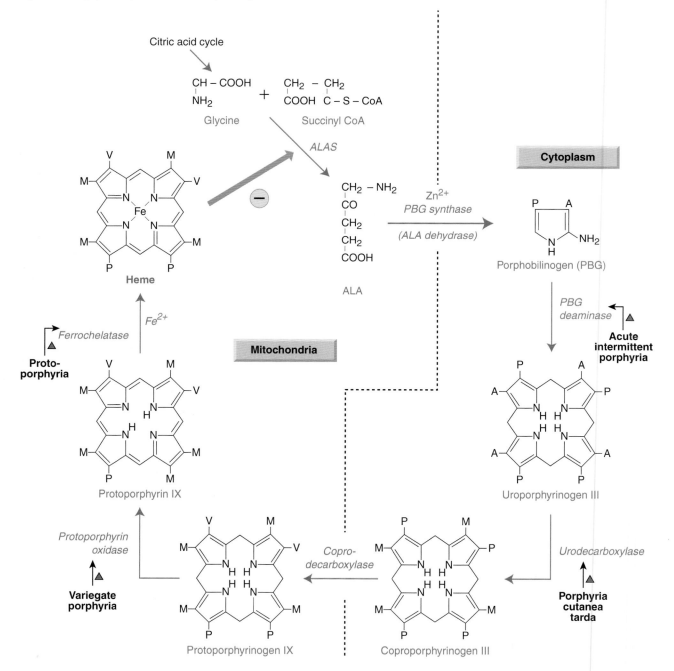

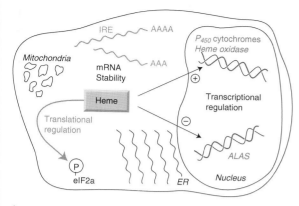

Figure 18.10 The multiple mechanisms regulating heme expression and metabolism. ALAS, aminolevulinic acid synthetase; ER, endoplasmic reticulum; IRE, iron-response element.

The porphyrias

Heterozygous mutations affecting hepatic and red cell heme-metabolizing ALAS pathways are responsible for the tissue-specific accumulation of heme manifesting as **hepatic porphyrias** and **erythropoietic porphyrias** respectively (Figure 18.9). These hereditary disorders may present with a variety of neurologic and/or dermatologic signs; the mutations exhibit incomplete penetrance, with the clinical severity depending on the functionality of the residual allele.

Acute porphyric presentations are often precipitated by drug ingestion. By inducing the expression of hepatic heme-biosynthetic enzymes, such drugs may precipitate exacerbations in porphyria patients who are already overproducing heme precursors. The skin manifestations of porphyrias are precipitated by sunlight, indicating the ability of porphyrins to absorb light (see below).

Phototherapy and antimalarial drugs

Malarial parasites parasitize red cells (i.e., they are intraerythrocytic, though some subtypes also have an exoerythrocytic phase) leading to hemoglobin degradation. Human cells can metabolize heme degradation products, but malarial parasites cannot. A potentially toxic heme metabolite, **ferriprotoporphyrin IX** (also known as β-hematin or hemozoin) therefore accumulates within the parasites. These molecules are not metabolized, but rather are sequestered and polymerized within malarial digestive vacuoles.

The quinoline-ring antimalarial drugs – including **quinine, chloroquine,** and **amodiaquine** – inhibit the enzyme **heme polymerase** which mediates polymerization (and hence detoxification) of ferriprotoporphyrin IX. Malarial parasites that are notoriously chloroquine-resistant (e.g., *P. falciparum*) fail to concentrate the drug within vacuoles due to rapid efflux – a mechanism of resistance similar to that occurring through overexpression of the multidrug transporter (**Mdr**) in human tumors (p. 191). Consistent with this, mutations affecting the homologous efflux pump in *P. falciparum*, **Pgh1**, induce chloroquine resistance.

Since porphyrins are light-activated, they are exploited therapeutically as photosensitizers for ablative photodynamic (laser) therapy of local neoplastic lesions. Oral administration of excess ALA leads to intracellular accumulation of the heme precursor **protoporphyrin IX**. As this metabolite accumulates in gastrointestinal mucosal cells, gut tumors can be endoscopically treated with 630 nm laser light for approximately 24 hours following a photosensitizing oral dose of ALA.

Bilirubin is a breakdown product of heme metabolism

Heme requires not only correct biosynthesis and utilization (Figure 18.10) but also appropriate degradation and excretion. This excretory process involves the following steps (Figure 18.11):

1. Conversion of heme to **biliverdin** (rate-limiting step)
   - Catalyzed by heme oxidase.
2. Conversion of biliverdin to **bilirubin**
   - Catalyzed by biliverdin reductase.
   - **Unconjugated bilirubin** may undergo biliary excretion.
3. Conjugation (and hence solubilization) of bilirubin
   - Catalyzed by glucuronyltransferases (see below).
   - **Conjugated bilirubin** is excreted by the kidneys.

Figure 18.11 Breakdown of heme to bilirubin. Unconjugated bilirubin is excreted in the bile, whereas conjugated (solubilized) bilirubin is excreted in urine.

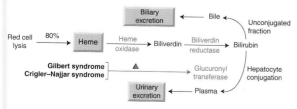

The liver sequesters heme obtained from the intravascular hemolysis of senescent or abnormal red cells. Such heme is derived from circulating complexes of either **haptoglobin-hemoglobin** or **heme-hemopexin**. This source accounts for about 70% of the 300 mg bilirubin normally produced daily by the human body. Bilirubin is a poorly soluble reddish-yellow hydrophobic tetrapyrrole, which circulates bound to albumin. In jaundiced neonates at risk of bilirubin-induced neurotoxicity – such as those with **hemolytic disease of the newborn** due to maternal rhesus (Rh) alloantibodies (p. 463) – drugs such as **penicillin** and **salicylates** may displace bilirubin from albumin-binding sites, thus increasing the risk of brain damage due to (free) hyperbilirubinemia.

Hyperbilirubinemia is recognizable clinically by a yellowish discoloration of the skin and sclerae termed jaundice. Hemolytic states such as **hereditary spherocytosis** can cause mild jaundice due to unconjugated hyperbilirubinemia; since this bilirubin remains insoluble, however, none is excreted in the urine, which retains its normal color. In contrast, obstruction of hepatic biliary outflow – due to, say, **pancreatic cancer** – leads to spillover of conjugated (soluble) bilirubin into the bloodstream, causing not only profound jaundice but also dark urine due to bilirubinuria. Bilirubin solubilization occurs when circulating bilirubin is taken up by hepatocytes, which conjugate the molecule via ester linkages to the sugar **glucuronide**.

MOLECULAR MINIREVIEW

Jaundice enzymes: glucuronyltransferases

Glucuronidation breaks intramolecular hydrogen bonds, reducing the parent molecule's hydrophobicity and thus increasing its solubility. The enzymes catalyzing this conjugation are termed **UDP glucuronyltransferases**; deficiency or dysfunction of these enzymes results in hyperbilirubinemia and jaundice. Mutations inactivating UDP glucuronyltransferases may cause severe inherited unconjugated hyperbilirubinemia (**Crigler–Najjar syndromes I/II**), which can be fatal in early life. However, mild UDP glucuronyltransferase deficiency (**Gilbert syndrome**) – which is detectable in 8% of the population – is treatable using drugs such as **phenobarbital** to induce expression of the deficient hepatic enzyme; (indeed, many patients do not require treatment). Gilbert syndrome is genetically heterogeneous, with milder forms associated with upstream mutations usually affecting the TATA box, namely an extra TA in the promoter, i.e., $(TA)_7TAA$ instead of the wild-type $(TA)_6TAA$. More severe phenotypes are linked to mutations affecting exon 1 of the UDP-glucuronyltransferase gene. Promoter polymorphisms cause jaundice more often when associated with other genotypic variants, e.g., **hereditary spherocytosis** or **glucose-6-phosphate dehydrogenase deficiency**.

Not all heritable hyperbilirubinemias are due to glucuronyltransferase mutations. **Dubin–Johnson syndrome** is a benign autosomal recessive hyperbilirubinemia caused by a loss-of-function mutation affecting an ATP-dependent bile canalicular organic anion transporter protein (MRP2). Mutations affecting a P-type membrane ATPase are responsible for **progressive familial intrahepatic cholestasis I** (PFIC I; Byler disease), and also for the milder syndrome of **benign recurrent intrahepatic cholestasis**. PFIC II and III arise due to mutations of Mdr efflux pumps (p. 191); since acquired biliary obstruction causes the transcriptional induction of Mdr, the pathogenetic significance is clear. Secondary changes of gene expression are seen in **primary biliary cirrhosis** (repression of the chloride-bicarbonate ion exchanger), **primary sclerosing cholangitis** (induction of organic anion transporters), and **biliary atresia** (repression of the sodium-taurocholate co-transporter).

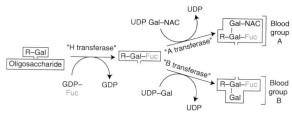

Figure 18.12 Formation of red blood cell A, B, and H antigens by UDP-galactosyltransferases (see text).

Blood groups

ABH antigens are red cell membrane carbohydrates

Red cell membranes contain glycolipids and glycoproteins, which in turn contain oligosaccharide chains. Specific carbohydrate epitopes within these oligosaccharides make up the major blood group antigens. These three major red cell carbohydrate antigens are termed **A**, **B**, and **H** (Figure 18.12):

1. **H antigen**
   - The precursor oligosaccharide for A and B antigens.
   - Consists of a fucose residue linked to galactose at the nonreducing end of the oligosaccharide chain.
2. **A antigen**
   - Formed by adding *N*-acetylgalactosamine to the H antigen galactose.
3. **B antigen**
   - Adds a galactose residue to the same H antigen precursor site.

Red cells not expressing A or B antigens are designated **blood group O**, though this phenotype actually represents HH antigen homozygosity. Despite this, the major red cell antigens are still termed **ABO antigens**.

A and B antigens are **immunodominant** over O(H) antigens, making AA and BB homozygotes serologically indistinguishable from AO and BO heterozygotes. The immunodominance of A/B antigens within the ABO system is responsible for the reputation of O-group individuals as universal donors (i.e., O red cells are not agglutinated by anti-A or anti-B) and for AB heterozygotes as universal recipients. However, whole blood from O-group individuals contains potentially hemolytic anti-A and anti-B in plasma – necessitating the use of washed (plasma-free) packed red cells – while AB individuals can receive only washed red cells from O-group donors.

> ### CLINICAL KEYNOTE
>
> #### Transfusion reactions
> Blood transfusions may be complicated by transfusion reactions if donor and recipient red cell antigens and/or plasma antibodies are incompatible. **Isoimmune hemolysis** occurs most often because of ABO incompatibility, reflecting the presence of complement-fixing IgM antibodies to nonself ABO antigens.
>
> Crossmatching an individual's blood for receiving a transfusion involves first typing the recipient's blood group for red cell A and B antigens using anti-A and anti-B, and then screening the recipient's plasma for red cell antibodies by checking agglutination in a panel of antigenic donor red cells incubated with recipient serum. A positive cross-match precludes transfusion.

Glycosyltransferase genes specify ABO blood groups

Serologic blood groups A and O are common among Caucasians – each occurring in 40–45% of the population – whereas group B is frequent in Asian (20–25%) and African (15–20%) kindreds. Group AB also occurs in 10–15% of Asians but in less than 5% of non-Asiatic individuals. The Mendelian inheritance of ABO antigens has enabled their use in assessing claims of consanguinity (though this approach has now been superseded by DNA fingerprinting; see Figure 22.3). Since A and B antigens are immunodominant, family pedigree analysis is required for serologic distinction of AA/BB homozygotes from AO/BO heterozygotes (direct genotyping, including sequence polymorphism analysis, is also possible). ABO antigens are not specified by antigen-synthesizing genes per se but rather by genes encoding enzymes – **glycosyltransferases** – which post-translationally modify erythrocyte membrane proteins (Figure 18.12). These epitope-creating enzymes, which are encoded on chromosome 9, include:

1. For blood group O(H)
   - α1-2 **fucosyltransferase**.
2. For blood group A
   - α1-3 *N*-**acetylgalactosaminyltransferase**.
3. For blood group B
   - α1-3 **galactosyltransferase**.

The differential activity of these enzymes determines the composition of the terminal trisaccharide – and hence the antigenicity – of these red cell carbohydrates. Transfused group-O erythrocytes may thus convert to group AB following ABO-incompatible allograft transplantation.

Organ transplants from pigs are rejected by xenoreactive antibodies to the carbohydrate epitope Galα1-3Galβ1-4GlcNAc-R (αGal), which is synthesized by a porcine glucosylgalactosyltransferase (αGT). Efforts are being made to knock-out pig αGT activity and thus to improve xenotransplant tolerance.

CLINICAL KEYNOTE

Secretors, nonsecretors, and *Helicobacter pylori*

ABH antigen expression is not restricted to red blood cells. About 80% of Caucasians also express ABH antigens in their secretions: such individuals (ABH **secretors**) appear more susceptible to respiratory viral infections than **nonsecretors**, whereas females with recurrent urinary tract infections are three times as likely to be nonsecretors. The latter may reflect the preferential expression in nonsecretors' vaginal epithelium of two glycosphingolipids that bind **uropathogenic** *Escherichia coli*. Hence, secretor genes are simply glycosyltransferases that determine patterns of cell-surface glycoprotein expression.

The long-standing observation that peptic ulceration is associated with blood group O is explained by the finding that the O-group erythrocyte antigen **Lewis b** (Le^b) – which is the main blood group antigen expressed on gastric epithelial cell surfaces in secretors – is a receptor for the gastritis-associated bacterium *Helicobacter pylori* which binds via **BabA** (blood group antigen-binding adhesin). The latter is a pathogenicity factor associated with both ulceration and gastric cancer, and hence a possible vaccination target. Substitution of the fucosyl residue by blood group A or B antigens confers a degree of protection against mucosal colonization by this organism.

The **Lewis a** (Le^a) determinant, on the other hand, is the dominant blood group antigen in nonsecretors, and may be a receptor for *Candida* spp. The sialylated **Lewis x** (Le^x) red cell antigen is a ligand for the cell adhesion molecules P-selectin and E-selectin.

Rh-negative recipients are alloimmunized by group-D donors

In addition to the ABO system, there are 20 other major blood groups which comprise over 400 red cell antigens. For example, fetal red blood cells can be distinguished from adult erythrocytes by expression of **i antigen**, rather than **I**

antigen in adults. Similarly, **glycophorins** (e.g., GPA) are red cell membrane antigens rich in sialic acid and hence negatively charged, thus inhibiting erythrocyte aggregation. The red cell **P antigen** (globoside) is a receptor for **human parvovirus B19**, whereas the **Duffy red cell antigen** is a receptor for *P. vivax* (as well as for endogenous chemokines; see below). All of these antigenic molecules seem likely to play important functional roles in normal life. Yet despite the existence of these numerous blood antigens, transfusional compatibility is routinely assessed on the basis of only three major immunogens:

1. Blood group A.
2. Blood group B.
3. Blood group **D – Rh antigen**.

Rh proteins are nonglycosylated sulfhydryl-containing hydrophobic molecules deeply embedded within the red cell plasma membrane. These polymorphic proteins are encoded by two homologous genes on chromosome 1: that encoding the Cc and Ee polypeptides, and that encoding the D protein. The D antigen is the major Rh antigen influencing transfusion compatibility, being the most immunogenic antigen after A and B: about 85% of the population is Rh-positive (DD or Dd) while 15% are Rh-negative (dd). This latter group is at risk of alloimmunization from repeated transfusions, a hazard most commonly encountered in the context of maternal–fetal incompatibility.

CLINICAL KEYNOTE

Rh disease

Rh (rhesus) **antigens** are best known as precipitants of **maternal–fetal incompatibility** (hemolytic disease of the newborn) in multiparous individuals. Rh-negative primiparous mothers having an Rh-positive pregnancy may develop Rh IgG alloantibodies during the peripartum period, and these antibodies can cross the placenta in subsequent pregnancies and cause hemolysis in Rh-positive fetuses. Rh-negative mothers routinely receive passive immunization with Rh antibody (IgG **anti-D**) immediately following Rh-positive births to prevent maternal alloimmunization. Fetal RhD genotyping may be noninvasively achieved using PCR-based analysis of second-trimester maternal plasma.

Not to be confused with common dd Rh-negativity – in which the RhD gene has been deleted (or else has not yet arisen by duplication of the Cc/Ee locus in some kindreds) – are rare null mutations affecting both Rh genes. Such mutations are associated with red cell membrane dysfunction and hemolytic anemia, suggesting that Rh proteins are required for membrane integrity – perhaps acting as lipid transporters (e.g., phosphatidylserine flippases). This is consistent with the predicted structure of the RhD antigen as a 13-transmembrane-domain protein (Figure 18.13). Other Rh antigens (C, E) may occasionally cause hemolytic disease, as may anti-Kidd or anti-Duffy antibodies.

Coagulation

Tissue injury activates platelets and hemostatic enzymes

Since blood loss can be rapidly lethal, the human body has evolved an efficient network of receptors and cytokines that act locally to stem bleeding. At least three variables modulate this hemostatic response in vivo:

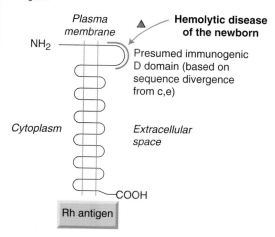

Figure 18.13 The Rh D antigen: a 13-transmembrane-domain protein. Maternal antibodies against the extracellular domain D antigen can trigger hemolysis in neonates. Letters c and e denote respective Rh antigens.

1. The efficiency of platelet activation.
2. The rate of peptide bond cleavage of procoagulant zymogens.
3. The availability and activity of circulating coagulation inhibitors.

Blood clotting is usually initiated by the activation of platelets at sites of tissue injury. Normal vessel endothelium secretes the platelet-inhibitory vasodilator **prostacyclin** (p. 294) which is antithrombotic. However, endothelial injury liberates **von Willebrand factor** which binds and activates the platelet integrin **glycoprotein Ib** (GPIb), thereby initiating platelet activation.

Subendothelial injury also releases **collagen**, which activates the constitutively expressed platelet **glycoprotein Ia/IIa**, leading in turn to expression of the integrin complex **glycoprotein IIb/IIIa** (GPIIb/IIIa; p. 224). GPIIb-IIIa is activated by the binding of its physiologic ligand **fibrinogen**, which is in turn cleaved by **thrombin** to form **fibrin** overlying the platelet plug. Many IIb-IIIa inhibitors are being evaluated in clinical trials, including antibodies (**abciximab**), peptides (**eptifibatide**) and small-molecule drugs (e.g., **tirofiban**, **lamifiban**). Of these, abciximab appears useful for preventing restenosis following percutaneous coronary angioplasty, and also for unstable angina.

As noted earlier, defective in vivo platelet adhesion (in vitro ristocetin-induced platelet aggregation) occurs in individuals with **Bernard–Soulier syndrome**, who have defective GPIb-IX complexes (i.e., reduced von Willebrand factor receptors). In contrast, impaired in vivo platelet aggregation is seen in individuals with reduced fibrinogen binding due to defective GPIIb/IIIa complexes (**Glanzmann thrombasthenia**).

MOLECULAR MINIREVIEW

Platelet activation

Platelets exert their hemostatic effects by undergoing separate adhesion and aggregation reactions. Activated platelets express **P-selectin** as well as **factor V receptors** and **factor VIII receptors** on their surface. The adhesion of neutrophils and monocytes to the platelet plug is mediated by P-selectin, while activation of the intrinsic coagulation pathway is induced by circulating factor VIII.

Bleeding into nonvascular tissue activates factor VII receptors (**tissue factor** – a catalytic glycoprotein constitutively expressed as an integral membrane protein by nonvascular cells) by blood-borne factor VII, with subsequent activation of factor X and the rest of the extrinsic coagulation pathway. Genetic polymorphisms of factor VII may be predictive of **myocardial infarction**: RR homozygotes for the R353Q polymorphism are at higher risk of infarction than are QQ homozygotes (who have lower factor VII levels). Similarly, patients with the A2 promoter polymorphism of factor VII appear protected from myocardial infarction.

Platelets also synthesize and release **ADP** (a cofactor for glycoprotein IIb-IIIa activation), **serotonin**, pro-aggregatory arachidonate derivatives such as **platelet-activating factor** and **thromboxane A_2**, adhesive glycoproteins such as **thrombospondin**, and the anti-angiogenic co-factor **platelet factor IV**. Finally, platelets promote healing by supplying mesenchymal growth factors such as **platelet-derived growth factor** and **transforming growth factor β**.

Cleaved von Willebrand factor affects coagulation and platelets

Tissue injury is a biological emergency in which the (solid) cell-adhesion and (liquid) blood-coagulation systems join forces to plug the hole; immune and inflammatory cells arrive on the scene later to organize more long-term

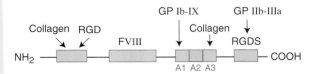

Figure 18.14 Von Willebrand factor (VWF), showing the RGD-binding domain, the factor-VIII-binding (FVIII) domain, and the GP-Ib-IX- and GP-IIb-IIIa-binding sites.

repairs. A key molecule mediating this cross-talk between the adhesion and coagulation pathways is **von Willebrand factor** (**VWF**), a circulating disulfide-linked multimeric adhesive glycoprotein that is synthesized by megakaryocytes and vascular endothelial cells (Figure 18.14). Following secretion into the plasma, the megadalton-size VWF polymer is cleaved between Tyr^{842} and Met^{843} by a cation-dependent metalloenzyme (**VWF-cleaving protease**). The resulting fragments exert three functions:

1. VWF transports **factor VIII** (FVIII, anti-hemophilic factor) as a noncovalent complex, thus protecting FVIII from activation by factor Xa (but not by thrombin) and from inactivation by protein C (pp. 470–1).
2. The type A domain of VWF modulates platelet adhesion to the vessel wall (and hence the initial phase of platelet plug formation) by attacking platelet GPIB (which, together with factor IX, forms a **VWF receptor**) to subendothelial tissues in response to vascular injury.
3. The RGD domain of VWF binds platelet GPIIb-IIIa (fibrinogen receptor) thus promoting platelet aggregation, the second phase of platelet plug formation (Figure 18.15).

VWF is released into plasma as a result of endothelial damage or disease. Release of exotoxin from *Shigella dysenteriae* or enterohemorrhagic *E. coli*, causes the release of VWF multimers from damaged endothelial cells and resultant intravascular platelet aggregation, particularly in the kidney (**hemolytic uremic syndrome, HUS**). A related syndrome with predilection for the nervous system, **thrombotic thrombocytopenic purpura** (**TTP**), involves excess release of unusually large VWF multimers. Consistent with these observations, familial TTP reflects a null mutation of VWF-cleaving protease, and nonfamilial TTP is linked to the presence of autoantibody inhibitors to this same enzyme. In contrast, VWF-cleaving protease activity is normal in HUS. Antiplatelet drugs such as **clopidogrel** and **ticlopidine** have been linked to TTP.

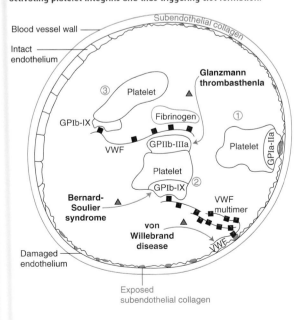

Figure 18.15 Function of von Willebrand factor (VWF) in mediating both platelet adhesion (to endothelium) and aggregation (to other platelets). Endothelial damage reveals subendothelial collagen, activating platelet integrins and thus triggering clot formation.

CLINICAL KEYNOTE

von Willebrand disease

The in vivo adhesive function of VWF can be assayed in vitro by mixing the plasma sample in question with normal platelets, adding a cationic antibiotic (ristocetin) that acts as a fibrin-like cofactor for GPIb adhesion, and assessing the resultant degree of platelet aggregation. Reduced aggregation indicates reduced or defective plasma VWF, as found in individuals with **von Willebrand disease** – a disorder that is usually autosomal dominant.

Families affected by this common condition may have histories of prolonged bleeding following dental extractions. However, severe inherited deficiency of VWF can be associated with secondary FVIII deficiency (see above) and hemophilia-like symptoms. VWD is very common, affecting as many as 1% of the population, with most cases arising from gene deletions.

Coagulation is catalyzed by a proteolytic cascade

Platelets alone do not ensure hemostasis. Blood coagulation requires a cascade of molecules that proteolytically activate one other in response to intrinsic and extrinsic cues related to bleeding or inflammation (Figure 18.16). These coagulation factors exert a variety of molecular functions:

1. **Circulating serine proteases**
   - Coagulation factors: factor II (prothrombin), VII, IX, and X.

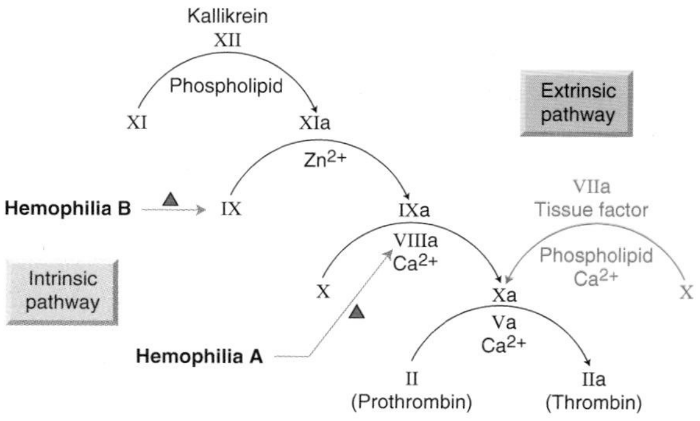

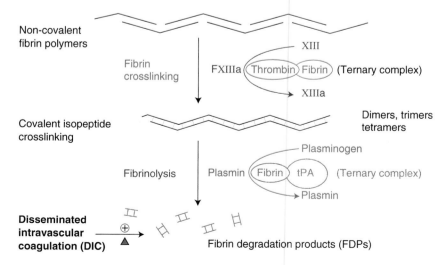

Figure 18.16 The coagulation cascade, summarizing the intrinsic and extrinsic components.

- Endogenous anticoagulants: protein C and protein S.
- Fibrinolytic enzymes: plasmin.

2. **Nonenzymatic cofactors**
   - Factor V (activates prothrombin).
   - Factor VIII (activates factor X).

3. **Transglutaminases**
   - Factor XIII (cross-links fibrin, VWF, fibronectin (see Figure 18.17)).

4. **Nonvascular membrane proteins**
   - Tissue factor (factor VII receptor).

Many structural motifs are shared by these multisubunit molecules. Trypsin-like catalytic domains containing the Asp-Ser-His active site (e.g., contributed by His[602], Asp[645], Ser[740] in plasmin) are found in all circulating serine proteases, as are glutamate-rich **Gla domains** (see below). **EGF-like domains** are found in vitamin-K-dependent serine proteases (except prothrombin) and also in urokinase and plasminogen activator. These EGF-like domains may bind calcium, and are believed to modulate protein-binding interactions. **Kringle domains** – triple-disulfide-bonded structures that bind proteins such as **fibrin** – occur in molecules such as plasminogen, plasminogen activators, prothrombin, and factor XII that are involved in fibrin polymerization and fibrinolysis (Figure 18.17).

CLINICAL KEYNOTE

Hemophilia

Dysfunctional mutations or inherited deficiencies of any of the coagulation factors lead to bleeding diatheses which may be life-threatening. Best-known among these are **hemophilia A** (75%) and **hemophilia B** (25%), which arise because of X-linked deficiencies of factor VIII and IX respectively. Affected males (1/5000) suffer repeated hemorrhages into joints – **hemarthroses** – among other complications, leading to joint deformities. The severity of the syndrome can be predicted by measuring the amount of residual clotting functionality associated with the affected factor. Treatment involves replacement therapy with factor concentrates: many hemophiliacs (about 75%) contracted HIV during the 1980s, prior to the advent of large-scale recombinant factor production, due to the use of contaminated concentrates. Despite the use of synthetic FVIII, approximately 20% of hemophilia A patients develop antibody inhibitors that prevent the effective use of FVIII: the

Figure 18.17 Fibrin polymerization and fibrinolysis. The fibrin-thrombin ternary complex promotes the former by activating factor XIII, whereas fibrin-tPA activates plasmin. tPA, tissue plasminogen activator.

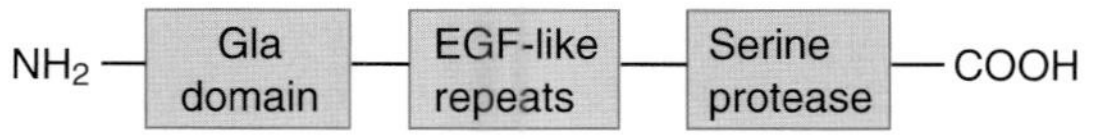

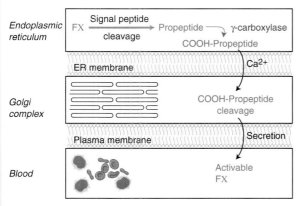

Figure 18.18 Generic structure of a serine protease coagulation factor, showing the glutamate-rich (Gla) domain, the calcium-binding EGF-like domain, and the catalytic domain. EGF, epidermal growth factor.

larger the gene deletion or protein truncation, the higher the probability (and severity) of such inhibitors. A bypass strategy for these patients, and also for hemophilia B patients, has involved the substitute use of recombinant FVIIa.

The FVIII gene comprises 26 exons extending over 180 kb; the protein consists of over 2000 amino acids. The sheer size of the FVIII gene accounts for the clinical heterogeneity of hemophilia A. At least 15 distinct FVIII deletions are recognized, even though these account for only 4% of cases (missense or nonsense point mutations account for 85%, with over a third of these affecting CG dinucleotides). Unlike its target serine protease (factor IX), FVIII is not an enzyme but a cofactor.

The factor IX gene is smaller, containing 8 exons ranging over 32 kb of genomic DNA. Genotype-phenotype correlations are better established: mutations (of which over 750 are known) generally aggregate in three or four hotspots, with more or less predictable clinical effects. Mild-to-moderate disease accompanies mutations affecting the EGF-like or Gla domains. An interesting pathogenetic variant is **factor IX Leyden** (not to be confused with **factor V Leiden**; p. 471) in which mutations disrupting the factor IX promoter lead to severe hemophilia in infancy but milder disease in adulthood due to testosterone-dependent enhancement of promoter activity. Severe disease is lifelong with catalytic or zymogen activation domain mutations – as well as with mutations that affect the propeptide domain, since these in effect abolish vitamin K-dependent γ-carboxylation of factor IX (see below). Unlike FVIII, FIX treatment may be complicated by **thromboembolism** and **disseminated intravascular coagulation** (Figure 18.17).

Vitamin K activates coagulation factors via γ-carboxylation

The activation of serine proteases involved in hemostasis is a multistep process requiring at least five post-translational modifications:

1. Signal peptide cleavage.
2. γ-carboxylation of glutamate residues.
3. Glycosylation (contributing almost 25% of the molecule's mass).
4. Disulfide bond formation.
5. Propeptide cleavage followed by secretion.

All circulating serine proteases – including the coagulation factors II, VII, IX, and X, and the endogenous anticoagulants proteins C and S – require **vitamin K** as a cofactor for activation. Dietary vitamin K is reduced by hepatic **vitamin K reductase** to the hydroquinone **vitamin KH_2**. Free energy of oxidation from this reaction powers the transformation of a weak base to a strong base, thus enabling conversion of specific clotting factor glutamic acid (Glu) residues to **γ-carboxyglutamic acid (Gla)** through proton removal by **γ-glutamyl carboxylase**. In this manner vitamin K permits the activation of serine proteases by transferring its free energy of oxidation to the deprotonating enzyme.

Vitamin-K-dependent coagulation factors initially undergo signal peptide cleavage within the endoplasmic reticulum. This cleavage makes the nascent propeptide domain accessible to γ-glutamyl carboxylase associated with the rough endoplasmic reticulum membrane; in effect, the propeptide domain says, "carboxylate me". Binding of the vitamin-K-dependent enzyme to the carboxylase-recognition site within the propeptide leads to γ-carboxylation of multiple (9–12) glutamate residues within the neighboring Gla domain (Figure 18.18). Glutamate γ-carboxylation adds CO_2-derived carbons to the Gla domain, thus providing additional carboxyl groups that permit chelation of calcium. The Ca^{2+}-bound γ-carboxylated factor is further modified by N-glycosylation and disulfide bond formation within the endoplasmic reticulum, then transported to the Golgi for propeptide cleavage and processing prior to secretion (Figure 18.19).

Figure 18.19 Activation of factor X (FX) by γ-carboxylation and proteolytic cleavage in the endoplasmic reticulum and Golgi respectively.

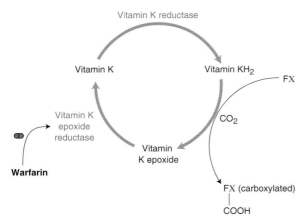

Figure 18.20 Mechanism of warfarin action. Inhibition of vitamin K epoxide reductase prevents the first of two vitamin K reduction reactions, thereby inhibiting γ-carboxylation and activation of factor X.

Abnormalities affecting any step in the vitamin-K-dependent coagulation pathway may disturb normal blood clotting. For example, the mutant propeptide sequences responsible for **factor IX San Diego** and **factor IX Cambridge** lead to the failure of signal peptide cleavage and reduced Gla domain γ-carboxylation, manifesting as severe **hemophilia B**.

PHARMACOLOGIC FOOTNOTE

Warfarin

Nonspecific therapeutic inhibition of vitamin-K-dependent coagulation using the rat poison **warfarin** is associated with potentially serious bleeding toxicity. Under normal circumstances active vitamin KH_2 is converted to the inactive oxide, which is subsequently reactivated by **vitamin K epoxide reductase** – the major therapeutic target of warfarin. Warfarin therefore does not directly inhibit γ-carboxylation of coagulation factors, but rather depletes the activated hydroquinone cofactor required for this post-translational modification (Figure 18.20).

An example of a more selective investigational reagent is a mutagenized **protein C** precursor, which is activated by thrombin in the absence of thrombomodulin. Such a molecule may be selectively activated in the presence of clotting plasma, hence preventing clot extension in individuals undergoing pathologic thrombosis.

Thrombin promotes clot formation via two distinct pathways

Thrombin is derived from its zymogen **prothrombin** (factor II) following limited proteolysis by factor Xa in the presence of calcium and activated factor V. Thrombin is the leading serine protease of the coagulation cascade, and has two mechanisms of procoagulant action:

1. Thrombin activates G-protein-coupled **thrombin receptors** by acting as a site-specific protease rather than as a typical ligand (Figure 18.21).
2. Thrombin proteolytically activates **fibrinogen** by cleaving the constituent fibrinopeptides A and B to yield soluble fibrin monomers, which polymerize to form insoluble fibrin clots (Figure 18.22).

Thrombin receptor activation causes not only platelet aggregation, but also monocyte chemotaxis, lymphocyte/fibroblast mitogenesis, neutrophil margination (vessel wall adhesion), and endothelial synthesis of prostaglandin I_2 (PGI_2), platelet-activating factor (PAF), platelet-derived growth factor (PDGF) and plasminogen activator inhibitors (PAIs). The binding of thrombin by **thrombomodulin** attenuates its procoagulant effects, as does complex formation with the circulating anticoagulant **antithrombin III**. The leech serpin **hirudin** also inhibits thrombin (Figure 18.23).

Blood clots need to be dissolved once they have served their hemostatic purpose. This process of clot dissolution, termed **thrombolysis**, is achieved via a biochemical cascade termed **fibrinolysis**, which is initiated by activation of the kringle-containing (and, hence, fibrin-binding) proenzyme **plasminogen** (see Figure 18.17). Conversion of plasminogen to the active (fibrin-degrading) enzyme **plasmin** is executed by plasminogen activators – either **tissue plasminogen activator** (tPA) or **urokinase-like plasminogen activator** (uPA). The latter protease is expressed by many human tumors, and is implicated in metastasis. Homozygous plasminogen deficiency presents in neonatal life with **ligneous (woody) conjunctivitis** in addition to tracheobronchial obstruction, impaired wound healing, and hydrocephalus.

Figure 18.21 Proteolytic activation of thrombin. Cleavage of the amino-terminal extracellular domain reveals a "tethered ligand", which autoactivates the G-protein-coupled receptor. Other protease-activated receptors may be activated by trypsin, factor VIIa, and factor Xa.

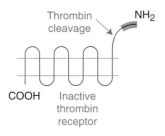

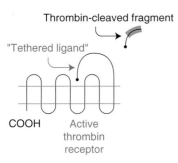

469

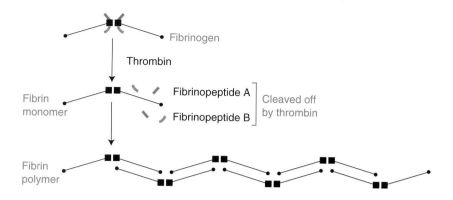

Figure 18.22 Thrombin-dependent conversion of fibrinogen to fibrin polymers.

MOLECULAR MINIREVIEW

Plasminogen activators and PAIs

The fibrinolytic cascade can be antagonized in two ways:

1. By α_2-**antiplasmin**, which directly inhibits plasmin activity, or
2. By serpins termed **plasminogen activator inhibitors** (PAIs).

α_2-antiplasmin is cross-linked to fibrin by the tetrameric transglutaminase **factor XIII**, and this stabilized fibrin then potentiates thrombin cleavage of XIII. Of note, a factor XIII mutation affecting the physiologic site of thrombin cleavage (Val34→Leu) appears protective against thrombosis and myocardial infarction.

Topical **fibrin glue** (sometimes used by surgeons to secure hemostasis of multiple bleeding points) consists of fibrinogen, factor XIII, and thrombin; use of recombinant factor XIII alone may inhibit fibrinolysis and accelerate the healing of **venous leg ulcers**. Similarly, the protease inhibitor **aprotinin** has been used to decrease postoperative bleeding, perhaps by inhibiting plasmin.

PAIs are bulky molecules (like most proteinase inhibitors), which act by restricting substrate accessibility to tPA/uPA catalytic sites. PAI–tPA complexes are cleared by internalization and degradation of the **low-density lipoprotein receptor-related protein** (LRP). Increased plasma levels of PAI-1 (the main PAI in human plasma) are seen in thrombotic disorders such as **hemolytic uremic syndrome**, and are predictive of poor survival in injured patients. Estrogen reduces PAI-1 levels, accounting in part for the postmenopausal increase in coronary disease.

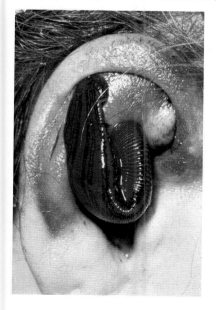

Figure 18.23 Leeches – the source of hirudin (Wellcome Medical Photographic Library, National Medical Slide Bank, no. 9031).

PHARMACOLOGIC FOOTNOTE

Thrombolytic therapy

Thrombi responsible for catastrophic arterial events such as **myocardial infarction** consist not only of the peripheral fibrin-rich portion (the red clot), but also of a solid platelet-rich core (the white clot). Unlike the red clot, the white clot cannot be readily lysed by the endogenous fibrinolytic system. Indeed, by releasing thrombin, fibrinolysis may accelerate white clot growth. A focus of future work is to test whether dissolution of white clots can be expedited by combining GPIIb/IIIa blockers with thrombolytic drugs based on fibrinolytic molecules:

- **tPA.**
- uPA (**urokinase**).
- **Streptokinase**

Use of thrombolytic drugs in acute coronary thrombosis may be associated with improved survival, reduction of infarct size, and preservation of ventricular function. The most selective of these drugs, tPA, cleaves plasminogen molecules on the surface of the fibrin clot: fibrin thus acts as an indirect activator of plasminogen by presenting fibrin-bound tPA to the zymogen.

Indiscriminate activation of both circulating and fibrin-bound plasminogen is induced by urokinase and streptokinase, resulting in widespread fibrinolysis with destruction of factor V, factor VIII, and fibrinogen.

The reduction in ischemic events associated with moderate red wine intake has been associated with morning-after increases in endogenous tPA levels.

Endogenous anticoagulants prevent thromboembolism

The human body's efficient antihemorrhagic system has a downside: thrombotic disorders such as myocardial infarction and stroke have become major causes of death. To counter this threat counter-regulatory molecules termed endogenous anticoagulants have evolved. These include **antithrombin III** (AT-III), **protein C**, and **protein S**.

Circulating serine protease inhibitors (serpins; p. 126) such as AT-III create inhibitory complexes with activated serine protease coagulation factors (e.g., factor Xa). The anticoagulant drug heparin acts via AT-III (see below). A second circulating anticoagulant related to AT-III is **heparin cofactor II**, the activity of which is potentiated by the proteoglycan dermatan sulfate.

Protein S is a cofactor that reorients the active site of protein C on the cell membrane. Under normal circumstances, binding of thrombin to its integral endothelial membrane receptor **thrombomodulin** leads to proteolytic activation of protein C which in turn leads to proteolytic inactivation of factor Va and VIIIa (Figure 18.24) and also, subsequently, of factor VIIIa.

Abnormalities of the endogenous clot control system may cause a 20-fold increased risk of thrombosis. Such pro-thrombotic predispositions, which may also be acquired from conditions such as malignancies, are termed **hypercoagulable states**. Mutation-induced functional deficiencies of AT-III, protein C or protein S account together for 5% of venous thrombosis cases. The following gene mutations also cause hypercoagulability:

1. **Prothrombin G^{20210}** (present in 5% of venous thromboses).
2. **Factor VIII promoter polymorphism** (high FVIII levels).
3. **Methylenetetrahydrofolate reductase** (*MTHFR*) **C^{677}→T** (homozygosity, leading to homocystinemia; p. 157).
4. **Factor V G^{1691}** (Factor V Leiden; see below).

Note that deficiency of the vitamin K-dependent **protein Z**, which potentiates factor Xa inhibition by the protein-Z-dependent proteinase inhibitor **ZPI**, has been linked to ischemic (arterial) stroke.

Although only a minority of thrombotic events can be traced to defects of the endogenous anticoagulant system, such cases are important to detect since treatment may require modification. Hypercoagulable states may also be acquired secondary to conditions such as disseminated cancer or severe endotoxic sepsis. In the latter eventuality, the inflammatory cascade (e.g., IL-6, IL-1α) may upregulate PAI-1 while downregulating thrombomodulin, thus inhibiting thrombin-dependent protein C activation and impairing fibrinolysis.

Recombinant activated protein C (drotrecogin alfa) may reduce plasma D-dimer levels (a marker of coagulation activation) and sepsis-associated mortality in dire emergencies such as **meningococcemia**.

Figure 18.24 Mechanism of action of the endogenous anticoagulant protein C. Thrombin-activated thrombomodulin activates protein C, inhibiting activation of factor V (FV) and thus interrupting the procoagulant conversion of prothrombin to thrombin by negative feedback.

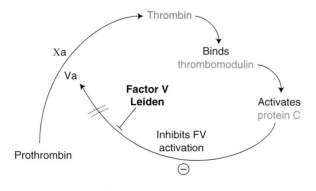

Factor V Leiden and protein C resistance

Subnormal response to the enzymatic action of activated protein C is the commonest phenotype underlying **familial thrombophilia** (a hereditary predisposition to venous thrombosis). Resistance to protein C is linked to mutations reducing the anticoagulant (protein C cofactor) activity of coagulation factor V. This procoagulable mutational phenotype, termed **factor V Leiden**, is present in 5% of Caucasians and in 30% of sporadic thromboembolism cases (thus being the commonest identified cause of hypercoagulability). The mutation conferring factor Va resistance to protein C is a single point mutation (G1691A) substituting Arg-506 by Gln in factor V, thereby removing the peptide bond normally cleaved by activated protein C. Hence, it is not a mutation of protein C itself that reduces endogenous anticoagulant activity in this condition, but a mutation of its substrate.

Like the G20210A prothrombin gene mutation (see above), factor V Leiden predisposes to **cerebral vein thrombosis**, particularly when associated with oral **contraceptive** use. The relative risk is about 10-fold for heterozygotes and about 100-fold for homozygotes.

PHARMACOLOGIC FOOTNOTE

Heparin

The naturally occurring glycosaminoglycan **herapin** is characterized by a strong negative charge. Lysine residues in antithrombin III (AT-III) are bound by heparin, leading to a conformational change that potentiates AT-III-mediated inactivation of factor Xa (and also factors XIa, XIIa, IXa, and thrombin). Inhibition of thrombin is due to an electrostatic interaction, whereas inhibition of Xa and the other factors is allosteric.

Low molecular weight heparin (e.g., **enoxaparin**) is a popular alternative to standard heparin for treating venous thrombosis. Low molecular weight heparin binds AT-III, thus reversing activation of factor Xa, but it does not directly inactivate thrombin since this requires formation of a larger ternary complex (Figure 18.17). The lower frequency of hemorrhagic complications with low molecular weight heparin may reflect this latter difference. The anticoagulant effect of heparin can be reversed using the antidote **protamine sulfate** (**protamines** are arginine-rich proteins expressed during postmeiotic spermatogenesis).

Individuals with inherited **AT-III deficiency** may become hypercoagulable and suffer from heparin-resistant venous thrombosis and/or life-threatening pulmonary thromboembolism. **Heparin-induced thrombocytopenia** (HIT) is a prothrombotic syndrome which may require treatment with thrombin inhibitors (e.g., **argatroban**), hirudin derivatives or heparinoids. Synthetic AT-III-binding sulfated pentasaccharides (e.g., **fondaparinux**) may neutralize factor Xa in a manner similar to low molecular weight heparin, but without the attendant hazards of platelet antibody formation, HIT, and paradoxical thromboembolism.

Summary

Oxygen acquires reactivity on entering cells. Hypoxia triggers a series of adaptive molecular responses.

Globin proteins transport oxygen to tissues. Hemoglobin gene clusters are switched on and off in utero. Tetramers of hemoglobin allosterically bind and release oxygen. Heme proteins are formed from porphyrin precursors. Bilirubin is a breakdown product of heme metabolism.

ABH antigens are red cell membrane carbohydrates. Glycosyltransferase genes specify ABO blood groups. Rh-negative recipients are alloimmunized by group-D donors.

Tissue injury activates platelets and hemostatic enzymes. Cleaved von Willebrand factor affects coagulation and platelets. Coagulation is catalyzed by a proteolytic cascade. Vitamin K activates coagulation factors via γ-carboxylation. Thrombin promotes clot formation via two distinct pathways. Endogenous anticoagulants prevent thromboembolism.

Enrichment reading

Library reference

Clerch LB, Massaro DJ (eds). *Oxygen, gene expression, and cellular function.* Marcel Dekker, New York, 1999

Stamatoyannopoulos G. *The molecular basis of blood diseases.* WB Saunders, Philadelphia, 2000

QUIZ QUESTIONS

1. Explain why oxygen is important to living cells.
2. How do cells sense oxygen? What cellular responses are triggered in response to a temporary shortage of ambient oxygen?
3. Describe how cyanide and carbon monoxide poison cells.
4. What is meant by the phrase hemoglobin switching?
5. How does hemoglobin deliver oxygen to tissues?
6. Explain the pathogenesis of thalassemias.
7. Which factors shift the oxygen dissociation curve of hemoglobin to the left and which to the right?
8. Describe the nature of the molecular defect responsible for sickle cell anemia.
9. What is meant by the terms ineffective erythropoiesis and iron-loading anemia?
10. Briefly explain the molecular pathogenesis of the hepatic and erythropoietic porphyrias.
11. What is the basis of chloroquine resistance in malarial parasites?
12. How do conjugated and unconjugated hyperbilirubinemia occur, and how do they manifest?
13. Describe the expected spectrum of clinical presentations in patients with mutations affecting glucuronyltransferase genes.
14. Explain the common molecular antecedents for incompatible blood transfusion.
15. What, if any, are the clinical consequences of ABH antigen expression in nonhematopoietic tissues?
16. How do platelets contribute to blood clot formation?
17. Explain how mutations affecting von Willebrand factor (VWF) lead to von Willebrand disease (VWD).
18. Describe the molecular role of vitamin K in the coagulation cascade.
19. How do warfarin and heparin work?
20. Which proteins are involved in fibrinolysis?
21. Name some genetic predispositions to venous thromboembolism, and explain their pathogenesis in molecular terms.

19 | Immunity

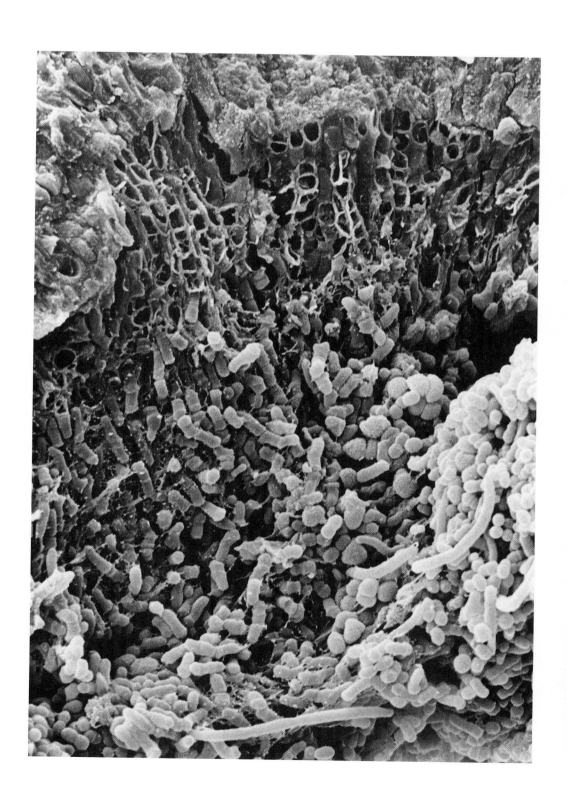

Antibody function

The basic structure of antigen receptors and their accessory molecules is discussed elsewhere (pp. 198–208). In the following section we consider the functional correlates of antigen receptor structure in human lymphoid cells.

Immunoglobulin specificity derives from V(D)J exon variation

Biological systems exploit variability. Bacteria and viruses, for example, use genetic variability to acquire resistance to host defense mechanisms. The human immune system deploys similar strategies to counter the threat posed by these noxious moving targets. There are two main mechanisms by which immunocytes generate antibody diversity:

1. **Germline V(D)J recombination.**
2. **Somatic hypermutation.**

Immunoglobulins are multisubunit proteins consisting of two heavy chains (each containing about 440 amino acids) and two light chains (each about half the size of a heavy chain). These subunits are encoded by genes at three loci: the κ light chain locus on chromosome 2; the λ light chain locus on chromosome 22; and the heavy chain locus on chromosome 14. Transcription of these genes is controlled by transactivating molecules that bind enhancers present within the respective genomic DNA sequences.

Light chains consist of constant (C), variable (V), and joining (J) domains, whereas heavy chains contain an additional diversity (D) chain. The tremendous range of immunoglobulin variation arises due to **V(D)J exon recombination** within these latter gene loci. As the name suggests, the constant (C) domain does not undergo recombinational modification.

Heavy chain gene expression begins in pre-B cells, and is followed by light chain synthesis in B cells (which express surface immunoglobulin) and in plasma cells (which release soluble immunoglobulin). Similarly, heavy chain recombination (D_H joins J_H, then D_HJ_H is joined by V_H to make $V_HD_HJ_H$) precedes κ chain recombination ($V_{\kappa L}$ joins $J_{\kappa L}$) which in turn precedes that of λ chain ($V_{\lambda L}$ joins $J_{\lambda L}$). Such recombination events may not occur with equal efficiency; for example, λ light chain rearrangements occur less commonly than those affecting κ chains. Secondary rearrangements (e.g., of V_H into previously rearranged $V_HD_HJ_H$ loci) may further expand the variety of immunoglobulins obtainable.

Genes encoding T cell receptors (TCRs) undergo germline V(D)J recombination in a manner analogous to immunoglobulin genes, though affecting the α/β and γ/δ chain TCR loci in place of the heavy chain (μ), κ and λ light chain immunoglobulin loci.

CLINICAL KEYNOTE

Abnormal immunoglobulins in human disease
Creating a normal immunoglobulin is a complex process fraught with error. It is therefore unsurprising that many human disorders involve abnormalities in immunoglobulin synthesis and/or regulation. Such disorders include:

1. Paraproteinemia, i.e., secretion of an excessive quantity of a monoclonal immunoglobulin, reflecting the presence of a neoplastic cell clone – such as may be responsible for **myeloma, primary amyloidosis** (Figure 19.2) or **lymphoma**.

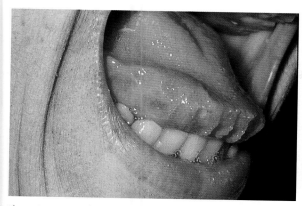

Figure 19.2 Macroglossia in primary amyloidosis, reflecting paraprotein deposition (Wellcome Medical Photographic Library, no. N0000331C).

Such immunoglobulins may be dysfunctional due to mutations affecting the flexible hinge region, leading to stiff molecules.

2. Heavy chain diseases, i.e., monoclonal immunoproliferative disorders causing excessive secretion of immunoglobulin heavy chains alone. For example, **α-heavy chain disease** typically affects the secretory IgA system.
3. Abnormal immunoglobulin gene recombination; for example, defective V(D)J recombination is implicated in the pathogenesis of **SCID (severe combined immunodeficiency)** and of human hematopoietic neoplasms.

Although it has been assumed that human neoplasms arise clonally, analyses of variable immunoglobulin heavy chain (V_H) regions from Reed–Sternberg cells in **Hodgkin lymphoma** suggest that this neoplasm may be polyclonal.

Germline immunoglobulin gene diversity is generated by RAGs

Normal recombinogenic processes give rise to the **naive immunoglobulin repertoire**, which is characterized by the following features:

1. Present in newborns.
2. Associated with the presence of virgin (non-activated) B cells.
3. Formed via an antigen-independent process in the germline.
4. Generated mainly by V(D)J recombination.
5. Composed predominantly of low-affinity antibodies.

Progenitor B cells and T cells utilize a common **V(D)J recombinase** activity that is expressed in a lymphoid-specific fashion (though genes other than those encoding antigen receptors may undergo rearrangement by this recombinase). The location of recombinationally competent V(D)J gene sequences is marked by flanking recombination signal sequences. Activation of V(D)J recombinase is induced by the concerted action of two **recombination-activating genes**: *RAG1* and *RAG2*. These genes are chromosomally located in tandem on 6q21.3, and both appear necessary for immunologic function. Loss-of-function *RAG* mutations may lead to autosomal recessive **SCID** (p. ***) or else to the lethal disorder **Omenn syndrome** (erythroderma, hepatosplenomegaly, hypereosinophilia, and hyper-IgE levels).

Since the number of B cells in the human body ($\sim 10^{10}$) is less than the number of germline antibody configurations ($\sim 10^{11}$), the naive immunoglobulin repertoire is immunologically incomplete at any one time. Hence, the threat of pathogen exposure following postnatal clearance of circulating maternal immunoglobulin means that the humoral immune system of any individual must be capable of rapid adaptation to new antigenic stimuli. The simultaneous induction of B cell clonal expansion and differentiation – termed **replication-recognition coupling** – is an integral feature of human antibody development following antigen exposure or immunization.

MOLECULAR MINIREVIEW

Immunoglobulin class switching

The **class** of a given antibody is specified by the identity of its heavy chain. Although each antibody-synthesizing cell produces immunoglobulins of a single antigenic affinity (defined by the three-dimensional structure of its antigen-binding site), changes may occur in the regulation of heavy chain expression. These changes are referred to as **isotype class switching** (Figure 19.3):

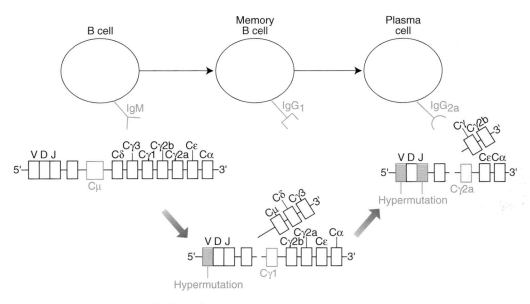

Figure 19.3 Affinity maturation of the humoral immune response. Both heavy chain isotype class switching and somatic V(D)J hypermutation are involved.

1. Virgin B cells expressing only surface IgM may later switch to mixed production of IgM and IgD, usually reflecting a reversible change in RNA processing.
2. On entering the secondary response phase to an antigenic challenge, IgM-expressing B cells undergo terminal differentiation to memory B cells or plasma cells that secrete IgG, IgA or IgE. This irreversible switch in isotype expression, termed **switch recombination**, reflects a deletional DNA modification affecting highly repetitive (hence recombinogenic) immunoglobulin **switch regions.** Prior to switch recombination, transcriptional activation of switch regions leads to the relaxation of surrounding supercoiled DNA; this relaxed configuration is maintained by the formation of RNA-DNA hybrids from nascent RNA transcripts.

Immunoglobulin class switching occurs when cytokines activate B cells. Switch regions are specified by particular cytokines, leading to production of the appropriate antibody subclass. Hence, the effect of class switching is to enhance the functional diversity of antibody-synthesizing cells: instead of being restricted to production of a single antibody, such cells can produce a variety of immunoglobulins with identical antigen specificity but varied immunologic characteristics.

Somatic hypermutation drives antibody maturation

Antigen ligation of surface immunoglobulin causes B cell differentiation to antibody-secreting factories (plasma cells) or to memory cells making up the germinal centers of lymphoid organs. In both cases isotype switching occurs such that the heavy chain C region changes from IgM/IgD (the usual surface immunoglobulin constituents of naive B cells) to IgG, IgA or IgE. Antigen-antibody binding selectively activates those naive B cells that happen to express an immunoglobulin with high antigen affinity, leading to clonal selection of B cells fated to differentiate into plasma cells (or memory cells in germinal centers). This antigen-dependent process of B cell selection, termed **affinity maturation**, is preceded by successive rounds of immunoglobulin variable (V) region mutation (Figure 19.3).

Germline V(D)J recombination is the main mechanism of antibody diversity. The number of unique V(D)J combinations is enhanced by the variability of editing: the junctions between the recombined gene regions are imprecisely located, resulting in additional length polymorphisms. Several other mechanisms contribute to antibody diversity, including immunoglobulin heavy chain class switching and alternative splicing of heavy chain mRNA to generate membrane-bound (B cell) and soluble (plasma cell) forms of the same antibody. Splicing and class switching modify the functional characteristics of the antibody; for example, membrane-bound IgM and IgD molecules contain a carboxy-terminal hydrophobic tag responsible for membrane insertion.

In contrast, affinity maturation fine-tunes the specificity of antibody binding via antigen-inducible V region gene mutations. Unlike in fetal life, the acquisition of immunoglobulin diversity in adult life reflects not only combinatorial but also error-prone processes. These errors or mutations take place within the immunoglobulin gene V region at a far higher frequency (approximately 1 error/kb DNA per cell division) than background somatic mutation (approximately 10^{-6} errors/kb DNA per cell division). This phenomenon – termed **somatic hypermutation** – represents a masterstroke of the immune system, creating as it does expanded B cell clones that initially express low-affinity (predominantly IgM) antibodies.

In mechanistic terms somatic hypermutation is induced by transcription-coupled double-strand DNA breaks which appear in immunogloblulin genes following completion of DNA synthesis. Antigen-driven somatic hypermutation of variable region (V_L and V_H) genes is followed by the selection of high-affinity subclones, which avidly bind target antigen and hence undergo further clonal expansion. This second (antigen-dependent) pathway of immunoglobulin diversification gives rise to the **mature immunoglobulin repertoire** which is:

1. Inducible via exogenous stimuli, e.g., infections and immunizations.
2. Associated with the presence of memory (long-lived) B cells.
3. Formed via an antigen-dependent process in lymph nodes.
4. Generated mainly by somatic hypermutation.
5. Inclusive of high-affinity antibodies.

The characteristics of the naive and mature immunoglobulin repertoires are thus distinct. Abnormalities affecting any step in the maturation of the immune response can result in clinical syndromes of impaired immunity. For example, maturation of the antibody repertoire (via both somatic hypermutation and class switching) is prevented by mutations in an RNA editing enzyme termed **activation-induced deaminase (AID)**; since the primary (RAG-dependent) repertoire is unaffected by AID mutations, AID inhibitors could prove useful in autoimmune disorders.

CLINICAL KEYNOTE

Primary human immunodeficiency syndromes
A variety of developmental abnormalities of the immune system are recognized:
1. **Severe combined immunodeficiency (SCID)**.
   - **X-linked SCID**. The severity of this syndrome reflects a mutation affecting the common **γ chain** of the IL-2, -4, -7, -11, -15 **receptors**. This pathogenesis accounts for up to 40% of SCIDs
   - **Autosomal recessive SCID** may be caused by mutations affecting the cytokine-inducible effector **Jak3**. Mutations disrupting the IL-12 receptor **β1 chain** or the IL-7 receptor **α chain** cause similar SCID-like syndromes. Autosomal recessive SCID may also arise due to deficiencies of purine-degrading enzymes such as **adenosine deaminase** (ADA) or **nucleoside phosphorylase**.

2. **Common variable immunodeficiency**. Denotes a distinctly uncommon and heterogeneous grouping of adult-onset hypogammaglobulinemias associated with **gastric cancer**, **lymphomas** (especially in women), **inflammatory bowel diseases** and **celiac disease**.
3. **Selective IgA deficiency**, a relatively common and mild immunodeficiency affecting 1/700 live births, arises because B cells fail to differentiate into plasma cells. Hence, surface IgA is present but secreted IgA is not.
4. **X-linked** (**Bruton**) **hypogammaglobulinemia** due to mutations affecting the cytosolic tyrosine kinase **Btk** which is essential for B cell development and function.
5. **Wiskott–Aldrich syndrome** arises due to a mutation affecting a gene at Xp11.23 encoding a proline-rich protein (**WASP**: Wiskott–Aldrich syndrome protein) which binds SH3-containing signaling proteins such as Nck. It causes frequent infections associated with low IgM levels, and is treated with **intravenous immunoglobulin**.
6. Hyper-immunoglobulin syndromes
   - **Hyper-IgM syndrome** is an AIDS-like syndrome due to a defective **class switch recombinase**; only IgM is produced.
   - **Hyper-IgE syndrome** is an autosomal dominant syndrome of skin and lung abscesses, craniofacial abnormalities, scoliosis and bone fractures.

PHARMACOLOGIC FOOTNOTE

Therapeutic antibodies

The treatment of human diseases using immune modalities is termed **immunotherapy**. The most direct immunotherapeutic approach is to synthesize antibodies against a putative therapeutic target, and then to infuse patients. This is a problematic undertaking from several viewpoints: intravenous access is required (being proteins, antibodies cannot be effectively administered by mouth), host immune reactions are common, and costs are high.

Most therapeutic antibodies are initially generated as mouse monoclonals. Because murine Fc domains are immunogenic to humans, the gene clone of desired specificity can either be modified to produce monomeric **Fab fragments** (as used in digoxin poisoning, for example) or they can be **humanized** by substituting human sequences. The latter approach is essential if bivalent antibody binding is required (for example, if dimerization of a receptor is required for therapeutic effect). The process of mouse monoclonal antibody humanization typically begins with substitution of human Fc domains, and may then be followed with additional smaller substitutions of the complementarity-determining regions in the Fab domain. Examples of commercially available therapeutic antibodies include **anti-CD20** (rituximab) which is used for refractory **B cell lymphomas**, **anti-ErbB2** (trastuzumab) which is licensed for use in **metastatic breast cancer**, and **anti-GPIIb/IIIa** (abciximab) which is used to prevent **coronary restenosis**.

Immune surveillance

T cells talk to B cells via reciprocal ligand-receptor interactions

Germline diversity of T cell receptors (TCRs) far exceeds that achieved by immunoglobulins. This partly reflects the extent of **junctional diversification** of TCRs caused by the addition of variable lengths of

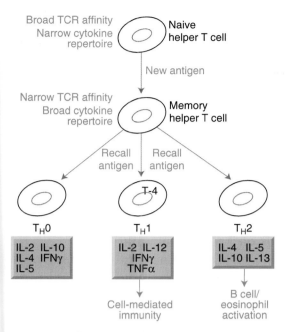

Figure 19.4 T cell receptor affinity maturation driving T cell subtype differentiation. The pattern of lymphokine release associated with each functional T cell subset is shown below. IFN-γ, interferon-γ; IL, interleukin; TCR, T cell receptor; TNF, tumor necrosis factor.

Figure 19.5 Helper T cell subspecialization into T_H1 and T_H2 subsets. The former "help" mainly in cell-mediated immunity, whereas the latter "help" the humoral immune response.

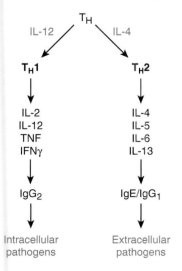

nucleotide (N regions) to intragenic VDJ junctions by **terminal deoxynucleotidyl transferase (TdT)** – a DNA-modifying enzyme also used as a non-B cell lymphocyte marker in hematologic pathology. As many as 10^{17} distinct TCR heterodimers appear possible, far exceeding the figure calculated for antibodies. However, TCRs do not undergo somatic hypermutation following exposure to antigen, presumably to prevent the clonal expansion of autoreactive T cell clones. Since affinity maturation does not affect expanding TCR clones, TCRs generally bind antigen with much lower affinity (approximately 10^{-5} M) than is obtainable with mature antibody (which may reach affinity constants of 10^{-10} M).

The immune response to an antigen generally involves four cellular phases: immunocyte adhesion; antigen recognition; co-stimulation of B and T cells; and immunocyte proliferation. Antigen capture by surface immunoglobulin initially leads to antigen internalization followed by endosomal processing. Degraded antigen peptide fragments are complexed with MHC class II molecules, which transport linearized antigens to the cell surface for presentation to T cells expressing receptors with specific antigen affinity. So-called **helper T cells** help (activate) B cells via a two-way pathway in which activated B cells reciprocate by alerting T cells to the presence of antigen. Communication between helper (T_H) T cells and B cells is transduced by two sets of signals:

1. The B cell receptor **CD40** and the T cell ligand **CD40L**
   - Enables B cells to be helped by activated T cells.
2. The T_H receptor **CD28**, and the B cell ligand **B7** (CD80)
   - Enables CD4$^+$ T cells to respond to activated B cells by releasing **lymphokines** which vary with the helper T cell subtype (Figure 19.4):
     – Activated T_H1 cells release tumor necrosis factor α (TNFα) IL-2, interferon-γ (IFNγ), and IL-12
     – Activated T_H2 cells release IL-5, IL-4, IL-3 (±IL-6, IL-10, IL-9).

Linking these two co-activation cascades is the CD28 homolog **ICOS** (inducible co-stimulatory molecule). Following the antigen-specific initiation of T cell activation, ligation of CD28 by B7 leads to T cell proliferation and lymphokine release. However, antigen-dependent B cell IL-4 release, germinal center formation and immunoglobulin class switching (particularly IgE) require ICOS activation by its B cell counter-receptor **B7RP** (B7-related protein). Interestingly, ICOS knockout mice appear prone to autoimmune demyelinating disorders.

Helper T cells: help or hindrance?

The functional division of CD4-expressing helper T cells into type 1 (T_H1) and type 2 (T_H2) cells depends not only on their pattern of lymphokine release, but also on their predominant mode of immune activity: the proinflammatory cytokine surge initiated by T_H1 cells mainly promotes cell-mediated responses, whereas T_H2 cells more potently trigger antibody release (Figure 19.5). In inflammatory bowel disease, **ulcerative colitis** features a predominant activation of T_H2 cells with increased IL-5, IL-10 and IL-4 release, whereas **Crohn disease (regional ileitis/colitis)** is associated with increased mucosal release of the T_H1 cell cytokines TNFα, IL-12, IL-2 and IFNγ. The latter disease may be treated with IL-10 (which can be delivered by **probiotics**, that is, by live microorganisms programmed to release IL-10 into the gut lumen) or by neutralizing antibodies to TNFα. Consistent with this rationale, IL-10 knockout mice develop a Crohn-like enterocolitis. Parasite-induced elevations of IL-10 in chronic **schistosomal infestation** are negatively associated with **atopy**, indicating a suppressive role for IL-10 in allergic states.

It is mainly the T_H1 system that is activated in the immune response of **rheumatoid arthritis** and **multiple sclerosis**, whereas the T_H2 system dominates in **systemic lupus erythematosus** and **pregnancy**. Female sex hormones enhance the latter response and (thus) dampen down the former, which may be why pregnancy seems to improve rheumatoid arthritis and multiple sclerosis, but not lupus. Drugs such as **suplatast tosilate** that selectively inhibit T_H2-related cytokines like IL-4 and IL-5 may reduce tissue eosinophilia in diseases such as **asthma**, as may recombinant IL-12, but such therapies have yet to demonstrate clinical efficacy.

Thymic cell fate depends on T cell signal duration

CD40 activation by CD4$^+$ cells leads in turn to clonal expansion of activated B cells; stimulation of immunoglobulin class switching; plasma cell differentiation of cell clones secreting the required antibody; and suppression of apoptosis in germinal-center B lymphocytes. Neutralizing antibodies to CD40 may thus reduce inflammation in autoimmune diseases.

The foregoing teaches us that CD40 activation (on B cells) by CD4$^+$ (helper) T cells induces the following effects.

1. Clonal expansion of activated B cells.
2. Stimulation of immunoglobulin class switching.
3. Plasma cell differentiation of antibody-secreting clones.
4. Suppression of apoptosis in germinal center B cells.

In contrast, signal transduction induced by the antigen cross-linking of surface immunoglobulins is associated with activation of the cytosolic B cell tyrosine kinase Lck. The resultant wave of tyrosine phosphorylation leads to internalization of antigen–receptor complexes at the cell surface. This sequence of signal transduction events is similar to that initiated by the activation of TCR.

Whereas helper (CD4$^+$, T_H) T cells seek MHC-II-bearing cells (macrophages and B cells), **cytotoxic-suppressor (CD8$^+$, T_S) T cells** bind the more ubiquitous MHC I molecules. MHC protein recognition is a dual function of the TCR and its accompanying CD4/CD8 coreceptor. The duration of TCR signaling influences whether thymic cell precursors mature into helper or suppressor T cells: longer durations (e.g., >12 hours) of signaling give rise to CD4$^+$ cells, whereas shorter durations (e.g., <2 hours) give rise to CD8$^+$ cells.

A late effect of TCR–antigen complex formation is that helper T cells release IL-2, causing the presenting B cell to differentiate into an immunoglobulin-secreting plasma cell. As with surface immunoglobulin in B cells, antigen binding by TCRs leads to a wave of tyrosine phosphorylation which results in the clonal expansion of T cells with identical antigen affinity.

MOLECULAR MINIREVIEW

SAP and SLAM

SLAM (signaling lymphocyte-activation molecule, or CDw150) is a 70-kDa lymphocyte transmembrane protein that is a receptor for the measles virus. Both T and

B cells express SLAM on their surfaces, forming a homotypic activating receptor–ligand pair which regulates the proliferation and function of both lymphocyte classes.

X-linked lymphoproliferative disease (XLP) arises because of null mutations of the X-chromosomal **SLAM-associated protein** (SAP). SAP is an intracellular SH2-containing protein which competes for the SLAM binding site of the SH2-containing tyrosine phosphatase SHP-2. Loss of SAP expression in XLP patients leads to a communication breakdown between T and B cells. This in turn causes profound dysregulation of B cell proliferation in response to **Epstein–Barr virus** (EBV) infection. Normal individuals with acute primary EBV exposure may have up to 10% of their peripheral B cells infected with the virus, leading to a strong T cell response which destroys most of the EBV-colonized cells. In XLP, however, the T cell response is unregulated by the normal SLAM-SAP cross-talk, leading to an overenthusiastic cytotoxic T cell response as well as unregulated polyclonal B cell proliferation, which culminates in **non-Hodgkin lymphomas**.

Immediate hypersensitivity reactions are caused by IgE

The term **allergy** denotes a clinical spectrum of immediate hypersensitivity disorders mediated by **IgE**. Allergic tendencies may have evolved as a defense against parasitic disorders, in which context IgE triggers the release of cytokines such as **histamine** from reactive leukocytes termed eosinophils. Other mediators in hypersensitivity responses include the leukotrienes, platelet-activating factor and chemokines such as **eotaxins 1–3**.

Individuals or families that have a predisposition to exogenous (nonparasitic) IgE-dependent responses are defined as atopic. A gene postulated to regulate serum IgE levels has been mapped to chromosome 5q31.1 in a cohort of individuals with **atopic asthma**. This locus includes the IL-4 gene; since helper T cells release IL-4 which activates B cells, IL-4 may cause B cells to switch immunoglobulin heavy chain production to the IgE subclass (Figure 19.6). Consistent with this, gain-of-function Gln576Arg mutations of the IL-4 receptor are also linked to atopy. Further loci implicated in IgE hyper-responsiveness are the Ile181Leu polymorphism for **FcεR1-β** and the Gln27Glu polymorphism of the β_2-adrenoceptor (in asthma).

If allergy is simply a matter of IgE hyper-responsiveness, why are some individuals allergic to some stimuli (e.g., **exercise-induced asthma**) but not others (e.g., **allergic rhinitis**)? A clue is suggested by an association between atopic eczema and a chromosome 14 gene polymorphism encoding a serine protease (mast cell **chymase**) produced by the skin. Organ-specific hypersensitivity may thus arise in part via genetic polymorphisms which govern detection sensitivity for ubiquitous antigens.

Figure 19.6 Modulation of the allergic response by T$_H$2 cells. B cells are reprogrammed to secrete IgE in response to IL-4 and IL-13 release by T$_H$2 cells, whereas IL-3 and IL-5 release prime basophils and eosinophils respectively to join in the allergic reaction.

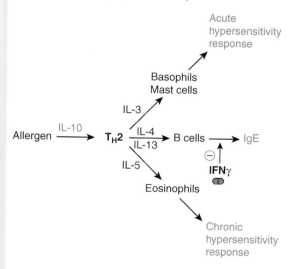

CLINICAL KEYNOTE

Delayed hypersensitivity reactions

T cells mediate **delayed hypersensitivity responses** such as contact dermatitis and certain types of leprosy. Such IgE-independent (nonallergic) hypersensitivity reactions involve T cell receptor activation which induces the chemotaxis of monocytes rather than eosinophils. Nonacute **graft rejection** in the clinical setting of organ transplantation is another common scenario for delayed hypersensitivity, and one that is minimized by the use of immunosuppressive drugs.

Xenobiotics such as metals can also cause hypersensitivity responses: examples include **nickel sulfate** (stabilizes TNFα mRNA), **mercuric chloride** (releases IL-1 from macrophages), and **dinitrochlorobenzene** (induces IL-1 transcription in and keratinocytes).

Innate immunity takes its *Toll* on microbes

Most of the human immune system is **adaptive** in nature: that is, the effectors are capable of being uniquely customized (i.e., selected from a diverse repertoire) to match the particular antigenic specificity required. In contrast, what has been termed **innate immunity** involves more primitive molecular effectors that only recognize invariant microbial structures such as those of bacterial lipopolysaccharide (LPS), lipoarabinomannan (LAM; in *Mycobacteria* spp.), teichoic acids, *N*-formylmethionine or peptidoglycan. Such innate immune effectors include:

1. *Toll*-**like receptors** (TLRs).
2. **Calcium-dependent lectins**.
3. **CD1** cell surface glycoproteins.

The *toll* gene product of *Drosophila* is a transmembrane receptor with cytoplasmic domain homology to the pro-inflammatory IL-1 receptor. Both of these receptors activate NFκB signaling via the TRAF/IKK pathway, leading to the activation of antimicrobial genes with NFκB-binding promoter sequences. Humans express at least ten *toll*-**like receptors (TLRs)**. Immune signaling in response to the lipid A component of bacterial LPS, or to bacterial contact, depends upon the recruitment of an adaptor protein (MyD88) to a patch-like TLR cytoplasmic domain containing a conserved proline residue.

Toll-like receptor 4 (TLR4) is the LPS receptor in Gram-negative bacteria, as shown by the resistance of TLR4-knockout mice to endotoxic shock; these mice also exhibit abnormally low resistance to Gram-negative bacterial infections. In contrast, TLR2-knockout mice fail to respond to bacterial peptidoglycan. Of note, the TLR9 receptor can selectively recognize hypomethylated CpG residues from bacterial DNA, leading to a strong helper T cell immune response to infection. TLR5 detects the bacterial **flagellin** virulence factor present in the flagella. A distinct (non-TLR) component of the innate immune system is the **TREM** receptor family which is present on neutrophils. Microbes such as *S. aureus* and *Ps. aeruginosa* activate TREM1, for example.

CLINICAL KEYNOTE

Medical relevance of innate immunity

Calcium-binding lectins are circulating opsonins that tag bacteria for complement attack. **Mannose-binding protein** is one such protein important for innate immunity in human infants, which may prove therapeutically relevant.

The CD1 orphan family of MHC-like glycoproteins captures and presents lipid (rather than peptide antigens) to T cells. Hence, CD1-restricted immunocytes recognize microbial lipids (e.g., those of *M. tuberculosis*, such as mycolic acid) as well as self ceramides (e.g., gangliosides). Of note, the latter process could contribute to the pathogenesis of **multiple sclerosis**.

The reported therapeutic benefits of stimulating the immune system with **probiotics** (such as *Lactobacillus* spp., for example) may be mediated via TLR2/4/9 via NFκB-dependent stimulation of T_H1 cells. The efficacy of htis strategy in **Crohn** disease may relate to the TLR-like **NOD2** protein which, when mutated, confers susceptibility to this disorder.

An advantage of innate immunity is that the simple and invariant effector system is not prone to misidentification of antigens. The innate system does not permit evolution of higher organisms, however; the pluralistic adaptive immunity required is prone to self-antigen recognition and hence **autoimmune disease**.

Unstable viruses and retroviruses evade the immune system

The **acquired immunodeficiency syndrome** or **AIDS** is caused by the retrovirus human immunodeficiency virus (HIV). Two strains of HIV are identified: **HIV1**, first identified in 1983 (but also detected in an African human blood sample from 1959), and the less common **HIV2** which was later isolated from West African AIDS patients seronegative for HIV1. Transmitted by sexual, parenteral, and perinatal routes, HIV may have originated when an ancient monkey virus – simian immunodeficiency virus (SIV) – leapt the species barrier. In support of this theory, there is strong sequence homology between the HIV2 genome and that of an SIV affecting West African sooty mangabey monkeys. A parallel exists with influenza – another virus that has successfully crossed species and, in doing so, caused lethal epidemics. Smallpox (from cowpox), Ebola and Hantaan viruses may be other examples of "nonequilibrium" cross-species viruses. Influenza and HIV are the most rapidly mutating microorganisms known: this high mutation frequency creates the threat of viral epidemics and complicates the development of vaccines.

The term HIV1 denotes a variety of viral strains, the largest of which is the **M** group (classified into ten subgroups, A to J, of which B predominates in the USA and Europe). The **O** group may represent monkey–human transmission, whereas other subtypes have been linked to localized HIV epidemics. This viral heterogeneity suggests the need for multivalent vaccines and/or combination chemotherapy (such as the simultaneous use of reverse transcriptase inhibitors and protease inhibitors).

HIV undermines the human immune system by destroying 10^8–10^{10} CD4$^+$ (helper) T cells per day. CD8$^+$ (cytotoxic) T cells respond by secreting anti-HIV β-chemokines such as macrophage inflammatory protein-1 (MIP-1) and RANTES. However, the virus exploits this response of the immune system by using chemokine receptors to expedite its own intracellular entry. Mutations affecting certain of these receptors, including the monocyte CCR5 and CCR3 receptors, confer de novo resistance to HIV (p. 222).

CLINICAL KEYNOTE

The molecular biology of AIDS

One of the five primate lentivirus families of retroviruses, HIV was exported from African monkeys to humans in the late 1950s (in contrast, HTLV1 has been infecting humans for at least 1500 years). The RNA genome of HIV is 9 kb in length. Many other retroviruses contain only three **polycistronic** genes, – i.e., containing more than one coding region – which together encode the viral protein core:

1. **Gag**
   - Core (nucleocapsid) proteins (including **p24**, **p17**).
2. **Env**
   - Envelope proteins (including **gp120** and **gp41**).
3. **Pol**
   - Enzymes (including **reverse transcriptase** and **HIV protease**).

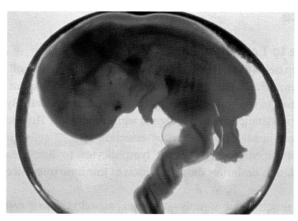

Figure 19.8 The fetus – why is it not rejected? (Wellcome Medical Photographic Library, no. N0010151C).

Conversely, induction of tolerance by mimicking self antigen expression may underlie the symbiotic potential of parasitic infestations.

CLINICAL KEYNOTE

The fetal graft

The immune systems of immunocompetent individuals reject most transplanted allografts. However, the human **fetus**, which expresses nonconsanguineous paternal antigens, is well tolerated by its maternal host (Figure 19.8). Why is it so?

Neither the syncytiotrophoblast nor the cytotrophoblast expresses MHC II antigens. A nonclassic MHC I molecule, **HLA G**, protects cytotrophoblasts from NK-cell-dependent cytolysis. HLA-G-expressing chorionic villi are the sole antigenic determinants present at the fetomaternal interface; since HLA G is nonimmunogenic, this may explain the immunologic privilege of the fetus. Defective MHC I protein expression by embryonic cells may also modulate fetal tolerance.

Trophoblasts express a tryptophan-catabolizing enzyme, **indoleamine 2,3-dioxygenase** (IDO). Since pharmacologic inhibition of this enzyme causes T-cell-dependent fetal rejection in laboratory animals, it is possible that tryptophan depletion leads to the local induction of T cell tolerance at the maternofetal interface. Another possibility is that transplacental passage of an IDO-dependent tryptophan metabolite leads to more general inhibition of T cell activity; if so, the implications for novel immunosuppressive and transplant-sparing therapies would be profound.

PHARMACOLOGIC FOOTNOTE

Vaccines

Immunization involves the controlled administration of antigen (whether purified or otherwise) to prevent infectious disease. Passive immunization consists of postexposure prophylaxis to a given microorganism using preimmune immunoglobulin (i.e., harvested from exposed individuals), whereas active immunization involves vaccination using antigens from target organisms: vaccination may be executed using bacterial vectors (e.g., BCG, *Salmonella* spp.), subunit vaccines (e.g., influenza surface glycoproteins hemagglutinin and neuraminidase, or the more invariant M2 protein), and polysaccharides (pneumococcal, *Hemophilus* spp.). A recent development has been the use of naked DNA from target organisms to engender an immune response (p. 599).

Future vaccine targets include **tuberculosis** (3 million deaths/year), **malaria** (2 million), *HIV* (1.5 million), and cancer. HIV vaccines have concentrated on envelope protein immunogens such as the third hypervariable (V3) loop; however, these have proven poorly immunogenic thus far, consistent with the minimal antiviral effect of B cell humoral responses to HIV.

The feasibility of a cancer vaccine is suggested by the observation that **malignant melanomas** may be accompanied by the development of vitiligo due to the generation of anti-melanin antibodies; vitiligo-associated melanomas of this kind have a better prognosis than similarly staged melanomas without vitiligo, implying that the antibodies have antitumor effects. Preventive cancer targets for vaccination include *Helicobacter pylori* (for gastric cancer), human **papillomavirus** (for cervix and penile cancer), and the epithelial tumor marker **carcinoembryonic antigen** (CEA).

Figure 19.9 Mechanism of action of the immunosuppressive drugs ciclosporin and tacrolimus (FK506). Binding of cyclophilin by these drugs inhibits activity of the serine-threonine phosphatase calcineurin; this leads in turn to increased phosphorylation and reduced activity of NFκB and NFAT, resulting in repression of IL-2 transcription and of T cell activation, respectively.

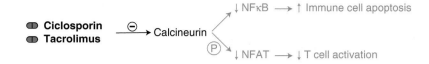

Figure 19.9 Mechanism of action of the immunosuppressive drugs ciclosporin and tacrolimus (FK506). Binding of cyclophilin by these drugs inhibits activity of the serine-threonine phosphatase calcineurin; this leads in turn to increased phosphorylation and reduced activity of NFκB and NFAT, resulting in repression of IL-2 transcription and of T cell activation, respectively.

Inhibition of calcineurin prevents graft rejection

Immunosuppressive drugs are used to manage organ transplantation and autoimmune diseases. Many pharmacologic drugs (e.g., cytotoxics) have broad immunosuppressant activity, whereas biological reagents (such as monoclonal anti-CD3 or anti-CD25 antibodies) may act by inhibiting T cell receptor function. Among the more specific pharmacologic immunosuppressants are two unrelated drug classes – both derived from soil microorganisms – with convergent targets:

1. **Ciclosporin**, a fungal cyclic undecapeptide.
2. **Tacrolimus** (FK506) and **rapamycin**, macrolide antibiotics.

These immunosuppressants act by binding endogenous proteins termed **immunophilins**: either cyclophilins (bound by ciclosporin) or FK506/rapamycin-binding proteins (FKBPs). **Cyclophilins A/B** and **FKBP 12** appear the most important for drug activity. These immunophilins have rotamase (**cis-prolyl isomerase**) activity in the absence of binding to these drugs. The ability of cyclophilins to isomerize proline residues may be important in the stabilization of red-green visual pigments (opsins; p. 514) in retinal photoreceptors, where cyclophilins act as chaperones.

However, it is not the inhibition of rotamase activity that is responsible for the immunosuppressive effects of these drugs. Rather, it is the secondary binding of the drug-immunophilin complex – either ciclosporin-cyclophilin or FK506-FKBP – to the T cell protein phosphatase **calcineurin** (also known as protein phosphatase 2B, PP2B) which appears critical. Inhibition of calcineurin activity leads to increased phosphorylation and reduced activation of its normal substrates: these include the pro-inflammatory transactivator NFκB and the IL-2 transactivator **NFAT** (nuclear factor of activated T cells; Figure 19.9), both of which remain in the cytoplasm when phosphorylated. NFAT transactivates a panel of genes involved in cardiac hypertrophy, leading to ciclosporin-inducible **hypertrophic cardiomyopathy** which may be mimicked by **minoxidil** or blocked by the L-type calcium channel blocker **diltiazem**.

Hence, ciclosporin and tacrolimus cause reduced IL-2 synthesis, inhibition of T cell activation, and immunosuppression. By binding calcineurin, the African swine fever viral protein A238L also represses cytokine expression in infected macrophages. However, not all immunosuppressant actions are mediated by this pathway; for example, rapamycin-FKBP binds to a molecule distinct from calcineurin termed **FRAP** (FKBP-rapamycin-associated protein) which has lipid kinase activity and blocks cell cycle progression in S phase. Similarly, ciclosporin-dependent immunosuppression may induce cancer progression via enhanced synthesis of transforming growth factor-β (TGFβ). Inhibition of calcium signaling is a feature of tacrolimus action, consistent with the FKBP-12 knockout phenotype of ventricular septal defects and cardiomyopathy due to ryanodine receptor dysfunction.

Immunosuppression may also be achieved using the inositine monophosphate dehydrogenase inhibitor **mycophenolate mofetil** to inhibit lymphocyte activation, thereby permitting the discontinuation of ciclosporin therapy in

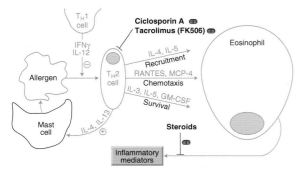

Figure 19.10 Immunosuppression by steroids. Unlike ciclosporin and tacrolimus, which act mainly on T$_H$2 cells, glucocorticoids act primarily to inhibit pro-inflammatory cytokine release from eosinophils. IFNγ, interferon-γ; IL, interleukin; GM-CSF, granulocyte-macrophage colony-stimulating factor; MCP-4, monocyte chemotactic protein-4; RANTES, regulated on activation, normal T cell expressed and secreted (cytokine).

renal transplant patients who have incurred nephrotoxicity. A novel therapeutic strategy for inducing tolerance in graft-versus-host disease (and also in **psoriasis**) involves the inhibition of T cell activity by the cytotoxic T lymphocyte antigen **CTLA-4**.

PHARMACOLOGIC FOOTNOTE

Steroids and immunosuppression

Glucocorticoids (such as **hydrocortisone** and the synthetic corticoids **prednisolone** and **dexamethasone**) are widely used as anti-inflammatory and immunosuppressive drugs. Corticosteroids have at least three mechanisms of action:

1. Direct complex formation between the ligand-activated glucocorticoid receptor (GR) and other transcription factors, leading to inhibition of the related pro-inflammatory signaling pathways (e.g., induced by TNF; p. 302)
   - Affects activator protein-1 (AP1) and NFκB.
2. Transcriptional repression of genes encoding inflammatory mediators
   - Affects the interleukins, chemokines, ICAM-1, inducible nitric oxide synthase (iNOS), cyclooxygenase-2 (COX2) and phospholipase A$_2$ (Figure 19.10).
3. GR-dependent induction of certain genes
   - Lipocortin-1, IL-1 receptor antagonist, IκB, β_2-adrenoceptor.

Of these mechanisms, the inhibitory effects are believed to be most important for the anti-inflammatory and immunosuppressive effects, whereas the transactivating effects of steroids appear to be responsible for most of the metabolic effects and side-effects. Hence, new steroids are being sought which transrepress, but do not transactivate, the above gene groupings.

The acceleration of fetal lung maturation induced by steroids during threatened premature labor has been linked to the induction of TGFβ_3 in fetal lung fibroblasts. **Nongenomic** activities of glucocorticoids such as methylprednisolone may be mediated via any non-GR-dependent pathway, including changes in ion channel or mitochondrial behavior.

Superantigens are non-MHC-restricted T cell activators

T cells may be activated by various stimuli, including:

1. Antigenic peptides.
2. Polyclonal T cell mitogens (e.g., **concanavalin A**).
3. **Superantigens** (monomeric ~ 25-kDa proteins).

Normal peptide antigens activate only 0.01–0.0001% of all T cells. In contrast, **superantigens** activate a high proportion (up to 5–25%) of T cells. The ability of superantigens to stimulate large numbers of T cells reflects the non-antigen-specific binding of these molecules to variable regions of T cell receptor β chains (V$_\beta$), rather than to the multidomain antigen receptor. They also bind to non-peptide-binding regions of MHC II receptors in a non-allele-specific fashion – that is, superantigen binding is not MHC-restricted (Figure 19.11). Moreover, unlike ordinary antigens, superantigens do not need to be processed for presentation to T cells. There are two types of superantigens:

1. **Foreign superantigens**
   - **Bacterial exotoxins**
     S. aureus toxins.
     Enterotoxins (A–E, especially B).
     Toxic shock toxin (TSST-1).
     Scalded skin (exfoliating) toxins A, B.
     Gp A streptococcal pyrogenic exotoxins (A–D).
     Yersinia and *Clostridia* enterotoxins.

Figure 19.11 MHC-unrestricted T cell activation by superantigens. Unlike conventional peptide antigens which require presentation to T cells by MHC proteins, superantigens bind directly to the β-chain variable region of the T cell receptor, obviating the need for MHC presentation.

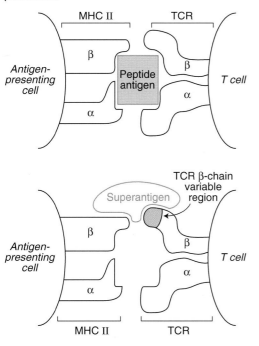

2. **Self superantigens**
   - Retrovirally encoded murine gene products such as the murine mammary tumor virus (MMTV)-encoded **minor lymphocyte stimulating** – Mls – gene products in rodents.

One hypothesis is that mice express self superantigens to activate potentially autoreactive T cells, thus causing clonal deletion via activation-driven cell death. A second possibility is that T cells expressing the appropriate TCR Vβ chain (i.e., those that can be activated by bacterial toxins, and thus mediate host tissue damage) are eliminated by self superantigens to minimize the risk of lethal bacterial infections (note that this clonal deletion mechanism predisposes to rodent transmission of MMTV). In addition to lineage deletions, however, superantigens may induce peripheral T cell anergy, perhaps by activating suppressor T cells – a possible pathogenetic mechanism for HIV.

CLINICAL KEYNOTE

Superantigens in human disease
Human diseases linked to bacterial superantigens include:
1. Diseases mediated by staphylococcal toxins
   - **Toxic shock syndrome** (also caused by *Streptococcus pyogenes*),
   - **Staphylococcal scalded skin syndrome**,
   - **Staphylococcal food poisoning**.
2. Diseases associated with mycoplasmal toxins
   - *Mycoplasma* **arthritis**.
3. **Rabies**
   - Involves a rabiesvirus nucleocapsid superantigen.
4. Drug-induced
   - **Toxic epidermal necrolysis** (Lyell syndrome).

Toxic epidermal necrolysis, fatal in one-third of cases, most often occurs because of **sulphonamide, nonsteroidal anti-inflammatory drugs** (NSAIDs) or **anticonvulsant** use. The "scalded skin" appearance is due to apoptotic epidermal cell death; the affected keratinocytes express Fas ligand. Blockade of the Fas receptor (CD95) using intravenous immunoglobulin may be effective.

Superantigens are also candidates for triggering autoimmune disorders such as **rheumatic** and **scarlet fevers, rheumatoid arthritis, Kawasaki syndrome** and perhaps **multiple sclerosis.** Synthetic peptide antagonists to the binding sites of superantigens have been used with therapeutic success in animal models.

Summary

Immunoglobulin specificity derives from V(D)J exon variation. Germline immunoglobulin gene diversity is generated by recombination-activating genes (RAGs). Antigen-driven affinity maturation of antibodies requires somatic hypermutation.

T cells talk to B cells via reciprocal ligand–receptor interactions. Thymic cell fate depends on T cell signal duration. Immediate hypersensitivity reactions are caused by IgE. Innate immunity takes its *Toll* on microbes. Unstable viruses and retroviruses evade the immune system.

Tolerance arises due to T cell clonal anergy or deletion. Inhibition of calcineurin prevents graft rejection. Superantigens are non-MHC-restricted T cell activators.

Enrichment reading

Library reference

Flint SJ (ed). *Principles of virology: molecular biology, pathogenesis and control.* American Society of Microbiology, 1999

QUIZ QUESTIONS

1. Briefly explain how the immune system generates antibodies capable of recognizing a potentially infinite number of foreign antigens.
2. What is meant by the following terms: (a) affinity maturation of the immune response; (b) somatic hypermutation; (c) isotype class switching; (d) switch recombination?
3. What is the molecular mechanism by which T cell subsets "help" B cells?
4. Explain the role of Tat and TAR in HIV pathogenicity.
5. Briefly describe the structure and function of the multisubunit T cell receptor.
6. What is the function of terminal deoxynucleotidyl transferase (tdt) in T cells?
7. How do $\gamma\delta$ T cell receptors differ from $\alpha\beta$ T cell receptors in terms of function?
8. Briefly explain how tolerance may arise.
9. What is the mechanism of action of the immunosuppressant drug ciclosporin A?
10. Define the term superantigen. What is the clinical significance of this?

Neurobiology

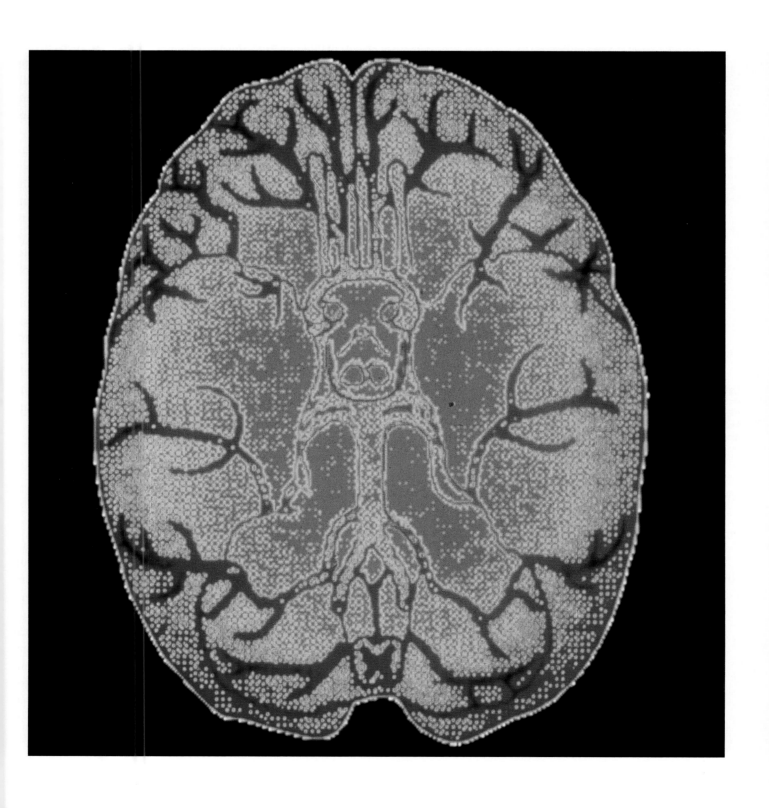

The most complex feature of the human body is the brain. Of all the genes in the human genome, as many as 50% may be exclusively expressed in the brain. In this section we consider the molecular basis of brain and nervous system function in health and disease.

Neurotransmitter molecules

Nerve impulses are propagated by membrane depolarization

Life is electric. Neurons, of which we each own approximately 10^{12}, conduct electrical signals to other nerve or muscle cells. To maximize the speed of conduction, certain human neurons are up to a meter long. The signal terminates in a specialized intercellular junction termed a synapse which, when electrically excited, releases neurotransmitter molecules into a cleft and thus chemically activates adjacent neurons. The long (transmitting) part of the nerve is called the axon, whereas the branched (receiving) parts are termed dendrites.

Differences between intracellular and extracellular ionic charge give rise to a transmembrane potential. Neuronal membrane resting potential is usually around -70 mV. Stimuli such as voltage or neurotransmitter release induce the depolarization of neural tissue – that is, conversion of the transmembrane potential to a less negative level such as 0 mV. Membrane depolarization activates voltage-gated sodium channels, leading to an inward flux of sodium ions (Na^+) down an electrochemical gradient. Since sodium influx leads to further depolarization, a self-amplifying wave of electrical excitation is created; nerve impulses triggered in this way are termed action potentials.

When action potentials reach the presynaptic terminal, transmembrane voltage changes cause an inward flux of calcium (Ca^{2+}) ions that triggers membrane fusion of exocytic vesicles. Neurotransmitter diffusion across the synaptic cleft is followed by activation of postsynaptic receptors, leading to further membrane depolarization and activation of voltage-gated sodium channels. The resultant action potentials are terminated by Na^+ channel inactivation and increased potassium (K^+) efflux leading to membrane repolarization (Figure 20.2). Neuronal ion channel subtypes include:

1. Voltage-gated ion channels
   - e.g., Voltage-gated calcium channels.
2. Mechanically-gated ion channels
   - e.g., Touch receptors, auditory receptors.
3. Ligand-gated ion channels (ionotropic receptors)
   - e.g., Nicotinic acetylcholine receptors, glycine receptors.

Ligand-gated ion channels should be distinguished from ion channels which are indirectly regulated by G-protein-coupled receptors. **GABA$_B$ receptors** are ligand-activated G-protein-coupled receptors that regulate adjacent K^+ channels, for example, whereas **GABA$_A$ receptors** consist of ligand-binding pentameric subunits surrounding a central Cl^- channel (see Figure 20.7).

Synaptic transmission of most human nerve impulses is an electrochemical (rather than electrical) process, occurring over a 30- to 50-nm cleft without any cytoplasmic connection. Rare exceptions include intercellular messages sent by glial cells via connexin-lined gap junctions, which effectively create cytoplasmic syncytia bridged by a 2-nm cleft. Such nonchemical synapses transmit bidirectional ion flux.

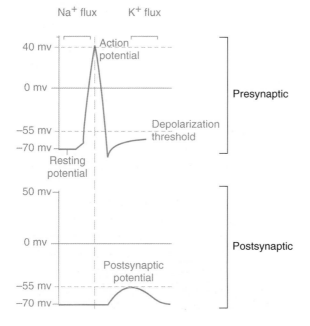

Figure 20.2 Molecular mechanism of neurotransmission. Once the resting potential exceeds the depolarization threshold, sodium influx is triggered, creating an action potential which in turn causes vesicle fusion with the presynaptic membrane, leading to postsynaptic signal propagation.

MOLECULAR MINIREVIEW

Voltage-operated calcium channels (VOCCs)

Calcium channels are oligomeric structures consisting of α, α_2/δ, β and γ subunits. These molecules are present in virtually all excitable cells, and are activated (opened) by depolarization to $+20$ mV within a millisecond of voltage sensing. Calcium channels are classified as either L-type, N-type, T-type or P-type:

1. Low-threshold (low-voltage-activated) calcium channels
   - **T-type calcium channels** are transient (rapid-closing, low-conductance, $Ca_v3.2$) ion channels that are abundant within the transverse tubules of skeletal muscle where they mediate excitation–contraction coupling. T-type channels – which are inhibited by the drug mibefradil – often coexist with L channels. Pacemaking functions are associated with T-type channels in cardiac nodal tissues.
2. High-threshold (high-voltage-activated) calcium channels
   - **L-type calcium channels** are long-lasting (slow – long opening – high conductance, $Ca_v1.2$) ion channels that are sensitive to dihydropyridine drugs such as the antianginal agent nifedipine; the α_{1c} subunit of the L-type channel is the dihydropyridine receptor. L-type channels occur in cardiac and smooth muscle. The selective effects of verapamil and diltiazem on slowing atrioventricular node conduction may indicate an additional effect of these drugs on T-type channels. Second-generation L-channel inhibitors, which include nicardipine and amlodipine, cause vasodilatation without inhibition of conduction or inotropy, suggesting a preference for noncardiac L-type channels.
   - **N-type calcium channels** are neither L- nor T-type channels (neuronal, medium conductance, $Ca_v2.2$). Sensitivity to **ω-conotoxin** defines a subtype of neuronal (N-type) channels which are autoantibody targets in the paraneoplastic **myasthenic (Eaton–Lambert) syndrome** associated with **small-cell lung cancer** (SCLC); the accompanying weakness reflects impairment of presynaptic acetylcholine release (Table 20.1).
   - **P-type channels** are also neuron-specific proteins, but are found predominantly in cerebellar Purkinje cells.

Neuronal G-protein-coupled receptors gate synaptic channels

Neuronal ion channels may be activated by voltage, mechanical stimuli or neurotransmitters. Synapse function is also regulated by neurotransmitter-dependent G-protein-coupled receptors that are secondarily linked to ion channels. Such channels alter their ground state (open or closed) following receptor-dependent release of second messengers such as cAMP, cGMP or inositol 1,4,5-trisphosphate (IP_3). The main categories of G-protein-coupled receptor within the brain include:

1. **Light-activated (photoisomerized) G-protein-coupled receptors**
   - cGMP-gated retinal ion channel closure.
2. **Odorant-activated G-protein-coupled receptors**
   - cAMP-gated olfactory ion channel opening.
3. **Neurotransmitter-gated G-protein-coupled receptors**
   - e.g., Muscarinic acetylcholine receptors, adrenergic receptors.

Unlike voltage-sensitive Na^+ and K^+ ion channels, which regulate action potential transmission along the nerve, G-protein-activated ion channels localize to the synapse. Some neuronal G-protein-coupled receptors require peptide ligands for activation – i.e., they are ligand-gated (as are some integral neuronal ion channels). Other brain receptors may be activated by ligand-independent processes such as photon absorption. The *N*-methyl-D-aspartate (NMDA) subtype of **glutamate receptor** is both ligand-gated and

Table 20.1. Paraneoplastic neural autoantibodies

Malignancy	Paraneoplastic syndrome	Autoantibody target	Autoantibody pathogenicity
SCLC	Myasthenic (Eaton–Lambert) syndrome	Voltage-gated calcium channels (neuro-muscular junction)	Yes
Thymoma	Myasthenia gravis	AChR (neuromuscular junction)	Yes
Ovarian cancer, Hodgkin disease	Cerebellar degeneration (ataxia, diplopia)	Yo (Purkinje cells), Tr	No
Ovarian cancer	Polymyositis (proximal weakness)	Jo-1 (muscle cells)	No
Testicular germcell tumors	Limbic encephalitis Brainstem dysfunction	Ma2 Ma1	?
Thymoma, Breast cancer	Encephalomyelitis (confusion, coma)	CV2 (oligodendrocytes) Amphiphysin (synapses)	No
Breast cancer, SCLC, Neuroblastoma	Opsoclonus-myoclonus (oscillopsia, vertigo)	Ri (neuronal nuclei) Hu (neuronal nuclei)	No
SCLC	Sensory neuropathy, encephalitis	Hu (neuronal nuclei)	No
Thymoma, SCLC	Neuromyotonia (myokymia, cramps)	Voltage-gated potassium channels (neuromuscular junction)	Yes

Notes:
SCLC, small cell lung cancer; AChR, acetylcholine receptor.

voltage-gated, consistent with a synapse-strengthening role for this receptor in learning (p. 519). Conversely, neurotransmitter ligands may activate more than one type of receptor: **glutamate**, **GABA**, **serotonin** and **acetylcholine** are all capable of activating both ligand-gated ion channels and ligand-gated G-protein-coupled receptors (Table 20.2).

MOLECULAR MINIREVIEW

Acetylcholine receptors

The neurotransmitter **acetylcholine** (ACh) is synthesized by **choline acetyltransferase** (ChAT), transported to secretory vesicles, and then released into the synaptic cleft where it activates two ligand-gated receptor classes named for their sensitivity to the alkaloids nicotine and muscarine **nicotinic** (nAChR), and **muscarinic** ACh receptors (mAChR) (Figure 20.3):

1. **Nicotinic AChRs** (N1, N2) are ligand-gated channels permeable to calcium/sodium, which have a pentameric $\alpha_2\beta\gamma\delta$ rosette structure. Nicotine receptors occur at neuromuscular junctions where the extracellular binding of two ACh molecules (one to the high-affinity $\alpha\gamma$ site, the other to low-affinity $\alpha\delta$ site) triggers the opening of a central pore (up to 200 000) within microseconds. About a million cations pass into the cell via each channel per ACh binding event, but this rapid ion transit is inhibited by the binding of **curare** (tubocurarine) to the $\alpha\gamma$ site. Note that the β_2 subunit of nicotinic receptors is required for nicotine addiction.

2. **Muscarinic AChRs** (M1–M5) are G-protein-coupled receptors that activate

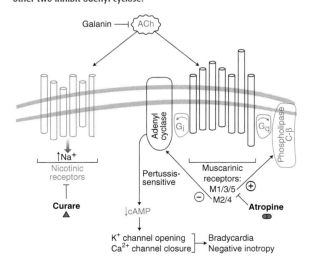

Figure 20.3 Nicotinic and muscarinic acetylcholine receptors. The former are ligand-gated cation channels, whereas the latter include five subtypes: three of these activate phospholipase C-β, whereas the other two inhibit adenyl cyclase.

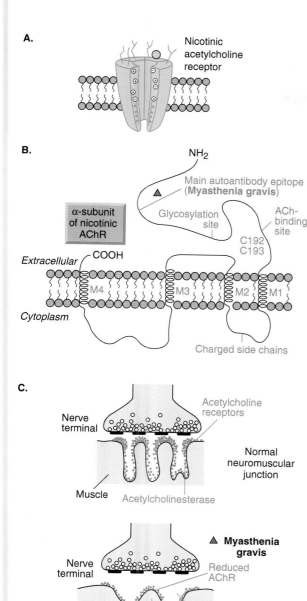

Figure 20.4 The nicotinic acetylcholine receptor (AChR). *A*, Domain structure of the channel, showing the high-affinity ACh-binding site on the α subunit. *B*, Fine structure of the nicotinic ACh receptor α subunit, showing the extracellular sites for ligand binding, glycosylation, and autoantibody binding in myasthenia gravis. *C*, Micropathology of myasthenia gravis. Under normal circumstances nicotinic ACh receptors are abundant in the neuromuscular junction (upper panel), but in myasthenia the autoantibodies deplete ACh receptors while also widening the synaptic cleft and blunting the postsynaptic folds.

cation channels (e.g., cardiac K^+ channels) via G-proteins, and are inhibited by **atropine**. Odd-numbered receptors (M1, M3, M5) activate phospholipase C, whereas even-numbered receptors (M2, M4) inhibit adenyl cyclase. Antimuscarinic drugs such as **oxybutinin** are used to reduce bladder tone and thus improve urinary incontinence.

ACh may thus act as a (fast-nAChR) neurotransmitter or a (slow-nAChR) neuro-modulator, depending upon which receptor is being activated. Cholinergic neuro-transmission is further modulated by a soluble glia-derived **ACh-binding protein** (**AchBP**) homologous to the nAChR ligand-binding domain.

PHARMACOLOGIC FOOTNOTE

Cholinergic agonists and antagonists

Within the synaptic cleft, ACh is hydrolyzed to choline and acetate by **acetyl-cholinesterase**. The actions of ACh may thus be potentiated using acetyl-cholinesterase inhibitors such as **physostigmine** and **neostigmine**. These drugs may be used to treat the clinical syndrome of **myasthenia gravis** in which autoantibod-ies to nicotinic AChRs (AChRAbs; sometimes produced by thymomas) cause fati-gability due to neuromuscular junction damage (Figure 20.4).

Irreversible acetylcholinesterase inhibition is inducible by organophosphates such as **parathion** which are used as insecticides. Snake venoms such as **α-bun-garotoxin** and **cobrotoxin** bind postsynaptically to nicotinic AChR at the neuromus-cular junction, but affect neither snakes themselves nor their adversary the mongoose (this invulnerability reflects a difference in four AChR amino acids that prevents toxin binding). **Botulinum toxin A** inhibits neuronal ACh release from cholinergic autonomic neurons and at neuromuscular junctions. When locally injected it is effective treatment for muscle spasm associated with spasticity, acha-lasia, and (even) unsightly forehead wrinkles.

The muscle relaxant **succinylcholine** is an ACh agonist that resists acetyl-cholinesterase hydrolysis. Since it is metabolized by circulating cholinesterases collectively termed **pseudocholinesterase**, inherited **pseudocholinesterase defi-ciency** may be associated with prolonged postanesthetic apnea.

Vesicle-membrane fusion triggers neurotransmitter release

Neurotransmitters come in different shapes and sizes. Peptide neurotrans-mitters such as opioids, calcitonin, luteinizing hormone releasing hormone (LHRH) and the brain-and-gut peptides are slow-acting neuromodulators that bind G-protein-coupled receptors. Purinergic neurotransmitters such as ATP and adenosine activate plasma membrane P_2 purinoceptors. The nitrergic neurotransmitter nitric oxide acts via its receptor, soluble guanylyl cyclase, to increase neuronal cGMP levels. Synapses and neuromuscular junctions, on the other hand, tend to be bridged by other ligand classes:

1. Amino acid neurotransmitters
   - e.g. Glycine, glutamate, GABA (γ-aminobutyric acid).
2. Amine neurotransmitters
   - e.g. Catecholamines (e.g., epinephrine, dopamine), ACh, serotonin.

How is presynaptic neurotransmitter release regulated? Rapid transneural propagation of the action potential is arrested at the synapse where voltage-activated calcium channels initiate calcium ion influx. Neurotransmitter storage vesicles then fuse with the presynaptic membrane – an interaction mediated by actin-binding proteins termed synapsins (see below). This vesicle-membrane fusion event releases neurotransmitter into the synaptic

Table 20.2. Ligand-gated versus receptor-gated neuronal ion channels

Ion channels which are directly ligand-gated	Ionic flux	Ion channels that are indirectly ligand-gated via G-protein-coupled receptors	Ionic flux
1. Nicotinic AChR	Cations (Na^+, Ca^{2+})	1. Muscarinic AChR	Cations (Na^+, Ca^{2+})
2. Ionotropic glutamate receptors	NMDA – Ca^{2+} AMPA/KA – Na^+	2. Metabotropic glutamate receptor	Ca^{2+}
3. $GABA_A$ receptor	Cl^- influx	3. $GABA_B$ receptor	K^+ efflux
4. $5HT_3$ receptor		4. $5HT_{1,2,4-7}$ receptors	

Figure 20.5 Neurotransmission via voltage-gated calcium channels. *A*, In the resting state, the presynaptic nerve terminal is replete with neurotransmitter vesicles. *B*, Delivery of an action potential (1) causes presynaptic membrane depolarization followed by calcium ion influx via voltage-gated channels (2); this calcium influx triggers vesicle fusion with the presynaptic membrane (3), leading to neurotransmitter release into the synaptic cleft (4). Vesicle discharge is followed by activation of postsynaptic neurotransmitter receptors (5) and membrane depolarization (6). *C*, Membrane depolarization causes sodium ion influx (7) followed by propagation of a postsynaptic action potential (8).

cleft (Figure 20.5). The postsynaptic clustering of neurotransmitter receptors adjacent to neuron terminals is mediated in due course by secreted neuronal clustering factors termed **agrins**. Activation of postsynaptic neurotransmitter receptors depolarizes the dendritic membrane, thereby activating postsynaptic voltage-gated sodium channels and propagating the action potential.

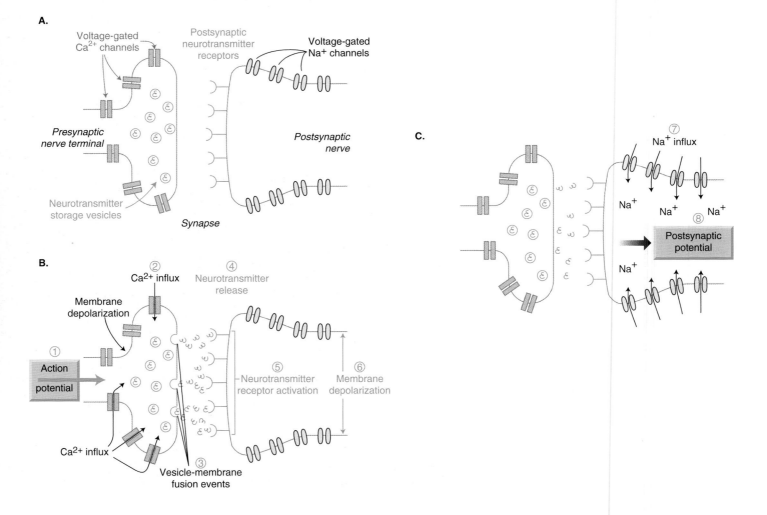

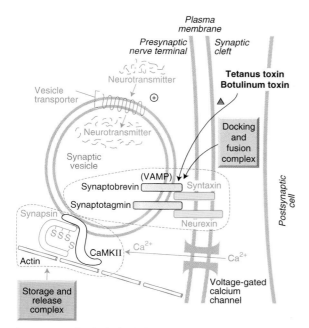

Figure 20.6 Molecular biology of neurotransmitter vesicle fusion and release. Voltage-gated calcium channels are activated by an action potential, leading to presynaptic calcium influx followed by activation of calcium/calmodulin-dependent kinase 2 (CaMKII). Phosphorylation of actin-bound synapsins then occurs, releasing the "grip" of synapsins on neurotransmitter vesicles. The latter migrate freely to the presynaptic nerve terminal where a SNAP-SNARE ineraction occurs (p. ***) between molecules such as syntaxin and VAMP. Microbial toxins such as tetanus and botulinum toxin inhibit this latter interaction, thereby paralyzing synaptic neurotransmission.

MOLECULAR MINIREVIEW

Synapsins

Release of neurotransmitters from axon terminals depends upon a family of neuron-specific actin-binding phosphoproteins termed **synapsins**. The following sequence of events occurs (Figure 20.6):

1. Nerve stimulation causes activation of voltage-gated calcium channels, leading to Ca^{2+} influx into the nerve terminal.
2. Increased cytosolic free calcium activates calcium/calmodulin-dependent protein kinases (CaM kinases).
3. Kinase activation causes phosphorylation of synapsins.
4. Synapsin phosphorylation leads to the mobilization of synaptic neurotransmitter vesicles within the presynaptic nerve terminal.
5. Liberated synaptic vesicles are escorted to the active zone of the presynaptic membrane by the calcium-sensing protein **synaptotagmin**, which binds to docking proteins termed **syntaxins**.
6. Membrane fusion and neurotransmitter release into the synaptic cleft follow, occurring within 200 μs of calcium ion influx.

Synapsin dephosphorylation inhibits neurotransmitter release by reducing the number of synaptic vesicles fusing with presynaptic membranes. This occurs because synaptic vesicles bind with high affinity to dephosphorylated actin-bound synapsins, preventing migration to sites of membrane vesicle fusion. Depolarization and repolarization of presynaptic nerve terminals thus correlate with synapsin phosphorylation and dephosphorylation, respectively.

Inhibitory neurotransmitters induce neuronal hyperpolarization

Just as membrane depolarization (due to Na^+ influx) initiates action potentials, so hyperpolarization (due to K^+ efflux) inhibits neurotransmission. Neurotransmitters can therefore be characterized as excitatory or inhibitory on the basis of their ion channel effects. Excitatory neurotransmitters include **glutamate, aspartate, acetylcholine, epinephrine (norepinephrine), serotonin**, and **ATP**; such neurotransmitters trigger cation influx, principally Na^+ or Ca^{2+}. The two main inhibitory neurotransmitters in the human nervous system are **GABA** (γ-aminobutyric acid, derived from decarboxylation of the excitatory amino acid glutamate by the enzyme **glutamic acid decarboxylase**; p. 430) and **glycine**. Inhibitory neurotransmitters induce neuronal hyperpolarization by causing either:

1. Anion influx – e.g., glycine receptor activation, leading to Cl^- influx.
2. Cation efflux – e.g., $GABA_B$ receptor activation leading to K^+ efflux.

$GABA_A$ receptors are GABA-gated Cl^- channels – the major mediators of inhibitory neurotransmission within human neurons and glial cells. Many different $GABA_A$ receptors have been identified, with at least 16 genes known to encode the five subunits ($\alpha, \beta, \gamma, \delta, \varepsilon$) of the pentameric receptor; ligand binding activates the central Cl^- channel. Four varieties of $GABA_A$ receptors can be distinguished on the basis of α subunits 1, 2, 3 and 5. The α_2 $GABA_A$ receptor subtype, which is abundant in the limbic system, mediates the anxiolytic effect of benzodiazepines, whereas their sedative (and perhaps also amnestic and anticonvulsant) effects appear dependent upon α_1 $GABA_A$ receptors. Hence, neurotic mice lacking the γ_2 subunit appear resistant to the calming effects of diazepam, whereas the α_1-specific benzodiazepine zolpidem acts mainly as a hypnotic. Surprisingly, cleft palate occurs in animals deficient in either GABA or the $GABA_A$ receptor, revealing a developmental role for this signaling pathway. **$GABA_B$ receptors** are

Table 20.3. Antiepileptic drug targets

Neural ion channel/ receptor subtype	Neuropharmacologic inhibitors
Voltage-gated sodium channels	Carbamazepine, lamotrigine
Voltage-gated calcium channels	Valproate
GABA receptors	Benzodiazepines, gabapentin

heterodimeric G-protein-coupled receptors that activate inward-rectifying potassium channels (Figure 20.7).

Glycine receptors cluster at inhibitory synapses because of anchoring by **gephyrin**, a cytoskeleton-attached protein required for the activity of molybdenum-containing enzymes. Gephyrin knockout mimics the phenotype of **strychnine** poisoning, which inhibits glycine-inducible chloride conductance. Inhibitory neurotransmitters may not inhibit every target cell type: for example, hippocampal neurons may be excited by GABA, leading to the synchronized recruitment of inhibitory interneurons. Of possible relevance to this, Pavlovian conditioning may convert certain synapses from inhibitory to excitatory.

PHARMACOLOGIC FOOTNOTE

GABA receptors

Epilepsy is a heterogeneous disorder characterized by episodic cerebral overactivity. Inhibitory neurotransmitter receptors such as $GABA_A$ receptors are thus an attractive target for therapeutic intervention (as are several other channels and receptors involved in neurotransmission; Table 20.3). The $GABA_A$ receptor contains multiple drug-binding domains:
1. The GABA-binding site.
2. The benzodiazepine-binding site.
3. The barbiturate-binding site.
4. The picrotoxin-binding site.

Benzodiazepines are $GABA_A$ receptor agonists with anticonvulsant activity for tonic-clonic seizures. In contrast, the antispasticity drug **baclofen** is a $GABA_B$ receptor agonist, which may actually exacerbate absence (petit mal) seizures. Endogenous ligands for $GABA_A$ receptor benzodiazepine-binding sites are termed **endozepines**. Benzodiazepine overdosage is treatable using the short-acting antagonist **flumazenil**, and GABA binding to $GABA_A$ receptors is competitively inhibited by the pro-convulsants **bicuculline** and **picrotoxin**. **Penicillin** can bind competitively to GABA receptors via its non-β-lactam moieties, and may thus cause convulsions if instilled into the intraventricular space.

Abnormal GABA metabolism is implicated in the pathogenesis of **myoclonus**, **startle disease** (hyperekplexia), **Huntington disease** (striatal deficiency) and

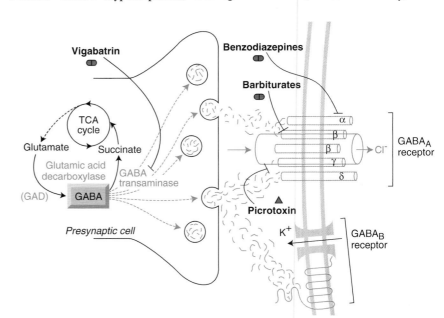

Figure 20.7 GABA signaling. Glutamate from the citric acid cycle is converted to GABA by GAD; the anticonvulsant vigabatrin inhibits reconversion (by transamination) of GABA to succinate and thence to reincorporation into the citric acid cycle. Synaptic release of GABA activates both $GABA_A$ (inward rectifying chloride channels) and $GABA_B$ receptors (outward-rectifying potassium channels); benzodiazepines and barbiturates act on the former receptor subtype. GABA, γ-aminobutyric acid; GAD, glutamic acid decarboxylase; TCA, tricarboxylic acid.

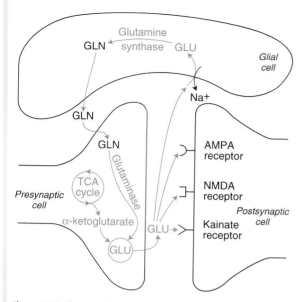

Figure 20.8 Glutamate biosynthesis and signaling. Glial cell uptake of glutamate is followed by conversion to glutamine, which is in turn reconverted to glutamate within presynaptic nerve terminals. Calcium-dependent release of glutamate-containing vesicles into the synaptic cleft is then followed by postsynaptic glutamate receptor activation. AMPA, amino-3-hydroxy-5-methyl-4-isoxazolepropionate; GLN, glutamine; GLU, glutamate; NMDA, *N*-methyl-D-aspartate; TCA, tricarboxylic acid.

Friedreich ataxia (cerebellar deficiency). **Premenstrual tension** may occur when declining progesterone levels cause a parallel decline in cerebral GABA function; either the GABA agonist **alprazolam** or the neurosteroid **allopregnanolone** (another GABA$_A$ receptor agonist) may be useful in treatment.

Excitatory molecules

Glutamate receptors may be both ligand- and voltage-gated

The most abundant excitatory neurotransmitter in the human central nervous system – present in millimolar concentrations – is the amino acid L-glutamate. Glial cells take up glutamate and convert it to glutamine, which is in turn reconverted to glutamate in presynaptic neurons by deamination via the citric acid cycle (Figure 20.8). Postsynaptic glutamate receptors fall into one of two main classes: metabotropic or ionotropic.

Metabotropic glutamate receptors (mGluR) are slow-acting G-protein-coupled receptors that activate phospholipase A$_2$ and, thus, the arachidonic acid cascade. In contrast, **ionotropic glutamate receptors** (iGluR) are heteromultimeric complexes that consist of any of 15 different subunits. Once activated, these receptors switch on fast-acting ligand-gated ion channels consisting of homotetrameric subunits resembling voltage-gated potassium channels. iGluR are named after the agonists by which they are selectively activated (Figure 20.9):

1. **NMDA receptors**
   - Agonist: *N*-methyl-D-aspartate (NMDA).
   - Consist of NR1, NR2A–D, or NR3 receptor subunits.
2. **Non-NMDA receptors**
   - **AMPA receptors**
     Agonist: amino-3-hydroxy-5-methyl-4-isoxazolepropionate (AMPA).
     Consist of GluR1–GluR4 receptor subunits.
     Targeted to synapses by the PDZ-interactive protein **stargazin**.
   - **Kainate (KA) receptors**
     Activated by kainic acid (KA).
     Consist of GluR5 – GluR7 and KA1–KA2 subunits.

NMDA receptors require the binding of a coagonist, **glycine**, to prevent desensitization and thus maintain receptor activation. This coagonist activity, which has been a target for neuroprotective therapies, must be distinguished from the inhibitory effects on neurotransmission caused by binding to the glycine receptor. Unlike the latter, the glutamatergic coactivating activity of glycine is insensitive to strychnine.

NMDA receptors do not fit neatly into paradigms of ligand- and voltage-gated receptors. Rather, they require both ligand (glutamate) and a change in neuronal voltage for activation. As detailed later, this characteristic of NMDA receptors as coincidence detectors is essential for learning. All glutamate receptors conduct sodium ions, but the properties of this ionic flow alter in response to the insertion of a single amino acid by RNA editing. Calcium-dependent processes involving NMDA receptors are implicated in **synaptic plasticity**, an adaptational neuronal response involved in learning.

Metabotropic glutamate receptors are classified into eight subtypes which in turn comprise three subgroups. These receptors may be activated not only by glutamate but also by elevations of extracellular calcium, reflecting sequence homology with the calcium-sensing receptor and also the pheromone receptor (which collectively make up the mGluR family). Binding of glutamate transforms the disulfide-bonded mGluR extracellular domain

riluzole slows progression of **amyotrophic lateral sclerosis**. Short-term **lithium** treatment can downregulate glutamate receptors and thus inhibit excitotoxic signaling; consistent with this, maintenance lithium treatment may cause radiological increases in cerebral grey matter. The neurotoxic effects of intraneuronal glutamate-induced calcium influx may be reduced by the L-type calcium channel antagonist **nimodipine**. Other blockers of glutamate function include the anticonvulsant **lamotrigine** and the recreational drug **ethanol** (though the latter is neurotoxic in its own right). The nucleoside neuromodulator **adenosine** is an inhibitor of glutamate release and a candidate neuroprotective drug, whereas the neuroprotective effects of **aspirin** relate to the prevention of glutamate-dependent NFκB transcription. The association of long-term **NSAID** (e.g., aspirin) usage with reduced risk of **Alzheimer disease** – but not with protection from vascular dementia – supports a role for cyclooxygenase in activating a neurotoxic calcium-dependent glutamate pathway. Conversely, NMDA receptor blockers (e.g., **phencyclidine** – angel dust – **amantadine**, and **ketamine**) may cause psychotic symptoms which necessitate the concomitant use of GABA agonists.

Nerve growth factors promote neurite sprouting

The developing human nervous system is sculpted from a vast excess of neurons – most of which die when they fail to make good connections. That this type of cell death is physiologic is indicated by transgenic mouse studies in which knockout of pro-apoptotic proteases induces widespread morphologic brain abnormalities and early mortality. So how does synapse formation prevent the death of developing nerve cells?

Depolarization of nerve cells may induce expression of and-or hypersensitivity to neuronal growth factors. These **neurotrophins** favor either nerve growth itself or neurite extension (i.e., sprouting of axonal or dendritic terminal processes, often occurring after nerve injury). The increased membrane depolarization frequency associated with synaptic development enhances the effects of such growth factors, whereas growth factor deprivation leads to apoptosis. Growth-factor-dependent circuit reinforcement of this kind may also play a role in the adult nervous system during learning and memory storage. Growth factors that promote nervous system development include:

1. **Nerve growth factor** (NGF).
2. **Brain-derived neurotrophic factor** (BDNF).
3. **NT3** (neurotrophin-3), **NT4** (neurotrophin-4).
4. **Glial-derived neurotrophic factor** (GDNF).

Three of these structurally related growth factors activate receptor tyrosine kinases encoded by the **Trk** (pronounced trek) proto-oncogene family: NGF binds TrkA, BDNF and NT4 bind TrkB, and NT3 binds TrkC, all of which are present in dorsal root ganglia. In contrast, GDNF binds the **Ret** proto-oncogene (p. ***). Like epidermal growth factor (EGF), NGF is found in male salivary glands, consistent with a role in wound healing. Despite its status as the first polypeptide growth factor to be discovered, NGF does not stimulate neuronal proliferation as such, but rather exerts a trophic activity. Ligation of TrkA by NGF activates GTPase-activating protein (GAP) and MAP kinase, promoting both nerve cell survival and axon extension (differentiation) in sympathetic and sensory neurons. Conversely, null mutations of TrkA cause the rare syndrome of **congenital indifference to pain and anhidrosis** (CIPA).

Like other neurotrophins, NGF binds a 75-kDa low-affinity receptor which constitutively induces neuronal apoptosis when unligated. Peripheral nerve injury induces NGF-dependent sprouting of pain fibers as part of a healing response: consistent with this, topical application of NGF produces skin hyperalgesia and promotes corneal ulcer healing. Sensory neuron function and survival depend upon NGF, BDNF and GDNF, whereas motor neuron survival and neuromuscular synapse development are promoted by BDNF and NT3 (and ciliary neurotrophic factor; see below). GDNF overexpression in muscle increases the number of innervating axons in muscle, whereas striatal overexpression augments dopaminergic neuronal function and thus improves **Parkinson disease** in animal models.

Developing nerve fibers contain subcellular structures called growth cones, which integrate both soluble and intracellular guidance cues. One of these soluble nerve chemoattractants is the **netrin-1** ligand which activates a receptor complex including the **DCC** ("deleted in colon cancer") receptor and the **adenosine A2b** receptor. Signaling from these receptors guides spinal commissural axon growth in a protease-sensitive manner

MOLECULAR MINIREVIEW

Eph receptors and ephrins

Another commissure-regulating molecular group is the **Eph** family of receptor tyrosine kinases which contains at least 15 members from two families (EphA and EphB). All such receptors are activated by membrane-bound (rather than soluble) ligands termed **ephrins** which repel axons, thereby directing growth cones. These repulsive forces are countered by cone-attracting cGMP signaling events, whereas intracellular calcium transients cause the stalling of embryonic axonal growth and retraction of growth cones. Protease-regulated cell-to-cell contact thus plays a key role in Eph-dependent neural pathfinding: consistent with this, Eph receptors signal in part via phosphatidylinositol 3'-kinase (which modifies cytoskeletal proteins and thus controls cell motility), as well as via the **Src-like adaptor protein** (**SLAP**). Alternative splicing of Eph receptors can interconvert ephrin-dependent axonal repulsion and adhesion, suggesting a mechanism for congenital craniofacial and neural tube defects.

CLINICAL KEYNOTE

Nerve regeneration

The only regenerating neuronal lineages in the adult central nervous system are the olfactory basal cells, and the stem cells of the hippocampus and retina. In contrast, the regeneration of vertebrate peripheral nerves can occur over distances of more than a meter. Part of this nerve injury response involves NGF release by Schwann cells, which synthesize the myelin nerve sheath of peripheral nerves; crush injuries causing nerve cell degeneration are accompanied by NGF loss and neuronal death. Lower vertebrates increase the expression of neuronal growth factors (and receptors) in response to nerve injury and denervation, suggesting the existence of neuromuscular sprouting factors with therapeutic potential. Similarly, the frog microtubule-binding protein **myoseverin** induces wound repair genes that may help initiate muscle (and perhaps also nerve) regrowth during amphibian limb regeneration.

The regenerative inability of central nervous system axons may in part reflect oligodendrocyte expression of a specific myelin-associated neurite outgrowth inhibitor of the **reticulon** family termed **Nogo**. A variety of other glycoproteins and proteoglycans inhibit axon growth. Hence, removing growth inhibition may be at least as important as neurotrophic factors for the medical treatment of neuronal loss syndromes (e.g., **macular degeneration, Parkinson disease**).

Sensory molecules

Tactile stimuli activate mechanically gated ion channels

The five human senses – vision, hearing, smell, taste, and touch – are heterogeneous at the molecular level, sharing only the common signaling mechanism of ion channel modulation. These sensory pathways differ in such fundamental respects as:

1. Detection molecules; for example:
   - G-protein-coupled receptors detect vision, smell and taste; these stimuli are transduced by sense-specific G-proteins such as G_t (transducin), G_{olf} (olfactory G-protein) and G_{gust} (gustducin).
   - Mechanically-gated ion channels detect auditory and tactile stimuli.
2. Stimulus modulation; for example:
   - Photons are detected by **chromophore absorption**.
   - Odorants are bound by **odorant-binding proteins**.
3. Specificity of signal detected; for example:
   - Color perception depends on **absorption spectrum**.
   - The tone heard depends on **vibrational resonance**.
4. Effect of sensory response on ion channel patency; for example:
   - Visual and gustatory sensing cause **ion channel closure**.
   - Olfactory, touch and auditory sensing cause **ion channel opening**.

Tactile perception can be subclassified as fine touch, thermal perception, pain (nociception), stretch perception, joint position sense (proprioception), and vibration sense. These sensations are transmitted to the central nervous system by different nerve fiber subtypes, e.g., myelinated and unmyelinated fibers of varying diameters. Hence, touch-receptor neurons differ from pain-receptor neurons, just as cerebral cortical representation of pain is distinct from that defining vibrotactile stimuli. Mutations affecting touch-receptor proteins can cause neurodegeneration in lower organisms; these proteins, termed **degenerins**, are structurally related to cation channels. Indeed, the brain Na^+ channel **BNC1** appears necessary for light touch sensation, suggesting the existence of a mechanosensory complex (Table 20.4).

Touch represents only the most ubiquitous variety of mechanotransduction. Plant cells, for example, are sensitive to mechanical stimulation by wind. However, tactile sensation is not always explained by mechanical stimulation; for example, individuals who have lost arms or legs may experience distressing phantom limb perceptions sometimes associated with pain.

Table 20.4. Sensory signaling pathways

Sense	Stimulus	Apical membrane receptor	G-protein	Effector	Second messenger	Intracellular ionic flux	Basolateral ion channel response
Touch, hearing	Mechanical					Cations	Opening
Salt/sour taste	Na^+/H^+			Na^+ (salt) H^+ (sour)	$\uparrow Na^+$ $\downarrow Na^+$	$\uparrow Ca^{2+}$	K^+ channel closure
Sweet/bitter taste	Sugars Amino acids	GPCRs	G_q (sweet) G_{gust} (bitter)	Adenyl cyclase	$\uparrow$ cAMP (sweet) $\downarrow$ cAMP (bitter)	$\uparrow Ca^{2+}$	K^+ channel opening
Smell	Odorants	GPCRs	G_{olf}	Adenyl cyclase, PLCβ	$\uparrow$ cAMP $\uparrow IP_3$	Cations	Ca^{2+} channel opening
Vision	Photons	GPCRs: opsins	G_t (transducin)	Phosphodiesterase	$\downarrow$ cGMP	$\downarrow Na^+/Ca^{2+}$	Ca^{2+} channel closure

Notes:
GPCR, G-protein-coupled receptors.

Hearing requires hair cell depolarization

Like touch, auditory sensation (i.e., acoustic neurotransmission) is initiated via mechanical stimuli. Hearing is not listening, however, as every spouse knows: functional imaging of brain activity in response to the same auditory stimulus reveals different neural responses depending upon the attention state of the sensor. Moreover, an enlarged cerebral response area is apparent in those trained to appreciate what is heard (e.g., musicians hearing music).

Sounds are sensed through the mechanical displacement of pivoting microvilli on cochlear hair cells termed stereocilia, which act as mechano-electrical transducers. The hundred or so stereocilia ("hairs") on each hair cell experience a shearing stress when sound waves cause the adjoining tectorial membrane to vibrate. Mechanotransduction occurs via the conversion of stereocilial kinetic energy to electrical energy: displacement of the sound-blown stereocilium by even a nanometer pulls open nearby K^+ and Ca^{2+} channels, which are connected thereto in a trapdoor-and-rope arrangement involving myosin-containing extracellular filaments termed tip links. The resulting cationic influx from potassium-rich cochlear endolymph alters hair cell membrane potential, activating a motor protein termed **prestin** which alters the length and stiffness of the "cochlear amplifier" or outer hair cell. Depolarization causes outer hair cell shortening, whereas hyperpolarization causes lengthening; the former results in the opening of cation channels and transmission of a receptor current, a process that depends upon the integrity of the tectorial membrane protein **α-tectorin**.

When the auditory impulse stops, potassium ions escape from the hair cell through ion-specific channels (**KCNQ4**) into adjacent supporting cells from where they recirculate via connexin-bound pores and then re-enter the endolymph through inward-rectifying potassium channels (**KCNQ1, KCNE1**). Hence, hair cells function both as sensory receptors and mechanical effectors. Cochlear vibrations are thus transduced to the inner hair cell which in turn provides the brain with auditory information.

CLINICAL KEYNOTE

Syndromic deafness

There are more than 30 known genetic causes of primary human deafness: these genotypes underlie most of the one in 800 cases of neonatal deafness, and contribute to many cases of age-related deafness (60% of those older than 70 have at least a 25-decibel hearing loss).

So-called syndromic deafness occurs in association with other abnormalities, such as in **Alport syndrome** (with renal failure), **Usher syndrome** (**myosin 7A** mutated in type 1B – the genetic defect responsible for *Shaker* mice – and the cochlear membrane protein **otogelin** in type C) and **Pendred syndrome**. The latter syndrome, associated with thyroid goiter, affects the prestin (see above) homolog **pendrin** – a sulfate/iodide/chloride transporter. This is consistent with the dual pathology of Pendred syndrome, since normal chloride transport is required for cochlear endolymph secretion, just as normal iodide transport is needed for thyroid hormone biosynthesis. **Connexin-32** is mutated in the deafness associated with **X-linked Charcot–Marie–Tooth disease**.

The symptoms and signs of **Waardenburg syndrome** (deafness with white forelock; p. 400) reflect impaired melanocyte migration. Relevant to this, melanocytes in the stria vascularis of the cochlear help to generate and maintain the high resting potential (70 mV) of the endolymph. Consistent with this, susceptibility to acquired deafness appears to vary with the ocular melanin phenotype (which presumably reflects cochlear melanocyte density). Hence, individuals with light-colored eyes (blue, green) are more prone to deafness following meningitis or loud noise than are those with brown eyes, whereas the reverse is true of ototoxic (e.g., cisplatin-induced) deafness.

MOLECULAR MINIREVIEW

Single-gene mutations causing deafness

Nonsyndromic (monogenic) deafness occurs because of gene mutations affecting **connexin-26** (gap junction protein β-2, *GJB2*) and **connexin-31**. Of these, connexin-26 mutations account for almost half of all recessive deafness cases in Ashkenazi Jews, and for 10–20% of such cases in other kindreds. Additional mutational targets in nonsyndromic deafness include **α-tectorin** (see above), **COCH**, **FGFR3**, and **POU 4F3** (all autosomal dominant), **myosin 15** (autosomal recessive), **POU 3F4** (Brn4; X-linked) and **12S RNA** (mitochondrial); mutations affecting the latter protein may predispose to aminoglycoside-induced hearing loss.

An extracellular matrix protein appears to be encoded by the *COCH* gene, mutations of which cause both progressive high-frequency hearing loss and **Meniere syndrome** (vertigo). Another unconventional (nonmuscle) myosin, **myosin 1B**, regulates stereocilia tip link tensions; together with **myosin 6**, it is a candidate mutational target in deafness, as are other stereocilial proteins such as **vezatin** and **harmonin**. Loss-of-function mutations affecting the inner hair cell molecule **otoferlin** – a synaptic vesicle recycling protein – may also cause autosomal dominant deafness, as can mutations affecting L-type calcium channels.

Mutations affecting the cochlear potassium channel encoded by the *KCNQ4* gene locus also give rise to **progressive high-frequency hearing loss** due to the failure of potassium ions to exit normally from the hair cell; indeed, disruption of endolymph homeostasis (high potassium, low sodium) is a general mechanism of deafness mutations. For example, mutations of other potassium channels (**KCNQ1, KCNE1**) that normally replenish endolymph potassium may cause the hearing loss associated with one variety of long-QT syndrome (**Jervell and Lange–Nielsen syndrome**; p. 184). The importance of normal mitochondrial function for hearing is suggested by the concurrence of deafness in syndromes such as **MERFF, MELAS** and **Kearns–Sayre** (pp. 39–40) which in some families may present with deafness alone.

Substance P mediates pain sensation

Pain sensation is a conserved mechanism for minimizing exposure to noxious stimuli, and is hence termed nociception. Normal postnatal mammalian development of pain fibers requires nerve growth factor, and this process results in two major types of pain fiber:

1. Small myelinated A δ fibers
   - Sense rapid-onset pain,
   - Are activated by glutamate (via NMDA receptors) and aspartate.
2. Cutaneous unmyelinated C fibers
   - Transmit lingering poorly localized pain
   - Are activated by substance P, somatostatin, calcitonin gene-related peptide (CGRP), cholecystokinin (CCK), vasoactive intestinal polypeptide (VIP), bradykinin, histamine, serotonin, and glutamate.

Spinal cord release of the pain-specific tachykinin neurotransmitter **sub-**

stance P elicits the sensation of pain. This undecapeptide is concentrated in the dorsal horn of the spinal cord; injection of substance P into the substantia gelatinosa triggers histamine release from mast cells, thus causing vasodilatation and pain. Substance P also causes the pain associated with smooth muscle contraction and the neurogenic inflammation induced by prostaglandins. Mice with blunted responses to intensely painful stimuli are produced by knockout of either the **protachykinin A** gene (which encodes the precursor molecule for substance P and its congener neurokinin A) or the **neurokinin-1 receptor** (with which substance P interacts). NMDA receptor antagonists such as the anti-influenza drug amantadine and the anesthetic agent ketamine likewise have analgesic properties.

Painful nerve impulses may be transmitted by other neurotransmitters such as CGRP, VIP, CCK or corticotropin-releasing hormone (CRH). Phenomena such as central (thalamic) pain – which is unrelated to peripheral nerve impulses – may be associated with the downregulation of thalamic GABA receptors. However, synaptic degeneration and excitotoxic reactions may also contribute to central sensitization.

Nociceptors are ligand-gated ion channels that may be activated by stimuli as diverse as heat, sunburn, or hydrogen ions. ATP – which is co-released with norepinephrine from sympathetic nerves and which binds nociceptive purinoceptors – also plays a role in the generation of pain signals. The pain associated with an over-full bladder is mediated via $P2X_3$ purinoceptors – selectively expressed on small-diameter sensory neurons – which are activated by extracellular ATP, leading to ion channel activation. Neurogenic (hyporeflexic) bladders can thus be induced in experimental animals by $P2X_3$ receptor gene knockout, whereas pharmacologic $P2X_3$ antagonists could prove useful for treating overactive bladders. $P2X_3$ knockout is also associated with thermal hyperalgesia due to chronic inflammation of the skin, but this nociceptive pathway is only operative between skin temperatures of 20°C and 40°C. Skin pain induced by temperatures above 45°C are mediated by **vanilloid receptors** instead (see below).

MOLECULAR MINIREVIEW

Capsicum and vanilla

Capsaicin is the spicy **vanilloid** that makes chilies taste anything but chilly. The lipophilicity of capsaicin explains why the painful sensation of ingesting too much cayenne pepper is more efficiently doused with fat than with water. Activation of the **VR1** vanilloid receptor by capsaicin, heat, inflammation (including **Crohn disease**) or endogenous ligands (e.g., **leukotriene B$_4$**) causes cation influx through vanilloid-gated cation channels; the subsequent release of neurotransmitters such as substance P and NMDA agonists triggers the pain sensation. Application of rubefacients (including capsaicin cream) to sore muscles may achieve the advertised analgesic benefit via VR1 receptor downregulation. Consistent with this, *VR1*-knockout mice can eat capsica all day, even though mucosal injuries still occur.

The molecular biology of itch
Pruritus, or itching, is a poorly understood phenomenon. Like pain, itch is sensed via the spinothalamic tracts and via unmyelinated C nerve fibers. Many receptors and mediators of itch have been implicated, including:
1. **Opioid μ-receptors** (see below).
2. **Histamine-1 (H1) receptors.**
3. Neuropeptide receptors for:
   - Substance P
   - Vasoactive peptide hormones: **VIP, CGRP.**
An inverse relationship between itch and pain sensation has been noted in certain contexts: activation of opioid μ-receptors relieves pain but provokes itch, whereas blockade of opioid receptors suppresses itch but worsens pain. Hence, patients with marked pruritus – due to **cholestasis** or **uremia**, say – may benefit from opioid receptor antagonists of the naloxone class.

Inhibition of H1 receptors by antihistamines may relieve itch – though not in the context of atopic eczema, a classic allergic disorder. The therapeutic contribution of central sedation is unclear in the setting of antihistamine antipruritic action.

Opioids prevent pain by inhibiting adenyl cyclase
The human brain contains endogenous pain inhibitors termed **endorphins** (Table 20.5, derived from the opioid precursors pro-dynorphin and pro-opiomelanocortin) and **enkephalins** (derived from pro-enkephalin). All contain a high-affinity receptor-binding domain consisting of a protonated amine next to an aromatic ring. These endogenous opioids bind at least three types of G-protein-coupled opioid receptors that act by inhibiting adenyl cyclase via receptor coupling to G_i:
1. **μ** opioid receptors
   - Preferred endogenous ligands: endorphins,
   - Preferred drug: morphine.
2. **δ** opioid receptors
   - Preferred endogenous ligands: enkephalins.
   - Preferred drug: deltorphins (contain D-amino acids)
3. **κ** opioid receptors
   - Preferred endogenous ligands: **dynorphins.**
None of the common narcotic analgesics displays absolute specificity for one class of opioid receptors, but lack of cross-tolerance between μ and κ opioids suggests that they have different mechanisms of action. The **μ receptor** mediates most of the classic morphine-like effects (analgesia, tolerance, and addiction), and mutations of this receptor cause **inherited codeine insensitivity.** Of note, the desensitizing protein β-arrestin-2 is required for morphine tolerance but does not mediate drug dependence. Morphine also causes the release of enkephalins, suggesting that these opioids (which bind δ receptors) partly mediate the effects of morphine. Heroin (diacetylmorphine) is more lipid-soluble than morphine, and equilibrates more rapidly in the brain.

Synergistic analgesia induced by opioids and aspirin reflects inhibition of GABAergic potassium channels in midbrain periaqueductal grey matter by activated μ opioid receptors linked to this signaling pathway via arachidonate (which is more abundant in the presence of cyclooxygenase inhibition). A potent side-effect of opiates is constipation: consistent with this, the antidiarrheal agent loperamide is a μ-receptor agonist, while another antidiarrheal drug (racecadotril) is an enkephalinase inhibitor.

Table 20.5. Endorphins: endogenous opioids

Endorphin	Amino acid sequence
met-enkephalin	Tyr-Gly-Gly-Phe-Met
leu-enkephalin	Tyr-Gly-Gly-Phe-Leu
β-endorphin	Tyr-Gly-Gly-Phe-Met-(3)- Lys-Ser-(21)
dynorphin	Tyr-Gly-Gly-Phe-Leu-(10)- Asn-Gln
nociceptin	Phe-Gly-Gly-Phe-(4)- Lys-Ser-(5)- Asn-Gln

κ **receptors** are so named because they were first activated in vitro by keto-cyclazocine. The addictive drug cocaine modulates the cAMP-PKA-CREB pathway in the brain's reward center), thereby altering dynorphin transcription and κ receptor function. Pharmacologic κ receptor agonists are being developed to treat itch, visceral pain, and inflammation.

Counter-irritation analgesic strategies (such as acupuncture and transcutaneous electrical nerve stimulation, or TENS) may work in part via endogenous opioids. This is not true for vibration therapy, since its effect persists following administration of opiate inhibitors such as naltrexone or naloxone. Opiate addiction is mediated in part via dopaminergic signaling within the basolateral amygdala, yet also appears to depend on co-expression in the ventral forebrain of the receptor for substance P. The amnesic effects of opiates, on the other hand, reflect impaired synaptic potentiation associated with reduced synapsin phosphorylation.

MOLECULAR MINIREVIEW

Nociceptin and galanin

Nociceptin is a dynorphin-like neuropeptide that causes hyperalgesia (rather than narcosis) when injected intraventricularly; this activity is mediated by a distinct receptor (ORL_1) similar to κ. The nociceptin precursor molecule contains an antagonist ligand termed **nocistatin**, which inhibits nociceptin-dependent pain and also reduces the allodynia (i.e., hypersensitivity to extrinsic pain) induced by prostaglandin E_2.

Direct inhibition of pain transmission at the spinal cord level is mediated by the 29-amino-acid neuropeptide **galanin**, which activates a G-protein-coupled receptor. Galanin may act synergistically with morphine, and is implicated in adaptive responses to nerve injury. Nerve injury also enhances the analgesic effects of galanin while permitting pain fiber excitation by adrenergic receptors, perhaps accounting for the analgesic effects of sympathectomy in pathologically indeterminate conditions such as **causalgia**. This also provides a rationale for the action of tricyclic antidepressants in relieving neuropathic pain, since these drugs block norepinephrine reuptake.

PHARMACOLOGIC FOOTNOTE

Anandamide – the endogenous cannabinoid

Like opioid receptors, the CB1 **cannabinoid** (δ-9-**tetrahydrocannabinol**, THC) **receptor** is a G-protein-coupled receptor in the brain that is normally activated by a fat-soluble endocannabinoid termed **anandamide** (*N*-arachidonoyl-ethanolamine) – a brain arachidonate derivative released together with **palmitylethanolamide** (PEA) from a phospholipid precursor.

As is true for morphine and its endogenous counterpart leu-enkephalin, structural homology between anandamide and THC is restricted to the receptor-binding domain. The analgesic effects of cannabinoids involve activation of a brainstem (rostral ventromedial medulla) circuit that is also targeted by opioids. Consistent with this, knockout of the **CB1 receptor** in mice reduces the addictiveness of opiates as well as impairing cannabinoid responsiveness. Synthetic cannabinoids are routinely used for the therapy of nausea (e.g., during cancer chemotherapy) or spasticity (e.g., associated with **multiple sclerosis**). CB1 receptors also mediate the biphasic effects of endogenous cannabinoids on bronchial responsiveness. In noncerebral tissues such as skin and lymphoid tissues, anandamide and PEA may cooperate to induce analgesia by binding peripheral CB1-like receptors as well as a second cannabinoid receptor, CB2.

Cannabis enthusiasts have long been aware of "the munchies" – the increase in appetite which accompanies pharmacologic stimulation of the CB1 receptor. This phenomenon is explained by the leptin-dependent downregulation of hypothalamic endocannabinoids (anandamide and **2-arachidonyl glycerol**) which normally contributes to reduced food intake. High levels of cannabinoids (endogenous or extrinsic) also make the endometrium less receptive to implantation. Perhaps offsetting this, THC-dependent CB1 receptor activation crosstalks with the progesterone and dopamine signaling systems to cause an aphrodisiac effect in females of lower mammalian species.

G_{olf} is the target of a smell receptor superfamily

The sense of smell is critical for survival in lower organisms, being required not only for food localization but also (via sex-seeking **pheromones**) for mate selection. This is the basis of the "armpit effect" in which hamsters sniff out genetically unrelated partners with whom to breed, and women find that sweaty T-shirts of unrelated men smell sexier (? less repulsive) than those of close relatives. Mammalian pheromones are sensitively detected (10^{-11} M) by two families of G-protein-coupled pheromone receptors (**V1R** and **V2R**) expressed in the vomeronasal organ which, together with the olfactory and taste tissues, is one of three chemosensory epithelia in the oropharyngeal region.

Odorants are volatile lipid-soluble ligands with detection thresholds as low as 10^{-17} M in certain mammals (e.g., dogs). Although not approaching this sensitivity, olfaction remains the most diverse of human senses. The variety of aromas detectable by the olfactory epithelium far exceeds that of any other sensory stimulus, reflecting the existence of over 1000 smell receptors (>1% of the entire genome's coding capacity). This G-protein-coupled receptor superfamily – which, being larger than the immunoglobulin and T cell receptor gene families combined, is the largest such superfamily – dwarfs the pheromone receptor superfamily, which numbers fewer than 200. In contrast, the human eye distinguishes thousands of hues using only three photoreceptors (p. 515). The molecular players mediating odorant signaling are:

1. **Odorant-binding proteins**
   - Mucus proteins that transport or sequester odorants.
2. **Olfactory G-protein-coupled receptors**
   - Homologous to sperm cell receptors; liberate cAMP.
3. **cAMP-gated ion channels**
   - Cause Na^+/Ca^{2+} influx, which is then amplified by a Cl^- efflux current.
4. **UDP-glucuronyltransferase**
   - The enzyme responsible for olfactory ligand inactivation.

Olfactory cells are ciliated neurons. Although few odorants have been paired with specific receptors, repetitive odorant exposure enhances olfactory sensitivity, suggesting that olfactory receptor expression is upregulated by intermittent stimulation. Even small changes in odorant structure may cause major perceptual differences: for example, L-carvone smells like spearmint, whereas its stereoisomer D-carvone smells like caraway seeds. A rare congenital syndrome of defective fetal synapse formation is characterized by the sensation of an aroma in response to visual perception of a color.

Odorants bind G-protein-coupled receptors that act via the heterotrimeric G-protein G_{olf} to activate adenyl cyclase within 40 milliseconds of exposure, leading to the synthesis of cAMP and the opening of cAMP-gated calcium channels (Figure 20.11). G_{olf} signaling is terminated following phosphodiesterase activation and ligand biotransformation by **UDP-glucuronyltransferase**. Signal termination is accelerated when odorant-induced calcium influx desensitizes cAMP-dependent signaling via calmodulin; prior to desensitization, however, calcium influx amplifies the cAMP-dependent signaling current by depolarizing a calcium-dependent chloride channel. Receptor polymorphisms affecting the fourth and fifth membrane helix are common, suggesting that the extracellular loop connecting these regions recognizes odorants.

CLINICAL KEYNOTE

Anosmia

Up to 100 000 olfactory neurons project their axons to a single glomerulus, and about 1000 such glomeruli comprise the olfactory bulb which in turn projects to the olfactory cortex. The brain does not have a topographic map for odors as it does for visual and somatosensory stimuli, though sorting of odoriferous information within the olfactory bulb may be analogous to retinal visual processing. In addition to their olfactory functions, odorant receptors may guide olfactory neurons to their targets in the developing brain. Of note, separate brain regions are activated by sniffing (olfactory exploration) and smelling (olfactory recognition).

Unlike vision and hearing (which grade stimuli by quantitative criteria such as wavelength and frequency) olfactory recognition is a qualitative process analogous to antibody recognition. Immunoglobulin diversity mainly reflects gene recombination, however, whereas olfactory receptor diversity reflects the number of sensors encoded. Discrimination between smells is thus made by the peripheral receptor rather than by the brain, and each olfactory neuron expresses only one receptor type, consistent with the numerous clinical disorders of odor recognition, or **anosmias**. However, the commonest cause of anosmia remains head trauma due to motor vehicle accidents.

Taste is transmitted by either ions or G-proteins

Ion channels on the surface of gustatory receptor cells transmit taste. About 50 taste receptor cells make up a single taste bud, which is punctuated by a

Figure 20.11 Depolarization of olfactory neurons by odorants. Olfactory G-protein-coupled receptors transduce signals via G_{olf}, activating either adenyl cyclase or phospholipase C-β effectors; cation influx results, leading to olfactory neuron depolarization and sensory propagation. IP_3, inositol 1,4,5-trisphosphate; PIP_2, phosphatidylinositol (4,5)-bisphosphate.

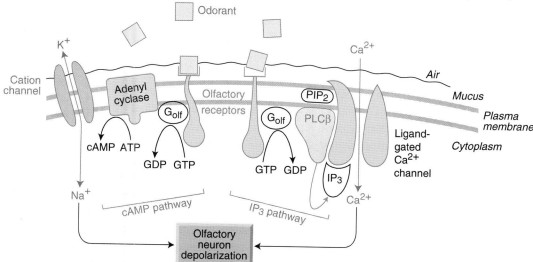

Figure 20.12 Gustatory signaling. Salty and sour tastants transmit sensation via ion channels, whereas bitter and sweet tastants act via G-protein-coupled receptors linked to gustducin. Sweet and bitter tastes may be transmitted via different receptors as shown. Unlike sugar-sweet tastes, however, saccharine-sweet tastes may be transmitted via the PLC-β pathway shown at left. AC, adenyl cyclase; PDE, phosphodiesterase; PKA, protein kinase A; PLC, phospholipase C.

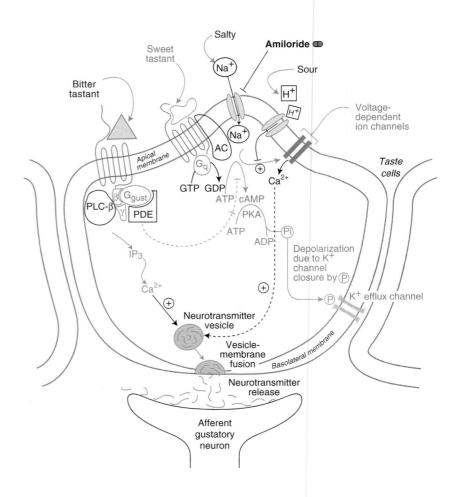

central pore containing the microvilli of the receptor cells. Taste-sensing papillae of the tongue contain up to 200 taste buds; unlike odorants, millimolar (high) concentrations of tastants are required for taste sensation. Individual taste buds vary in their specificity, leading to the perception of complex tastes. The basic taste-sensing mechanisms are

1. Ionic
   - Salty (Na^+)
   - Sour (H^+)
2. G-protein-coupled-receptor-mediated
   - Sweet (caloric)
   - Bitter (noxious)
   - Umami (monosodium glutamate)

Such mechanisms may trigger voltage-gated K^+ channel closure in the basolateral membrane when activated (Figure 20.12).

Salty and sour tastes are transmitted via monovalent (Na^+, H^+) cation influx. Salty (Na^+) stimuli enter gustatory epithelial cells by passing through apical amiloride-sensitive Na^+ channels, whereas sour (H^+) stimuli block amiloride-sensitive Na^+ channels. These ionic fluxes determine whether the taste cell becomes depolarized (activated) or hyperpolarized (inhibited): depolarization leads to K^+ channel closure which then triggers neurotransmitter release. Sodium chloride tastes saltier than sodium acetate or sodium gluconate (the anion paradox) because the smaller chloride ions follow sodium through the tight junctions of the gustatory epithelium, thereby neutralizing the positive charge (i.e., the chloride itself is not responsible for the taste). In contrast, the slower transit of acetate or gluconate ions causes a net positive (Na^+) charge within the epithelium – leading to hyperpolarization followed by inhibition of neurotransmission.

Good taste and bad taste receptors

Sweet and bitter tastes are sensed by two superfamilies (40 to 80 members) of G-protein-coupled receptors which are structurally homologous to the V2R and V1R pheromone receptor families respectively. Since sweet tastes are attractive and bitter tastes aversive, this homology suggest that the respective pheromone receptor families could also mediate attractive and aversive responses. Sweet tastant receptors are few in number, consistent with the relatively homogeneous structure of carbohydrate ligands, whereas the structural diversity of bitter tastants – e.g., cyanide, quinine, caffeine, propylthiouracil, alkaloids, cycloheximide – implies the existence of numerous bitter receptors (see below). Sucrose triggers activation of the G-protein-coupled receptor **T1R3** which is encoded within the *Sac* locus on chromosome 4; subsequent activation of the G-protein G_q transduces adenyl cyclase, cAMP-dependent K^+ channel closure, and nerve depolarization. In contrast, nonsugar sweeteners increase levels of IP_3, calcium, and PKC, perhaps explaining their unique saccharine-like flavor.

Bitter tastant receptor activation stimulates the G_i (adenyl cyclase-inhibitory) G-protein alpha-subunit family member **G_{gust} (α-gustducin)**, which reduces cellular cAMP levels by activating phosphodiesterase. Of note, however, G_{gust} is also implicated in sweet taste transmission. Most bitter tastants trigger an intracellular influx of calcium, thus triggering vesicle fusion and neurotransmitter release. Such tastants are sensed by a mammalian superfamily of 40–80 **T2R** taste receptors, many of which are expressed by a single taste cell. The umami flavor enhancer, monosodium glutamate, activates an alternatively spliced form of the metabotropic glutamate receptor (mGluR), leading to the opening of large cation conductance channels in gustatory epithelial cells. Fatty acids may transmit "nonconventional" taste sensations via distinct ion channels and/or transporters.

Light is sensed by 11-cis-retinal bound to rhodopsin

The eye contains two types of photoreceptor cells – rod cells (about 100 million) and cone cells (about 10 million) – which contain G-protein-coupled receptors of differing subunit composition. Rods are responsible for scotopic (low-illuminance, starlight) vision, and are thus of most importance in dark adaptation where they distinguish shades of gray (Figure 20.13). In contrast, cones are responsible for photopic (high-illuminance, daylight) vision and thus mediate visual acuity and color vision. Dark-dependent activation of mGluR amplifies cone signaling to "on" bipolar cells, whereas "off" bipolar cells are desensitized by activation of kainate (ionotropic) glutamate receptors. By preventing signal saturation, the latter permits the continued detection of small, graded light stimuli even in the dark. Key molecules involved in light sensing include:

1. **11-cis-retinal**
   - Light-absorbing prosthetic group derived from vitamin A.
2. **Rhodopsin**
   - G-protein-coupled receptor occurring exclusively in retinal rods.
3. **Transducin** (G_t)
   - Retina-specific G-protein that activates cGMP phosphodiesterase.

Figure 20.13 Scanning electron micrograph of a retinal rod cell, adjacent to a capillary (Wellcome Medical Photographic Library, no. B0001051C07).

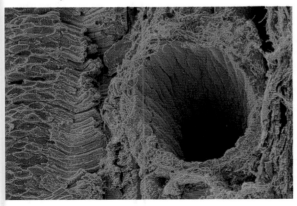

Unlike most G-protein-coupled receptor ligands which are soluble or circulating, the visual chromophore 11-cis-retinal is covalently bound to a pocket within the transmembrane helix (specifically, at Lys^{296} in helix VII) of the 40-kDa 495-nm-wavelength photoreceptor **rhodopsin** in rod cells. Molecules regulating the availability of 11-cis-retinal include retinaldehyde-binding protein and interphotoreceptor retinol-binding protein. In its ground state 11-cis-retinal lies cradled in a pocket of the rhodopsin transmembrane domain, maintaining it in an inactive conformation. Absorption of light catalyzes flipping (isomerization) of 11-cis-retinal to ***all*-trans-retinal** (vitamin A aldehyde). This extracellular flipping reaction initiates movements of rhodopsin transmembrane helices that trigger torsional conversion to metarhodopsin within 200 femtoseconds ($2 \cdot 10^{-13}$ seconds) of illumination. Activated rhodopsin in turn activates hundreds of copies of a retina-specific G_α-protein termed **transducin** (G_t) – a cGMP phosphodiesterase activator which mediates the first stage of visual stimulus amplification (Figure 20.14).

MOLECULAR MINIREVIEW

Opsins

Light-sensing rhodopsin evolved from color-sensing cone cell visual pigments termed **opsins** – integral membrane proteins formed from the covalent binding of 11-cis-retinal to retinal cone apoproteins. There are three such visual pigments in humans (Figure 20.15): blue-sensitive (426 nm peak absorbance wavelength), green-sensitive (530 nm) and red-sensitive (either of two polymorphisms: 552 nm or 557 nm). The latter two proteins are encoded by opsin genes located together at the tip of the long arm of the X chromosome (Xq28) near the genes for factor VIII and glucose-6-phosphate dehydrogenase; this region of the human genome contains more known genetic disease loci than any other. The perception of color vision is based on differential spectral absorbances from retinal bound to these different cone receptor proteins, though limited color vision is detectable in rare individuals possessing only one set of cones. Color discrimination is also facilitated by the interaction of 11-cis-retinal with key residues in rhodopsin which determine the maximally absorbed wavelength.

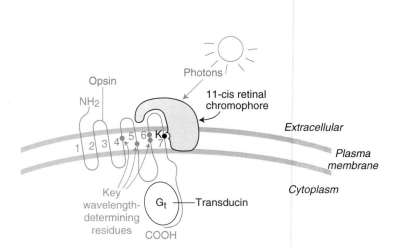

Figure 20.14 Light sensation by retinal G-protein-coupled receptors (opsins or rhodopsin). The 11-cis-retinal chromophore absorbs radiant light energy, transmitting a conformational change to the transmembrane receptor and thereby activating transducin. The positions of transmembrane residues affecting the specificity of color wavelength are indicated.

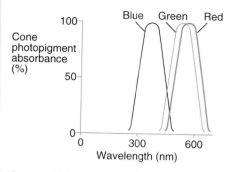

Figure 20.15 Representation of the normal visual pigment wavelengths, illustrating the proximity of the red and green spectra.

Retinal pigments absorb light at different wavelengths

Most nonprimate mammals express only a single yellow-green (550 nm) opsin gene and are constitutively colorblind for red and green hues, whereas at the other extreme a few vertebrates have tetrachromatic (four-color) vision. Normal primate vision is **trichromatic** – i.e., tuned to peak wavelengths of 430 nm, 535 nm, and 562 nm – perhaps reflecting evolutionary pressures relating to the need for distinguishing leaf (and perhaps fruit) color.

Three amino acid substitutions are responsible for the 30-nm spectral shift between red and green color vision. These pigment genes are thought to have arisen by duplication, and their extensive sequence homology (>90%) favors frequent misalignments during homologous recombination. This tendency to unequal crossing-over has genetic consequences:

1. Further gene duplication events, often leading to supernumerary opsin genes positioned in tandem on the X chromosome.
2. Formation of fusion genes containing coding sequences normally present in both green and red opsins.
3. Frequent gene deletions.

Red and green pigment genes contain six exons, the first and last of which are identical. Since exons 2 to 5 of the red and green pigment genes contain most of the coding differences, **colorblindness** usually results from unequal homologous recombination occurring in the intervals between these exons. The severity of red-green confusion varies with the microanatomy of the molecular lesion: major spectral shifts often accompany exon 5 mutations, whereas nonconserved amino acid substitutions due to exon 4 mutations tend to be more subtle in their visual consequences. As many as 8% of males (but fewer than 1% of females) have some degree of red-green colorblindness.

A rare presentation of colorblindness is **incomplete achromatopsia**. This syndrome, which is caused by inactivation of both long-wavelength opsin genes, may arise due to the deletion of an upstream element situated more than 40 kb upstream from the green pigment gene promoter. Clinically this manifests with the rare (1/100 000) X-linked syndrome of **blue cone monochromacy** associated with central retinal degeneration and poor visual acuity.

CLINICAL KEYNOTE

Red-green colorblindness

Two-thirds of colorblind males exhibit **anomalous trichromacy**: such individuals express all three pigments, one of which has a spectral sensitivity between normal red and green. Spectral shifting of this kind results from the creation of a red-green fusion opsin that shifts the anomalous pigment absorption towards that of the remaining (normal) long-wavelength opsin. Anomalous red pigment spectral sensitivity (G$^+$R') gives rise to **protanomalous trichromacy**; anomalous green (G'R$^+$) gives rise to **deuteranomalous trichromacy**. Since X chromosomes often contain two or more green pigment genes, the latter variety of colorblindness is twice as common as the former.

One-third of affected males exhibit **dichromacy**; that is, these individuals (**dichromats**) completely lack red or green pigment spectral sensitivity. Human dichromats have the evolutionary advantage of being able to detect camouflage better than ordinary trichromats – perhaps explaining their genetic success. Complete lack of red pigment sensitivity (G^+R^-) gives rise to **protanopia**, whereas complete lack of green pigment sensitivity (G^-R^+) is termed **deuteranopia**. Autosomal dominant **tritanopia** manifests with blue light insensitivity.

Rod cell cation channels are active in the dark

During darkness, cation (Na^+ and Ca^{2+}) channels within rod cells remain open because of the binding of cyclic GMP (cGMP). Light causes rhodopsin to activate transducin, leading to negative-feedback activation of **cGMP phosphodiesterase**. Rod cGMP levels therefore decline by hydrolysis in response to light-induced **rhodopsin bleaching**, causing the closure of rod cGMP-gated sodium channels, reduced Na^+ and Ca^{2+} influx, and consequent rod cell hyperpolarization. Prolonged light exposure thus switches rod sensing off.

The rod cell photoreceptor system is ultrasensitive, with each absorbed photon reducing transmembrane influx by several million Na^+ ions per rod cell. Dark-adapted rod cells readily admit sodium ions to their outer segments, but ion flow slows once light is sensed. Light-inducible inhibition of rod function occurs relatively slowly, taking several hundred milliseconds. Key molecules regulating the stimulus-reversal of light/dark adaptation include:

1. **Rhodopsin kinase**
   - Homologous to the desensitizing kinase βARK (pp. 280–1).
2. **Arrestin**
   - Cytoplasmic protein that binds phosphorylated rhodopsin.
3. **Recoverin**
   - Guanylate cyclase activator involved in dark adaptation of rods.

Rhodopsin activity is attenuated following its phosphorylation by **rhodopsin kinase** – an event that competitively inhibits transducin binding by promoting the interaction of phosphorylated rhodopsin with **arrestin**. Inactivated rhodopsin is hydrolyzed to opsin and all-trans-retinal, necessitating photoreceptor regeneration on dark exposure. When lights are switched off, the hydrolyzed opsin moiety of rhodopsin is dephosphorylated, increasing its affinity for 11-cis-retinal (regenerated from all-trans-retinal in the retina).

Dark adaptation of rhodopsin coincides with the activation of guanylate cyclase by a small calcium-inhibited enzyme termed **recoverin**. Light-induced reduction of rod calcium levels (from ~500 μM to ~50 μM) enhances recoverin activity, thus (1) activating guanylyl cyclase which (2) replenishes cell cGMP thus (3) restoring Na^+ influx and (4) depolarizing rods in readiness for (5) a renewed cycle of rhodopsin photoactivation. Recoverin is thus a functional antagonist of transducin-activated cGMP phosphodiesterase which helps the cell recover from light-induced hyperpolarization (Figure 20.16).

Not all human vision requires intact peripheral nerve pathways: visual field scotomas (blind spots), for example, may be actively filled in by cerebral cortical compensatory mechanisms. Such "blindsight" may arise because of residual function within the primary geniculostriate visual pathway, or through secondary retinotectal or subcortical visual pathways. Milder defects of visual information processing are implicated in the pathogenesis of **dyslexia**. The variability of retinal–cortical synaptic connections during development – referred to as **visual cortical plasticity** – may be prolonged by rearing animals in the dark.

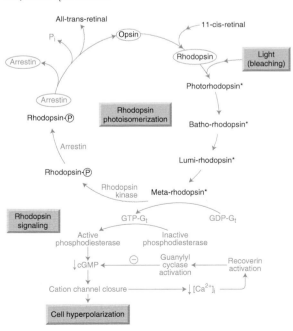

Figure 20.16 Cartoon of rhodopsin photoisomerization and dark adaptation. G_t, transducin.

Synaptic plasticity of this kind is mediated by glutamate-activated NMDA receptors which govern the neurophysiologic process of **long-term potentiation** (p. 519).

CLINICAL KEYNOTE

Retinitis pigmentosa

Just as loss of cone cell function is characterized by colorblindness, so loss of rod cell photoreceptivity is characterized by night blindness (**nyctalopia**) and progressive loss of peripheral acuity (tunnel vision). This syndrome, termed **retinitis pigmentosa** affects two million people (1/4000) worldwide. The clinical features of retinitis pigmentosa are caused by photoreceptor cell death, which leads to migration of the underlying pigment cell layer into the retina (ophthalmoscopically visible as a pigmentary retinopathy).

Mutations of the 5-exon rhodopsin gene on chromosome 3q21-q24 occur in about 20% of subjects with the autosomal dominant (i.e., least aggressive) form of retinitis pigmentosa. Single-base mutations affecting codon 23 – a conserved proline common to all rhodopsins and opsins – have been reported in up to 12% of such cases. Highly dysfunctional mutations include those leading to abnormal protein folding with retention in the endoplasmic reticulum; intracellular export mutants of this type have also been described for the cystic fibrosis transmembrane conductance regulator and the low-density lipoprotein receptor gene. Overall, more than 50 different rhodopsin mutations have been associated with retinitis pigmentosa. These include not only rhodopsin-misfolding mutations but also opsin-activating mutations in which opsin is constitutively activated in the absence of light, leading to congenital night blindness.

Degeneration of rod photoreceptors is the pathophysiologic hallmark of retinitis pigmentosa. Since rods are present mainly in the peripheral retina, this manifests as narrowing of the visual field. Cone degeneration (loss of central vision, color discrimination and daytime acuity) eventually supervenes in most subjects, however, suggesting that rhodopsin mutations are neither necessary nor sufficient for retinitis pigmentosa – in other words, the syndrome displays genetic locus heterogeneity. Other genes implicated in this phenotype include those encoding peripherin, recoverin, arrestin and transducin.

Neuronal biorhythms are set by oscillators

Neurons are capable of generating rhythmic activity, as exemplified in vivo by cardiac pacing. Similarly, breathing rhythms are controlled by a brainstem pacemaker, giving rise to **Cheyne–Stokes respiration** (periodic breathing) in individuals with brainstem injury. The **circadian pacemaker**, which lies within the 10 000 neurons of the hypothalamic suprachiasmatic nucleus (SCN), is light-sensitive: detection of light-dependent activity in isolated neurons suggests that changes in membrane conductance may contribute to such regulation. Since light synchronizes the transcription of immediate-early genes in both the visual cortex and in the SCN, photoreceptor stimulation also appears central. Experimental ablation of both rod and cone function can be associated with the retention of circadian hormone responses, however, suggesting the existence of nonrod noncone ocular photoreceptors. Of note, age-related degeneration of circadian pacemaker function occurs independently of photoreceptor dysfunction.

Trans-regulatory molecular oscillators generically termed **Clock** proteins underlie these 24-hour rhythms. Such clocks are set or **photoentrained** by ionotropic glutamate receptors which control calcium influx into the SCN in response to nocturnal dimming. The light cycle thus sets the primary (input) circadian pacemaker or clock, leading to the activation of **secondary oscillators**. The latter include gene repressors such as the heterodimeric nuclear proteins **Tim** and **Per**, originally characterized in fruitflies as *Period* and *Timeless*. *Per* and *Tim* switch on in the morning, accumulate in the cytoplasm during the day, then by evening reach a critical concentration culminating in heterodimerization, nuclear translocation, and transcriptional autorepression. Additional genes such as *Clock* and *Cryptochrome*, which also encode transcription factors, influence this process.

Reciprocal diurnal cycling of growth hormone and somatostatin expression is consistent with the operation of a neuroendocrine (central) transcriptional oscillator located in the SCN; changes in temperature, as well as light, may modulate the timing of this rhythm. Circadian oscillators also exist in tissues outside the SCN (such as the liver, kidneys, and heart), but these peripheral timing mechanisms are set by endogenous glucocorticoids. Moreover, not all body clocks are circadian. For example, the timing of parturition by a placental clock is linked to free levels of corticotropin-releasing hormone (CRH).

MOLECULAR MINIREVIEW

Sleep substances

The mammalian sleep-wake cycle is regulated by endogenous sleep substances such as **muramyl peptides** and **delta sleep-inducing peptide** (DSIP). Release of such hormones is related to light exposure via effects on the light-inhibited pineal hormone melatonin (p. 323). Synthesis of the latter is controlled in turn by circadian variation of the pineal enzyme **arylalkylamine *N*-acetyltransferase** which is itself regulated by noradrenergic stimulation of the cAMP-dependent transcription factor CREM.

Mutations affecting the small GTP-binding **Rab3a** protein, which regulates synaptic neurotransmission, may abbreviate circadian rhythms by inducing non-REM delta wave (1–4 mHz) thalamocortical oscillations. Since the Rab3a gene locus on chromosome 19p13 is adjacent to the **neuropeptide Y** gene locus, and the HLA-DQ-linked compulsive sleep disorder narcolepsy is associated with null mutations of the orexigenic type 2 **hypocretin receptor**, a link between circadian timekeeping and appetite regulation seems plausible.

Thinking molecules

Long-term potentiation of synapses enhances learning

The human nervous system comprises a low-voltage battery (the brain) with numerous wires (neurons) which make connections (synapses) within and outside it. This electrical circuit comprises around a thousand billion neurons, each with about 1000 synapses – that is, as many as 10^{15} synapses in all. Given this structural complexity, it is not surprising that many gene abnormalities can give rise to nervous system defects. Cerebellar dysfunction, for example, is inducible by mutations affecting *Hox*, *Wnt* and calcium channel genes.

The organization of the central nervous system into flexible cell networks differs from traditional hard-wired paradigms of brain organization. How are these cobweb-like networks integrated? Synapses that repeatedly fire in a synchronous pattern get stronger (the **Hebb rule**), especially when reinforced by brainstem neuromodulators. Hebbian synapses may also interact in a retrograde fashion, however, leading to reduced synaptic efficiency. The synaptic plasticity of the brain so defined thus arises via at least two mechanisms:

1. **Long-term depression** (LTD)
   - Implicated in cerebellar motor learning.
2. **Long-term potentiation** (LTP)
   - Implicated in hippocampal memory acquisition.

The acquisition of motor coordination by cerebellar learning requires the concurrent glutamate-dependent excitation of climbing and parallel cerebellar fibers, mediated via metabotropic glutamate receptors. This conjunctive stimulus brings about long-term depression of neurotransmission (i.e., synapse elimination) along Purkinje cell parallel fibers. Animal studies using microinjections of the mushroom-derived GABA$_A$ receptor agonist **muscimol** have suggested that memory traces of conditioned cerebellar responses are localized within the cerebellum itself.

A distinct variety of synaptic plasticity, LTP, mainly affects the CA1 cells of the hippocampus. LTP is implicated as a mechanism of long-term (declarative) memory storage in the hippocampus, and takes place following repetitive calcium entry into hippocampal postsynaptic membranes following NMDA receptor activation. Animal studies confirm that learning and memory are enhanced by the overexpression of forebrain NMDA receptors, though synaptic reinforcement via this mechanism is also accompanied by an increase in pain sensitivity.

LTP may be reinforced at the presynaptic level by the synapse-strengthening **retrograde messenger**, nitric oxide, which increases glutamate release and thus enhances spatial and olfactory memory (Figure 20.17). Other candidate retrograde messengers modulating LTP include the guanylyl cyclase activator **carbon monoxide**, a product of heme breakdown by neuronal heme oxygenase. Endorphins are implicated as retrograde inhibitory neurotransmitters that block LTP induction in animal models, possibly promoting amnesia; the same is true of cannabinoids, which reduce GABA release from hippocampal synapses. Though best characterized in the hippocampus and cerebellum respectively, LTP and LTD probably occur to some extent throughout the neocortex.

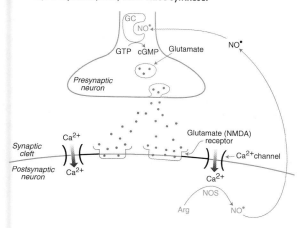

Figure 20.17 Activation of nitric oxide (NO•) as a retrograde messenger for synaptic neurotransmission. GC, guanyl cyclase; NMDA, *N*-methyl-ᴅ-aspartate; NOS, nitric oxide synthase.

CLINICAL KEYNOTE

Learning molecules

Only gross behavioral changes are likely to be demonstrable in animal models of learning. Such phenotypes have been observed in gene knockout experiments (p. 585) involving transgenic animals:

1. Gene targeting of **calcium/calmodulin-dependent** (CaM) **protein kinases** impairs memory in animals.
2. Mice expressing a defective protein kinase isoform, **protein kinase C-γ**, exhibit selective impairment of LTP with associated learning and memory defects.
3. Inactivation of the **Fyn** nonreceptor tyrosine kinase also antagonizes LTP and spatial learning; in addition, neonatal Fyn knockout mice exhibit impaired suckling responses. These deficits probably reflect a critical developmental role for Fyn in the initial events of CNS myelination.

4. Knockout of the adhesion molecule **N-CAM** causes difficulties in negotiating mazes, indicating impaired spatial learning.

Caution should be exercised in extrapolating these crude experimental observations to human physiology.

Memory requires calcium/calmodulin-dependent kinase II

Memories vary, depending upon who is remembering. Defective memories are likewise heterogeneous: some human diseases impair the acquisition of new memories, others impair the retention of recent memories, while still others impair the retrieval of old memories. Neurophysiologists (who think about these things more than most of us) distinguish two groups of memories:

1. **Implicit** (conditioned) memories such as fear of the dark are localized in the amygdala and striatum, where the **memory trace** remains constant.
2. **Explicit** memories such as telephone numbers are localized to the hippocampus and medial temporal lobe. The anatomical location of the memory trace may change within several weeks of initial learning, and formation of such memory traces requires de novo neurogenesis within the subgranular zone of the adult hippocampus. Memory retrieval of this kind is termed **reconstructive**, i.e., involves learning in reverse gear.

Storage of both types of memory requires **calcium/calmodulin-dependent kinase II** (CaMKII; Figure 20.18). This enzyme, which regulates glutamate receptor density by phosphorylation, plays several roles in brain function:

1. Directs the developmental migration of embryonic neuronal growth cones
   - Defects impair intelligence and future learning ability.
2. Modulates LTP within hippocampal CA1 cells
   - Defects impair explicit learning.
3. Modulates the synaptic strength of memory traces within the amygdala
   - Defects impair implicit learning.
4. Modulates the synaptic plasticity of hippocampal CA3 pyramidal neurons
   - Defects impair spatial learning.

LTP stimulation is accompanied by a 30% increase in nerve CaMKII levels within 5 minutes. The electrical activity across the synapse triggers the microtubular translocation of CaMKII mRNAs from the cell body to the dendrites, where protein synthesis occurs. Heterozygous knockout of α-CaMKII drastically reduces mouse brain function in terms of learning, memory, and spatial behavior; that is to say, they learn normally but forget very fast. Constitutive α-CaMKII overexpression within the forebrain or amygdala also induces defects in explicit and implicit memory respectively, however, implying that induction of LTP is not simply a function of CaMKII expression. Hence, speculation that this or other genes represent intelligence genes for eugenic purposes appears premature. Other synapse-strengthening pathways (such as the positive feedback loop between protein kinase C and MAP kinase) could also contribute to LTP in hippocampal CA1 cells. Indeed, numerous memory-associated proteins have been identified, including **calexcitin**; the NMDA-receptor-associated protein **postsynaptic density-95** (PSD95); and even intraventricular (soluble, secreted) forms of the infamous **amyloid precursor protein**.

The mechanisms underlying short-term (working) memory remain contentious. Working memory may be thought of as analogous to the random-access memory of a computer, unlike declarative memory which is written to

Figure 20.18 Longterm potentiation (LTP) of synaptic signaling. A, Interplay of glutamate-dependent postsynaptic calcium influx (anterograde messenger) and calcium-dependent NOS activation leading to nitric oxide activation of presynaptic cGMP-dependent glutamate vesicle release. B, Similar sequence of events in central nervous system CA3 (presynaptic) and CA1 (postsynaptic) hippocampal neurons, leading to LTP and learning.

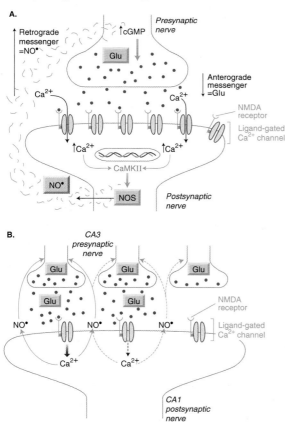

disk. Clinical amnestic conditions such as **Wernicke–Korsakoff syndrome** (thiamine deficiency affecting the mamillothalamic tracts, resulting in loss of short-term memory) illustrate that short- and long-term memory can be dissociated. This view is supported by experiments showing that protein synthesis is necessary for long-term (but not short-term) memory, and that glucocorticoid treatment impairs retrieval of long-term memory.

MOLECULAR MINIREVIEW

Higher center function

Complex biological attributes such as temperament and emotional stability may be influenced by expression patterns of specific molecules. For example, social behaviors involving the territoriality of lower vertebrates are regulated by hormone-secreting cells within the nervous system. When it comes to human higher center functions such as learning and memory, however, understanding remains rudimentary.

Cognitive functions are localized within the brain during development (Figure 20.19). Anatomically distinct brain regions are activated during closely related activities such as hearing words, seeing words, and speaking words. Even nouns and verbs are independently represented in the cerebral cortex, whereas consciousness itself – more accurately regarded as a process than a trait – seems to be a function of the neocortex.

Specification of cortical areas depends upon neuronal patterning genes analogous to the *Drosophila* fate-determining gene *prospero*. **Fate mapping** of neurons reveals that cortical patterning proceeds in an orderly sequence determined by multiple factors, including **cell birthday** (temporal sequence of neurogenesis during ontogeny), microenvironmental cues (such as expression of chemotaxins and cell adhesion molecules) and cell growth phase.

Trinucleotide inserts in neuron DNA are prone to amplification

The specificity of heritable **trinucleotide repeat disorders** (p. 82) for the central nervous system is remarkable. The commonest of these disorders are the CAG-repeat disorders, in which the coding region of the target gene is invaded by glutamine-encoding codons. These CAG-repeat disorders and their target proteins, sometimes termed **polyglutaminopathies**, comprise:

1. **Huntington disease**
   • **Huntingtin.**
2. **Spinal and bulbar muscular atrophy** (SBMA; Kennedy disease)
   • **Androgen receptor.**
3. **Spinocerebellar ataxia type 1**
   • **Ataxin-1.**
4. **Dentatorubral and pallidoluysian atrophy** (DRPLA; in Japanese kindreds)
   • **Atrophin-1.**
5. **Machado–Joseph syndrome.**

These neurologic phenotypes are inducible in mice either by expression of the expanded protein, or by higher-level overexpression of the normal protein. Hence, some property of the wild-type protein that is amplified by the mutant appears to trigger neuronal toxicity (see below).

Unlike wild-type huntingtin, which binds calmodulin, the polyglutamine-expanded mutant huntingtin complexes with the polyglutamine-containing transcriptional coactivator CREB-binding protein (CBP). Similar transcriptional

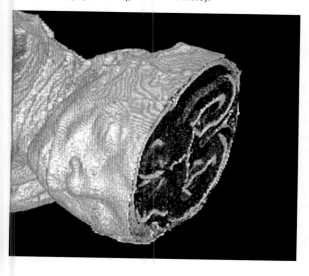

Figure 20.19 High-resolution magnetic resonance imaging (HRMRI) scan of a human fetus showing head and brain. (N. Jeffery; Wellcome Medical Photographic Library, no. B0001014C05).

inhibition occurs in DRPLA mice expressing the mutant atrophin-1 gene product, as well as in CAG-expanded androgen receptor SBMA models. Moreover, CBP-dependent gene products such as brain-derived neurotrophic factor (BDNF), enkephalin, and Jun are downregulated in these neurodegenerative models, whereas experimental overexpression of CBP rescues neuronal toxicity. Interference with CBP-dependent transcription may thus contribute to the pathogenesis of CAG-repeat disorders.

In striking contrast to the CAG-repeat disorders, CTG, CGG or GAA repeats (which give rise to **myotonic dystrophy**, **fragile X syndrome**, and **Friedreich ataxia**, respectively; Table 3.1, p. 83) may insert into introns or untranslated regions. Hence, the proclivity of neuronal genes to accumulate trinucleotide repeats suggests selection occurring at the nucleic acid level. Relevant to this issue, CTG repeats have been noted to form hairpin secondary structures within Okazaki fragments which may predispose to double-strand breaks and thus to further amplification. Alternatively, long (>350 bp) repeat sequences composed of other trinucleotides could create architectural "cis-morphisms" prone to homologous recombination (and hence to deletion, inversion or duplication). The latter possibility of repeat-induced genetic destabilization is supported by the hypermutability of homopolymeric nucleotide runs that encode membrane proteins in antibiotic-resistant bacteria such as *C. jejuni*.

MOLECULAR MINIREVIEW

Huntingtin

The autosomal dominant neurodegenerative disorder **Huntington disease** manifests with involuntary movements (chorea). This disease is caused by the expansion of a polyglutamine-encoding CAG repeat sequence exceeding 40 repeats within the first exon of the gene encoding the 350-kDa **huntingtin** protein. Creation of a transgenic mouse model of Huntington disease by expression of the CAG-expanded gene has confirmed the direct pathogenicity of this mutation. The length of the expanded sequence varies inversely with the age of onset, the average being around 40 years, and directly with disease severity. Curiously, although polyglutamine tracts are pathologically aggregated in the cerebral cortex of affected individuals, neuronal cell death occurs mainly in the corpus striatum of Huntington patients.

Normal protein degradation is needed for neuron survival

A consistent observation relating to human neurodegenerative conditions is that they often arise due to gain-of-function mutations – as opposed to large gene deletions or nonsense mutations, for example. This is illustrated by the failure of mouse models to reproduce the disease phenotype when the gene of interest is inactivated by targeting. Gain-of-function mechanisms responsible for such neurodegenerative diseases, and the putative target proteins affected thereby, include:

1. Abnormal neural proteolysis/degradation:
   • **Alzheimer disease (β-amyloid precursor protein)**.
2. Increased neural oxidative DNA damage:
   • **Familial Parkinson disease (α-synuclein**; see below).
   • **Familial amyotrophic lateral sclerosis (superoxide dismutase 1)**.
3. Neural protein misfolding:

- **Prion disorders (PrP^C).**
- **Polyglutaminopathies** (see above).

As recognized for mutant prion disorders (p. ***), protein misfolding may prove to be a common mechanism mediating this toxic gain-of-function. In Alzheimer disease, for example, the formation of β-amyloid clumps – whether due to increased β-amyloid synthesis, as in familial disease, or secondary to reduced neprilysin-dependent degradation, as may be plausible in old age – is directly implicated in the neuropathogenesis. Similarly, in the polyglutaminopathies CAG-repeat length varies directly with the severity of target protein misfolding, as demonstrated for both huntingtin and **ataxin-1** (encoded by the *SCA1* gene). Selective cleavage of the misfolded mutant huntingtin by caspase-3 might thus initiate an Alzheimer-like enzymatic cascade in which the truncated huntingtin fragments activate the caspase-8 pathway, leading to neurotoxic cell death. The analogy between prion disorders and the polyglutaminopathies may be prescient: misfolded neuronal proteins could yet prove to transmit conformational abnormalities to adjacent wild-type proteins via a seeding mechanism.

The accumulation of both the normal (overexpressed) and expanded proteins in nuclear inclusions accompanies many of these neurodegenerations. For example, wild-type huntingtin protein localizes to the cytoplasm, whereas the mutant form appears in the nucleus. This accumulation of neuronal nuclear inclusions may occur secondary to impairments of ubiqutin-dependent proteasomal degradation caused by the abnormal protein aggregates. Consistent with this, components of the ubiquitin-proteasomal (**E1-E3**) system are implicated as modifiers of disease severity within and between affected kindreds. Furthermore, the overexpression of scavenger proteins such as **Hsp40** can suppress the phenotype of these gain-of-function disorders in model systems such as the Huntington fly.

CLINICAL KEYNOTE

Mutational antecedents of Parkinson disease

Familial Parkinson disease is an uncommon entity that affects patients younger than those affected by sporadic parkinsonism. Mutations of several genes have been implicated in familial Parkinson disease:

1. **Autosomal dominant familial Parkinson disease** (rare)
   - α-**Synuclein** (on chromosome 4).
   - Onset around age 40–50; rapid progression.
   - α-Synuclein is the main component of Lewy body neuropathology in the substantia nigra (also contributes to other synucleinopathies such as **neurodegeneration with brain iron accumulation type 1**).
   - The A53T (and also A30P) *α-synuclein* mutations trigger Lewy body-like fibril formation in early-onset Parkinson disease.
   - Extensive **nitration** of α-synuclein tyrosine residues implicates oxidative/nitrative damage in the pathogenesis.
2. **Autosomal recessive juvenile Parkinson disease** (less rare)
   - **Parkin** (on chromosome 6q; affected by deletions).
   - Responsible for about 50% of early-onset Parkinson disease.
   - Onset around age 20–30; dystonia and hyperreflexia common.
   - No Lewy bodies; progression tends to be gradual.
   - Good response to L-DOPA, but high incidence of dyskinesias.

Aggression and depression are influenced by serotonin

Many psychiatric and psychosocial conditions, including **schizophrenia** and **bipolar affective illnesses**, are associated with genetic predispositions: schizophrenia has been linked to susceptibility loci on chromosome 1q21 and 13q32, for example. Like the dopamine receptor system, **serotonin receptors** are heavily implicated in the pathogenesis of such disorders. A biogenic amine structurally related to melatonin, serotonin (5-hydroxytryptamine, 5HT) modulates neuronal activity in both the central and peripheral nervous systems. There are two broad groups of serotonin receptor:

1. The $5HT_3$ receptor:
   - Is a serotonin-(ligand)-gated ion channel.
   - Causes rapid neuronal depolarization when activated.
   - Is inactivated by the marine snail venom **α-conotoxin**.
2. The $5HT_1$, $5HT_2$ and $5HT_3$ receptors
   - Are serotonin-activated G-protein-coupled receptors.
   - Modulate slow neuronal responses via second messengers.

Serotonin is implicated in the pathogenesis of various psychiatric disorders, including abnormal aggression. Indeed, $5HT_{1B}$ knockout mice are not only highly aggressive but also display a striking dietary preference for 20% ethanol over tap water. $5HT_{1A}$ knockouts, on the other hand, are prone to anxiety (who moved my cheese?), hinting that small-molecule agonists targeting this receptor subclass should make useful anxiolytic drugs. Children with **attention-deficit hyperactivity disorder** may have an abnormally low serotonin:dopamine ratio in the brain, an imbalance that may be corrected by treatment with the amphetamine **methylphenidate**.

Anxiety-related personality traits and endogenous depression have been linked to polymorphisms affecting the **serotonin transporter gene**. Control sequences upstream of this gene contain a polymorphism: the short variant leads to decreased transcription. This polymorphism accounts for 5–10% of the variance in inherited anxiety traits. Variations in the length of an intron 2 tandem repeat polymorphism in this gene have also been linked to **puerperal psychosis (post-partum depression)**. Other alleles that have been implicated in personality traits include the serotonin receptor variants $5HT2_A$ $His^{452}Tyr$, $5HT2_C$ $Ser^{23}Cys$, and the $5HT2_A$ -1438G/A polymorphism associated with **anorexia nervosa**.

Selective serotonin reuptake inhibitors (SSRIs) such as **fluoxetine** (Prozac™) are effective antidepressant drugs. Consistent with this, suicide risk in depressive patients is associated with low cerebrospinal fluid concentrations of the serotonin metabolite **5-hydroxyindoleacetic acid** (5-HIAA). Of diagnostic relevance, plasma 5-HIAA levels are elevated in patients with **carcinoid syndrome**; such patients may develop "serotoninergic" fibrotic complications such as **cardiac valvular stenosis**. It is intriguing to note that the $5HT_2$ receptor-blocking anti-migraine drug **methysergide** can also cause the fibrotic complications of **retroperitoneal fibrosis**.

Serotonin, sumatriptan, and sickness

Vascular serotonin receptors control blood vessel caliber. This pathway is strongly implicated in the pathogenesis of **migraine** headaches, which may begin with activation of the vascular serotonin receptors $5HT_{2B}$ and $5HT_7$. Different 5HT receptor subtypes populate different blood vessels: cranial arteries such as the basilar, mid-cerebral, temporal, and dural express mainly $5HT_1$ receptors (subclasses 1a–1e), whereas extracranial vessels such as the coronary, femoral and mesenteric vessels express $5HT_2$ and $5HT_3$ receptors. Drugs that selectively activate **$5HT_{1D(1B/1F)}$ receptors**, termed triptans (e.g., sumatriptan), can thus constrict $5HT_1$-receptor-expressing arteries, reversing the vasculogenic pain associated with meningeal vasodilatation in **migraine** headaches.

$5HT_3$ receptor antagonists such as ondansetron and granisetron – which selectively antagonize the direct ligand-gated ion channel activity of serotonin in the central nervous system – are potent antinausea drugs used to treat patients undergoing cancer chemotherapy. Of note, triptans also reduce emesis associated with migraine, while the prokinetic properties of $5HT_4$ agonists may be useful in nausea associated with gastroparesis of functional dyspepsia.

Ecstasy – the recreational wrecker
The illicit drug **MDMA** (methylenedioxymethamphetamine, "Ecstasy") wrecks serotoninergic neurons in the brains of users, reducing the numbers of 5HT-containing axons in the striatum, hippocampus, and cortex. Structurally similar to amphetamine and mescaline, MDMA is thus a serotonin neurotoxin (particularly in females) which acts initially by triggering brain release of monoamines (i.e., serotonin or dopamine). Tolerance develops fast: chronic MDMA users are thus at high risk for **depression** secondary to low serotoninergic drive. The causality of this relationship is controversial, however, since individuals with low premorbid serotonin levels in the brain may be predisposed to impulsivity, thrill-seeking and hence to MDMA addiction. Long-term MDMA use (read, brain serotonin deficiency) can be complicated by thermoregulatory disorders, manifesting on occasion with lethal episodes of hyperthermia, and may also cause cardiac dysfunction, memory defects, and eating disorders.

Dopamine and serotonin are degraded by monoamine oxidases

Brain monoamines include dopamine, serotonin, and norepinephrine. These are degraded by two isozymes (A and B) of **monoamine oxidase** (MAO). Unlike dopamine and serotonin, however, norepinephrine is also metabolized by the catechol-*o*-methyltransferase (COMT) enzyme pathway. Monoamine oxidase inhibitors (MAOIs) are second-line antidepressant drugs.

Smoking reduces brain MAO-B levels by about 40%. Since MAO-B metabolizes dopamine, this pleasurable molecule becomes more bioavailable in the brains of smokers. The likely importance of dopamine in cigarette addiction is illustrated by the suppressive effects of the antiepileptic drug vigabatrin on both nicotine-induced brain dopamine elevations and on cigarette craving (anhedonia).

Parkinson disease (also known as paralysis agitans, shaking palsy) arises because of the loss of cerebrostriatal dopaminergic cells, and is associated with reduced expression of dopamine transporters (Figure 20.21). Local injection of the GABA agonist muscimol into the globus pallidus appears temporarily effective. The antiparkinsonian drug selegiline (L-deprenyl) inhibits MAO-B and raises cognitive alertness, similar to cigarettes. Selegiline is not addictive, however, suggesting that addictive behavior may result from an interaction between nicotine and MAO-B suppression, leading to high brain dopamine levels. An inverse relationship between cigarette smoking and the incidence of

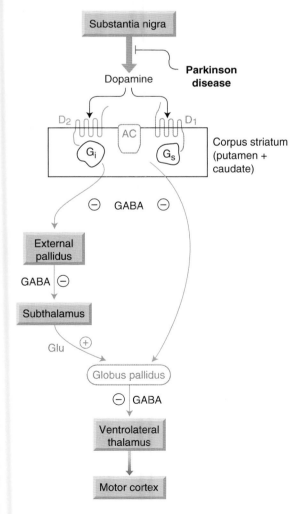

Figure 20.21 Dopamine signaling in the basal ganglia. Following release of dopamine from the substantia nigra, dopamine receptors in the corpus striatum differentially transduce signals to the external pallidus and globus pallidus. Glutamate may enhance, and GABA inhibit, certain dopamine signaling pathways.

Parkinson disease has long been suspected: chronic MAO-B suppression in the brain could be the explanation, although nicotine does not appear responsible for this. Improved cognitive functioning may occur in **Down syndrome** patients treated with nicotine patches.

Coffee drinking is also negatively associated with Parkinson disease, though whether this reflects caffeine-induced elevation of dopamine levels (or whether coffee drinkers have higher dopamine levels to begin with, explaining their "novelty-seeking" pursuit of the perfect espresso) is not clear.

PHARMACOLOGIC FOOTNOTE

MAOIs and hypertensive crises

Drug inhibitors of MAO (called **MAOIs**) are used in refractory (tricyclic- and tetra-cyclic-resistant) **depression**. Inadvertent ingestion of certain amine-containing foods during MAOI treatment may cause **fulminant hypertension**. This complication occurs with tyramine-containing foodstuffs such as red wine (e.g., Chianti), mature cheeses, soya bean, and pickled herring. Importantly, other drugs – notably **fluoxetine, pethidine**, and the cold remedy **pseudoephedrine** – can induce such crises. Treatment of MAOI-induced hypertensive crisis may involve intravenous administration of the α-adrenergic blocker **phentolamine**, which is otherwise rarely used.

Summary

Nerve impulses are propagated by membrane depolarization. Neuronal G-protein-coupled receptors gate synaptic channels. Vesicle-membrane fusion triggers neurotransmitter release. Inhibitory neurotransmitters induce neuronal hyperpolarization.

Glutamate receptors may be both ligand- and voltage-gated. Excess glutamatergic neurotransmission triggers neuronal necrosis. Nerve growth factors promote neurite sprouting.

Tactile stimuli activate mechanically gated ion channels. Hearing requires hair cell depolarization. Substance P mediates pain sensation. Opioids prevent pain by inhibiting adenyl cyclase. A smell receptor superfamily drives G_{olf}. Taste is transmitted by either ions or G-proteins. Light is sensed by 11-cis-retinal bound to opsins. Retinal pigments absorb light at different wavelengths. Rod cell cation channels are active in the dark. Neuronal biorhythms are set by oscillators.

Long-term potentiation of synapses enhances learning. Memory storage requires calcium/calmodulin-dependent kinase II. Trinucleotide inserts in neuron DNA are prone to amplification. Normal protein degradation is needed for neuron survival.

Dopamine receptors regulate reward-seeking behaviors. Aggression and depression are influenced by serotonin. Dopamine and serotonin are metabolized by monoamine oxidases.

Enrichment reading

Bedtime reading

Eckstein G. *The body has a head*. Harper & Row, London, 1970

Barondes SH. *Molecules and mental illness*. WH Freeman, New York, 1999

Cheap'n'cheerful

Levitan IB, Kaczmarek LK. *The neuron: cell and molecular biology*. Oxford University Press, Oxford, 1996

Library reference

Martin JB (ed). *Molecular neurology*. Scientific American, 1998

Shepherd GM. *Neurobiology*. Oxford University Press, Oxford, 1997

QUIZ QUESTIONS

1. Explain in molecular terms how neuronal ion channel patency may be regulated.
2. Describe the differences between the various kinds of acetylcholine receptors. What is the clinical significance of these differences?
3. Briefly state the function of the following molecules: (1) agrins; (2) synapsins; (3) syntaxins.
4. Name some excitatory and some inhibitory neurotransmitters. How does their mechanism of action vary?
5. What sorts of neuronal receptors are activated by the glutamate analog NMDA?
6. Define the term excitotoxicity.
7. What are the functions of neural growth factors?
8. Explain in molecular terms the mechanism of transmission of (1) the sense of touch, and (2) the sense of hearing.
9. How is pain caused and therapeutically relieved?
10. Describe the molecular pathway involved in olfaction.
11. Contrast the sensory events mediating sour and bitter tastes.
12. Explain how absorption of light photons leads to the sensation of sight.
13. What is meant by long-term potentiation?
14. What are some of the molecules which have been implicated as important for learning, memory and intelligence? What might they do?
15. How do the behavioral effects of dopamine receptors and serotonin receptors differ?
16. What is the clinical significance of drugs which inhibit monoamine oxidases?

V

From molecular physiology to human molecular biology

Genetic experimental systems

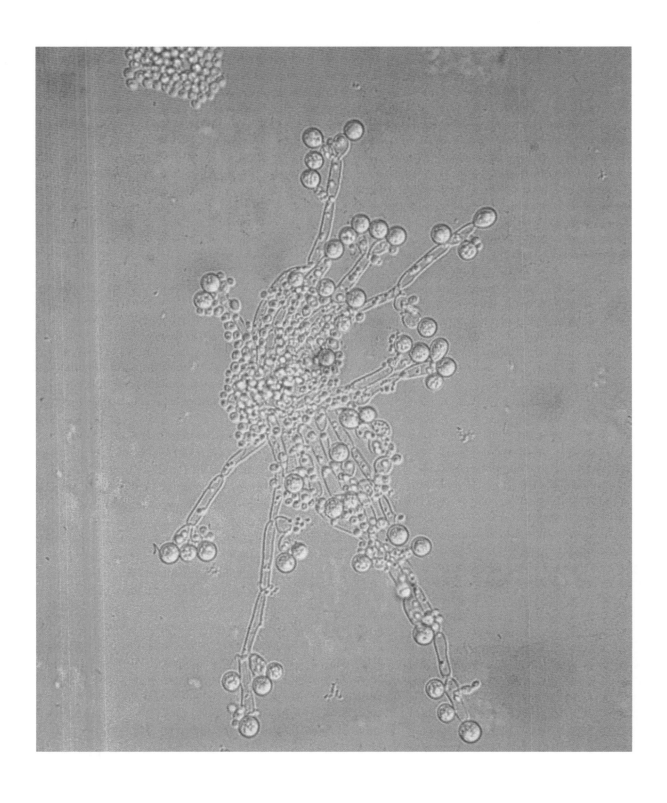

Figure 21.1 (*previous page*) Yeast – the fundamental eukaryotic organism (Wellcome Medical Photographic Library, no. 13851).

Great ideas in molecular biology are like babies – easy to conceive but hard to deliver. Biological theories require experiments to be confirmed or refuted, and experiments require techniques for generating reproducible data. Direct human experimentation is often impractical or unethical; for this reason most biomedical research is undertaken using model test systems. In this section we consider the most popular research systems for investigating problems relevant to human health and disease.

Unicellular test systems

Genetic analysis demands a variety of test systems

The complexity of higher organisms derives not from the number of genes, but from the reutilization of ancient molecular processes operative in less advanced organisms (Table 21.1). By virtue of their simplicity, these latter "lower" organisms provide attractive test systems for cell and genetic analysis. Examples of common experimental systems in biology include:

1. Viruses (e.g., phage λ, SV40) are amongst the simplest genetic models, but require independent host cells for their propagation.
2. Bacteria (e.g., *Escherichia coli*) are prokaryotic systems for genetic manipulation, analysis and protein expression.
3. Yeast (e.g., *Saccharomyces cerevisiae*, or bread mould) provide a plasmid-bearing unicellular eukaryotic system.
4. Multicellular insects such as *Drosophila melanogaster* fruit-flies are a high-turnover system for analyzing tissue patterning.
5. The roundworm *Caenorhabditis elegans* is used to investigate the development of invertebrate brain and nervous system.
6. The frog *Xenopus laevis* produces large eggs (2 mm diameter) that facilitate research into vertebrate embryonic development.
7. Both rodent (e.g., 3T3) and human (e.g., HeLa) cultured cell lines are useful for mammalian cell studies.
8. Transgenic mice are a graphic means of illustrating the functional consequences of gene overexpression, mutation, or knockout.
9. Clinical trials are used for testing or comparing therapeutic interventions in living individuals.

A key difference between these systems is the time-scale upon which biological events play out (Figure 21.2). Even relatively small differences in organism replication time, for example, can make a large exponential difference in genetic evolution over a few generations. The choice as to which system to use therefore depends on the endpoints of the experiments.

Viruses are an inevitable accompaniment of DNA-based living systems. Since isolated viruses are not strictly alive – being genomic parasites that usurp the replication machinery of cells for their propagation – they are used experimentally in conjunction with eukaryotic or bacterial cell systems. The relevance of viruses to biomedical research lies partly in their ability to act as gene delivery modules for human cells (pp. 597–8).

Phages (bacteriophages) such as lambda (λ) are viruses that infect bacteria. Phage λ has a two-phase lytic/lysogenic life cycle and is a popular cloning vector (p. 563). Its linear DNA sequence terminates in two cohesive-end sites (**cos sites**) that permit the derivation of larger **cosmid** vectors by subcloning into pBR322 plasmids. Bacteriophage C1 expressing a hydrolase termed **lysin** has been used to eradicate pathogenic group A *Streptococci* spp. in mice, perhaps presaging an approach for preventing rheumatic and/or scarlet fever.

Table 21.1. Genome sizes and gene number across species

Species	Genome size (Mb)	Putative gene number
Human	3 000	32 000
Mouse	3 000	32 000
Rice	450	48 000
Fruit-fly	150	13 600
Worm	100	18 000
Yeast	12.5	5 800
E. coli	5	4 400

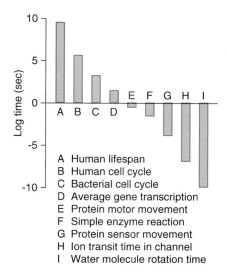

A Human lifespan
B Human cell cycle
C Bacterial cell cycle
D Average gene transcription
E Protein motor movement
F Simple enzyme reaction
G Protein sensor movement
H Ion transit time in channel
I Water molecule rotation time

Figure 21.2 The range of molecular biological time-scales.

MOLECULAR MINIREVIEW

Prokaryotic gene transfer

Unlike humans, bacteria engage in lateral gene transfer via three distinct processes:

1. **Transduction**
   - The incorporation of host bacterial DNA sequences into phage DNA.
2. **Transformation**
   - The experimental incorporation of exogenous DNA (usually plasmids) into bacteria permeabilized in vitro by rubidium chloride.
3. **Conjugation**
   - Heterosexual-like gene transfer between two bacteria, one of which contains fertility genes.

These processes require distinction from cell transfection, in which exogenous genes are expressed de novo in eukaryotic cells (see Figure 23.4).

Rapid growth and gene transfer promote bacterial selection

Bacteria are the most successful cells on Earth, having arrived here some three billion years before plants and animals. Hence, it is no coincidence that bacteria also provide the foundation for modern molecular biology. There are many advantages of using bacterial experimental systems:

1. The noncompartmentalized structure of the prokaryotic genome offers unparalleled accessibility to genetic events.
2. The absence of introns and pretranslational RNA processing enhances the ease of genetic analysis.
3. The ability to propagate plasmids bearing antibiotic-resistance genes confers the ability to select for genes co-expressed on the same plasmid.
4. Less efficient repair of the bacterial genome encourages rapid mutability of replicated DNA, facilitating mutant outgrowth.
5. Population doubling times as short as 20 minutes permit the generation of an enormous quantity (milligrams) of target DNA for analysis.

A common experimental bacterium is the Gram-negative coliform bacillus *E. coli* – approximately 10^{10} of which grow every day within the human gut. The *E. coli* genome is organized as a single chromosome which, unlike eukaryotic DNA, is located immediately subjacent to the cell exterior.

Plasmids resemble circular mini-chromosomes that contain drug-resistance genes which are readily taken up by bacteria and yeast. Host cell growth is accompanied by plasmid replication, thus expediting horizontal gene transfer. Approximately 5–20% of *E. coli* DNA consists of plasmid DNA.

Plasmids may also contain **jumping genes** which facilitate the transfer of genetic material to host cell chromosomes. Certain bacteria such as *Borrelia burgdorferi* and *Mycoplasma genitalium* contain hundreds of extrachromosomal genes within conserved plasmids; for example, there are 17 linear and circular plasmids in *Borrelia*, in addition to its 1-megabase linear chromosome. This suggests that such microorganisms have substituted plasmid genes for chromosomal genes as a mechanism for promoting antigenic variation and thus evading immune surveillance.

Bacterial research dominates many areas of biology: transcriptional regulation and DNA repair are two examples. Human cells are biochemically distinct from bacteria, however, being richer in protein and lipid and correspondingly less concentrated in terms of DNA and RNA. Such differences prevent bacte-

A.

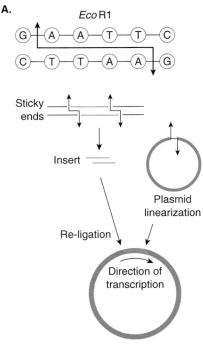

B.

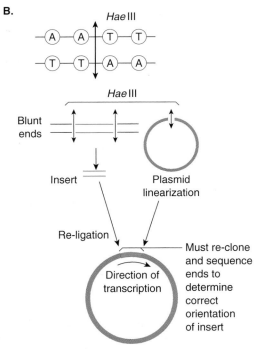

Figure 21.3 Restriction enzyme function. *A*, Action of a sticky end-cutter, *Eco*R1. *B*, Action of a blunt-end cutter, *Hae*III. Because the orientation of the reintegrated insert cannot be assumed correct, it must be re-sequenced within the plasmid minipreps.

ria from being a perfect model system for human biology, and mandate the use of other experimental systems.

MOLECULAR MINIREVIEW

Restriction endonucleases

The synthesis of DNA-sequence-specific enzymes by bacteria evolved as a defense against phages. Historically, phage co-incubated with one strain of bacterium were noted to thrive, whereas identical phage incubated with another strain were **restricted** in their growth. This phenomenon was traced to the expression of **bacterial endonucleases** which nicked the viral DNA, thereby preventing its replication (bacteria protect their own genomes from autodigestion via **DNA methylation**). **Restriction endonucleases** are thus bacterial enzymes that cut specific DNA sequences, enabling the selective cutting-and-pasting of genes in the laboratory. A subtype of restriction endonucleases known as **type II enzymes** – the sort used for everyday molecular cloning – recognize and cleave palindromic 4- to 6-bp motifs in duplex DNA (in contrast, type I enzymes cleave DNA nonspecifically at sites 1–5 kb away from the recognition sequence, and hence are not useful for genetic manipulation). These palindromes are only truly reversible when read across duplex DNA, i.e., they are defined by an axis of **rotational symmetry**: the sequence AGATCT, for example, provides such an axis since the complementary strand reads the same backwards as does the sense strand forwards (Figure 21.3). A **six-cutter** enzyme will on average cut duplex DNA once every 4^6 bp – i.e., once every 4096 nucleotides. The repetitive DNA sequences known as Alus are so-called because they are cut by *AluI*, whereas LINEs (sometimes called Kpn sequences) are cut by *KpnI*. Other popular restriction enzymes include:

1. *Eco*RI
   - From RI plasmid of *E. coli*; cuts at G-AATTC.
2. *Hin*dIII
   - From dIII serotype of *Hemophilus influenzae*; cuts at A-AGCTT.
3. *Bam*HI
   - From *Bacillus amyloliquefaciens* H; cuts at G-GATCC.

Cutting double-stranded DNA with such enzymes may leave either **sticky ends** (e.g., a 4-bp 5′ overhang; Figure 21.3*A*) or **blunt** (even) **ends** which in turn require ligation (by the action of **DNA ligase** on a similar DNA end). Alternatively, the sticky end stagger of 3′ cutters such as *Pst*I can be filled in by enzymes with nonspecific 5′→3′ DNA polymerase activity such as **T4 polymerase** (from T4 phage) or the **Klenow fragment** of *E. coli* DNA polymerase I. Each restriction enzyme requires a specific pH (buffer) to maximize its activity. DNA fragments that are subcloned into blunt-ended regions require sequencing across the join to confirm the orientation of the insert (Figure 21.3*B*).

Established gene sequences are characterized by a **restriction map** that identifies DNA fragments of known size following endonuclease digestion. Abnormalities of such restriction analysis may reflect either deleterious gene mutations or harmless **restriction fragment length polymorphisms** (RFLPs; pronounced "rifflips").

A.

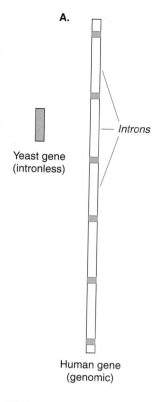

Yeast gene
(intronless)

— Introns

Human gene
(genomic)

B.

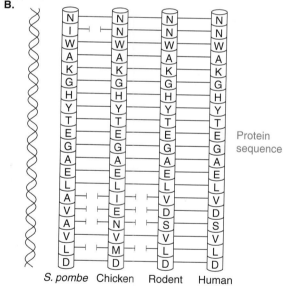

S. pombe   Chicken   Rodent   Human

Protein
sequence

Figure 21.4 Sequence homology between yeast and mammalian cells. *A*, Genomic DNA comparison of a hypothetical human gene and its yeast homolog. *B*, DNA sequence comparison of a yeast gene with its mammalian homologs.

CLINICAL KEYNOTE

Bacterial genomics in medicine

The availability of complete genome sequences for many bacterial species – *H. influenzae, B. burdorferi, Helicobacter pylori, M. pneumoniae, E. coli* O157, *Chlamydia trachomatis, Ureaplasma urealyticum*, for example – has huge implications for medicine and biology. Genomic analysis of the bacterium *Pseudomonas aeruginosa* reveals a large ($6.3 \cdot 10^6$ bp) genome incorporating numerous genes involved in chemotaxis, metabolic regulation and molecular efflux, consistent with the opportunistic behavior of this notoriously drug-resistant pathogen. Similarly, the 4-megabase *Vibrio cholerae* genome provides insights into the evolution of this organism: it consists of two circular chromosomes (the smaller of which resembles a plasmid in its ability to capture genes from host cells) and contains many virulence factors and toxins. The notorious clinical problem of methicillin-resistant *Staphylococcus aureus* (MRSA) can likewise be better understood by genomic analysis: the MRSA genome has acquired up to 70 virulence factors by lateral gene transfer, contains pathogenicity islands comprising exotoxin, enterotoxin, and toxic shock syndrome (TSS) toxin gene clusters, and exhibits superantigen gene reduplication.

"Chip-based" diagnostic capabilities, enhanced characterization of pathogenicity and virulence, gene-based prediction of antibiotic sensitivity and resistance, availability of cross-genomic comparisons, rational opportunities for vaccine development – these are some of the opportunities for exploiting microbial genomic data. In the case of *H. pylori*, for example, strain-specific variations in outer membrane protein (e.g., porin) genes appear to be fewer than expected, enhancing the prospect of using such targets for vaccine development. Conversely, the notorious O157:H7 *E. coli* strain responsible for hemorrhagic colitis has been found to possess 1387 genes: compare this with non-enteropathogenic *E. coli*, which expresses only 528 genes.

Yeast cells mimic the genetic machinery of higher eukaryotes

The yeast *Saccharomyces cerevisiae* – best known for its role in the genesis of bread and beer – is a single-cell eukaryote that exhibits remarkable genetic homology with mammalian cells (Figure 21.4). *S. pombe* is an unrelated strain with larger chromosomes. The *S. cerevisiae* genome is highly compacted with few introns, and its 16 chromosomes contain only one-tenth the DNA of a single human chromosome. Although yeast reproduction is largely asexual, chromosomal exchanges between yeast can be detected under some circumstances, suggesting an origin for sexuality.

Unlike bacteria, many of the processes by which yeast express genes and replicate chromosomes mimic those found in human cells. An exception relates to yeast mating, which is strongly regulated by pheromones. Adjacent yeast colonies can signal to each other via ammonia release, on the other hand, leading to growth inhibition.

Many human genes remain functional when expressed in yeast – an example is the human *Ubiquitin* gene, which encodes a protein 96% homologous to the yeast form. Hence, yeast generally provide a more interpretable model system for human genes than do bacteria. Although yeast grow more slowly than bacteria, they adapt to environmental changes with comparable speed. Since *S. cerevisiae* grow at about half the rate of *E. coli* despite having fivefold higher DNA content, these organisms are ideal for selective studies, whether in vitro or in vivo (Table 21.2). Human gene systems that have been elucidated in yeast include those relating to:

Table 21.2. In vitro and in vivo. There are two main ways to analyze human molecular biology: either in an artificial test system (in vitro – literally, in glass) or in living organisms (in vivo). Such terms may take on different meanings depending upon whether molecules, drugs or cells are being analyzed.

Analysis of:	in vitro	in vivo
Prebiotic molecules	Cell-free system	Cells (including bacteria, yeast)
Proteins	Cell culture	Multicellular test systems, e.g., fruit-flies, animals
Genes	Cell transfectants	Transgenic systems
Toxic chemicals	Cell culture	Laboratory animals
Proprietary drug therapies	Cell culture	Animals Clinical trials

1. Cytoskeletal proteins
   - Especially actin (89% identical) and tubulin (75% identical).
2. GTP-binding proteins
   - e.g., Ras (60% identical).
3. Cell-cycle control genes
   - e.g., Cdk1 (homologous to yeast p34^{cdc2}).

In multicellular organisms such as mice and humans, germline mutations affecting important genes tend to be embryonic-lethal and hence difficult to characterize in functional terms. In contrast, even the most critical yeast genes may be phenotypically defined with relative ease. Abnormal yeast phenotypes can be characterized by complementation studies in which a normal gene (or genes) reverts the phenotype when reinserted; for example, human *Ras* genes complement yeast *Ras* mutants. Variant phenotypes can thus be categorized into genetic **complementation groups**.

Identification of the specific gene underlying a mutant phenotype can be achieved by experimental strategies involving gene cloning (Chapter 23). Conversely, the function of the cloned gene may be clarified using recombination of a defective gene copy to create a null mutant – an approach termed gene targeting or knockout (Chapter 24).

Multicellular test systems

Worms provide a defined multicellular analytic system

Complex biological processes may defy investigation in single-cell systems such as bacteria or yeast. Such processes include:

1. Embryonic development of normal tissues.
2. Multicellular functioning of organs such as the eye.
3. Higher neurologic processes such as memory and learning.

The nematode *Caenorhabditis elegans* measures less than half a millimeter in length, yet provides a superb experimental system for characterizing nervous system development at single-cell resolution. As with yeast, the phylogenetic distance between invertebrates and *Homo sapiens* does not preclude using this model to clarify broad principles of human molecular development. The attraction of *C. elegans* lies in its combination of functional complexity and structural simplicity: with only six chromosomes,

10 000 genes, a 10^8-bp DNA genome, a nervous system comprising 302 neurons (compared to 100 billion in humans), a complete adult organism of 959 cells, and a life-cycle of three days, the self-fertilizing metazoan's compaction of function is attractive when compared with the huge redundancy of human physiology. Given that it boasts a complete physical gene map, a library of ordered cosmid clones, a comprehensive embryogenetic fate map, and a full neuronal wiring diagram, *C. elegans* can be justifiably described as a defined biological system.

C. elegans research has also contributed to the molecular understanding of apoptosis. About a quarter of embryonic *C. elegans* neurons undergo apoptosis induced by **Ced** (cell death) genes, suggesting a model for human neurodegenerative conditions such as Alzheimer and Parkinson diseases. The effector gene products are calcium-activated **deathases**, which are potential drug targets. A distinct area of worm investigation has been that of genital development, which has been shown to depend upon epidermal growth factor receptor-dependent activation of the Ras signaling system.

In contrast to the elegance of *C. elegans*, the foot-long human parasitic roundworm *Ascaris lumbricoides* does not lend itself to embryogenetic studies. It does, however, provide a useful in vitro model for analyzing RNA processing and translation – as do RNA-editing protozoans such as *Trypanosoma* and *Leishmania* spp.

MOLECULAR MINIREVIEW

Vertebrate embryogenesis in frogs

Human oocytes measure approximately 0.1 µm in diameter – an order of magnitude smaller, that is, than most other human cells – whereas amphibious oocytes from the frog *Xenopus laevis* may be as large as 2 mm across. This 2000-fold size difference underlies the popularity of the *Xenopus* oocyte system for developmental studies (albeit not without competition from, say, zebrafish). Extensive use of this system has been directed to the following objectives:

1. Localization of cytoplasmic information within the oocyte.
2. Elucidation of growth factors (e.g., activins, fibroblast growth factors) responsible for embryonic induction.
3. Application of oocyte microinjection technology.

Information from *Xenopus* studies has helped clarify how vertebrate embryos establish polarity and induce embryonic tissue differentiation. Oocyte microinjection studies mimic an in vivo test-tube, which is useful for analysis of mRNA translation since *Xenopus* chromosomes (like those of *Drosophila*) permit unusually detailed ultrastructural investigation. These **lampbrush chromosomes** grow during oocyte meiosis – which may last months – and contain about 10 000 highly extended chromatin loops, each of which corresponds to an invariant DNA sequence. Chromatin assembly in *Xenopus* may also be studied using cell-free (actually broken-cell) systems.

Mutational phenotypes are readily characterized in fruit-flies

Genetic analysis of *Drosophila melanogaster* fruit-flies has been in progress for a century. Although the 165-million bp *Drosophila* genome contains only 5% of the DNA content of a human genome, the rapid reproductive rate of these insects makes them genetically informative. Sick flies do not see the doctor, but efficient screening for mutant phenotypes can nonetheless permit the analysis of complex processes.

Insects containing recessive mutations are easily maintained, making it easy to produce lethal or infertile homozygotes for study. These mutant phenotypes – which fruit-fly investigators have accorded names such as *spotted dick* (in which condensed brain cell chromosomes resemble the British fruit pudding), *stuck* (in which male flies experience difficulty withdrawing their sex organs), *engrailed, hunchback, knirps* and *sevenless, notch, disheveled* – include aberrant sex determination, reduced sensory perception, and abnormal circadian rhythms. Elucidation of complex embryogenetic signaling networks relevant to human health and disease – such as the *Wnt-armadillo* and *smoothened/hedgehog-patched* cell fate pathways – has been crucially expedited by fruit-fly research.

Over 3000 gene mutations have so far been characterized in *Drosophila*. Many wild-type genes have human homologs, including:

1. Transcription factors
   - e.g., *Hox* gene products, zinc finger proteins.
2. Neuronal proteins
   - e.g., Acetylcholine receptors, sodium channels.
3. Cell adhesion molecules
   - e.g., Laminin.
4. Proto-oncogene products
   - e.g., Src, Abl, Myb; Wnt-1 (*wingless*), Rel (*dorsal*).
5. Polypeptide growth factors and receptors
   - e.g., Transforming growth factor β, epidermal growth factor receptor.

The salivary glands of *Drosophila* larvae contain gigantic polytene chromosomes, reflecting the occurrence in these cells of up to a dozen DNA-synthetic cycles without cell division (polyploidy). The haploid chromosome number is four, and the largest of these is equivalent in size to the smallest human chromosome. Transcriptional activation of genes within these cells (e.g., by the insect steroid hormone ecdysone) induces the formation of chromosome puffs, reflecting band decondensation due to the accumulation of RNA and protein. Chromosomal bands visible by light microscopy may contain as little as 10 kb DNA, making the resolution of cytogenetic analysis orders of magnitude greater than that obtainable using mammalian nuclei.

Gene identification in *Drosophila* may be carried out using either traditional cloning approaches, or else by an approach termed **transposon tagging**, in which a transposable **P element** mutagenizes a target gene which is then identifiable by the insertion. There are more than 50 different mobile (transposable) elements in the *Drosophila* genome, but no *Alu*-like small interspersed nuclear elements as in humans.

CLINICAL KEYNOTE

Fly diseases

Like worms, fruit-flies are useful for elucidating complex human genetic traits and diseases in vivo. This approach has yielded particular benefits in the understanding of neurodegenerative disease. Transgenic expression of mutant genes encoding defective **α-synuclein** (Ala30Pro or Ala53Thr; p. 523), for example, has permitted the development of **Parkinson disease** models in the fruit-fly. Similar models have been created for the polyglutaminopathies **Huntington disease** (128-glutamine insert – 128Q – versus 16Q wild-type) and **spinocerebellar ataxia type 1**.

In the latter example, creation of a fly with an 82Q expansion of the *ataxin-1* gene causes progressive neuronal degeneration, as does high-level overexpression of the wild-type (30Q) gene product; whereas knockout of the *SCA1* gene has no such effect. Remarkably, these latter inset models also illustrate the defects of locomotion and coordination that characterize the respective human diseases.

Single-gene defects may be modeled in animals

If it does not worry you to know that we humans are all genetically 99.9% identical, the knowledge that you are also sharing 99.3% of your DNA sequences with chimpanzees perhaps should. Moreover, of the 30 000-plus homologous genes common to you and the chimp, fewer than 200 are expressed at levels differing by more than two-fold. Reassuringly, much of the latter difference is found in the brain (where more than 1% of genes are discordantly expressed) rather than in, say, the liver or blood (where fewer than 0.5% of genes differ in expression). Yet despite this genetic similarity, many common human diseases rarely affect other primates; these include asthma, rheumatoid arthritis, Alzheimer disease, epithelial carcinomas (unlike leukemias, which affect humans and apes with comparable frequency), and malaria.

The term animal model usually refers to a mammalian species, most commonly a mouse. Although at first glance humans may not resemble mice, the molecular similarities between the two species are more striking than the differences. An advantage of using animals such as mice for research purposes is that their gestation and generation times are short, enabling far more rapid phenotypic analysis of genetic traits than is feasible in humans.

When both the phenotype and genotype of an animal disease are homologous to that of a human disease, an animal model is said to exist; such models are useful for studies of pathophysiology and treatment (see also p. ***). Naturally occurring (spontaneous) animal models of human single-gene defects include:

1. Gunn rat
   - **UDP-glucuronyl transferase** mutation.
   - Simulates **Crigler–Najjar syndrome**.
2. Watanabe heritable hyperlipidemic (WHHL) rabbit
   - Low-density lipoprotein (**LDL**) **receptor** mutation,
   - Simulates **familial hypercholesterolemia.**
3. *Mdx* mouse
   - **Dystrophin** mutation, but few symptoms (cf. golden retrievers).
   - Muscle samples have characteristics of **Duchenne muscular dystrophy.**
4. Irish setter
   - **Factor VIII** mutation (**hemophilia A**),
5. Beagle
   - **Factor IX** mutation (**hemophilia B**).
6. Cone-head mouse
   - **β-glucuronidase** mutation.
   - Simulates **Sly syndrome** (lysosomal storage syndrome).
7. Sparse-fur mouse
   - **Ornithine transcarbamylase** mutation.
   - Causes urea-cycle dysfunction.

Human diseases are often caused by dysfunction of more than one cell lineage. In diseases of uncertain etiology – rheumatoid arthritis and non-insulin-dependent diabetes are examples – the nature of the primary abnormality may be unclear. Certain murine polygenic disorders have been proposed as models for human disease. These include NOD mice (**diabetes mellitus**), NZB/NZW mice (**systemic lupus erythematosus**), SJL mice (**Hodgkin disease**) and MRL/Mp mice (**rheumatoid arthritis**). Mice may develop a syndrome termed experimental autoimmune encephalomyelitis (EAE) – a condition that mimics **multiple sclerosis** – following autoinoculation with **myelin basic protein** (MBP). In contrast, homozygous deletion of the MBP locus is associated with the demyelinative *shiverer* phenotype, which is characterized by **epilepsy**. Another popular animal model is the **SCID-hu** immunodeficiency mouse, which is used in viral (including HIV) studies. Additional models of **AIDS** include the monkey infected with simian immunodeficiency virus (SIV).

CLINICAL KEYNOTE

Problems with animal models

The limitations of animal models are numerous. The mouse heart weighs 100 mg and discharges its tiny stroke volume (10 μl) 600 times per minute, for example, whereas the 300-g human heart beats tenfold less often.

The **cystic fibrosis** (CF) mouse develops a different pattern of disease compared to the human CF patient; for example, meconium ileus in the mouse affects the small (rather than large) intestine, whereas lung disease in CF mice mainly affects the lower airways and causes minimal secretion with rare infections.

Similarly, the Apc^{Min} mouse model of **familial polyposis** develops mainly small intestinal polyps, and the number of polyps varies with the strain of the mouse (C57BL, B6, etc.) used.

Human genomes can be analyzed by computational biology

The sequencing of the human genome is one of the outstanding achievements of human history – comparable in scale and significance to the circumnavigation of the oceans and the exploration of interplanetary space. What has been the rationale of this massive international initiative? No prospective hypothesis has required testing. Rather, the long-term fruits of the Human Genome Project will be reaped from retrospective data mining and computer-generated associations.

Similar seismic shifts in the culture of human biological research are taking place. High-throughput techniques permitting the simultaneous analysis of thousands of molecules have begun to erode the dominance of traditional low-yield benchtop approaches. Powerful resources such as molecular databases are now posted on public websites, allowing immediate access to the accumulated knowledge base. In short, computerized information management has become a prerequisite for biological research.

The base sequence of the human genome has now been mapped out. A number of surprises have been forthcoming – not least the anticlimactic finding that the total gene number is not much larger than 32 000. Since even the 900-cell flatworm *C. elegans* requires 18 000 genes for its daily functions, the finding that *H. sapiens* requires only a few thousand more genes has been a jolt to the self-esteem of many who had hitherto prided themselves on their biological complexity. Solace has been provided by the proposal that the average human gene might encode three or four distinct protein isoforms;

though whether this can atone for the political damage of a low gene number remains to be seen.

Fortunately, genome analysis has also revealed that the architecture of human proteins is more complex than that of their homologs in lower organisms. Although only a minority (<10%) of all known protein domains are vertebrate-specific, humans and their closer relatives cobble together more domains per protein – usually by tacking them on to the amino- or carboxy-terminal – than do flies or worms. The human homolog of the fly *Trithorax* protein contains an additional four domains, for example; a similar comparison can be made between the worm *lin-49* and human **peregrin** gene products. Domain accretion of this kind facilitates protein multitasking within human cells, thus enhancing regulatory flexibility and evolutionary adaptation. The functional dynamism of human life thus appears to result not from gene number per se, but from additional layers of structural complexity.

Many further discoveries are promised from comparison of the human genome sequence with those of other species. This growing field of interspecies genetic analysis, termed **comparative genomics**, is based on the phylogenetic footprinting of similar genes (orthologs) and similar chromosomal regions (synteny; p. 579). This approach can help to identify cryptic regulatory sites outside the open reading frame. Remarkably, at least two hundred human genes appear to have originated by direct horizontal transfer from bacteria, i.e., without any homologs detectable in yeast, flies or worms. Such genes (many of which now contain introns) include those encoding **metal-binding proteins**, **monoamine oxidase**, **epoxide hydrolase**, and the **glucose-6-phosphate transporter**.

Since countless revelations are in store regarding the rich circuitry of switches underlying genome function, it is premature to label the twenty-first century as the postgenomic (or even postsequencing) era. Genomic analysis remains in its infancy, and the large-scale sequencing of nonhuman genomes will provide unique insights into the dynamic nature of genetic networks. The "race to the starting line" has now begun.

MOLECULAR MINIREVIEW

Secrets of the human genome

Analysis of the genome sequence has generated many new insights into human evolution. Unexpectedly, the chromosomal terrain is highly uneven: some areas are gene-rich, while others are remarkably gene-poor. Chromosome 19 (and 17) is the veritable USA (and Europe) of the genome, being packed with genes; whereas chromosome 21 (and 18 and 13) more closely resembles Siberia (or Greenland or Australia). Indeed, the relative barrenness (low gene density) of these latter chromosomes may well account for the selective viability of their trisomies, reflecting as it does the least potent gene-dosage effects.

Another revelation concerns gender-dependent mutation rates. Based on studies of Y chromosomal *Alu* evolution – and perhaps reflecting the requirement of many more cell divisions for spermatogenesis than for oogenesis – it now appears that male DNA sustains approximately double the mutation rate of female DNA. This means that males are likely to have contributed two-thirds of all disease mutations. On a more positive note, this pro-mutagenic propensity means that males can also claim genetic credit for two-thirds of evolutionary progress.

But perhaps the greatest revelation of the Human Genome Project has been that humans are genetically pretty much equal (there goes that old pipedream of cloning a supertribe of like-minded nonconformists) and that beauty really is only skin deep. Still, that itty-bitty 0.1% of interindividual genomic variation leaves 3 million base pairs of divergent sequence which could yet give rise to a surprising number of polymorphic variants and point mutations . . .

PHARMACOLOGIC FOOTNOTE

Clinical trials

Advantages of using research systems in preference to human experimentation include greater accessibility, flexibility, reproducibility, quantitation, and economy – not to mention significantly fewer (though far from insignificant) ethical and legal concerns. Some of the areas in which basic research leads may culminate in medical progress include disease locus mapping and/or cloning, prenatal disease screening, presymptomatic disease prevention, and disease treatment. Disease screening and prevention require the development of predictive and/or diagnostic assays: this applies to conditions such as **chronic granulomatous disease**, **phenylketonuria** and **hemochromatosis**, for example, in which specific biochemical assays have revolutionized disease detection and monitoring. The contribution of basic research to medical progress in this setting can be rapid and dramatic.

However, the biggest gap between basic and clinical research is in the area of treatment. Irrespective of how much preparative work is conducted beforehand – whether it be molecular analysis, cell culture studies, or studies in animal models – the final arbiter of therapeutic efficacy remains the controlled clinical trial. Early phase clinical trials – **phase** I and **II** – assess the toxicity (dosing) and efficacy (appropriate disease spectrum) of a new treatment, respectively, whereas **phase III** trials compare the efficacy of a new treatment with that of the standard therapy for that condition. All such studies require careful design, ethical appraisal, informed consent, monitoring of treatment-related side-effects, and interim analyses of measurable endpoints. The main target of such empirical studies are the common (usually polygenic) diseases such as **atherosclerosis** and **cancer**, for which incremental advances are keenly sought.

The above summarizes the basics of some commonly used biological systems in research practice. In the next section, we consider the laboratory techniques needed for analyzing these experimental systems.

Enrichment reading

Bedtime reading

Bernard C. *An introduction to the study of experimental medicine.* MacMillan, London, 1927

Library reference

Harper DR. *Molecular virology.* Springer-Verlag, Berlin, 1998

Summary

Genetic analysis demands a variety of test systems. Rapid growth and lateral gene transfer promote bacterial selection. Yeast cells mimic the genetic machinery of higher eukaryotes.

Worms provide a defined multicellular analytic system. Mutational phenotypes are readily characterized in fruit-flies. Single-gene defects may be modeled in animals. Human genomes can be analyzed by computational biology.

QUIZ QUESTIONS

1. What is a phage? How can they be experimentally useful?
2. How much larger, approximately, is a human genome than an *E. coli* genome: 100, 1000, 10000, 100000 or a million-fold?
3. Explain why bacteria may be more useful than human cells in performing some kinds of genetic analysis.
4. Describe what a restriction endonuclease does (a) in vivo, and (b) in vitro.
5. What is the meaning of the term complementation group when used in the context of yeast studies?
6. Explain what it is about the nematode *C. elegans* system that makes this an attractive experimental model for analyzing cell function.
7. What is the difference between lampbrush and polytene chromosomes, and for which kinds of experimental analysis are they respectively useful?
8. Give some examples of animal models of human diseases. How can these be useful?
9. What kinds of questions can be asked using clinical trials?
10. Propose examples of ethical issues that might preclude a clinical trial from being performed.

Gene and protein analysis

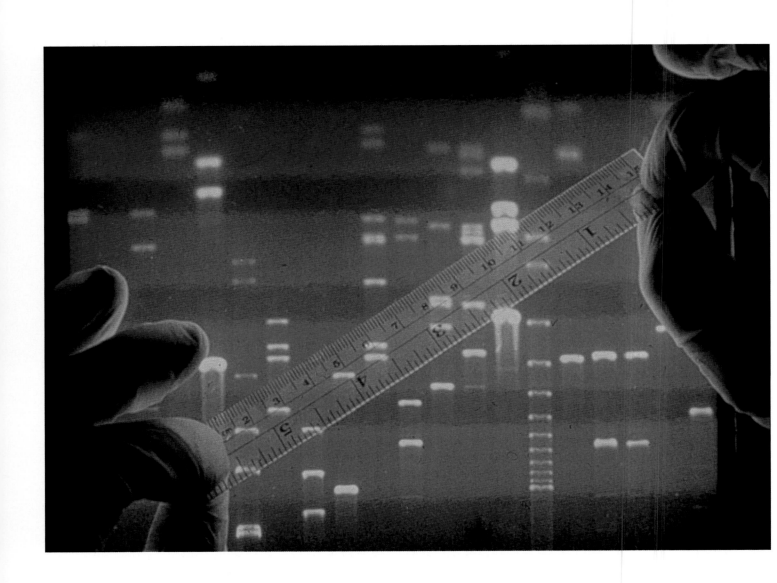

It can be difficult to appraise the significance of research findings without some familiarity of the procedures used. Such knowledge enables the validity of the data to be assessed. In this section we discuss some basic principles underlying laboratory analysis of protein and DNA.

Gels and membranes

Proteins and nucleic acids can be separated within gels

Experimental biology depends on two principles of molecular recognition that underlie the specificity of assay detection:

1. Linear nucleic acids are identified by **sequence-specific hybridization** with synthetic complementary DNA sequences (oligonucleotide probes).
2. Three-dimensional or denatured protein structures are identified by **epitope-specific antibody binding**.

Most assays detecting these phenomena involve the electrophoretic separation of molecules using porous jelly-like slabs termed **gels**. Indeed, for the last two decades, many scientific manuscripts have contained few data other than those involving visualization of molecules within gels. There are many different gel compositions, with the most common being **agarose gels** (used for separating nucleic acids) and **polyacrylamide gels** (used for separating proteins).

Gels are modified for specific purposes; for example, formaldehyde is often added to urea-containing agarose gels when RNA is being electrophoresed. Nucleic acids can be visualized on agarose gels by adding the intercalating agent **ethidium bromide**, which fluoresces on absorbing ultraviolet light. Similarly, the detergent **sodium dodecyl sulfate (SDS)** is added to protein gels when polypeptide denaturation is desired – denaturation destroys the noncovalent secondary structure of proteins, permitting linearization and hence more accurate electrophoretic measurement of molecular weight. Specialized applications of gel electrophoresis include capillary electrophoresis and pulsed-field gel electrophoresis.

Figure 22.2 Protein gel electrophoresis. Prestained molecular weight markers, consisting of proteins such as albumin or transferrin, are shown in the left lane. Addition of a protein denaturant such as the detergent sodium dodecyl sulfate (SDS) will destroy any secondary structure in loaded proteins, thus retarding the rate of gel migration to a maximal extent. Similarly, the addition of reductants such as dithiothreitol (DTT) or β-mercaptoethanol will eliminate cystine bonds in folded proteins, again tending to retard electrophoretic speed.

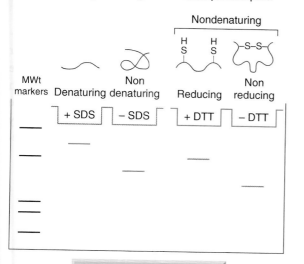

MOLECULAR MINIREVIEW

Electrophoresis

Following cell lysis, covalent cysteine–cysteine intermolecular links (i.e., cystines) within proteins can be destroyed by reduction of disulfide (S–S) bonds to free cysteines (−SH, −SH) using reducing agents such as **dithiothreitol** or **β-mercaptoethanol**. Apparent differences in molecular weight between reduced and nonreduced protein samples indicate the effect of cystine bonds on higher-order protein structure (Figure 22.2). Similarly, the contribution of *N*-glycosylation to a protein's size can be determined by treating cells with the galactosyltransferase inhibitor tunicamycin. The speed at which a given molecule electrophoreses (its electrophoretic mobility) therefore depends on a number of factors:

1. Molecular weight
   - Large molecules migrate slowly, small molecules quickly.
2. Conformation
   - Supercoiled (circular) DNA migrates quickly.
   - Relaxed (nicked circles, or linearized) DNA migrates slowly.
   - Denatured, reduced or glycosylated proteins migrate more slowly.
3. Gel concentration

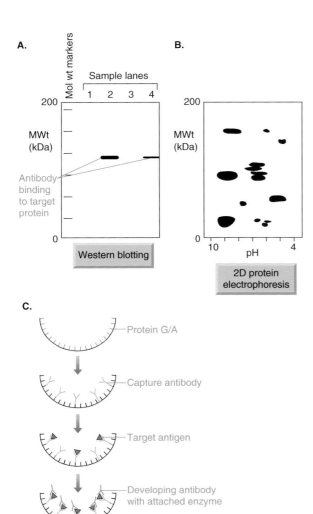

Figure 22.5 Protein detection assays. *A*, Western blotting (immunoblotting). Proteins are gel-electrophoresed, separated by molecular weight, transferred to a membrane, then identified by antibody binding. *B*, 2D protein electrophoresis. Proteins are first separated on the basis of charge then, in the second dimension, on the basis of molecular weight. *C*, ELISA. Microwells are first coated with protein A or protein G beads which bind polyclonal or monoclonal (capture) antibodies respectively. Following the adsorption of target proteins to these antibodies, the well is washed, and a second (developing) antibody conjugated to an indicator molecule (e.g., enzyme or fluorochrome) is added prior to development.

3. **Pulsed-field gel electrophoresis**
   - Used for analysis of large DNA regions during gene mapping,
   - Detects deletions such as those that follow chromosome breakage.

DNA sequences are further analyzed by computer programs that identify reading frames, restriction sites, and sequence homologies with known genes. The reading frame determines which trinucleotide groups form the codon sequence (cf. a frameshift mutation which disrupts the reading frame, thus terminating transcription) and where the codon sequence begins and ends. Bioinformatic analysis of this kind can also predict whether a given sequence encodes functional motifs such as a transmembrane region, nuclear localization sequence, glycosylation site, leader sequence, and so on. The choice of DNA sequencing modality depends in turn on the endpoint (Table 22.1).

Polymerase chain reactions amplify primed DNA sequences

A central problem in gene diagnostics is the difficulty of obtaining suitable quantities of target DNA – or mRNAs converted to cDNAs – for analysis. Cloning technology (see below) permits the production of large DNA quantities in proliferating cells such as bacteria or yeast, but such cloning is labor-intensive and slow. The **polymerase chain reaction** (PCR) is an in vitro process that enables cell-free production of abundant DNA (microgram quantities) for sequencing and other studies. This ingenious technology has made it possible to amplify any known nucleic acid sequence (between 100 bp and 2 kb in size) up to a million-fold within hours. In this way it is possible to harvest analyzable quantities of a single-copy target DNA sequence from a single cell.

The perpetual-motion-machine characteristics of PCR relate to the use of cyclic DNA denaturation and renaturation in the presence of an enzyme called *Taq*I **DNA polymerase**. This enzyme is produced by the thermophilic bacterium *Thermus aquaticus* which normally lives in hot springs. A unique property of *Taq*I polymerase is its heat-stability, which allows it to function through multiple (as many as 60) rounds of heat-induced DNA denaturation. Unlike, say, *E. coli* polymerase, *Taq*I tolerates temperatures above 90°C and functions best at 70–75°C. PCR is a cyclical two-temperature process: initially, the duplex DNA sequence of interest is rapidly denatured at around 97.5°C for 15 seconds. Following cooling to 75°C, the chain reaction begins: synthetic oligonucleotides termed **nested primers**, complementary to sequences flanking the duplex target, anneal to the now-denatured DNA. *Taq*I polymerase then bidirectionally extends the target DNA in opposite directions, with each duplex replication product undergoing sequential rounds of heat-induced denaturation (Figure 22.7). In this manner the products act as templates for sequential rounds of replication initiated by the other primer, culminating in the exponential production of 2^n sequence copies (where n = the number of cycles). In theory, 20 cycles of PCR should cause a million-fold sequence amplification, whereas 40 cycles should cause 10^{12}-fold amplification. PCR is used for:

1. Prenatal diagnosis of gene mutations
   - e.g., **Sickle-cell anemia, phenylketonuria, hemophilia, cystic fibrosis**.
2. Diagnostic detection of target DNA sequences
   - e.g., **HIV, HTLV1, tuberculosis**, *Legionella*, **Whipple disease**.
   - Also as a marker of residual disease in (say) **leukemias**.
3. Genome scanning for mutations, repetitive DNA sequences, etc.

A.

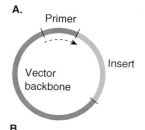

B.

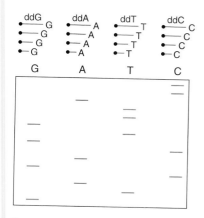

Figure 22.6 Dideoxy DNA sequencing. *A*, Vector into which primers are inserted. *B*, The DNA to be sequenced is used as the template for a series of in vitro polymerase reactions in which chain-terminating nucleotides are used to randomly terminate DNA synthesis; these dideoxynucleotides (e.g., ddG) lack the 3′-hydroxyl group of normal deoxynucleotides (e.g., dG). A DNA primer corresponding to the beginning of the desired sequence is first incorporated into the plasmid. The randomly synthesized fragments accruing from each dideoxy incorporation reaction are then electrophoresed, revealing a ladder of fragments separated by single-nucleotide lengths. Hence, the sequence shown would read, from above, as CCATTGTGC, etc.

Table 22.1. Gene and DNA characterization techniques

1. Determination of the linear base sequence of a DNA fragment
   – **DNA sequencing** (usually dideoxy)
2. Localization of a sequence within a much larger DNA fragment
   – **PCR** (see below), **Southern blotting** or **restriction analysis** (Figure 22.4)
3. Chromosomal localization of a known DNA sequence
   – **In situ hybridization**
4. Expression of a specific gene sequence in a given tissue or individual
   – **RT-PCR** (see below)
5. Comparison of inherited RFLPs between two individuals
   – **DNA fingerprinting**
6. Assessment of gene copy number in chromosomal DNA
   – **Southern blotting**

4. Forensic matching of scanty cellular DNA with individual suspects
   • e.g., Identification (in 1994) of the Russian Tsar's family remains following their execution by the Bolsheviks (in 1918).

Many variations of PCR (e.g., anchored PCR, inverse PCR) have been developed, as have alternative techniques such as the **ligase chain reaction** (LCR). Although the invention of PCR ranks as one of the great thought-experiments of all time, most PCR techniques retain certain problems in common.

MOLECULAR MINIREVIEW

Problems with PCR

Despite its remarkable abilities, PCR has its limitations. The main problems relate to:
1. Contamination
   • i.e., False-positive results from oversensitive detection of, say, aerosolized DNA or previous sample carry-over.
2. Accurate quantification
   • e.g., Of gene expression (RNA PCR). The latter technique, also termed RT-PCR, involves the use of reverse transcriptase (RT) to convert RNA to DNA. The technique is regarded as only semiquantitative, since it is difficult to control the efficiency of sequence amplification when comparing different samples.
3. Primer requirement
   • Makes it impossible to amplify any gene lacking the sequence data required to generate primers.

Gene chips create barcodes of mRNA expression patterns

The monitoring of gene expression by direct quantification of mRNA is complicated by the infamous in vitro susceptibility of RNA to degradation by contaminating ribonucleases. For this reason mRNAs are converted by reverse transcriptase to cDNAs for analytic purposes. Gene expression assays have now been developed that involve the quantitative hybridization of cDNAs to complementary gene sequences spotted on glass slides. This **gene chip** assay system – more correctly termed **DNA microarray** – can routinely define expression patterns for 4000–6000 mRNAs/cm^2 bound to cDNA sequence tags of known specificity, and such chips can survey an entire (yeast) genome in a single step. Newer chips may contain up to 400000 probes covering 30 kb DNA. Chips may come to be superseded by **wafers** containing up to 40 million probes covering 3 Mb DNA, however, enabling the entire human genome to be covered by as few as 300 such wafers.

Creating an informative array is the most labor-intensive step of gene chip technology. The identity of probes to be attached to the chip may be chosen from databases such as Genbank; oligodeoxynucleotide sequences (0.5–2.5 kb in length) from the target genes are then printed onto the slide or membrane (nitrocellulose or nylon). Such sequences may be obtained synthetically or by amplification of genomic DNA. The target material for analysis in a DNA microarray experiment is usually a pooled mRNA sample purified over an oligo-dT column that has been converted to cDNAs by reverse transcriptase. This latter reaction is carried out in the presence of fluorescence-labeled nucleotide precursors, leading to incorporation of fluorescent tags into the reverse transcripts. Since the object of the analysis is to compare two different mRNA expression patterns, a green fluor (fluorescein) may be used to tag one

Table 22.2. Analytic techniques for higher protein structure

1. Amino acid sequence analysis
   - Computational prediction
2. Indirect physical techniques
   - **Gel electrophoresis**
   - **Binding studies** (e.g., radiolabeled ligands, antibodies)
   - **Spectroscopy** (e.g., infra-red, Raman, circular dichroism)
   - **Chromatography** (e.g., paper, thin-layer, column, HPLC)
3. Direct physical techniques
   - **X-ray crystallography**
   - **Nuclear magnetic resonance** (NMR; p. 559)

properties, knowledge of this higher structure is a prerequisite for understanding molecular biology.

Random amino acid sequences are not usually associated with a stable three-dimensional structure. In contrast, the evolutionary conservation of a functional protein implies that the amino acid side-chains fit into a stable structure. The importance of **side-chain packing**, as opposed to main chain conformation, merits emphasis in this context. Deleterious mutations act most often by causing local derangements of side-chain packing with minimal (~1 Å or 0.1 nm) main chain rearrangements. In general, buried (hydrophobic) residues tend to be more important for protein integrity than are surface (hydrophilic) residues.

Proteins tolerate most single amino acid substitutions, but the exceptions are instructive: an example of a catastrophic mutation is the substitution of hydrophilic glutamate by hydrophobic valine in sickle-hemoglobin (p. 456). Techniques for determining protein structure are summarized in Table 22.2. The gold standard for structural studies involves the development of a **crystal** which, once created, permits determination of the structure by **X-ray diffraction**. The scattering of ionizing radiation passing through a crystal enables reconstruction of the irradiated molecule's atomic image to a sensitivity as high as 0.1 nm (1 Å) (Figure 22.12); this is how the double-helical structure of DNA was deduced. Examples of crystallized proteins range from hemoglobin and tRNA to pancreatic lipase, nerve growth factor, and SV40 virus: albumin has been characterized as a heart-shaped molecule, whereas TATA-binding protein (pp. 86, 373) is saddle-shaped. Progress in this field depends upon development of crystal structures for mutant molecules with known amino acid substitutions; for example, insertional mutagenesis of hemoglobin may generate a bulge in the otherwise smooth helix. A novel approach for characterizing the structure of proteins difficult to crystallize involves X-ray diffraction analysis of anti-idiotypic antibodies.

The quickest route to three-dimensional prediction involves finding sequence homology with proteins or domains already crystallized and structurally represented within a public protein database. This structure-solving strategy, termed computerized **homology modeling**, is of greatest utility for proteins exhibiting greater than 60% amino acid homology. For proteins exhibiting lesser degrees (30–50%) of homology with characterized molecules, the amino acid sequence provides a limited opportunity for remodeling the structure using variables such as amphipathicity, electrostatic analysis, energy minimization, and hydrophobic moments. However, since this involves predicting the best side-chain arrangement for the protein from millions of possibilities, such modeling is often inaccurate.

Homology modeling of protein structure involves assigning one or more folded structures to each target protein domain. "Doing it in silico" in this manner is starting to replace more direct analytic techniques such as crystallography. Computer modeling of this kind may be useful for docking studies of heterologous protein binding – as well as for excluding junk conformations or steric nonsense – but may not reliably solve the structure when used alone.

Figure 22.12 Modeling of three-dimensional protein structures (Wellcome Medical Photographic Library, no. B0000443C02).

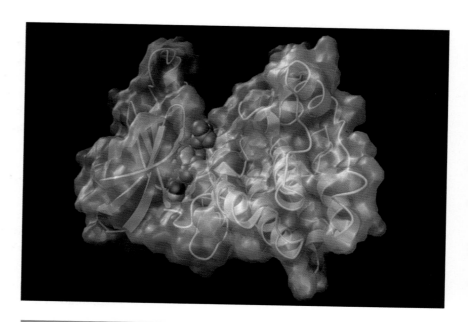

Nanotechnology

The term **nanoscale** broadly applies to anything less than 100 nm in diameter. Since the physical properties of matter change at sizes less than 20 nm or so – for example, self-replication may become easier – the nanoworld has become tantalizingly attractive to technopreneurs. **Nanotechnology** refers to anything built to work from the atomic level upwards, rather than the other way around; hence, any manufactured item that works at the submicron level would be an example. In practice, most nanotech devices tend to be electrochemical and other microelectronic gadgets in which nanoparticles are either structural components or substrates. Atomic-scale structures of this size may be imaged using scanning tunneling electron microscopy (see below).

The basis of this vogue for miniaturization is the use of **nanomaterials**. An example is the use of topical zinc oxide to prevent solar skin damage: old-fashioned zinc oxide consists of large particles that are readily visible as white streaks on the skin, whereas nanofied zinc oxide consists of particles so small that the cream (which still blocks the Sun) appears clear on the skin. The production of carbonaceous **nanotubes** from buckminsterfullerene is another such application. These "buckytubes" are one hundredfold stronger than steel per unit mass, while having the electrical conductivity of copper or silicon and the thermal conductivity of diamond.

Nanomachines may be inspired by natural nanostructures. The synthetic aramid textile Kevlar™ was designed to mimic the intermolecular hydrogen bonding of silk. Other organic materials worthy of emulation include the antifreeze proteins of fish, abalone shell nacre, wood, and the bacterial flagellum; the latter could inspire the design of nanomachines equipped with rotary robotic arms.

Isotopic and ultrastructural analysis

Radioisotopes are used to label target molecules

Laboratory analysis of biological molecules often depends on radioactive studies involving unstable **isotope** tagging. Isotopically labeled forms of many biomolecules (e.g., oligonucleotides, amino acids, ligands, antibodies) are routinely synthesized and used for quantitative incorporation or binding studies. The principal radioisotopes and their half-lives are:

1. ^{32}**P**
   - Used mainly for radiolabeling nucleic acid probes.
   - Also used for functional phosphoprotein studies in vitro or in vivo.
   - $t_{1/2}$ 14 days.
2. ^{35}**S**
   - Mainly used for labeling methionine or cysteine residues, which are then incorporated into nascent proteins.
   - $t_{1/2}$ 87 days.
3. ^{14}**C**
   - Useful as a control marker in radioactive turnover studies.
   - $t_{1/2}$ >5000 years.
4. ^{3}**H** (tritium)
   - Often used in thymidine labeling of proliferating cells to determine cell DNA replication activity, and hence growth fraction.
   - $t_{1/2}$ 12 years.
5. ^{125}**I** (or ^{131}**I**)
   - Commonly used for custom radiolabeling of ligands or antibodies.
   - $t_{1/2}$ 1–2 weeks.

Isotopes undergo nuclear disintegration and thus emit subatomic particles measurable as either **β-** or **γ-radiation**. Apart from ^{125}I (a γ-emitter), most common isotopes emit mainly β-radiation.

Radioactive ^{32}P-labeled nucleic acid hybridization tags ("probes") are prepared by gel-purifying a short DNA sequence of interest (the **insert**) and then incorporating the isotope in vitro using a procedure termed **end-labeling** (Figure 22.13). The radiolabeled probe is then boiled to denature the duplex DNA, thus allowing hybridization to complementary target sequences immobilized on membranes. The DNA double helix denatures at high temperatures (or pH>13) but renatures when the temperature drops below 65°C; this is the basis of the polymerase chain reaction (PCR; see above).

When isotopes are localized in microtiter plates, scintillation vials or membranes, emitted radiation can be quantified. Nonisotopic emissions such as fluorescence, phosphorescence and colorimetry are also used, though these methods tend to be less quantitative. Different isotopes have different half-lives, emission distances and shielding needs that dictate the safety measures needed for their use and disposal.

Figure 22.13 Preparation of a radioactive nucleic acid probe using nick-translation (see text for details).

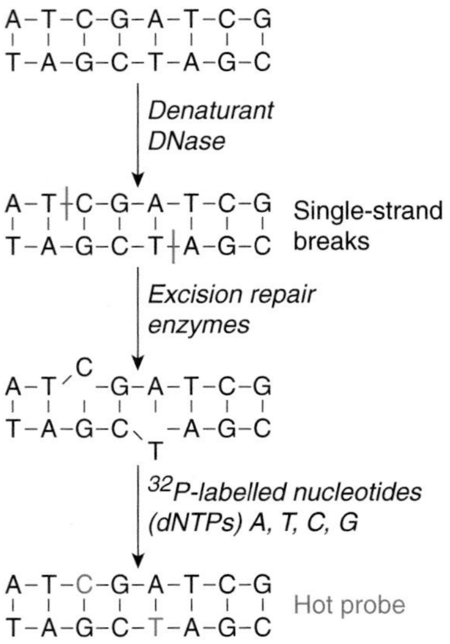

CLINICAL KEYNOTE

PET imaging

Assessment of tissue function – e.g., in the brain, heart or in tumors – has been revolutionized by the advent of the functionally dynamic isotopic imaging technologies **positron emission tomography** (PET) and **single-photon emission computed tomography** (SPECT), both of which visualize molecular function. **PET** enables direct visualization of metabolic tracers labeled with positron-emitting isotopes such as ^{18}F, ^{15}O, ^{11}C, and ^{13}N. For example, [^{18}F]**fluorodeoxyglucose** (^{18}FDG) is used for glucose utilization studies, and is thus useful in evaluating cancer patients with suspected occult disease or residual masses of uncertain significance. This reflects the fact that (hypoxic) tumors generally engage in increased glycolysis. Similarly, [^{11}C]methionine has been used for measuring amino acid metabolism in gliomas, whereas alterations in blood–brain barrier permeability may be assessed using [^{68}Ga]EDTA. Other tracers enable the measurement of variables such as cerebral blood flow after stroke, oxygen utilization ($^{15}O_2$), neurotransmitter release, and even attentiveness or consciousness. PET scanning may thus be useful in distinguishing neuropathologic conditions such as dementia (hypometabolic) and depression (normal); cerebral radiation necrosis (hypometabolic, hypoperfused) and recurrent brain tumor; or a primary refractory epileptic focus (hypometabolic, hypoperfused) and a secondary focus (hence, not suitable for excision). Imaging of human tumors following initial chemotherapy may also prove predictive of chemosensitivity and hence of long-term therapeutic benefit.

SPECT is used with more readily available isotopes such as ^{201}Tl (thallium), ^{99m}Tc, and ^{123}I, and hence does not require an on-site cyclotron. The information supplied by SPECT complements that of PET: whereas PET is used for imaging metabolism, SPECT is used mainly for perfusion studies such as those assessing myocardial vascularization.

Cell metabolism is measurable using NMR spectroscopy

Nuclear magnetic resonance (NMR) spectroscopy provides both a noninvasive way of determining the structure of proteins and other macromolecules, and an approach to metabolic analysis of living cell function. Nuclei most often used for the latter application are ^{31}P, ^{13}C, ^{15}C, and ^{1}H. Bombardment of such nuclei with radiowaves causes these molecules to recover their equilibrium alignment, leading to the emission of radiofrequency radiation.

Cells stressed by hypoxia supplement their threatened ATP stores by using **creatine kinase** (CK) to add high-energy phosphate groups to creatine; the **phosphocreatine** so formed can in turn transfer this high-energy group to ADP. This explains why elevations of tissue-specific CK isoforms are used diagnostically following suspected myocardial infarction, and why lower concentrations of ATP, creatine, and creatine phosphate are demonstrable within ischemic myocardial regions. NMR studies of cell metabolism using ^{31}P can thus detect metabolic changes during (say) **cardiac ischemia** by quantifying differential changes in molecules such as ATP, ADP, phosphocreatine, inorganic phosphate, lactate, and choline (as well as pH alterations). These metabolites are identified by their characteristic frequency of emitted radiation relative to a control signal, or **chemical shift** – a measurement from which the 2D NMR spectrum (a 3D fingerprint of the molecule) is determined. Such analyses can be used to define protein domain structure (e.g., lysozyme, myoglobin) and may be of diagnostic value in conditions such as **McArdle syndrome** (myophosphorylase deficiency) of muscle weakness.

Magnetic resonance imaging (MRI) depends on radiowave absorption by hydrogen nuclei (in H_2O) within living cells, and permits noninvasive imaging of tissue anatomy and function. Unlike computed tomography, MRI imaging does not require ionizing (X-) radiation. Strong magnetic fields of up to 2 tesla are needed to align the atomic nuclei for anatomic imaging (by comparison, the Earth's magnetic field is less than 0.0001 tesla, i.e., 20 000-fold weaker). Within this field, radiofrequency coils transmit and receive radiowaves, leading to the generation of nuclear relaxation times termed T1 (spin-lattice) and T2 (spin-spin) recovery curves. The combination of proton density, T1, T2, and blood flow leads to generation of the image. **Gadolinium** – a contrast agent that also causes T1 shortening – is used to illuminate enhancing tumors on T1-weighted images.

Functional magnetic resonance imaging (FMRI)

The capabilities of MRI have been magnified by the advent of **ultrafast** (single-shot) MRI, which permits measurement of small signal fluctuations caused by changes in the ratio of oxygenated to deoxygenated hemoglobin, so-called blood oxygenation level dependent (**BOLD**) imaging: neuronal activity within the brain causes an increase in blood flow that exceeds any associated rise in oxygen consumption, leading to a net increase in the BOLD image signal. Mental activities such as thinking and planning can be neuroanatomically mapped by direct visualization using this approach. Local areas of brain hypoperfusion have thus been demonstrated in **Alzheimer disease** (temporoparietal region) and in **schizophrenia** (frontotemporal region). Another use of this approach is in the presurgical evaluation of intractable **epilepsy**. BOLD MRI is also being used in sickle-cell disease, in which context abnormal blood deoxygenation may be detectable.

Other kinds of **functional MRI** (FMRI) explore the molecular behavior of the brain. Like PET, FMRI can detect metabolic alterations in human tissues using tracers such as [^{13}C]glucose; for example, FMRI can detect sexual arousal by localizing increased activity to the anterior cingulate gyrus near the frontal lobe. Hence, both FMRI and PET can measure flow-related alterations in brain energy consumption that correlate with brain cell activity. A further FMRI variation involves the in vivo assessment of neuronal viability using proton magnetic resonance spectroscopic imaging (MRSI) of the neuronal marker **N-acetyl-aspartate**.

Electron microscopy

Genetic, biochemical, and other nanoscale events may be clarified using the visualizing power of electron microscopy. High-voltage electron beams have tiny wavelengths, permitting ultrafine resolution approaching 0.1 nm or 1 Å – about 1000-fold finer than that achievable with the best light microscopes. There are a number of different varieties of electron microscopy, including:
1. **Transmission** electron microscopy.
2. **Scanning** electron microscopy.
3. **Scanning tunneling** electron microscopy.

The most common type of electron microscopy (EM) in biomedical research is transmission electron microscopy. This is used to investigate crystal structure (resolution to about 0.2 nm or 2 Å) or to characterize biological tissues. For the latter indication, specimens are fixed with glutaraldehyde and osmium tetroxide before ultrathin sectioning (about 10^{-7} m) to enable electron penetration. This enables good visualization – resolution typically ~1 nm – of subcellular organelles that cannot normally be distinguished by light microscopy. Specific antigens can be identified by coupling antibodies to electron-dense **colloidal gold** particles, while cell membrane interiors can be displayed using a technique called **freeze-fracture**.

Scanning electron microscopy is used for visualizing whole cells and tissues with magnifications up to 20 000 and resolution down to 10 nm. A cruder device than transmission EM, the scanning EM nonetheless provides stunning 3D pictures complete with depth of focus and shadow. Unlike the scanning EM, scanning tunneling EM resolves molecular surfaces with atomic-scale resolution, and is thus usually used in the physical sciences.

Enrichment reading

Bedtime reading

Martin C. *The thirteen steps to the atom: a photographic exploration.* Harrap, London, 1959

Cheap'n'cheerful

Clark DP, Russell LD. *Molecular biology made simple and fun.* Cache River Press, Vienna, IL, 1997

Durbin R (ed). *Biological sequence analysis: probabilistic models of proteins and nucleic acids.* Cambridge University Press, Cambridge, 1999

Turner PC (ed). *Instant notes in molecular biology.* Springer-Verlag, Berlin, 1998

Library reference

Banaszak LJ. *Foundations of structural biology.* Academic Press, New York, 2000

Griffiths A, Miller JH, Suzuki DT. *An introduction to genetic analysis.* WH Freeman, New York, 2000

Wilkins MR, Williams KL, Hochstrasser DF, Appel RD (eds). *Proteome research: new frontiers in functional genomics.* Springer-Verlag, Berlin, 1997

Summary

Proteins and nucleic acids can be separated within gels. Molecules within gels are transferred to membranes by blotting.

DNA structure can be assayed directly or indirectly. Polymerase chain reactions amplify primed DNA sequences. Gene chips create barcodes of mRNA expression patterns.

Proteins are identified by immunologic and physical methods. Proteomics connects cell behavior and protein function. Three-dimensional protein structures can be solved in silico.

Radioisotopes are used to label target molecules. Cell metabolism is measurable using NMR spectroscopy.

QUIZ QUESTIONS

1. What are gels used for in laboratory practice? How does their composition affect their uses?
2. Explain what is meant by the term (a) reducing gel, (b) denaturing gel.
3. Name some different kinds of blotting, and explain their various purposes.
4. What are some of the ways in which DNA sequence can be obtained? Under what circumstances would you choose to use one method in preference to another?
5. Describe briefly the principle behind (a) radioimmunoassay, and (b) ELISA.
6. Explain what is measured by spectrophotometry.
7. What is chromatography?
8. Which techniques are available to determine three-dimensional protein structure? Why might this information be important?
9. Name some different radioisotopes, their approximate half-lives, and their different experimental uses.
10. Distinguish the principles underlying PET imaging from those of MRI imaging.
11. How does nuclear magnetic resonance give information about cell metabolism?

23 | Genetic engineering, gene mapping, and gene testing

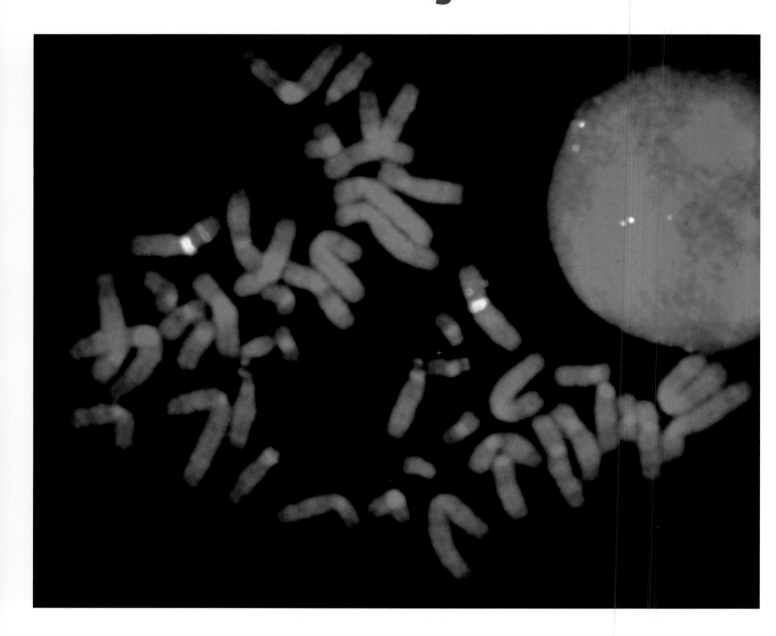

Figure 23.1 (*previous page*) Example of a FISH lacking Duchenne muscular dystrophy: human karyotype probed by fluorescent in situ hybridization. (Wellcome Medical Photographic Library, no. B0000325C06).

People say that the human genome is now sequenced, but what exactly do they mean? Your genome or mine?

Hard as it may be to believe, you share 99.9% of your genetic structure with other people you see on the street. In other words, only 0.1% of your genome is uniquely "you". This 0.1% consists of repetitive DNA variations, gene polymorphisms, intronic variants, splice junction aberrations, imprintings, and perhaps a few amplification and missense mutation events. These latter anomalies may manifest in some instances as disease phenotypes, but may also predispose to disease susceptibilities that only become manifest in conjunction with other genetic variations or environmental exposures.

Sequencing the genome thus provides a reference point for interpreting variations – many of which may have little if any functional significance. Equally, however, many apparently functionless polymorphisms may prove to have genetic significance. The next generation of biomedical scientists will grapple with the complexities of correlating gene structure with (human) function. A prerequisite for this challenge will be the basic tools of molecular biology, as described briefly in this section.

Constructs and vectors

Genes are packaged into vectors for expression in vitro

Isolating a gene of interest is only a first step towards characterizing the gene's function. The structure of the gene may provide clues as to its function – marking it, for example, as a member of a particular gene superfamily – but the cellular context in which normal gene expression occurs is also likely to be important. Hence, a useful initial exercise is to seek a differential pattern of gene expression in adult tissues, and to compare this with fetal tissue patterns.

More direct analysis of gene function requires expression of the target gene in a cell culture system. This involves permeabilizing cells to enable entry of exogenous genes – a process termed DNA **transfection**. The inefficiency of this process demands incorporation of a gene (linked to the target gene) that acts as a **selectable marker** for successful transfection; such markers provide the selectivity required for **gene cloning**. Cloning requires two ingredients: the DNA sequence to be cloned (often a gene) and the cutting and pasting of that DNA into a suitable cloning **vector**. Common vectors include:

1. **Plasmids**
   • Usually bacterial but occasionally yeast.
2. **Phage**
   • Nonpathogenic bacterial viruses; usually phage lambda (λ).
3. **Cosmids**
   • Hybrid vectors derived from crossing plasmids with phage λ.
4. **Yeast artificial chromosomes** (YACs; see below)
   • Used for packaging large inserts.

Plasmids are unsuitable for genomic mapping studies since insert size is restricted (100 bp to 15 kb). Moreover, large plasmids are deselected by fast-replicating smaller plasmids during cloning. *Escherichia coli* is the plasmid host most commonly used in laboratory work. Plasmid vectors are linearized (cut) by incubating with a restriction enzyme predicted to cleave at a specific sequence within the vector's cloning site. This allows ligase-dependent incorporation of target insert into this site prior to re-annealing and circularization (Figure 23.2).

Phage lambda (λ), a viral particle that parasitizes *E. coli*, is also a popular

Figure 23.2 Use of plasmids for cloning DNA inserts. *A*, Excision of the target DNA (insert) using the sticky end-cutter *Eco*RI. *B*, Cleavage of the plasmid cloning site using the same restriction enzyme, permitting the unambiguous insertion of target DNA in the correct orientation. Ligation is completed by the addition of DNA ligase.

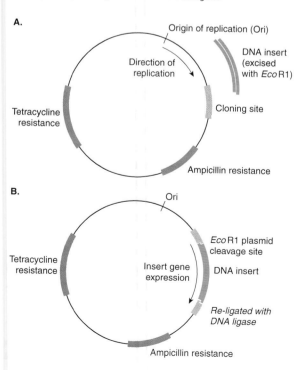

A.

Origin of replication (Ori)

DNA insert (excised with *Eco*R1)

Direction of replication

Cloning site

Tetracycline resistance

Ampicillin resistance

B.

Ori

*Eco*R1 plasmid cleavage site

Insert gene expression

DNA insert

Tetracycline resistance

Re-ligated with DNA ligase

Ampicillin resistance

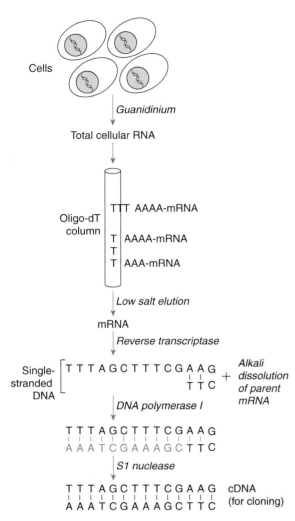

Figure 23.7 Preparation of a cDNA expression library. Total cellular RNA is first prepared from target cells, then the mRNA purified over an oligo-dT column. Reverse transcription of these mRNAs into cDNAs creates the library.

inserts in terms of both size and sequence. These recombinant plasmids can then be used to transform permeabilized bacteria. Since the plasmid vector contains an antibiotic-resistance gene, bacterial clones containing plasmids (and hence inserts) can in turn be rapidly isolated by treating with the relevant antibiotic. This assemblage of plasmid-transformed bacterial clones constitutes the library.

Most clones within a genomic DNA library will not contain transcribable DNA. A popular strategy for enriching the gene content of libraries is to isolate the target cell's mRNA using an oligo-dT column to bind poly-A-containing species. These transcripts are then treated with reverse transcriptase to yield cDNA clones which are in turn used to generate recombinant plasmids and libraries (Figure 23.7). This **cDNA library** is likely to contain clones encoding gene products that are highly expressed by the target cell population; for example, a cDNA library from a liver extract might be expected to be enriched for albumin gene clones. Prior enrichment of this library could be engineered by initially using an antibody to immunoprecipitate polyribosomes attached to nascent albumin molecules, thereby purifying for the attached albumin mRNA. A second method of enrichment, termed **subtractive hybridization**, involves using mRNA from two cell populations, only one of which expresses the gene of interest. A PCR-based cDNA subtraction technique termed **suppressive subtractive hybridization** (SSH) is a newer version of this approach. Similarly, mRNA **differential display** and DNA microarray may be used for this purpose.

MOLECULAR MINIREVIEW

Library screening

Selectable markers for plasmid expression in *E. coli* typically contain the **β-lactamase** (ampicillin-resistance) gene. Mammalian transfectants, on the other hand, most often contain the **neomycin-resistance** gene, which provides selective pressure for cells treated with the cytotoxic antibiotic G418.

Libraries are **screened** to identify recombinant inserts of interest using a variety of approaches. The most direct form of screening is to use a radioactively labeled (nick-translated) oligonucleotide probe matching some of the target gene sequence – as predicted, for example, by amino acid microsequencing of part of the protein of interest – to hybridize with replica-plated filters. A second screening approach involves initial cloning of the library using an expression vector that promotes synthesis of the protein; expression libraries of this kind can then be probed using a suitable antibody.

Localized genes may be cloned by function or position

The first step in cloning a disease gene is often that of identifying affected families. **Cytogenetic analysis** of such families may occasionally provide genetic clues in the guise of a localizing chromosomal deletion or translocation. Affected families (both cases and normals) are then genotyped for the presence of polymorphic markers (up to 300) throughout the genome. Co-inheritance of the disease and a marker sequence may implicate nearby alleles of appropriate function in the pathogenesis. This cloning strategy, termed the **candidate gene** approach, may be realized by finding mutations or deletions affecting the target gene in affected families, and may be further supported by transgenic knockout experiments in which the disease is simulated in an animal by loss of candidate gene function. The drawback with this approach is that the location and the function of the candidate gene need to be known, as do some details of disease pathophysiology.

Such combinations of chromosomal and linkage studies in affected families often provide the starting point for the next phase of disease gene identification. An illustrative cloning strategy is that used for identifying the gene for **chronic granulomatous disease** which was initially mapped to Xp21 by linkage. Chromosomal microdissection of the Xp21 region was used to create a genomic library; to screen the library, mRNA was prepared both from dysfunctional polymorphonuclear leukocytes (presumed to lack the target cDNA) and from unaffected cells. Subtractive hybridization enriched for the defective cDNA clone, which was then used to screen the Xp21 library.

An alternative gene hunting strategy is **positional cloning**. Using this approach, gene identification is only the first step; once cloned, the real task of working out the function of the new gene begins. The Rosetta stone for the latter exercise is a computer database (e.g., GenBank) containing most of the human genome. Examples of positional cloning include those involving the genes for **cystic fibrosis** and **Duchenne muscular dystrophy**.

MOLECULAR MINIREVIEW

Positional cloning of dystrophin

Duchenne muscular dystrophy (**DMD**) is the commonest fatal X-linked disorder of childhood, affecting one in 5000 live male births. X-autosome translocations resulting from postmeiotic nonhomologous recombination during spermatogenesis may occasionally lead to inactivation of the normal X chromosome with resultant expression of the disease in females. Characterization of the responsible gene product, **dystrophin**, represented the first success of positional cloning.

The X-linked pattern of DMD inheritance has been recognized for half a century. Cases involving chromosomal translocations and deletions implicated the Xp21 band as a probable disease gene locus. Approximately two-thirds of DMD cases arise due to deletions of one or more exons within the *DMD* gene. There are two mutational hotspot within the coding region of the gene: one at the 5′ end, and the other about midway along. This clustering enables multiplex PCR to examine a few specific exons (1–8) for mutations, detecting up to 98% of deletion mutants. However, such deletion-duplication detection strategies fail to diagnose about 30% of DMD patients with regulatory sequence defects or inactivating point mutations; linkage analysis using nearby RFLPs is required for diagnosis in such cases. A reasonable sequence of investigations for a child with suspected DMD might be:

1. Plasma creatine phosphokinase (CPK) and electromyography.
2. Muscle biopsy:
   - Histology.
   - Dystrophin immunofluorescence in females (patchy dystrophin absence due to mosaic germ-cell X-inactivation may be diagnostic.
   - Dystrophin immunoblotting (the diagnostic test of choice in males).
3. Genetic studies for family screening and prenatal testing
   - PCR and/or Southern blotting for deletion/duplication detection.
   - RFLP linkage analysis in probands with negative PCR/Southern blots.

polymorphisms of the genes encoding **factor VII** and **cholesteryl ester transfer protein** are respectively linked to **myocardial infarction** frequency and clinical benefit from **statin** treatment. Germline polymorphisms within coding regions are less frequent than in noncoding regions, but nonetheless accumulate at a rate between 10^{-4} to 10^{-7} per generation.

Additional areas of difficulty in the clinical interpretation of gene mutations include the issue of **genotype-phenotype correlation**. For a few genes, the power of such correlations is established: an example is the *Ret* gene in which certain gain-of-function mutations cause **familial medullary thyroid cancer** (exons 13–15), **MEN 2A** (exons 10, 11) or **MEN 2B** (exons 15-16), whereas other (loss-of-function) mutations may cause congenital aganglionic megacolon (**Hirschsprung disease**). Hence, similar understanding of phenotypic correlations for other discrete gene defects should greatly enhance the clinical utility of genetic testing.

A third area of interpretational difficulty is **age-specific mutational penetrance** – that is, the interindividual variation in age at which the same gene mutation may cause clinical problems. Such differences in mutational penetrance may signify an interplay with confounding environmental or genetic factors. These considerations are important when assessing the likely benefits and risks of prophylactic interventions such as surgery or drug treatment for at-risk individuals who are so labeled on the basis of mutational testing.

A final area of confusion relates to the high **de novo mutation frequency** of many heritable disorders. **Familial retinoblastoma** and **MEN 2B** arise de novo in 50% of cases, for example, whereas **familial adenomatous polyposis** arises in the absence of a family history in 30% cases. Having a sibling with a genetic diagnosis may thus not consign the rest of the family to indefinite mutation screening in the absence of a multigenerational family history of disease.

Modifier genes regulate occurrence of polygenic diseases

Good genetics requires good phenotypes; in other words, ascertaining the genetic basis of a given trait is easier if the trait is readily detectable. This point is most often made in the context of animal model development – including transgenic, knock-in and knockout models (Chapter 24) – but is equally applicable to the genetic basis of diseases variously designated as complex, multifactorial or **polygenic**. The genetic component of such diseases typically involves:
1. Large numbers of genes.
2. High-prevalence genetic variations (polymorphisms).
3. Small phenotypic effects of individual polymorphisms.
4. Critical additive effects of environmental interactions.

Genetic mapping of complex diseases thus involves a search for **modifier genes** that may be suppressors or enhancers of the disease phenotype. By definition, modifier gene products do not contribute directly to the main pathway of disease pathogenesis. Conversely, such genes do not usually accumulate drastic gain-of-function or loss-of-function mutations, but rather tend to be polymorphic variants. Common functions of modifier genes include transcriptional regulation, nuclear import/export, RNA processing, protein degradation, and cell detoxification.

An intriguing example of the influence of modifier genes occurs in the APC^{Min} mouse model of colorectal carcinogenesis. This model, which was induced by ethylnitrosourea-induced truncation of murine APC at codon 850, differs from the human **familial adenomatous polyposis** phenotype by virtue of its association with anemia and small bowel polyposis. The number of polyps varies widely both within and between APC^{Min} kindreds, suggesting an interaction with other genetic and/or environmental variables. This view is supported by the finding that the efficiency of adenoma growth varies with the functional state of heterologous genes such as *PLA$_2$*, *COX2*, or *Smad4*.

Modifier genes are difficult to map, reflecting their genetic heterogeneity. One method of expediting such mapping is to identify **endophenotypes** – measurable traits (e.g., atypical physical responses or biochemical stigmata) that segregate with the disease. **Schizophrenia** provides an example: it is difficult to monitor delusional thinking (particularly in animal models), whereas the associated endophenotypes of olfactory dysfunction, startle inhibition, and smooth pursuit eye movements are easy to detect.

MOLECULAR MINIREVIEW

SNPs

Single-nucleotide polymorphisms or SNPs (pronounced "snips") are the commonest variant sequences in the human genome, occurring as often as once every 500 bp (i.e., about ten million SNPs per diploid genome). Each SNP reflects a single mutation that has (probably) occurred only once in the history of the human race. In general, the more common the SNP – i.e., the higher the population frequency – the more ancient the founding mutation is likely to be.

A high-density genomic **SNP map** incorporating over a million sequence variants will in time be developed for the analysis of linkage disequilibrium in case–control studies; this number of SNPs would permit localization of disease target genes to within 3 kb upstream or downstream of the marker in question. The more informative of such SNPs might be expected to be located within coding sequences (i.e., **cSNPs**), intron-exon boundaries, or upstream or downstream control regions. Homology modeling of the encoded protein should indicate whether a given SNP-associated missense mutation is expressed within the core of the molecule (or in the active site, P-loop, or DNA-binding domain, say), under which circumstances it is more likely to be phenotypically significant. The **lipoprotein lipase** gene contains over a hundred SNPs, for example, but only a minority of these directly affect the coding sequence.

The advent of genotyping arrays (nanochips or "snip chips") will assist linkage studies of diseased families as well as help locate new disease genes in isolated population studies. This latter application reflects the persistence of linkage disequilibrium between most genomic loci closer than 100 kb: about 60 kb in European lineages but much shorter in Africans, suggesting a major demographic divergence 50 000 years ago. The phenomenon of linkage disequilibrium reflects the comparatively small number of human generations, and hence the relative lack of recombinational disruption of such linkage.

SNP analysis has identified genetic susceptibility loci for diseases such as **HIV infection** (via identification of the *CCR5* gene), **migraine with aura** (19p13), **non-insulin-dependent diabetes** (12q), **psoriasis** (3q21) and **Alzheimer disease** (apoE: 19q13). Genes identified as susceptibility markers may not necessarily prove to be drug targets, however. Rather, they may be nonmutated modifier genes relevant to the pathogenetic pathway of interest. Nonetheless, a major application of SNP technology is anticipated to be in the field of pharmacogenomics, permitting the customized prescription of effective and nontoxic drug dosages.

Enrichment reading

Bedtime reading

Ridley M. *Genome: the autobiography of a species in 23 chapters*. Harpercollins, New York, 2000

Cheap'n'cheerful

Brown TA. *Gene cloning*. Stanley Thomas, London, 1995

Nicholl D. *An introduction to genetic engineering*. Cambridge University Press, Cambridge, 1994

Library reference

Cantor CR, Smith CL. *Genomics: the science and technology behind the human genome project*. John Wiley & Sons, New York, 1999

Haines JL, Pericak-Vance MA (eds). *Approaches to gene mapping in complex human diseases*. Wiley-Liss, New York, 1998

Imura H, Kasuga M, Nakao K. *Common disease – genetic and pathogenetic aspects of multifactorial diseases*. Elsevier, Amsterdam, 1999

Liu, B. *Statistical genomics: linkage, mapping and Qtl analysis*. CRC Press, Boca Raton, FL, 1997

Setubal JC, Meidanis J. *Introduction to computational molecular biology*. PWS Publishing Co, New York, 1996

Summary

Genes are packaged into vectors for expression in vitro. Promoter choice influences recombinant gene inducibility.

Reporter genes monitor the efficiency of target gene expression. Green fluorescent protein localizes target molecules in vivo.

Genes are hunted using different mapping strategies. In situ hybridization localizes gene sequences to chromosomes.

Gene cloning depends on the detection of rare events. Chromosome-localized genes can be cloned by function or position.

Normal gene function is elucidated by mutational analysis. Genetic polymorphisms may have functional significance. Modifier genes regulate occurrence of polygenic diseases.

QUIZ QUESTIONS

1. Explain how the polymerase chain reaction works. What are some of its clinical uses and technical limitations?
2. What is a vector? What is it used for?
3. Describe what attributes you would seek in a promoter for a gene you wish to express selectively in the adult thyroid gland of an experimental animal.
4. Distinguish what is meant by (a) cell transformation, (b) cell transfection.
5. Name some common reporter genes. What are they used for?
6. Why are mutations important in characterizing normal gene behavior?
7. Describe two experimental uses of in situ hybridization.
8. Explain the difference between how a genomic library and a cDNA library are made.
9. How does a candidate gene approach to cloning differ from that of a positional cloning strategy?

24

Gene knockouts, transgenics, and cloning

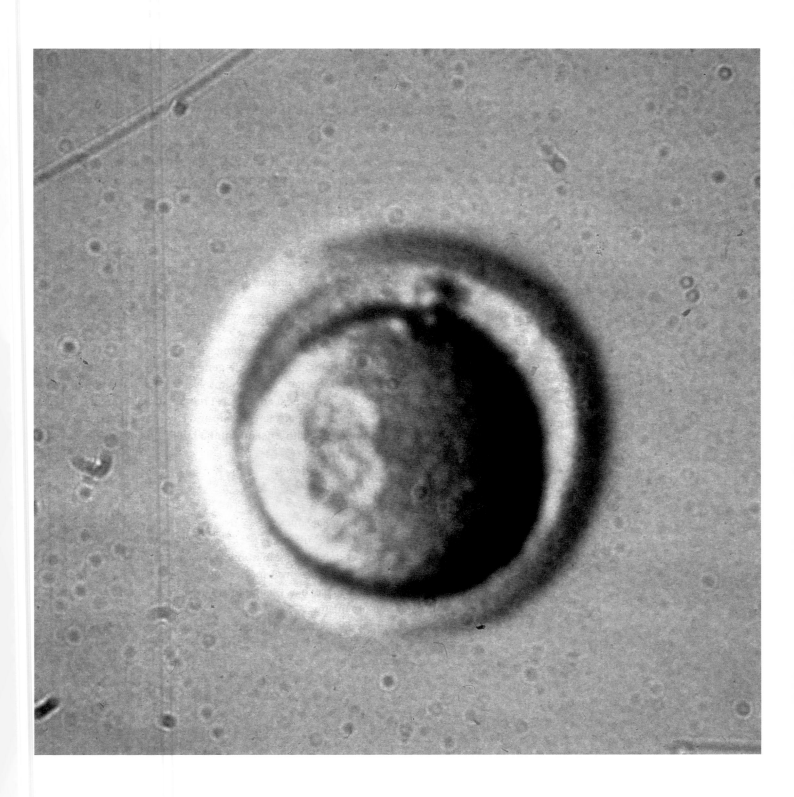

MOLECULAR MINIREVIEW

Dominant negatives and knock-ins

Knockout of a normal gene by a null mutation is one approach to gene targeting. An alternative approach involves co-expression of a gene with a missense mutation. The encoded molecule is characterized as a **dominant negative** (i.e., interfering) if its expression blocks function of the wild-type protein. Such molecules may prevent correct oligomerization or DNA binding of wild-type receptor molecules, for example, thereby competitively inhibiting wild-type function. Phenotypic characterization of such mutations in transgenic animals can be effected using so-called **knock-in** gene transfer strategies (any mutant phenotype can be expressed in vivo by this approach). Examples of dominant negative molecules include:

1. Mutations affecting the **p53** molecule which contribute to the genetic instability, drug resistance, and clinical progression of many common cancers.
2. The **HbS** mutation (an A to T transversion in the sixth codon of the β-globin gene; Glu→Val). Knock-in of this mutation causes the **sickle cell disease** phenotype in animal models co-expressing the wild-type allele.
3. Mutations of the **α1(I) collagen** gene may cause the bone fragility syndrome **osteogenesis imperfecta**, reflecting interactive effects on wild-type collagens.

A clinical model of a dominant negative is **piebaldism** characterized by mutation of the hemopoietic Kit receptor, leading to defective melanocyte migration. Homozygosity for this mutation is embryonic lethal, whereas heterozygotes present with white forelock, deafness, and constipation.

Our efforts to mimic nature remain at an early stage of development. We are now able to create custom-made animal models, and also to clone identical copies of certain mammals from their parents. In the next and final section, we consider the future of recombinant DNA technology and gene therapy.

Summary

Gene defects may cause similar syndromes across species. Homologous mutations support animal model relevance.

Transgenes may be propagated in germ cells, zygotes or embryos. Mammals can be cloned by somatic cell nuclear transfer.

Gene function is assessable in vivo using transgenic models. Gene targeting knocks out gene function in vivo.

Enrichment reading

Cheap'n'cheerful

Joyner AL. *Gene targeting: a practical approach*. Oxford University Press, Oxford, 2000

QUIZ QUESTIONS

1. Which criteria would you use to assess whether a mouse strain provided a useful model for analyzing a human disease?
2. What is meant by the term chromosomal synteny?
3. Name a human disease which corresponds to a mouse phenotype due to a genetically homologous mutation.
4. Explain how transgenic animals are made.
5. What assessment(s) would you make in a new transgenic animal which appears normal?
6. Define the following terms: (a) founder, (b) bigenic.
7. Explain how homologous recombination is used to knockout target gene expression.
8. What is meant by the term dominant negative? How is this concept relevant either experimentally or clinically?
9. Describe the sequence of events during somatic cell nuclear transfer, and discuss the potential medical value of this approach.
10. Discuss some of the regulatory safeguards which might be desirable once human cloning becomes routinely possible.

25

Gene therapy and recombinant DNA technology

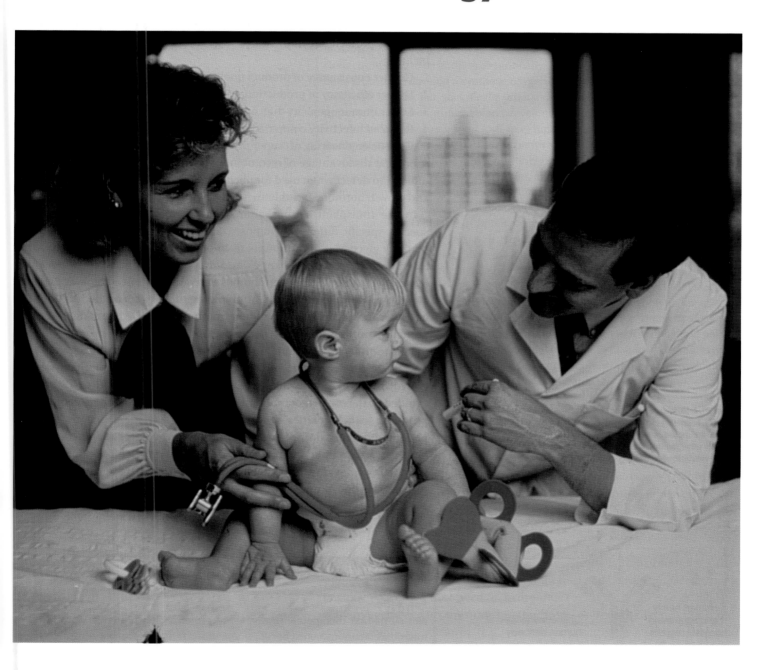

target gene to be amplified by exposing transfected cells to rising concentrations of the DHFR inhibitor methotrexate.

A gene that arises from a mixture of other genes is termed a **chimera** – or to be more prosaic, a mosaic. Unlike dicistronic genes, chimeric gene design involves substituting a domain of one gene for that of another gene. Hence, the DNA-binding domain (D) of protein X, say, can be fused with the ligand-binding domain (L) of protein Y to yield a hybrid (D)X(L)Y **fusion protein**, which is activated by ligand L but binds to sequence D. In vivo creation of fusion proteins using intracellular delivery of chimeric RNA-DNA oligonucleotides is one approach to correcting mutational defects such as sickle cell anemia. The success of fusion protein expression can be measured by raising a specific antibody to the fusion site. This is similar to the technique of **epitope tagging** wherein a nonfunctional but immunogenic protein domain is grafted onto a target protein, facilitating antibody detection of the parent molecule.

PHARMACOLOGIC FOOTNOTE

Therapeutic fusion genes

Researchers involved in drug development – the search for the magic bullet – are often preoccupied with issues of substrate selectivity and binding affinity. These problems may be solved by constructing a fusion gene encoding a chimeric protein that incorporates domains for selective binding and efficient catalytic activity. Examples of fusion proteins engineered with therapeutic intent include:

1. The **GM-CSF/IL-3** fusion protein
   - Designed to maximize the marrow-stimulatory effect of the two hemopoietic growth factors in a single recombinant.
2. Anticancer **ligand-toxin conjugates**, e.g.,
   - *Pseudomonas* toxin linked to interleukin-6 or fibroblast growth factor.
   - Diphtheria toxin linked to IL-2 or to melanocyte-stimulating hormone.
3. Immunosuppressive targeting of the IL-2 receptor by **IL2-IgM** conjugates.
4. An **FSHβ-HCGβ** fusion protein, where FSH is follicle-stimulating hormone and HCG is human chorionic gonadotrophin.
   - Creates a long-acting fusion protein by adding to FSH the carboxy-terminal *O*-glycosylated peptide which confers long plasma half-life on HCGβ.
5. A **protein C** precursor containing a **thrombin** activation site, allowing it to be selectively activated in the presence of thrombosis.

Some fusion genes occur in human diseases as a result of chromosomal translocations (e.g., Bcr/Abl, RARα/PML, Tpr/Met). Proteins encoded by hybrid genes are potential therapeutic targets by virtue of their unique fusion sequences which distinguish them from wild-type molecules. The encoded mRNA fusion sequences provide disease-specific targets for antisense oligonucleotides and ribozymes.

Recombinant protein expression systems vary in efficiency

The principles by which genes encode proteins are similar throughout the evolutionary tree. Recombinant proteins are thus capable of being produced in a variety of different expression systems, including:

1. *E. coli.*
2. Yeast.
3. Baculovirus-infected insect (Sf9) cells.
4. Transgenic animals (e.g., secreting transgenic proteins into milk).

The choice of expression system partly depends on the production requirements. Until recently, high-quantity protein expression was best suited to microbiological synthesis in yeast or *E. coli*, with animal cell systems or baculovirus-infected insect cells reserved for post-translational emergencies. However, the efficiency of animal cell production systems has greatly improved, and mammalian cell lines such as CHO (Chinese hamster ovary) and BHK (baby hamster kidney) cells are now often used for recombinant protein synthesis. Target proteins usually need to be secreted for efficient production. Recombinant immunogens are an exception, since even intracellular synthesis may provide sufficient antigen for successful vaccination.

In the commercial setting, rates of protein production need to be monitored: nonproducing cells may take over the culture system, necessitating the re-cloning of expressing cells. Another problem is that excessive cellular lactate production can limit culture growth. Developing and maintaining the growth (biomass) of the bioprocessing system requires appropriate inputs of glucose, glutamine, other amino acid nutrients, and supplements such as choleratoxin, heparin (which binds fibroblast growth factors), and thrombin.

Recombinant production of functional human proteins involves a number of technical hurdles, such as maintaining protein solubility. Similarly, bacterial production of proteins such as factor IX is not feasible since *E. coli* are incapable of γ-carboxylation (p. 467). A common problem with bacterial production systems is the failure to mimic human protein glycosylation, with variable functional and immunogenic consequences. Correct disulfide bonding of recombinant molecules may be essential for proper folding and function, although genetically engineered changes in disulfide bonding may in some instances enhance protein stability.

Small proteins and genes may now be synthesized de novo using solid-phase methodology. These include immunogens such as **hepatitis B surface antigen** (HBsAg) which is produced in situ by genetically engineered vaccinia virus. Recombinant human **insulin** has generated unexpected controversy, however, having proven no less immunogenic than porcine insulin while being linked to frequent clinical episodes of hypoglycemic unawareness.

PHARMACOLOGIC FOOTNOTE

Peptides and peptidomimetics

The functional (wild-type) forms of most proteins have evolved over hundreds of millions of years, eliminating many dysfunctional mutants by natural selection. Accordingly, it is easier to design a recombinant protein antagonist than an agonist which mimics normal function. The simplest approach for synthesizing a synthetic agonist is to reproduce the wild-type protein or part thereof (Table 25.2).

Informative human molecules contain peptide sequences which govern their biochemical reactivity. Reactive peptides are flexible, however, and in solution may not resemble the native conformation of the active protein. A central problem with recombinant peptides and proteins is that they cannot be administered orally: the recipient's stomach sees the expensive peptide medicament as just another piece of meat. For this reason most recombinant drugs need to be administered by injection. Additional problems with peptide-based drugs include poor bioavailability, low stability, high immunogenicity, and excessive production costs.

These drawbacks of peptide pharmacology are the focus of much research into **peptidomimetic drugs**. Nonproteolyzable small-molecule drugs that can be administered orally are the chief target of pharmaceutical development strategies, and improved protein modeling capabilities may permit the rational design of agonists or antagonists (e.g., developed by combinatorial chemistry). Peptide therapies may

Table 25.2. Examples of key biopharmaceuticals

Recombinant protein	Clinical scenario for therapy
Enzymes:	
DNase	Cystic fibrosis (viscid sputum)
Glucocerebrosidase	Gaucher disease
Tissue plasminogen activator	Thrombosis prevention
Peptide hormones and growth factors:	
Erythropoietin	Anemia
G-CSF, GM-CSF	Neutropenia
Growth hormone	Growth retardation
Insulin	Diabetes mellitus
Antibodies:	
Anti-CD3	Transplant rejection
Anti-CD20 (rituximab)	Lymphoma
Anti-IL-2 receptor (anti-CD25; daclizumab, basiliximab)	Transplant rejection, lymphoma
Anti-ErbB2 (trastuzumab)	Breast cancer
Anti-GPIIb/IIIa (abciximab)	Thrombosis prevention
Anti-TNFα (infliximab)	Crohn disease, rheumatoid arthritis
Immunogens:	
Hepatitis B surface antigen	Hepatitis B vaccination
Interferons:	
Alpha	Chronic myeloid leukemia, hepatoma
Beta	Multiple sclerosis
Gamma	Chronic granulomatous disease

Notes:

G-CSF, granulocyte colony-stimulating factor; GM-CSF, granulocyte-macrophage colony-stimulating factor, TNFα tumor necrosis factor α, IL-2, interleukin-2

still be used: the finding that the core PQPQLPY peptide sequence of α-gliadin is the target antigen for T cells in celiac disease suggests strategies for inducing tolerance in such patients, for example, whereas the QYNAD peptide sequence appears relevant to treatments targeting sodium channels. Of note, cytokines such as IL-10 have been delivered in intact form to gastrointestinal mucosa via oral administration of "packaging" acid-resistant bacteria, permitting topical treatment of inflammatory bowel disease in rodent models.

Antisense oligonucleotides

Ribozymes are RNA gene shears that kill the messenger

Enzymes are popular proteins for recombinant production strategies, reflecting the frequent involvement of this molecular class in inherited single-gene disorders. A good example is **α₁-antitrypsin deficiency**, an enzymopathy which predisposes to early-onset pulmonary emphysema and liver cirrhosis. Catalytic proteins are not the only molecules which are enzymatic, however; the conserved catalytic activity of RNA has made it possible to custom-design DNA shears made of RNA. These RNA scissors or **ribozymes** are metalloenzymes that catalyze the sequence-specific cleavage of phosphodiester bonds within mRNA molecules (Figure 25.3). Ribozymes are thus oligoribonucleotides that hybridize and cleave complementary mRNAs.

The sequence-specificity of ribozyme cleavage reflects complementary base-pairing. Accordingly, novel ribozymes can be systematically created to

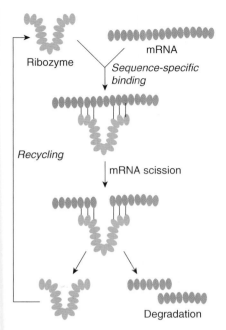

Figure 25.3 A day in the life of a ribozyme. On locating its complementary target mRNA, the enzyme binds, prepares for action, cuts and detaches – leaving the fragmented RNA to degrade while the ribozyme returns to the fray.

interfere with target messages – unlike development of enzyme-specific inhibitors, for example, which remains highly empirical. Indeed, custom ribozymes can selectively inhibit rogue genes which differ from wild-type genes by even a single nucleotide. Targets for ribozyme cleavage include:

1. Intracellular mRNA.
2. RNA viral genomes.

The specificity of ribozyme-substrate interactions depends critically upon the higher-order structure of the ribozyme. For example, the catalytic activity of the viroidal **hairpin ribozyme** is constrained by the nucleotide composition of the substrate. **Hammerhead ribozymes** contain a self-cleaving domain (the hammerhead) that consists of three helical regions binding 13 conserved nucleotides: such ribozymes may have therapeutic potential in HIV-associated diseases and other viral infections. Catalytic rates of ribozyme-dependent reactions may be up to 10^5-fold greater than uncatalyzed reactions.

Ribozymes are effective therapeutic reagents in plant diseases, yet remain investigational as medical reagents. Favored therapeutic targets include the *Bcr/Abl* fusion gene in **chronic myeloid leukemia**, the mutant *Ras* gene in **colorectal cancer**, and the *ErbB2* gene in **breast cancer**. Ribozymes may also be engineered to repair mutant gene transcripts (e.g., in **sickle cell disease**) or to carry out ribosome-like peptidyltransferase reactions.

MOLECULAR MINIREVIEW

The triple helix

Sequence-specific hybridization is a central principle of human biology. Either synthetic or endogenous strips of DNA – oligodeoxynucleotides, or oligos – can be targeted to hybridize with complementary nucleic acid sequences (sense sequences) of disease genes in two ways:

1. By forming a nontranslatable **double-stranded mRNA** with a critical region of the target message, thereby promoting nuclease degradation of the message.
2. By forming a nontranscribable **DNA triple helix** with a critical genomic region of the target gene, thus preventing transcription.

DNA triple helix strategies have one major therapeutic advantage over mRNA-targeted oligonucleotides: most genes are present in the genome at a copy number of one, whereas there may be 1000 copies or more of an average mRNA transcript. Furthermore, mRNA molecules are consistently replenished by transcription whereas gene sequences are only replicated once per cell cycle. The stoichiometry of antisense therapy is thus more attractive for gene-based than transcript-based approaches. Triple helix-forming oligos may be targeted to gene promoter sites with the aim of preventing transcription factor binding or RNA polymerase II progression. Such triplexes can also incorporate scrambled sequences that induce site-specific mutations into genomic DNA.

Whereas the stability of double helix formation depends on the combination of **base stacking** and **Watson-Crick hydrogen bonding** between complementary bases in the minor groove of DNA (triple helix formation involves a process termed **Hoogsteen hydrogen bonding**, which occurs between the single-stranded oligonucleotide (typically a polypyrimidine) and duplex Watson-Crick base pairs (ideally a homopurine) in the major groove. This constraint severely limits code recognition of the triple helix approach, since target sequences may be limited to purine (adenine, guanine) 15-mers. Moreover, accessibility to the target sequence is less predictable in chromatin than in cytosolic transcripts.

Catalytic antibodies

The abilities of antibodies are not confined to antigen recognition. Antibodies share a fundamental quality with enzymes: both protein groups exhibit fine discrimination for binding target molecules. Complementarity of binding sites between a ligand and its substrate does not ordinarily suffice for enzymatic activity, since complementarity of enzymatic active sites and the substrate reaction site is also desirable. However, binding alone can cause moderate catalysis under some circumstances.

The catalytic potential of certain immunoglobulins was recognized when antibodies raised against tetrahedral phosphate and phosphonate transition state analogs were noted to hydrolyze weak chemical bonds in carbonates and esters. Catalytic antibodies (also called **abzymes**) do not act in the same manner as enzymes: the latter function by binding (and hence stabilizing) the transition state of a biochemical reaction, whereas most noncatalytic antibodies bind the ground state of a reaction, thereby inactivating or neutralizing the target molecule. The creation of catalytic antibodies thus depends in principle on altering the specificity of antibody binding to the transition state – a strategy which could eventually enable the custom design of catalytic reagents for specific chemical reactions. Existing abzymes catalyze numerous biochemical reactions including pericyclic rearrangements, sulfide oxidations, and ester hydrolysis.

Catalytic antibodies have not yet matched the catalytic potency of conventional enzymes, some of which may accelerate biochemical reactions by as much as a billion-fold. Newer substrates for catalytic antibodies include peptide bonds, aminoacylation sites, and prodrugs. An alternative approach to producing catalytic antibodies involves raising anti-idiotypic antibodies to enzymatic active sites, thereby reproducing a three-dimensional image of the activating ligand.

Antisense therapies neutralize critical nucleic acid sequences

Bacteria and viruses transcribe some sequences bidirectionally. Despite tantalizing reports, antisense transcription in mammalian cells has not been shown to stabilize mRNA transcripts or otherwise influence message function. Antisense therapeutic strategies have focused on two major delivery systems:

1. Cellular instillation (e.g., by microinjection) of **synthetic antisense oligodeoxynucleotides**
2. Intracellular production of endogenous antisense mRNAs following the delivery and expression of genetically engineered **antisense genes**.

The latter approach involves expressing a gene sequence consisting of a correctly orientated promoter preceding a reversed (i.e., complementary, or antisense) gene, thereby tricking the cell into transcribing an mRNA sequence complementary to that encoded by the sense DNA strand. The untranslated antisense mRNA hybridizes with the target sequence – typically designed to be mutation-specific, or a critical sequence such as the 5′ cap, AUG initiation codon or exon-intron splice junction – thus sterically preventing ribosomal translation of the target protein (Figure 25.4). Oligonucleotide binding also appears to render transcripts more vulnerable to ribonuclease degradation.

The appeal of antisense technology lies in the affinity and specificity of sense-antisense nucleic acid hybridization. An average 15-base oligonucleotide binds to only one site per chromosome, representing a million-fold enhancement of site-specific binding compared to (say) a restriction enzyme

Figure 25.4 Antisense theory. A nondegradable single-stranded synthetic oligonucleotide binds in a sequence-specific fashion to the target (complementary) mRNA, preventing its translation. Alternatively, oligos may bind the template strand of the encoding gene, thus forming a triple helix and obstructing transcription.

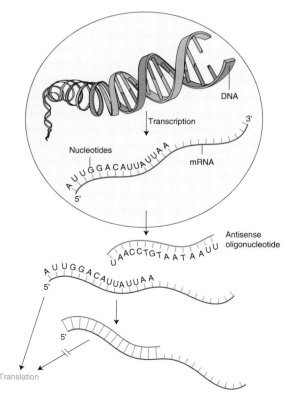

six-cutter. Of note, hybridization stability is greater for RNA:RNA duplexes than for either RNA:DNA or DNA:DNA duplexes.

The main problem with antisense therapy is delivery of the oligo to the cell, whether by cellular microinjection (ex vivo), retroviral delivery or direct intravascular inoculation (in vivo). The latter approach relies on nonselective receptor-mediated endocytosis and fails to deliver 99% of the injected dose to target nucleotide sequences. Whether in peripheral blood or endocytic vesicles, naked DNA sequences are efficiently lysed by nucleases – thus necessitating high initial (micromolar) plasma oligonucleotide concentrations and hence prohibitive production costs. Substitution of sulfur (for O_2) or methyl groups (for phosphate) in the oligonucleotide backbone yields more stable **phosphorothioates** and **methylphosphonates**, which protect oligos from digestion by exonucleases (in serum) and endonucleases (in cells). Such modifications also protect target mRNAs from nuclease digestion, however, and thus reduce therapeutic efficacy. Moreover, these synthetic modifications may cause toxic effects in recipients.

Variations on this recombinant theme include the replacement of DNA backbone sugar-phosphate groups with repeating polyamide (2-aminoethyl-glycine) modules to form so-called **peptide nucleic acids** (PNAs) – which, in fact, are neither peptides nor acids. The artificial structure of PNAs confuses both nucleases and peptidases, thus prolonging intracellular activity. Tight binding occurs between PNAs and complementary cDNAs, making these reagents potent gene inhibitors (i.e., assuming that import to the cell nucleus can be ensured). As with other gene-based therapies, target cell delivery is a major technical hurdle for PNA development.

Antisense is not nonsense. Despite its technical problems, the antisense approach provides a powerful strategy for selectively manipulating host gene expression without altering cellular genotype. Different problems are encountered when seeking to alter host cell genomes in human diseases – an approach termed **gene therapy**.

PHARMACOLOGIC FOOTNOTE

Candidate molecules for antisense therapy

One field in which antisense therapy already appears effective is plant biology: fruit ripening has been enhanced, flower color altered, and viruses such as CMV (denoting, in this context, cucumber mosaic virus) inhibited. Of greater commercial significance are the prospects for using antisense therapy in human diseases using the following targets:

1. Oncogene expression, e.g.,
   - Proliferation-associated genes such as *Myc* (e.g., in **Burkitt lymphoma**) and *Ras* (e.g., in **colorectal carcinoma**).
   - Chimeric genes such as the unique *Bcr/Abl* fusion gene expressed in Philadelphia chromosome-positive **chronic myeloid leukemia**.
2. Viral diseases, e.g.
   - **Herpes simplex virus** (HSV).
   - **Human papillomavirus** (HPV).
   - **Cytomegalovirus** (again, CMV).
   - **Human immunodeficiency virus** (HIV).

Antisense targets for antiviral therapies include the generic genes *Gag, Pol, Env*, reverse transcriptase and long terminal repeats (LTRs). More specific genes – such as the *Tat* gene of HIV which encodes the TAR transcript – are also attractive targets.

Antisense oligos have been used investigationally for other applications including the correction of thalassemic β-globin splicing defects and glutamate receptor downregulation to minimize ischemic neurotoxicity.

Gene therapy

Gene therapy complements tissue deficiency of a given protein

Gene therapy was originally inspired by the plight of young children with single-gene disorders such as **sickle cell anemia** or immunodeficiency due to **adenosine deaminase deficiency**. Replacement of the wild-type gene product in these disorders – whether by gene expression or by replacement of normal cells or proteins – reverts the clinical phenotype. This notion of gene therapists as genetic repairmen has since been applied to adult-onset disorders such as **familial hypercholesterolemia** (expression of the wild-type LDL receptor) and the common carcinoma (expression of wild-type p53).

A more creative application of gene therapy involves expression of a protein where no protein has gone before. The induction of collateral vessels in ischemic myocardium by epicardial inoculation of genes encoding the angiogenic growth factor VEGF is an illustrative example. Other examples include the introduction of so-called suicide genes into cancer cells, and expression of the multidrug efflux pump in bone marrow stem cells as a chemoprotective strategy. In the latter case, high chemotherapy dose intensities may be achieved that would ordinarily be limited by normal marrow tolerance, thus enhancing tumor cell killing.

The efficacy of gene therapy may be enhanced via bystander effects that affect surrounding cells: for example, expression of p53 secondarily reduces VEGF expression and hence inhibits new blood vessel formation. Bystander effects of this kind may help to offset persistent shortcomings in the efficiency of target gene delivery.

CLINICAL KEYNOTE

The technical problems of gene therapy

Some experts say that there are only three problems with gene therapy: delivery, delivery, and delivery. In fact there are more problems than this, including:
1. Efficient delivery of the vector to target cells.
2. Persistence of gene expression.
3. Appropriate control of gene expression.

Many approaches have been tried in an effort to optimize the efficiency of target gene delivery. Transcription efficiencies of introduced genes vary between experimental systems, with expression often detectable in fewer than 0.1% of transduced cells. Complete shutdown often occurs over time, reflecting either transgene deletion or incorrect genomic positioning. Housekeeping gene promoters (e.g., dihydrofolate reductase) may be incorporated into constructs in an effort to sustain gene expression.

Just as troublesome (albeit less frequent) is constitutive gene expression. When bone marrow stem cells are programmed ex vivo to express the red blood cell growth factor erythropoietin, for example, patients may find themselves requiring venesection to reduce the rising hematocrit. Lack of negative feedback control is even more hazardous in the context of insulin gene expression for **type I diabetes** – an otherwise prime gene therapy goal. Specificity of expression can be achieved to

Table 25.3. Tumor-specific gene promoters

Tumor type	Gene promoter
Prostate cancer	Prostate-specific antigen (PSA)
Breast cancer	MUC 1 (mucinous glycoprotein)
Adenocarcinoma	Carcinoembryonic antigen (CEA)
Hepatocellular carcinoma	Alphafetoprotein (AFP)
Melanoma	Tyrosinase

some extent using tissue-specific promoters such as prostate-specific antigen (Table 25.3). The inducibility of erythropoietin gene expression has been achieved in vivo using a fusion gene containing a binding site to the antibiotic rapamycin.

Proteins can be induced in proliferating cells using retroviruses

In vivo delivery and expression of an exogenous gene to a selected cell type is termed **somatic gene therapy**. Gene therapy remains an investigational approach which as yet has no place in routine medical management. The main strategies for gene therapy differ in the way the genes are packaged for delivery:

1. **Viral gene transfer** (Figure 25.5)
   * Retroviruses.
   * DNA viruses.
2. **Direct plasmid inoculation** into recipient tissue
   * Injection.
   * Aerosol inhalation (into lung tissue).
3. **Cell-based** gene therapy, e.g.,
   * Stem cell transplantation.
   * Myoblast transfer.
   * Skin fibroblast or endothelial cell delivery systems.
4. Other approaches
   * e.g., Use of mobile **group II introns** to insert into target DNA.

Retroviral RNA genomes are converted intracellularly to proviral DNAs capable of insertion into the host genome. The integrated provirus is then transcribed by endogenous cellular DNA-dependent RNA polymerase II; this is followed by translation of viral proteins that catalyze the replication of infectious viral particles from the retroviral genome. Expression in target cells may be stably induced by retroviruses, but the efficiency of delivery to nondividing cells remains a key problem. Retroviruses of this type can be produced recombinantly and maintained in **packaging cell lines**.

Retroviral integration only occurs during host cell mitosis, restricting targets to growing tissues; for example, retroviral integration into host liver cell genomes requires partial hepatectomy to induce hepatocyte division. This drawback of retroviral vectors has been exploited to enable selective delivery of the neurotropic herpes simplex thymidine kinase (HS-tk) gene to proliferating rodent **gliomas** – these tumors retain sensitivity to the anti-herpetic drug ganciclovir, whereas the nondividing (nontransduced) ambient neural tissue is spared. Slow-growing retroviruses termed lentiviruses – HIV being an example – may overcome this problem via the ability to infect nondividing cells and simultaneously to evade host immune detection.

Germline gene therapy involves introducing new or repaired genes into periconceptual or embryonic tissue. Although the problem of efficient delivery may be less daunting than in somatic gene therapy, the ethical issues are greater.

Figure 25.5 Viral gene therapy. Following insertion of the gene of interest into a viral expression vector, tissues can be inoculated directly (e.g., using a gene gun) or cells can be infected prior to reimplantation.

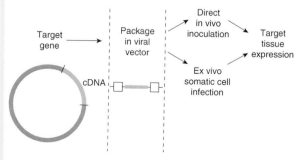

MOLECULAR MINIREVIEW

Retroviral safety issues

The species-specificity of retroviral cell targets is determined by envelope proteins – viruses encoding **ecotropic** envelope proteins infect rodent cells whereas human cells are infected only by **amphotropic** retroviruses. Serious safety concerns have been raised over the use of amphotropic retroviruses in human subjects. Such viruses are first attenuated by deletion of ψ sequences in the 5′ untranslated RNA region, thereby preventing the generation of infectious particles without affecting the translation of retroviral proteins. Although disabled in replicative terms, such retroviruses remain (theoretically) tumorigenic because of the possibility of insertional mutagenesis affecting normal genes via random retrotransposition of proviral DNA throughout the host cell genome.

The possibility that normal genes may be disrupted by nonhomologous gene incorporation – leading to insertional mutagenesis – is also a long-term safety concern. Deaths in clinical trials have occurred following the injection of large viral inocula (e.g., adenovirus), serving as a reminder that such viruses may be immunogenic. This problem of immunogenicity is avoidable by using nonviral delivery methods such as plasmid transfer using cationic liposomes. This approach can be equally applied to dividing and nondividing cells.

DNA viruses deliver genes to nondividing cells

Unlike retroviruses, DNA viruses are capable of infecting postmitotic cells, thereby permitting gene therapy of nonproliferating target tissues. The commonest DNA viruses used for gene therapy are:

1. Adenoviruses.
2. Herpesviruses.
3. Reovirus.

Adenoviruses (e.g., adenovirus type 5) structurally resemble "cannonballs with spikes", and preferentially infect bronchial epithelium. Diseases associated with lung phenotypes – such as **cystic fibrosis** and α_1**-antitrypsin deficiency** – are therefore promising targets for adenovirus-based gene therapy. Adenovirus vectors may be rendered replication-defective by replacing the E3 region and the transforming *E1A* gene (p. 371) with a gene cassette including the E1A enhancer and adenovirus major late promoter linked to the desired gene. One clever therapeutic strategy (Onyx-015™) has involved deletion of a gene essential for replication in normal (but not p53-null) cells, thus encouraging selective viral replication in tumor (p53-null) cells.

Adenoviruses are not confined to lung expression systems, being also used for gene transduction in tissues such as muscle, endothelium, liver, and central nervous system. The immunogenicity of adenovirus – i.e., the plasma level of blocking antibodies – can be reduced by substituting the parvovirus **adeno-associated virus** (AAV), which requires a helper adenovirus to replicate.

Herpesviruses infect neuronal cell bodies. Vectors such as herpes simplex must be rendered nonpathogenic and replication-defective prior to human use by eliminating the expression of immediate-early genes, latency genes, and genes involved in activating lytic potential. Prolonged expression of the **latency-associated transcript** (**LAT**) in herpesviruses may also provide a therapeutic opportunity since foreign genes downstream of the LAT promoter exhibit sustained expression in the nervous system. Selective herpesvirus growth in tumor cells can be encouraged by deleting nucleotide-synthesizing genes, since ambient nucleotide pools are generally higher in tumor cells.

Reovirus growth is tumor-selective without engineering, since only cells with an activated Ras will permit reovirus growth. However, some symptoms may emerge following viral replication in the rapidly dividing cell compartments of lung and bowel.

Gene guns and DNA vaccines

Vaccination is one of the most effective public health interventions of all time. Most vaccines contain microorganisms (killed or attenuated) or synthetic immunogenic proteins from such infective agents. In recent years, however, the injection of target organism DNA has been pursued as a new approach to creating effective vaccines. **Direct gene transfer** techniques include transfection, lipofection, electroporation, microinjection, microcell-mediated gene transfer, and chromosome-mediated gene transfer. Although these approaches may be useful for ex vivo treatment of cells destined for reimplantation (see below), none are ideal for in vivo gene therapy. Surprisingly, plasmid DNA may be directly injected into target tissues and expressed. Using this approach, plasmid genes have been successfully expressed in many tissues including muscle, endothelial wall, heart, liver, and lung – the latter by aerosol inhalation. Some such genes even appear to be appropriately regulated by microenvironmental stimuli. Direct gene transfer of this type is executed by the use of a so-called **gene gun**.

A variation of this approach involves inoculation of naked DNA into subcutaneous tissues, inducing a vaccination-like immune response to the encoded protein. This is reminiscent of the use of vaccinia virus to express large quantities of recombinant immunogen in situ, but without the viral expression machinery. Intravenous injection of plasmid DNA has no such immunizing effect, indicating the involvement of local tissues in expressing the plasmid. In theory, antitumor immune responses may be maximized by co-transfecting target cells with the granulocyte-macrophage colony-stimulating factor (GM-CSF) gene ex vivo.

Reimplanted host cells permit cellular gene therapy

Cell-based gene therapy approaches are applicable to diseases where cells can be removed from the body, manipulated in vitro, then reimplanted in the individual requiring treatment. A simple example is that of microencapsulated cells engineered to secrete proteins of interest – enzymes, hemoglobin, growth factors, hormones, clotting factors, opioids – through a semipermeable membrane following transplantation into the recipient. Other varieties of cellular gene therapy are more analogous to conventional organ transplantation – and, like ordinary transplants, the graft (or the expressed foreign protein) may be rejected. Cell transfer techniques include:

1. Stem cell transplantation.
2. Transfer of cell types: myoblasts, skin fibroblasts, keratinocytes, hepatocytes or endothelial cells.

These cell-based approaches often involve viral gene transfer to target cells following the temporary removal of cells from the body. Such ex vivo treatment is ideal for retroviral gene transfer since the problems of cell delivery and growth phase are reduced.

Stem cell transplantation is used for diseases involving inborn errors of metabolism such as **adenosine deaminase deficiency** (though lymphocytes are often used in place of stem cells), **Lesch–Nyhan syndrome** (HPRT deficiency) and **Gaucher disease** (glucocerebrosidase deficiency). Stem cells are useful for ex vivo gene transfer in view of their high replicative potential and multilineage developmental capacity. To isolate immortalized stem cells for long-term gene expression, recipient bone marrow is enriched using CD34 monoclonal antibodies. Marrow harvested for conventional autologous transplantation following ablative leukemic therapy may be **gene-marked** ex vivo, allowing confirmation of relapse from the reinfused (inadequately purged) cells. Indeed, gene-marking with reporter genes can be used to check the efficiency of tissue localization and/or expression of any gene therapy approach.

Myoblast transfer involves gene introduction into embryonic muscle cells. This approach has been used for muscle disorders such as **Duchenne muscular dystrophy**, as well as for systemic protein delivery and even intracerebral cell transplants for **Parkinson disease**. Well-vascularized target cells can act as protein factories that release the molecule of interest into the peripheral circulation. This approach should work best for diseases which require replacement of a missing plasma protein, but which do not require fine regulation of gene transcription or strict tissue-specific expression. To achieve the latter, the optimal constellation of upstream gene regulatory elements must be independently determined for each somatic tissue. Genes that integrate into the native (endogenous) chromosomal site by homologous recombination tend to be better expressed and controlled.

CLINICAL KEYNOTE

Diseases in search of effective gene therapy

Inherited human diseases arising from single-gene mutations – especially recessive mutations, since these often involve severe deficits of protein expression which may benefit from even minor augmentation – are good candidates for gene replacement therapy. Such diseases include:

1. Hemoglobinopathies (especially β-thalassemia).
2. Duchenne muscular dystrophy.
3. Cystic fibrosis.
4. α_1-Antitrypsin deficiency.
5. Hemophilias (especially hemophilia B).
6. Familial hypercholesterolemia.
7. Immunodeficiencies (e.g., severe combined immunodeficiency, leukocyte adhesion deficiency).
8. Inborn errors of metabolism:
   - Lysosomal storage diseases.
   - Lesch–Nyhan syndrome.
   - Phenylketonuria.
   - Urea cycle disorders.
9. Huntington disease.

These diseases all involve replacement of an abnormal gene product; for example, adenosine deaminase (responsible for about 25% of **SCID** cases), CD18 in **leukocyte adhesion deficiency**, the LDL receptor in **familial hypercholesterolemia**, or factor IX in **hemophilia B**. Some of these molecules have already been the subject of gene therapy attempts in animals and in selected human recipients.

Diseases such as **β-thalassemia** (which requires the balanced production of both globin chains) or severe lysosomal storage diseases such as **Niemann–Pick** or **Gaucher disease** (which may require intracerebral gene product replacement to prevent mental retardation) are problematic. Even more difficult are diseases such as **sickle cell anemia,** in which the β sickle gene needs to be knocked out by homologous recombination with the normal β-globin gene to prevent sickling. For now, however, palliative attempts to reduce HbS production are confined to overexpressing either β or γ chains. Novel gene therapy strategies include the transfer of drug-resistance genes to normal host cells (e.g., to minimize iatrogenic toxicity in the setting of high-dose cytotoxic therapy), and the transfer of histocompatibility genes to transplant recipients receiving mismatched grafts.

Enrichment reading

Bedtime reading

Khoury MJ, Burke W, Thomson E (eds). *Genetics and public health in the 21st century: using genetic information to improve health and prevent disease.* Oxford University Press, Oxford, 2000

Library reference

Greene JJ, Rao VB (eds). *Recombinant DNA principles and methodologies.* Marcel Dekker, New York, 1999.

Gordon EM, Kerwin JF. *Combinatorial chemistry and molecular diversity in drug discovery.* Wiley-Liss, New York, 1998

Meager A (ed). *Gene therapy technologies, applications and regulations: from laboratory to clinic.* John Wiley & Sons, New York, 1999

Stephanopoulos G, Aristidou A, Nielsen J, Nielson J. *Metabolic engineering: principles and methodologies.* Academic Press, New York, 1998

Wu-Pong S, Ronanasakul Y (eds). *Biopharmaceutical drug design and development.* Humana Press, Totowa, NJ, 1999

The benefit of such experimental treatments will not be known for some time. Luckily this doesn't matter all that much, since experts tell us that time will eventually end with the Big Crunch in another 14 billion years or so, which will bring us back to where we started. In the meantime, most human diseases will remain best treated by small-molecule inhibitors of receptors and enzymes, and immortality will continue to elude most of us.

So on we beat, boats along the river, run past Eve and Adams . . .

Summary

Synthetic human proteins are useful therapeutic agents. Chimeric molecules can be genetically engineered. Recombinant protein expression systems vary in efficiency.

Ribozymes are RNA gene shears that kill the messenger. Antisense therapies neutralize critical nucleic acid sequences.

Gene therapy complements tissue deficiency of a given protein. Proteins can be induced in proliferating cells using retroviruses. DNA viruses can deliver genes to non-dividing cells. Reimplantation of modified host cells permits cellular gene therapy.

QUIZ QUESTIONS

1. Explain why it is easier to produce recombinant human insulin than it is to produce recombinant human vitamin D.
2. Imagine you succeed in producing a recombinant protein intended for therapeutic use. What sort of problems might prevent the product being as useful as you would like?
3. Describe some hypothetical circumstances in which you might wish to synthesize a chimeric protein for therapeutic use.
4. What is a ribozyme?
5. List some pros and cons of antisense technology as a therapeutic prospect.
6. Distinguish the purpose of somatic gene therapy and germline gene therapy.
7. How do retroviruses and DNA viruses differ in their abilities to be used as gene therapy vectors?
8. What sorts of safety issues are of concern with respect to retroviral gene therapy?
9. What is a gene gun used for?
10. Under what circumstances would cell-based gene therapy be an attractive therapeutic option?

This is not the end
It is not even the beginning of the end
It is, however, the end of the beginning

Winston Churchill, 1943

Index

Numbers in *italics* indicate tables or figures. Major references are prioritized in bold.